DIAGNOSTIC *and* OPERATIVE GYNECOLOGIC LAPAROSCOPY

DIAGNOSTIC *and* OPERATIVE GYNECOLOGIC LAPAROSCOPY

VICTOR GOMEL, M.D.

Professor
Department of Obstetrics and Gynecology
University of British Columbia
Vancouver, British Columbia,
Canada

PATRICK J. TAYLOR, M.D.

Professor
Department of Obstetrics and Gynecology
University of British Columbia
Vancouver, British Columbia,
Canada

with 259 illustrations, 38 in full color

Mosby

St. Louis Baltimore Berlin Boston Carlsbad Chicago London Madrid
Naples New York Philadelphia Sydney Tokyo Toronto

Mosby
Dedicated to Publishing Excellence

Editor: Susie Baxter
Developmental Editor: Ellen Baker Geisel
Project Manager: John Rogers
Production Editor: Chuck Furgason
Designer: Renée Duenow
Manufacturing Supervisor: Linda Ierardi

Printed in the United States of America
Composition by the Clarinda Company
Printing/binding by Maple-Vail Book Mfg. Group, York

Mosby-Year Book, Inc.
11830 Westline Industrial Drive
St. Louis, Missouri 63146

Library of Congress Cataloging–in–Publication Data

Diagnostic and operative gynecologic laparoscopy / [edited by] Victor Gomel, Patrick J. Taylor.
p. cm.
Includes bibliographical references and index.
ISBN 0-8016-7823-4
1. Generative organs, Female—Endoscopic surgery. 2. Laparoscopy. I. Gomel, Victor. II. Taylor, Patrick J.
[DNLM: 1. Genital Diseases, Female—surgery. 2. Genital Diseases, Female—diagnosis. 3. Surgery, Laparoscopic—methods. 4. Laparoscopy—methods. WP 660 D536 1994]
RG104.7.D53 1994
618.1′059—dc20
DNLM/DLC
for Library of Congress 94-36442
CIP

95 96 97 98 99 / 9 8 7 6 5 4 3 2 1

CONTRIBUTORS

***James F. Daniell,* M.D.**
Clinical Professor
Department of Obstetrics & Gynecology
Centennial Medical Center
Nashville, Tennessee

***Alan G. Gordon,* F.R.C.S., F.R.C.O.G.**
Honorary Consultant Gynaecologist
Princess Royal Hospital
Hull, England

***Bryan R. Kurtz,* M.D.**
Clinical Assistant Professor
Department of Obstetrics and Gynecology
Vanderbilt University
Nashville, Tennessee

***Eric Leblanc,* M.D.**
Department of Obstetrics and Gynecology
Centre Oscar Lambret
Lille, France

***John M. Leventhal,* M.D.**
Clinical Instructor
Harvard Medical School
Cambridge, Massachusetts

***Carl J. Levinson,* M.D.**
Associate Professor
Department of Obstetrics and Gynecology
Stanford University
Stanford, California

***Malcolm G. Munro,* M.D.**
Associate Professor
Department of Obstetrics and Gynecology
University of California, Los Angeles
Los Angeles, California

***Camran Nezhat,* M.D.**
Clinical Professor, Department of Obstetrics & Gynecology
Stanford University, Stanford, California and
Mercer University, Macon, Georgia

***Farr Nezhat,* M.D.**
Clinical Professor, Department of Obstetrics & Gynecology
Stanford University, Stanford, California and
Mercer University, Macon, Georgia

***Denis Querleu,* M.D.**
Professor of Obstetrics and Gynecology
University of Lille
Roubaix, France

***Harry Reich,* M.D.**
Wyoming Valley Gynecology Associates
Kingston, Pennsylvania

***Theirry G. Vancaillie,* M.D.**
Center for Gynecologic Endosurgery
San Antonio, Texas

To our children
Monique and David Gomel
and
Sarah Howard and David Taylor

PREFACE

In an ideal world illness would never occur, or if it did, would be amenable to diagnosis and cure by noninvasive means. Regrettably, we do not live in such a world and with our present stage of knowledge must frequently have recourse to surgery to reach a diagnosis or to effect a cure or palliation.

The performance of surgery requires that four conditions be fulfilled: the patient must be spared the pain of the operation, the surgeon must be able to gain access to the site of surgery, the operation, be it extirpative or reconstructive, must be technically feasible without exposing the patient to undue risk, and the procedure must be justifiable.

Modern methods of anesthesia, narcolepsy, and analgesia have satisfied the first condition admirably. The technical feasibility of all gynecologic procedures has been established by the work of earlier surgeons who gained access to the operative site by means of abdominal incisions or through the vagina.

Modern laparoscopic equipment provided an alternative method of access to the internal female reproductive organs. In the 1970s the diagnostic role of laparoscopy gained wide acceptance. Even at this stage laparoscopic tubal sterilization, in part in response to consumer demand, was increasingly being performed.

In the last decade the pioneers of our discipline have shown that almost any gynecological operation can be performed laparoscopically. It must be stressed that the fundamental nature of the procedure is no different. Laparoscopy simply provides a means of access to the operative site. No more. No less. Inevitably the trauma caused by large abdominal incisions is avoided; it has been recognized that our patients experience less postoperative pain and more rapid recovery time.

These advances have not been achieved without cost. The surgeon must develop a new set of skills. Operating times tend to be prolonged. The laudable desire to spare patients pain and discomfort has led to a perception that minimal access operations are minor procedures, a perception fostered by those who would, inaccurately describe the field as "minimally invasive". A procedure is still invasive, still hazardous, whether it is performed abdominally or by using laparoscopic access.

This decade has seen a major change in the way that medicine is practised. No longer does the physician recommend treatment and the patient passively accept the advice. The new consumer of health care demands to be actively involved in the decision making process. Premature dissemination of information about, and hyperbolic descriptions of the virtues of, "minimally invasive surgery" may be causing unrealistic perceptions. This is not unusual in our discipline. The same phenomenon was seen when lasers were first introduced. It is our responsibility to offer our advice based on the most current and reliable data, and not be swayed by consumer demand when, in our best professional opinion, a laparoscopic procedure is contraindicated.

This is particularly so when many of these laparoscopically assisted procedures have been introduced without careful analysis, without demonstrating beyond reasonable doubt that the new approach is as safe as the old, and produces comparable or better outcomes.

Furthermore, the indications for many procedures were not rigorously established prior to the advent of minimal access surgery. That they can be performed by laparoscopic means does not make their true place in the surgeon's repertoire any more valid.

It is apparent that the time is ripe for critical reappraisal of many gynecologic surgical procedures so that their true value can be established, and for prospective trials of older, proven methods with similar operations effected by laparoscopic access. This has already been established for the management of tubal pregnancy.

Pregnancy rates were improved by the implementation of the microsurgical techniques and principles that were painstakingly developed by the pioneers of this field. Similar results can be obtained when repair of distal tubal occlusion is effected by means of minimal access.

Introduction of microsurgical tenets had more wide ranging effects than for reconstructive surgery alone. It made gynecologists aware of the critical need to treat the female reproductive organs with great delicacy, particularly if subsequent fertility was to be preserved. It is to be hoped that this recognition of the need for meticulous attention to detail will not become lost in the rush to embrace minimal access surgery.

It is not surprising that with the meteoric speed with which new operations have been introduced, a large number of textbooks of laparoscopic surgery have been or are about to be published. Why then the need for another? It is our hope that the reader will find within these pages a comprehensive description of all the facets of modern gynecologic laparoscopic practice from the very simple to the most complex.

For the interested reader, a short history precedes the rest of the work. Because many gynecologists must learn new skills, a chapter describing training and credentialling has been included: there is also a guide to the basic equipment needs of the laparoscopist. Modern laparoscopic surgery is dependent on the use of energy, be it mechanical, electrical, or laser. Sailors will not embark on a cruise in uncharted waters without a thorough understanding of all the equipment of their vessel. It would seem prudent that the laparoscopic surgeon should pay the same attention to understanding the details of the energy sources that are integral to the safe performance of operative endoscopy.

Certain fundamental principles are common to all kinds of gynecologic laparoscopy and these are described in the second section of the book.

Despite advances in modern imaging techniques, recourse to laparoscopy must often be made before a final diagnosis can be achieved. The third section of the book provides extensive discussions of the application of diagnostic laparoscopy to patients who may present with common gynecologic symptoms or conditions. A surgeon who is not a skilled diagnostic laparoscopist should not consider performing surgery by this means.

The fourth section examines the operations, beginning with the simplest and progressing to the more complex. Each chapter not only describes the technical details by which a specific procedure is performed but also provides a critical appraisal of the efficacy and the safety of these interventions; these appraisals are based on the currently available published data. Because the field is so new, it has not always been possible to define with any accuracy the true place of a given technique. If such is the case, we have so indicated.

Prophesy has always been an inexact science, but it would not have been proper to conclude without a chapter that attempts to see what the future holds. Not only gynecology, but all of the surgical disciplines, are daily expanding the horizons of minimal access surgery. The dam burst less than 10 years ago. The pressure that overran the ramparts came from the ingenuity of the instrument industry which has married technological advances to the needs of innovative surgeons. We now stand on the banks of a rapidly flowing river whose new course is not entirely predictable. We must decide whether to be swept along by the current or to try to channel the stream by means of the flood gates of continuous assessment of new techniques and the levees of follow up studies.

Because of the enormity of the subject no single surgeon can possibly be expert in all areas. Recognizing this, it was decided to ask some of our friends, who are internationally respected authorities, to contribute chapters describing their areas of expertise. To them we offer our sincere thanks.

It is hoped that the reader will find that our efforts and those of the contributing authors have provided clear guidance in those areas that seem to be well understood and have offered current information about the frontiers of modern gynecologic laparoscopy.

Victor Gomel
Patrick J. Taylor

ACKNOWLEDGMENTS

This book could not have been produced without the encouragement, dedication, and hard work of many individuals to whom we wish to express our most sincere appreciation. Stephanie Manning developed the concept and nourished the text through its initial phase. Susan McRae and Cherri Buckler faithfully processed the manuscript through its numerous revisions. Laurie Vaskalis illustrated the words with meticulous drawings. Finally the cooperative and attentive editorial and production staff of Mosby brought the project to completion with unfailing good humor.

CONTENTS

Part I INTRODUCTION

1 History of Laparoscopy, ***1***

2 Training and Credentialling, ***6***
Carl J. Levinson

3 Equipment and Instrumentation, ***13***

4 Energy Sources for Operative Laparoscopy, ***26***
Malcolm G. Munro

Part II PRINCIPLES OF GYNECOLOGIC LAPAROSCOPY

5 Principles of Diagnostic Laparoscopy, ***57***

6 Indications and Contraindications of Diagnostic Laparoscopy, ***68***

7 Principles of Operative Laparoscopy, ***71***

8 Documentation: Technical and Legal Considerations, ***89***
John M. Leventhal

Part III DIAGNOSTIC LAPAROSCOPY

9 Infertility, ***99***

10 Pelvic Pain, ***115***

11 Endometriosis, ***133***

12 Neoplasia, ***137***
with Denis Querleu and Eric Leblanc

Part IV OPERATIVE LAPAROSCOPY

13 Tubal Sterilization, ***149***

14 Tubal Pregnancy, ***157***

15 Fertility-Promoting Procedures and Assisted Reproductive Technology, ***169***

16 Pelvic Inflammatory Disease and Tubo-Ovarian Abscess, ***181***
with Harry Reich

17 Ovarian Surgery, ***189***

18 Endometriosis, ***201***
with Camran Nezhat and Farr Nezhat

19 Myomectomy, ***219***
Alan G. Gordon

20 Ablation of the Uterosacral Ligaments and Presacral Neurectomy, ***229***
James F. Daniell and Bryan R. Kurtz

21 Uterine Displacements, ***236***

22 Hysterectomy, ***241***

23 Appendectomy, ***259***

24 Urogynecologic Procedures, ***265***
Thierry G. Vancaillie

25 Gynecologic Cancer, ***277***
Denis Querleu and Eric Leblanc

26 Complications and Their Management, ***299***

Part V EPILOGUE

27 Future Directions, ***309***

Chapter 1

HISTORY OF LAPAROSCOPY

"Why look through the keyhole when you can open the door?" was a disparaging remark made by an eminent member of the gynecologic establishment following the presentation of some observations by one of this century's pioneers of laparoscopy. Laparoscopy is now the most frequently performed gynecologic procedure. In the past two decades, the possibilities of operative laparoscopy have been explored, the frontiers constantly expanded, and procedures once thought to be impossible through laparoscopic access are now in routine use.

The wish to peer into the body is as old as recorded history. The Babylonian Talmud (Niddah Treatise)[1] describes an instrument that was used for observation of the cervix. Clearly recognizable bivalve speculi recovered from the ashes of Pompeii can be seen in the Institute Rizzoli in Bologna. It was not until 1799 that Recamier, who also introduced the curette, reinvented the speculum.[2]

In 1805, Bozzini described his technique of examining the interior of the urethra of a living human being.[3] He reflected the light from a candle with a mirror, directing the rays along a metal tube. Imagine his chagrin when the august body to whom he reported, the Medical Faculty of Vienna, promptly censured him for "undue curiosity." Desormeaux[4] (1865) fared rather better. He had designed a functioning cystoscope. The Academie Impériale de Medecine de Paris rewarded him with a share of the Argenteuil prize.

Gynecologists were slow to enter the field. Although Panteleoni[5] (1869) did manage to visualize the uterine cavity of a woman with postmenopausal bleeding, little attention was paid to his report. The urologists were more ready to advance. Nitze (1879) replaced the cumbersome external alcohol-fueled lamp with an incandescent platinum filament that was sited on the distal tip of the cystoscope.[6] When brought to white heat it provided reliable illumination, the heat being dissipated by a continuous stream of water.

As is so often the case, medical progress was being driven by technological advances that were occurring in the wider scientific community. Thomas Edison developed the incandescent light bulb (1880). Newman quickly capitalized on this invention, adapting it for cystoscopic use by 1883.[7]

Despite increasing enthusiasm for laryngoscopy, bronchoscopy, and esophagoscopy, closed body cavities remained hidden from endoscopic view. The first direct inspection of the peritoneal cavity was made by von Ott in 1901. He passed a speculum into the abdominal cavity of a pregnant woman through a small culdotomy incision and used a head mirror to reflect light. He called the procedure "ventroscopy."[8]

To Kelling must go the credit for the development of one of the key steps of modern laparoscopy, the distension of the peritoneal cavity with gas.[9] In 1901 he used a needle to introduce room air. His early experiments in dogs, which he termed "celioscopy," were rapidly followed by the application of this technique to the human by Jacobaeus in 1910.[10] He first introduced a trocar and cannula. Room air was passed through the cannula. Once the abdomen was suitably distended, a cystoscope was inserted through the cannula. Jacobaeus was perhaps less well-grounded in the classical languages. He eschewed the terms "ventroscopy" (Latin-venter, belly) and "celioscopy" (Greek-koilia, belly) and coined the term "laparoscopy" (Greek-lapar, flank), the term is still used today. (As if the taxonomic minefield was not sufficiently cluttered, Steiner (1924) described his experience with "abdominoscopy"[1] and Redi (1935) reported several cases of "splanchnoscopy."[12])

By the end of the first decade of the twentieth century the fundamental principles of diagnostic laparoscopy had been established. Advances came rapidly. Nordentoft[13] (1912) demonstrated the value of placing the patient in deep Trendelenburg position to display the female pelvic organs, and Zollikofer[14] (1924) began using carbon dioxide as the insufflating gas. As was to be expected, the purely diagnostic application of the equipment did not satisfy surgeons for long.

In 1929 Kalk[15] began to perform liver biopsies through a second puncture under laparoscopic observation, and Fervers[16] (1933) designed instruments with which intra-abdominal adhesions could be cauterized. Of particular interest to gynecologists was the work of Boesch[17] (1936) in Switzerland and Anderson[18] (1937) in the United States. They proposed the performance of laparoscopic female tubal sterilization by fulguration. It is claimed that the first actual sterilization was performed by Power and Barnes in 1941.[19] The day of operative laparoscopy had dawned.

As the indications expanded, so the instruments were improved. Ruddock (1934) designed a single-puncture operating laparoscope and its accompanying instruments with which biopsies could be taken.[20] Veress (1938) adapted the spring-loaded needle, which at that time was used to induce a pneumothorax in tuberculosis sufferers, for use in establishing the pneumoperitoneum.[21] The spring-loaded inner blunt probe was intended to protect the abdominal contents from the outer, sharp sheath.

The most important advances of the fifties were technical. In 1952, Fourestier, Gladu, and Vulmiere[22] introduced a method of transmitting an intense light by means of a quartz rod, and the same year the application of fiber optics to endoscopy by Hopkins and Kapany[23] (1952) was described. This meant that the light source could be kept external to the peritoneal cavity. Today's routine use of video equipment would not be possible without the availability of these bright sources of illumination.

Even before the development of the cold light source, European gynecologists were enthusiastically embracing this new technique. Raoul Palmer of Paris should be regarded as the father of modern gynecologic laparoscopy. As early as 1946 he had collected over 250 personal cases.[24] In Germany, Hans Frangenheim who learned the technique from Palmer published a textbook of laparoscopy in 1959.[25] He paid particular attention to complications and their avoidance. In 1962 Albano and Cittadini[26] in Italy and Thoyer-Rozat[27] in France also published texts in their respective languages.

The first report of laparoscopy in the United States was from Bernkeim[28] in 1911. Although in 1941 there were over 300 laparoscopes in use in America,[7] the popularity of the technique went into eclipse for two decades. The English-speaking world seemed to have lost interest.

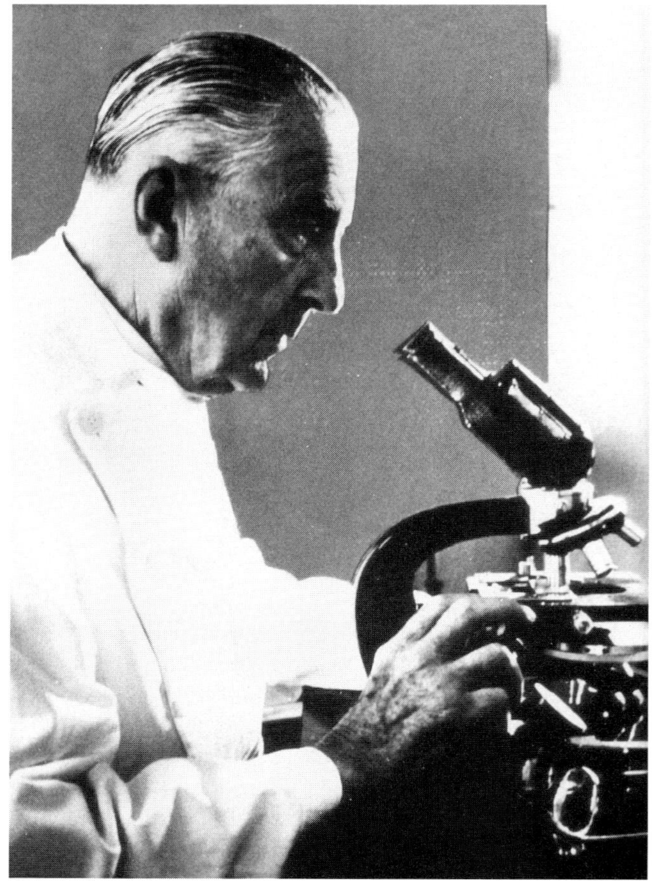

Fig. 1. Raoul Palmer.

"The inspiration to write this book largely stems from the infectious enthusiasm of Dr. and Madame Raoul Palmer, to whom I am especially indebted. I am also grateful to Dr. Hans Frangenheim for his contribution and for his personal communications, which have given me encouragement and valuable suggestions." Thus begins the "Acknowledgements" of the 1967 text, "Laparoscopy in Gynecology" by Patrick Steptoe.[29] The publication of this work in England and a similar book, "Laparoscopy, Culdoscopy, and Gynecography" by Melvin R. Cohen,[30] in the United States in 1970, signalled the reawakening of interest in the English-speaking countries. Perhaps the authors of this text can be forgiven if we remark with some pride and a very deep sense of gratitude that one of us was privileged to learn laparoscopy from Palmer (Fig. 1-1) and the other from Steptoe (Fig. 1-2).

Although interest had been piqued, many gynecologists seemed reluctant to embrace the new technology. Two events occurred in the early 1970s that led to a dramatic increased in the use of laparoscopy. The innovators were moving from using the equipment in a purely diagnostic mode to its application for performing female sterilization, a procedure that until then had required laparotomy or colpotomy, and the American Association of Gynecologic Laparoscopists (AAGL) was founded.

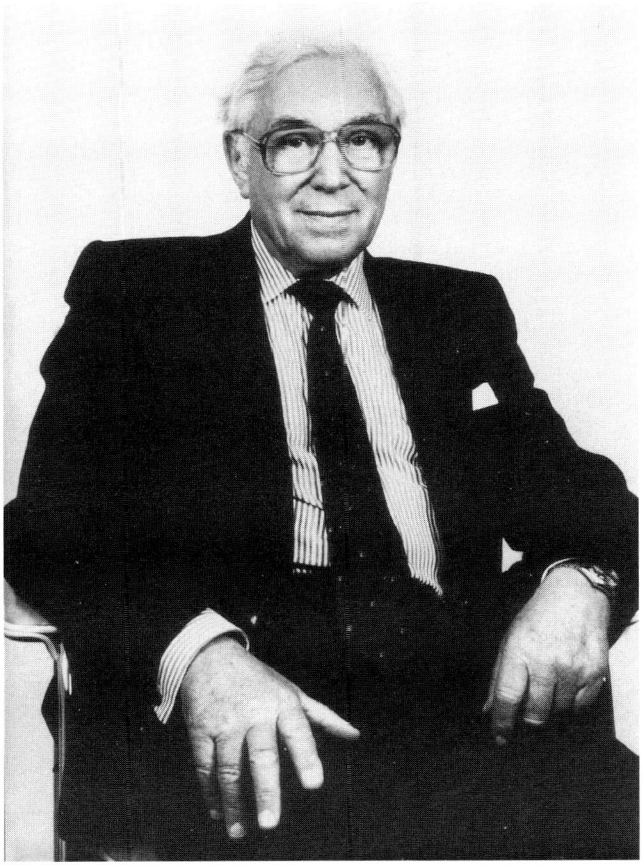

Fig. 2. Patrick Steptoe.

Following experiments by Boesch[17] and Anderson,[18] Power and Barnes[19] used a laparoscopic method of tubal sterilization by fulguration as early as 1941. Palmer[31] designed an ingenious instrument. It was a unipolar pair of grasping blades. The blades were surrounded by a cylindrical sheath, on the distal end of which was a sharp "cookie cutter." Once the tube had been grasped in the blades and desiccated, the cookie cutter was advanced with a screwing motion to sever the tube. Steptoe included a description of this technique in his monograph.[29] In 1969, Neuwirth[32] and Liston et al.[33] in 1970 both reported large series of female sterilizations. Wheeless[34] demonstrated the cost effectiveness of outpatient laparoscopic sterilization.

In Canada in 1970 two hands-on courses in laparoscopy were given independently, one in the University of British Columbia in Vancouver, directed by Victor Gomel, and the other in Laval University in Quebec City directed by Jacques Ricux. We believe that these were the first such hands-on workshops presented in North America.

Gynecologists were eager to learn this new and increasingly consumer-demanded technique. In 1972 Jordan Phillips, a man with extraordinary foresight and organization skills, founded the American Association of Gynecologic Laparoscopists (AAGL), a society dedicated to dissemination of the skills and knowledge of laparoscopy. The thirst for this information can be recognized when it is noted that at the first meeting of the AAGL, in Las Vegas in November 1972, over 600 registrants were in attendance. The AAGL gave innumerable hands-on courses in North America, established a flying squad of teachers who spread their knowledge in developing countries, and by 1980, began a long-standing relationship with the People's Republic of China.

During this stage of the evolution of gynecologic laparoscopy, most practitioners were satisfied to be able to carry out diagnostic procedures and female sterilization. Just as the introduction of laparoscopy itself had begun with the efforts of a few committed individuals so too was the exploration of the operative possibilities being conducted by a few enthusiasts.

Steptoe[29] had described division of adhesions using a diathermy knife, aspiration, and incision of ovarian cysts, ventrosuspension, and multiple punch biopsy of polycystic ovaries. Although not truly surgical laparoscopy, he and Edwards[35] were the first to aspirate mature human oocytes successfully, the first step toward today's ever-expanding practice of assisted reproduction.

In the 1970s use of laparoscopic access for the performance of other gynecologic procedures was being explored in many centers around the world. Prominent among these are Kiel in Germany and Vancouver in Canada. Semm and co-workers reported oophorectomy, salpingectomy, and adnextomy in 1979.[36,37] They introduced a ligation technique using a modified Roeder's loop, produced several new laparoscopic instruments through Semm's own company,[39] and developed endocoagulation.[40] Gomel presented his initial experience with operative laparoscopy in 1973[41] and demonstrated the value and safety in this approach for salpingo-ovariolysis, fimbrioplasty, and salpingostomy[42-46] and tubal pregnancy[47,48] managed by segmental excision.

Shapiro and Adler published a case report in 1973 describing the laparoscopic management of a tubal pregnancy by electrodesication.[49] In 1975 Soderstrom reported excision of tubal pregnancies in five patients using an electrical snare technique.[50] In 1980 Bruhat and co-workers reported the treatment of tubal pregnancy by tubal aspiration (for distal locations) and salpingostomy.[51]

By the end of the decade the CO_2 laser was being used in Clermont-Ferrand where a prominent endoscopic group was being established by Bruhat.[52] Thus by the end of the 1970s the principles of operative laparoscopy using electrical (unipolar and bipolar[53]), thermal, and laser energy, sharp and blunt dissection, and ligation and suturing[54] techniques were already established, and the value and advantages of this approach for several gynecologic procedures was recognized.

Performance of more extensive procedures was spearheaded in the first half of the 1980s by gynecologists focusing on endometriosis, most of whom favored using laser energy. These workers included Martin,[55,56] Feste,[57] Daniell,[58] Nezhat,[59] and Davis.[60]

Gynecologists promoted the use of operative laparoscopy by general surgeons and other surgical specialities. In 1983 Semm reported the performance of appendectomy by laparoscopy.[6] The recognition by general surgeons of the potential of laparoscopy for diagnosis and treatment of acute appendicitis, and especially the access it provided to perform cholecystectomy,[62] dramatically changed the surgical scene. After a long phase of indifference, surgeons embraced operative laparoscopy and rapidly expanded its applications in their own field.

These developments were largely catalyzed by general technical advances in optics and silicon chip technology, resulting in the development of small beam splitters and especially light weight video cameras and high-resolution television monitors. These advances permitted surgeons to perform procedures while viewing the operative field on the monitor. Although this approach had been tried in the 1970s,[63] the heavy weight of the video cameras and the limited resolution of the monitors then available made it impractical. Nezhat was an enthusiastic proponent of "video laparoscopy" in the latter half of the 1980s.[64]

The tide generated by the general surgeons in their newfound technology carried the gynecologist on to explore further applications including removal of dermoid cysts[65] and cystic ovarian tumors,[66,67] even in the postmenopausal women.[68] The publication of the first case report "Laparoscopic Hysterectomy" by Reich and co-workers[69] led to extensive use of this approach worldwide and introduction of a multitude of variations in technique and terminology. Suprapubic bladder neck suspension was performed laparoscopically.[70] Urinary and intestinal complications that resulted from the performance of more extensive surgery began to be treated by laparoscopy.[71,72] Gynecologic surgeons became more adventuresome in treating conditions that affected the bowel,[73] bladder, or ureter.[74] More recently, laparoscopic access has been used in gynecologic oncology for pelvic[74] and para-aortic[75] lymphadenectomy and radical hysterectomy.[76]

It is now apparent that almost every gynecologic procedure can be effected by means of laparoscopic access. The work of the modern surgical innovators has only been possible because of the efforts of the early pioneers both in the medical and the technologic spheres. The answer to the question, "Why look through the keyhole when you can open the door?" has been resoundingly answered by the next question, "Why open the door at all?"

REFERENCES:

1. Semm K. History in operative gynaecologic endoscopy. In Sanfilippo JS, Levine RL, editors: Operative Gynecologic Endoscopy. New York, 1989, Springer Verlag.
2. Recamier R: Curette. In Le Grand Dictionaire Encyclopedique Medical. 1979, Flammarion.
3. Bozzini P: Lichtleiter. Eine Erfindung zur Anschauung innerer Teile und Krankheiten. *J für Prak Heilkunde* 24:107, 1806.
4. Desormeaux AJ: De L'endoscopie et de des ses Applications au Diagnostic et au Traitement des Affections de L'urethre et de la Vessie. Paris, 1865, Bailliere.
5. Pantaleoni D: On endoscopic examination of the cavity of the womb. *Med Press Circ* 8:26, 1869.
6. Nitze M: Uber eine neue Behandlungs—methode der Höhlen des menschlichen Körpers. *Wien Med Wochenschr* 24:851, 1879.
7. Gunning JE: History of laparoscopy in laparoscopy. In Phillips JM, editor: Baltimore, 1977, Williams and Wilkins.
8. von Ott DO: Ventroscopic illumination of the abdominal cavity in pregnancy. *Zhurnal Akrestierstova I Zhenskikh Boloznei* 15:7-8, 1901.
9. Kelling G: Ueber Oesophagoskopie, Gastroskopie und Koelioskopie. *Munchner Medizinische Wochenschrift* 49:22-24, 1902.
10. Jacobaeus HC: Über die Möglichkeit, die Zystoskopie bei Untersuchung seröser Höhlungen anzuwenden. *Münch Med Wochenschr* 57:2090-2092, 1910.
11. Steiner OP: Abdominoscopy. *Surg Gynecol Obstet* 38:266, 1924.
12. Redi R: Über ein neues endoskopisches chirurgisches Instrument, das Splanchnoskop. *Zentralbl Chir* 558, 1935.
13. Nordentoeft S: Uber Endoskopie geschlossener Kavitaten mittels meines Trokar-Endoskopes. *Verhandlungen der Deutschen Gesellschaft Für Gynäkologie* 41:78-81, 1912.
14. Zollikoffer R: Zur Laparosckopie. *Schweizerische Medizinische Wochenschrift* 5:264-265, 1924.
15. Kalk H: Erfahrungen mit der Laparoskopie. *Zeitschrift für Klinische Medizin* 111:303-348, 1929.
16. Fervers C: Die Laparoskopie mit dem Cystoskop. Ein Beitrag zur Vereinfachung der Technik und zur endoskopischen Strangdurchtrennung in der Bauchhöhle. *Med Klin Chir* 178:288, 1933.
17. Bosch PF: Laparoskopische sterilization. Schweizerische Zeitschrift Für Krankenhaus und Anstaltswesen, 1936.
18. Anderson ET: Peritoneoscopy. *Am J Surg* 35:136-139, 1937.
19. Power FH, Barnes AC: Sterilization by means of peritoneoscopic tubal fulguration. *Am J Obstet Gynecol* 41:1038-1043, 1941.
20. Ruddock JC: Peritoneoscopy. *West J Surg* 42:392, 1934.
21. Veress J: Neues Instrument sur Ausfuhrung von Brust-oder Bachpunktionen und Pneumothoraxbehandlung. *Deutsche Medizinische Wochenschrift* 64:1480-1481, 1938.
22. Fourestier N, Gladu A, Vulmiere J: Perfectionnements a l'endoscopie medicale. Realisation bronchoscopique. *Presse Med* 60:1, 292, 1952.
23. Hopkins H: Optical principles of the endoscope. In Berci G, editor: Endoscopy. New York, 1976, Appleton-Century-Crofts.
24. Palmer R: Technique et instrumentation de la coelioscopie gynecologique. *Gynecol Obstet* (Paris) 46:420, 1947.
25. Frangenheim H: Die Laparoskopie und die Culdoskopie in der Gynaecologie. Stuttgart, 1959, Georg Thieme.
26. Albano V, Cittadini E: La Celioscopia in Ginecologia. Palermo, 1962, Denaro.
27. Thoyer-Rozat J: La Celioscopie, Paris, 1962, Masson et Cie.
28. Bernkeim BM: Organoscopy: cystoscopy of the abdominal cavity. *Ann Surg* 53:764-767, 1911.
29. Steptoe PC: Laparoscopy in Gynaecology, Edinburgh, 1967, E&S Livingston.
30. Cohen MR: Laparoscopy, culdoscopy and gynecography. Philadelphia, 1970, WB Saunders.
31. Palmer R: Essais de sterilisation tubaire celioscopique par electrocoagulation isthmique. *Bull Fed Soc Gynecol Obstet Lang Fr* 14:298, 1962.
32. Neuwirth RS, Cejas M: Sterilization by tubal cauterization and transection at laparoscopy. *Am J Obstet Gynecol* 105:632, 1969.

33. Liston WA, Downie J, Bradford W, Kerr MG: Female sterilization by tubal electrocoagulation under laparoscopic control. *Lancet* 1:683, 1970.
34. Wheeless CR: A rapid, inexpensive and effective method of surgical sterilization by laparoscopy. *J Reprod Med* 3:65, 1969.
35. Steptoe PC, Edwards RG: Laparoscopic recovery of preovulatory human oocytes after priming of ovaries with gonadotropins. *Lancet* 1:683, 1970.
36. Semm K: New methods of pelviscopy (gynecologic laparoscopy) for myomectomy, ovariectomy, tubectomy and adnexectomy. *Endoscopy* 11:85-93, 1979.
37. Mettler L, Giesel H, Semm K: Treatment of female infertility due to tubal obstruction by operative laparoscopy. *Fertil Steril* 32:384, 1979.
38. Semm K: Tissue-puncher and loop-ligation—new aids for surgical therapeutic pelviscopy (laparoscopy) = endoscopic intraabdominal surgery. *Endoscopy* 10:119-124, 1978.
39. Semm K: Suction pump—a new aid for pelviscopy. *Endoscopy* 7:85-88, 1975.
40. Semm K: Endocoagulation: a new and completely safe medical current for sterilization. *Int J Fertil* 22:238-242, 1977.
41. Gomel V: Experience with operative laparoscopy. Presented at the 20th Annual Meeting of the Canadian Fertility Society, Vancouver, June 1973. Published by the Canadian Fertility Society. Program, p3.
42. Gomel V: Laparoscopic tubal surgery in infertility. *Obstet Gynecol* 46:47-48, 1975.
43. Gomel V: Salpingostomy by laparoscopy. *J Reprod Med* 18:265, 1977.
44. Gomel V: Reconstructive surgery of the oviduct. *J Rep Med* 18:181-190, 1977.
45. Gomel V: Fertility surgery. In Phillips JM, editor: Laparoscopy. Baltimore, 1977, Williams & Wilkins.
46. Gomel V: Recent advances in surgical correction of tubal disease producing infertility. *Curr Probl Obstet Gynecol* 1:10 15-16, 1978.
47. Gomel V: Laparoscopy in the diagnosis and treatment of ectopic gestation. *Gine Dips* 2:85, 1978.
48. Stangel J, Gomel V: Conservative surgery of tubal gestation. *Clin Obs Gyn* 23:1221, 1980.
49. Shapiro HI, Adler DH: Excision of an ectopic pregnancy through the laparoscope. *Am J Obstet Gynecol* 117:290, 1973.
50. Soderstrom RM: Unusual uses of laparoscopy. *J Reprod Med* 15:77, 1975.
51. Bruhat MA, Mahnes H, Mage G, Pouly JL: Treatment of ectopic pregnancy by means of laparoscopy. *Fertil Steril* 33:411, 1980.
52. Bruhat MA, Mage G, Pouly JL: Use of the CO_2 laser in laparoscopy. In Laser Surgery: Kaplan I, Ascher PW, editors: Proceedings of the 3rd International Symposium on Laser Surgery, Tel Aviv, 1979, OT-PAZ Press.
53. Rioux JE, Cloutier D: A new bipolar instrument for laparoscopic tubal sterilization. *Am J Obstet Gynecol* 119:737, 1974.
54. Clarke HC: Laparoscopy: New instruments for suturing and ligation. *Fertil Steril* 23:274-277, 1972.
55. Martin DC: CO_2 laser laparoscopy for the treatment of endometriosis associated with infertility. *J Reprod Med* 30:409, 1985.
56. Martin DC: CO_2 laser laparoscopy for endometriosis associated with infertility. *J Reprod Med* 31;1089, 1986.
57. Feste JR: Laser laparoscopy a new modality. *J Reprod Med* 40:413, 1985.
58. Daniell J: Operative laparoscopy for endometriosis. *Semin Reprod Endocrinol* 3:353, 1985.
59. Nezhat C, Crowgey SR, Garrison CP: Surgical treatment of endometriosis via laser laparoscopy. *Fertil Steril* 45:778, 1986.
60. Davis GD: Management of endometriosis and its associated adhesions with the CO_2 laser laparoscope. *Obstet Gynecol* 68:422, 1986.
61. Semm K: Endoscopic appendectomy. *Endoscopy* 15:59-64, 1983.
62. Dubois F, Berthelot G, Levard H: Coelioscopic cholecystectomy. *Ann Surg* 211:60-63, 1990.
63. Soderstrom RM: Personal observation.
64. Nezhat C: Videolaseroscopy: A new modality for the treatment of endometriosis and other diseases of reproductive organs. *Colp Gynecol Laser Surg* 2:221-224, 1986.
65. Nezhat C, Winer WK, Nezhat F: Laparoscopic removal of dermoid cysts. *Obstet Gynecol* 73:278, 1989.
66. Hasson HM: Laparoscopic management of ovarian cysts. *J Reprod Med* 35:863-7, 1990.
67. Mage G, Canis M. Manhes H, Pouly J-L, Wattiez A, Bruhat MA: Laparoscopic management of adnexal cystic masses. *J Gynecol Surg* 6:71, 1990.
68. Parker WH, Berek JS: Management of selected cystic adnexal masses in postmenopausal women by operative laparoscopy: A pilot study. *Am J Obst Gynecol* 163:1574-1577, 1990.
69. Reich H, DeCaprio J, McGlynn F: Laparoscopic hysterectomy. *J Gynecol Surg* 5:213-216, 1989.
70. Vancaille TG, Scheussler W: Laparoscopic bladder neck suspension. *J Laparendo Surg* 1:169, 1991.
71. Gomel V, James C: Intraoperative management of ureteral injury during operative laparoscopy. *Fertil Steril* 55:416-419, 1991.
72. Reich H, McGlynn F, Budin R: Laparoscopic repair of full-thickness bowel injury. *J Lapar Surg* 1:119-122, 1991.
73. Nezhat C, Pennington E, Nazhat F, Silfern SL: Laparoscopically assisted anterior rectal wall resection and reanastomosis for deeply infiltrating endometriosis. *Surg Lapar Endo* 1:106-108, 1991.
74. Nezhat C, Nezhat F, Green B: Laparoscopic treatment of obstructed ureter due to endometriosis by resection and ureteroureterostomy: A case report. *J Urol* 148:865-868, 1992.
75. Querleu D, LeBlanc E, Castelain B: Laparoscopic lymphadenecomy in the staging of early carcinoma of the cervix. *Am J Obstet Gynecol* 164:579-81, 1991.
76. Nezhat CR, Burrell MO, Nezhat FR, et al: Laparoscopic radical hysterectomy with paraaortic and pelvic node dissection. *Am J Obstet Gynecol* 166:864-5, 1992.

Chapter 2

TRAINING AND CREDENTIALLING

Carl J. Levinson

The vast majority of practicing gyncologists and senior residents are fully trained in diagnostic laparoscopy and in the performance of sterilization procedures. Because the introduction of advanced laparoscopic surgery has been so rapid many established physicians are presently striving to master the new techniques, and not all residency programs have the facilities to train their graduates fully in these approaches. Until such time as all residents qualify as laparoscopic surgeons, and all those in practice who wish to become trained have done so, training of the individual and conferring of hospital privileges (credentialling) by medical institutions will be challenging.

It is the purpose of this chapter to suggest to physicians how they might most effectively introduce new laparoscopic procedures into their practices and to assist the heads of hospital departments and boards of directors to determine how best to ascertain the competence of a surgeon who wishes to use these techniques. This general discussion is based on three appendices. The first describes the guidelines of the Society of Reproductive Surgeons, the second is an approach that has been implemented in one hospital in the United States, and the third has been adapted from the recommendations of the Society of Obstetricians and Gynaecologists of Canada.

HISTORIC BACKGROUND

Until recently most major gynecologic surgery was performed by laparotomy or by the vaginal route. In the last decade the shift has been toward a laparoscopic approach. Indeed as many as 50% of cases that previously would have required laparotomy are now carried out laparoscopically. This figure is expected to increased in the near future. This rapid change has been driven by many factors, which include advances in technology, economic considerations, impetus from the instrument manufacturers, the introduction of new methods of energy delivery (lasers, Argon beam), use of video and, not the least, consumer pressure.

The entry of these endoscopic approaches to the North American continent in many ways parallels the introduction of vaginal surgery, although the rate of change has been much more widespread and much more rapid.

The early gynecologists were general surgeons who developed a special interest in the surgery of the female genital tract. Many of them had come from, or had studied in, Europe—particularly in Germany and Austria. Many were excellent abdominal surgeons. When vaginal surgery began to be developed it was not immediately embraced by all surgeons. Schools that did wish to pursue this approach evolved, for example, the one in Chicago. The techniques were taught by professor to student and by partner to partner. The facility of a given surgeon was often an accident of geography. Gradually the technique spread until it became universal practice.

This process was repeated in the early laparoscopy era as developments in France, Germany, and England were adopted in North America. In much the same way the early American pioneers of operative laparoscopy tended to be found in certain geographic areas. The American Association of Gynecologic Laparoscopists has played a very important part in rapidly disseminating the techniques. Today neither residents nor established practitioners can afford the luxury of gradually acquiring skills. There is an urgent need for effective training.

Many residency programs do not offer formal instruction, lacking as they do instructors who possess the necessary skills. Some have been able to arrange for residents to spend elective time in other institutions where the techniques can be learned. It is to be hoped that this deficiency will soon be rectified as more surgeons become trained. In some units learners are exposed to the simpler operations including only tubal ligation, lysis of minor adhesions, and fulguration of minimal endometriosis. This frequently is the level of expertise possessed by practitioners who wish to upgrade their skills.

TRAINING

It must be stated firmly that possession of surgical ability and/or attendance at a 2-day course does not constitute adequate preparation for undertaking more complex laparoscopic procedures.

In both the United States and Canada much thought has been given to how best to ensure that gynecologists can receive satisfactory training and how this training can be recognized by the institutions in which they practice. Although there are differences in detail, very similar principles have emerged. The trainee must possess a basic level of entry skills (described in the appendices), complete a theoretical course, observe video tapes of procedures, and devote time to hands-on practice both with models and with animal tissues.

The pelvitrainer is a transparent box into which a telescope and ancillary instruments can be passed. The learner can practice the use of the ancillary instruments for suturing, dissecting, knot tying, and the applications of various energy sources. Initially the manual skills are acquired by observing through the plexiglass without using a laparoscope. When these have been mastered an opaque covering is placed over the pelvitrainer, a laparoscope inserted, a video camera attached to the telescope, and the trainee repeats the exercises now working from the images displayed on the television screen. The pelvitrainer will accommodate both inanimate material and extirpated organic tissue. It is an excellent method of developing the hand-eye coordination necessary for the performance of endoscopic surgery. It is also a gentle way of demonstrating to those unfortunate individuals who seem to be unable to master this new approach that perhaps they should not be pursuing matters further.

Although use of the pelvitrainer is an excellent way to acquire the basic steps, it cannot fully replicate the experience that can be gained when working with live tissue. This is particularly important if the surgeon wishes to develop the skills necessary to perform the more complex procedures. The anesthetized pig and especially the goat are excellent models in which the gynecologist can practice dissection, securing hemostasis, suturing, using energy sources and stapling devices, and removing extirpated tissue. Many institutions have the necessary animal laboratory facilities to which gynecologists may gain access by either personal arrangement or by enrolling in a formal workshop.

The trainee should first master the less complicated procedures before moving on to the next level. It is recommended that surgeons do work in the animal laboratory, become experienced in the human, and return to the animal laboratory before moving on to the next level of complexity.

Prececeptorships can be arranged in institutions where a large volume of laparoscopic surgery is performed. Certain obstacles might make this impractical, however. It is often difficult to obtain privileges for a limited duration, so that while learners may observe they may not be permitted to operate. Furthermore, most gynecologists cannot spend extended amounts of time away from their practices. Hands-on human experience may be obtained in the physician's home institution under the supervision of an experienced preceptor. This can pose subtle difficulties. Who will "teach, certify, or credential"? Often the teacher and the student are both members of staff. It may be difficult for the preceptor to judge the skills of a colleague, particularly if in the opinion of the former the latter has not met the required standard of expertise. One solution is to arrange for a skilled endoscopist from another institution to be granted temporary privileges, either to supervise the training process or to attend a final evaluation session when the learner feels that a suitable level of competence has been achieved. Irrespective of the method used, the certifying surgeon must be scrupulously honest in making the appraisal.

These steps should be undertaken over a reasonable period. Every learner must be certified at one level of competence before moving on to learning at a higher level.

CREDENTIALLING

From the institution's point of view it is probably wise to grant temporary privileges initially, asking for a final report from the preceptor after the surgeon has carried out a number of cases unsupervised. On receipt of a satisfactory final report the department head should be then comfortable in recommending to the Board that active privileges be awarded. It is further recommended that all surgical privileges and complications should be kept under ongoing review by the department head, who should have clearly defined powers to revoke the privileges of any surgeon whose performance is judged to be unsatisfactory.

It is hoped that this advice will be of value to both those who wish to learn and those charged with the responsibility of determining competence. The detailed American and Canadian recommendations now follow as Appendices I, II, and III.

APPENDIX I
GUIDELINES FOR ATTAINING PRIVILEGES IN GYNECOLOGIC OPERATIVE ENDOSCOPY OF THE SOCIETY OF REPRODUCTIVE SURGEONS, AN AFFILIATE OF THE AMERICAN FERTILITY SOCIETY*

These guidelines presuppose the following:

1. The applicant is eligible or certified by the American Board of Obstetrics and Gynecology and is a member in good standing in the Department of Obstetrics and Gynecology of the hospital/institution to which the application is being directed.
2. The applicant has been granted privileges to perform diagnostic laparoscopy, laparoscopic tubal sterilization, and/or diagnostic hysteroscopy and has demonstrated competence in these techniques.
3. Privileges will be granted for laparoscopic and hysteroscopic skill levels as outlined in the Appendix.

The following guidelines are suggested for institutions that grant privileges for gynecologic operative endoscopy.

1. The applicant will request privileges for the use of: 1) a specific endoscope (e.g., laparoscope, hysteroscope or resectoscope), 2) a specific energy source or modality (e.g., electrosurgery, specific wavelength laser, harmonic scalpel); 3) a designated laparoscopic or hysteroscopic skill level (see boxes on pp 8 and 9).
2. For each requested privilege the applicant must submit evidence of the satisfactory completion of:
   A. A recognized (CME accredited) formal didactic course(s) of at least 16 hours duration that includes at least 4 hours of supervised inanimate laboratory experience (e.g., pelvic trainer or hysteroscopic models) and at least 4 hours of supervised laboratory experience with laparoscopic surgery in live animal models.
   B. Viewing of and/or assistance in several endoscopic operations at the designated clinical skill level.
   C. A preceptorship with a physician who is credentialled to perform the procedures designated at a particular skill level. The preceptor should be recognized in the community at large or nationally as someone who possesses the necessary experience and skills to function as a tutor and preceptor. The preceptorship experience should consist of tutoring both as the first assistant and as the principal surgeon. The hospital should provide an appropriate record-keeping system for the credentialling process and the preceptor should verify that the tutorial experience took place. The applicant should provide a case list that includes:
      Patient's name, medical record number, and date of surgery
      Preoperative and postoperative diagnosis
      Endoscopic surgical procedure performed
      Type of endoscope used
      Energy modality used
      Outcome and complications of the procedure.
      It is recommended that at least five and preferably 10 procedures be performed satisfactorily under supervision at each skill level before privileges in full are granted.
3. A periodic review of newly granted privileges to individual surgeons should be performed by the parent institution at annual or biannual intervals. Each credentialled physician should provide to the hospital credentialling committee a case list of endoscopic procedures performed and complications encountered during the time interval to be reviewed. Recertification will require demonstration of continuing performance of endoscopic procedures with an acceptable rate of complications.
4. A letter from the director of an approved residency training program can take the place of 2 A, B, or C if the required training criteria have been fulfilled during residency.
5. If there are no surgeons on the staff of the parent institution who can act as preceptors, then supervised preceptorships can be arranged by scheduling a number of appropriate cases in conjunction with other interested surgeons and inviting a visiting expert to serve as the preceptor.
6. Any surgeon already performing procedures for which privileges are being requested at the time the credentialling process is initiated will be required to submit a summary of his or her training and practical experience for each endoscopic skill level. In addition the surgeon will submit to the Chairman of the Credentialling Committee a case list for the past year, which contains the same information as in 2 C. The committee may grant privileges without completion of all the criteria stated in 2 C.

Stratification of hysteroscopic procedures

Procedures not requiring additional training (level 1)

Diagnostic hysteroscopy

Procedures requiring additional training (level 2)

Endometrial resection or ablation
Division/resection of uterine septum
Endoscopic surgery for Ashermans syndrome
Resection of uterine myomas
Fallopian tube cannulation

*These guidelines were approved by the American Fertility Society (AFS) Practice Committee, October 30, 1993 and the AFS Board of Directors, December 17, 1993.

Stratification of laparoscopic procedures

Procedures not requiring additional training (level 1)

Laparoscopic sterilization
Needle aspiration of simple cysts
Ovarian biopsy
Minor adhesiolysis
Partial salpingectomy for ectopic pregnancy
Linear salpingostomy for ectopic pregnancy

Procedures requiring additional training (level 2)

Laparoscopic division of uterosacral ligaments
Adhesiolysis for moderate and severe adhesions or adhesions involving bowel
Laser/diathermy drilling to ovaries for polycystic ovarian syndrome
Neosalpingostomy for hydrosalpinx
Salpingectomy/salpingo-oophorectomy
Endoscopic management of endometrioma and ovarian cystectomy
Laparoscopically assisted vaginal hysterectomy
Endoscopic surgery for AFS Stage III and IV endometriosis
Appendectomy

Procedures requiring significant additional training (level 3)

Pelvic lymphadenectomy
Extensive pelvic side-wall dissection
Presacral neurectomy
Dissection of an obliterated pouch of Douglas
Bowel surgery
Retropubic bladder neck suspension
Hernia repair
Ureteral dissection

APPENDIX II
STANDARD GUIDELINES FOR TRAINING IN OPERATIVE ENDOSCOPY IN ONE HOSPITAL IN THE UNITED STATES

The physician must be licensed to practice medicine and surgery and in good standing at the institution. Background must include experience in a range of medical and surgical therapies (including documented resident experience). The physician should be board certified, or eligible, with extensive experience in diagnostic laparoscopy and privileges for the same surgical procedure by laparotomy.

In the event that there are physicians already performing endoscopic procedures for 2 years or longer, they may be "grandfathered" for procedures at Level 1 and Level 2 with required proctoring for three cases.

Level 3 privileges cover advanced and complex procedures that are essentially "new" as performed by endoscopy. Each such procedure shall be credentialled separately. Requirements include attendance at a course for the special procedure, animal practice, and human work as an assistant surgeon. The procedure itself must be accepted as safe and appropriate with concurrence from those surgeons who performed the procedure by laparotomy. Complex procedures are best performed by a group of surgeons who perform them on a regular basis. These procedures are gener-

Definition of privileges

Level 1 privileges are automatically extended to all surgeons applying who may have met the basic requirements, have sufficient pelvitrainer experience, have attended appropriate courses of appropriate length, and have assisted at five cases. Privileges will be continued if good judgement is exercised and consultation sought when appropriate.

Level 2 privileges are extended to those surgeons with Level 1 privileges who have completed the required number of proctored cases. (Proctors should not be associated with the surgeon and it is preferable to have more than one Proctor.)

Level 1—Basic procedures

Lysis of adhesions not involving bowel
Lysis of filmy adhesions involving bowel
Removal of ectopic pregnancy with conservation of the tube
Endocoagulation
Use of Endoloops:
  Hemostasis
  Removal of pedunculated tumors
Application of clips
Puncture, enucleation, and removal of simple benign cysts

Level 2—Major procedures

Procedure	Required number of cases
Adhesion lysis:	
dense bowel adhesions	2
mid-upper bowel adhesions.	2
Myomectomy	2
Oophorectomy and cystectomy	2
Salpingo-oophorectomy	2
Salpingectomy	2
Appendectomy	
Intra-abdominal suturing	1
Intra- and Extra-corporeal knotting	3
Laser division of uterosacral ligaments	2

Level 3—Advanced procedures	Required number of cases
Retroperitoneal dissection with ureter dissection	2
Total hysterectomy (where the uterine artery is occluded laparoscopically)	3
Subtotal hysterectomy	1
Suspension of bladder/urethra	2
Presacral neurectomy	2

ally specialty specific and the surgeon must have privileges within that speciality.

In the event that there is a low volume of endoscopic surgical procedures and/or there is an inadequate number of proctors, it becomes the responsibility of the Chief of Service, with concurrence with the Board of Trustees, to determine how the surgeons may be credentialed for new procedures. Specialized training, proctoring, and careful evaluation are required.

TRAINING

For Levels 2 and 3, the trainee must have privileges for laparoscopic surgery, having demonstrated expertise in the same in the area of the body under consideration. In questionable cases, proctors may be assigned.

Training may be "in-house" if the department has developed a full training program. "Outside" training may be obtained via a preceptorship or by attending courses. Under a "preceptor program," the preceptor must attest to the competence of the preceptee. Training courses include the following:

Basic laparoscopy techniques
Laser physiology and safety
Electrosurgical principles and techniques
Approved faculty quality
Adequate didactic time
Adequate time with tissue or animals.

For Level 3 procedures, the courses must be procedure specific.

EXPERIENCE

In addition to the foregoing, the surgeon must act as an assistant to experienced surgeon(s) for cases that increase in complexity.

After having obtained the required training and experience, the surgeon must undergo the proctoring procedure. The proctor should be an experienced surgeon in the area who is unbiased and will act as a reviewer and evaluator of the surgical management. Specifically, the following items must be checked:

Familiarity with equipment
Familiarity with the operative procedure
Time involved
Knowledge of anatomy
Complications
General approach

The number of cases required is suggested but may be amended by the local institution.

FOLLOW-UP EVALUATION

Privileges should be reviewed every two years but complications should be reviewed annually.

APPENDIX III
GUIDELINES FOR TRAINING IN OPERATIVE ENDOSCOPY IN CANADA*

An Ad Hoc Committee of the Society of Obstetricians and Gynaecologists of Canada was formed to examine the need to standardize training in operative laparoscopy and to produce recommendations for guidelines. This committee was formed both in response to the numerous requests that had been received for such guidelines and also to what appeared to be a very rapid spread of the practice of these procedures. There have been various problems associated with the rapid spread of such procedures in many countries, including a number of deaths in the United States and the United Kingdom. Furthermore, a number of major complications have already been identified in Canadian centers. With these problems in mind, it was felt that a framework should be provided for training in order to provide the maximum support to clinicians while they endeavor to gain new skills.

Establishing guidelines for practicing gynecologists is a difficult concept. Most gynecologists are already accomplished diagnostic laparoscopists and have an excellent working knowledge of pelvic anatomy. The vast majority of physicians apply a high degree of clinical judgment to case selection and are aware of their own limitations. Operative endoscopy, however, requires new skills and techniques that have to be learned. The learning curve will differ markedly between individuals and there will be a range of aptitudes. Therefore, there should be a degree of flexibility in any training program.

A preceptorship has been included as an integral part of the training for certain endoscopic procedures (levels 2 and 3). It is recognized that trained gynecologists require supervision in acquiring new skills such as with radical hysterectomy and tubal microsurgery, and similarly operative endoscopy necessitates the acquisition of new skills. One of the most important points made within this document it that it is imperative for any gynecologist undertaking operative endoscopy to have appropriate experience in the normal range of alternate medical and surgical therapies. Furthermore, they must understand the pathology of the organ being operated upon. Important examples of an adverse outcome resulting from inexperience in these fields are the reproductive consequences of inappropriate ovarian surgery in which physiologic changes are misinterpreted during routine appendectomy.

PREREQUISITES

A physician wishing to be granted privileges in operative endoscopy must demonstrate the necessary additional training and competence in performance of the proce-

*Modified from J Soc Obstet Gynaecol Canada 14:101-107, 1993.

dure(s). Also to be taken into account are departmental needs and adequate facilities.

Prior to undertaking operative endoscopy at any level (see box on p. 9), the individual should have demonstrated proficiency in performing diagnostic procedures with the same instrument. The individual must be certified in the specialty of Obstetrics and Gynaecology by the Royal College of Physicians and Surgeons of Canada and/or Provincial College of Physicians and Surgeons and have privileges (see boxes on pp. 9 and 11) for the same procedures when performed by laparotomy.

Attendance at an appropriate course

The individual shall have completed a course especially designed for level of surgery performed. Such a course must be accredited for Continuing Medical Education (CME) and will include:

1. Didactic materials to enhance understanding of the operation of the endoscopic equipment and auxiliary equipment. If electrosurgery or laser is to be used, it is important to understand the physical principles of the equipment, including safety factors.
2. There shall be a "hands-on" aspect in the laboratory for a minimum of 10 hours, of which 6 shall be spent working with tissue and/or animal models.
3. The course shall include the use of video for demonstration purposes.

Preceptorship

The individual shall then usually proceed to a preceptorship. First, this will involve observation in the operating room in order to:

1. Understand all the equipment and acquire the capability of operating it.
2. Learn the role of nurses, including both the scrub and circulating nurses.
3. Observe surgery of the level of accreditation that is sought by the gynecologist by watching live video.

After the initial period of observing surgery, the individual shall operate as the first assistant to an experienced gynecologist and/or perform surgery with preceptor acting as first assistant. However, the final phase of the training requires the physician to perform surgery with the preceptor acting as first assistant, until a preceptor is satisfied that the surgeon is competent to operate on his or her own. During training, cases should initially be simple, increasing in complexity with the aptitude demonstrated by the trainee. When sufficient experience has been obtained, the preceptor may then recommend to the department head that procedural privileges be granted. During training, it is mandatory to use video equipment. However, an experienced endoscopic gynecologist may exercise his or her decision about the use of video equipment during clinical practice.

If no gynecologist is available for preceptorship at the community hospital, two (2) experienced gynecologists who have been performing laparoscopy for more than 3 years can be given temporary privileges by the Department Head. These gynecologists must then operate together on at least ten (10) cases of level 2 complexity before each can operate alone. Procedures should initially be simple and there should be slow progress through the levels of complexity. A record must be kept of all procedures, including adverse outcomes, which must be made available to the credentialling body. These temporary privileges should be formally reviewed after an initial 6 month period.

EVALUATION

It will be necessary for the individual to have ongoing experience in the performance of the procedures. It is recommended that the departmental head review the privilege(s) on an annual basis.

Stratification of laparoscopic procedures in Canada

Procedures not requiring additional training (Level 1)

Laparoscopic sterilization
Needle aspiration of simple cysts
Ovarian biopsy
Minor adhesiolysis
Laser/diathermy to endometriosis—AFS stages I and II
Laser/diathermy to ovaries for polycystic ovarian syndrome
Linear salpingostomy and/or salpingectomy for ectopic pregnancy

Procedures requiring additional training (Level 2)

Laparoscopic division of uterosacral ligaments
Adhesiolysis for moderate and severe adhesions or adhesions involving bowel
Salpingostomy for infertility
Salpingectomy/salpingo-oophorectomy
Laparoscopic ovarian cystectomy
Endoscopic management of endometrioma
Endoscopic surgery for AFS stages III and IV endometriosis
Laparoscopically assisted vaginal hysterectomy

Procedures requiring a subspecialist or advanced/tertiary level endoscopic skills (Level 3)

Myomectomy
Pelvic lymphadenectomy
Pelvic side-wall dissection
Ureteral dissection
Presacral neurectomy
Dissection of obliterated pouch of Douglas

STRATIFICATION OF AND PRIVILEGES IN OPERATIVE ENDOSCOPIC PROCEDURES

Operative laparoscopic procedures are stratified by level of complexity (see box on p. 11). This to promote gradual progression through levels of difficulty and to prevent gynecologists from being placed under pressure to undertake more complex cases before they have attained the necessary skills. Furthermore, this stratification emphasizes that complex endoscopic procedures are best undertaken by a group of individuals who regularly perform these procedures and who therefore possess a high level of skill. Level 3 procedures must be undertaken by a subspecialist or an individual who has advanced endoscopic skills. This also stresses the need to have a high level of skill in undertaking the alternative conventional form of surgery and the value in having an in-depth knowledge of the relevant field.

GRANDFATHER CLAUSE

At the introduction of these new guidelines, it will be necessary to "grandfather" a number of Level 2 and 3 gynecologic endoscopic surgeons who have a proved track record and have performed a large number of procedures at that level. Individuals who obtain level 2 or 3 privileges at the introduction of these new guidelines must have a clearly proved track record in this field. These individuals should have many years of experience with these procedures, have shown leadership in their respective hospitals or communities, and/or have been involved in teaching, research, and publication in the field of operative endoscopy.

LASER PRIVILEGES

Possession of any level of endoscopic privileges does not automatically confer the right to use a laser in either the abdominal or uterine cavity. To obtain endoscopic laser privileges, it will be necessary to demonstrate appropriate previous experience (grandfather) or be appropriately trained. The criteria for grandfathering regarding laser privileges should be as previously outlined. The initial phase of training requires attendance at a course that explains the physical principles of the laser, laser safety, and both equipment and technique used in laser endoscopy. During the next phase of training, a preceptorship should be undertaken as previously outlined. Where no preceptor is available in the community hospital, two experienced gynecologists can work together as defined in the preceptorship section. They should initially gain experience in the use of the laser in open procedures, before progressing to laser endoscopy.

Chapter 3

EQUIPMENT AND INSTRUMENTATION

A glance through the catalog of any instrument manufacturer can be confusing to say the least; the instruments available are bewildering in their diversity. Yet it is possible to perform all diagnostic laparoscopy and most operative laparoscopy with relatively few, well-chosen pieces of equipment. This chapter will describe the instruments that the authors have found to be indispensable and currently use. There is no intent to promote any specific manufacturer. Usually similar instruments are produced by several companies. A specific instrument may occasionally be unique to one producer. Our goal is to give the reader an understanding of what instruments and equipment are available, our preferences, and guidance in how to select equipment.

Since most surgical departments are now very involved in endoscopic surgery, it may be advisable to discuss with them what equipment is already available to avoid unnecessary duplication. Indeed, many hospitals have introduced endoscopy committees to coordinate instrument purchases.

The equipment that will be required is either of a general nature, including operating tables, storage facilities, and suction apparatus, or is specific to the performance of laparoscopy. In this latter category fall insufflators, light sources and cables, the external manipulators, pneumoperitoneum needles, principal trocars and cannulas, telescopes, energy sources (which will be described in Chapter 4), ancillary trocars, cannulas, and instruments. Video equipment is integral to the effective performance of operative laparoscopy (see Chapters 7 and 8). It is virtually impossible to perform laparoscopic surgery without recourse to their use. Each will be described.

GENERAL EQUIPMENT

The operating table and its attachments, storage facilities for the laparoscopic equipment, and suction fittings may not fall under the direct control of the gynecologist. Laparoscopists may have to adapt existing facilities to meet their needs.

Operating tables and their attachments

The various intra-abdominal structures are visualized with the patient in specific positions. The pelvic organs are best seen with the patient in the Trendenlenburg position, whereas the upper abdominal structures require the patient to be in the Fowler (head-up) position with varying degrees of right or left lateral decubitus used to display specific organs. To facilitate such positioning with the least amount of effort, automatic electrical operating tables would obviously be ideal but are available to few.

Although gynecologic laparoscopy invariably requires the use of the Trendelenburg position, the operating table must permit manual adjustment of its height, varying degrees of Trendelenburg and Fowler positions, as well as lateral rotation. In addition, it must accommodate stirrups to place the patient in the lithotomy position to provide access to the external genitalia, vagina, and cervix. The modified Lloyd-Davis stirrups are most suited since they provide support under the lower thigh, knee, and upper calf. Simple stirrups can be used, especially for short procedures. Padding can be used to prevent compression of leg vessels. The placement of the stirrups and the height and position of the knees are very important since erroneous placement may hinder the ability of the surgeon to manipulate the ancillary instruments (see Chapter 5).

Armboards are of great help to the anesthetist, but can get in the way during laparoscopy and can be responsible for damage to the bronchial plexus if incorrectly positioned. They should be removable so that once anesthesia has been induced the arm can be placed by the patient's side. Simi-

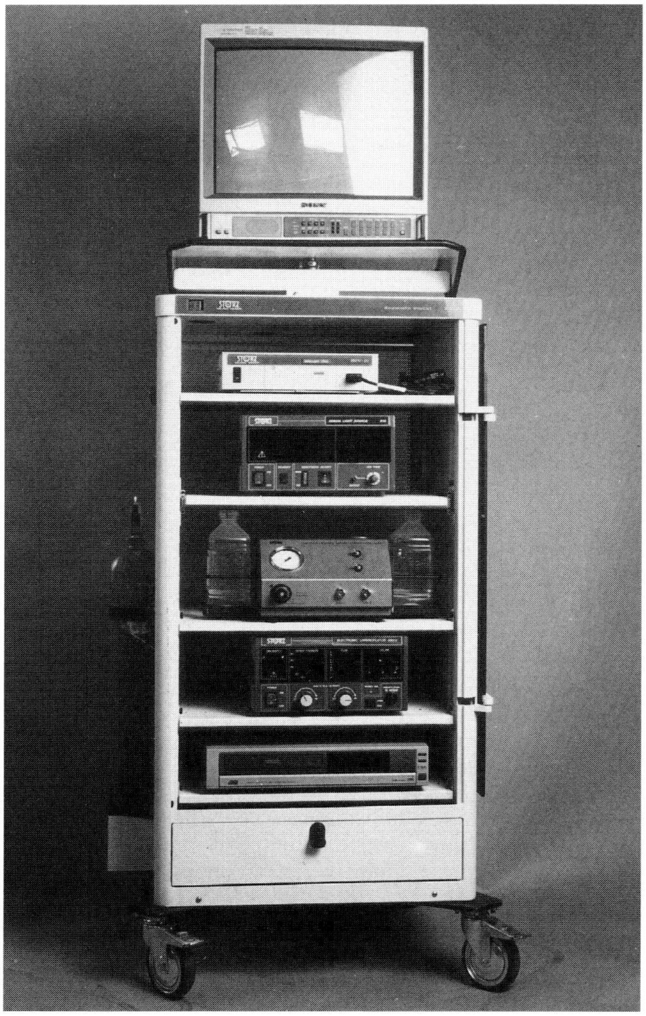

Fig. 3-1. Mobile equipment storage unit. (Courtesy Storz Instruments.)

larly shoulder braces can cause nerve damage when the table is placed in the deep Trendelenburg position. A non-slip underpad is preferable. As many operative procedures can take several hours, patients can be at risk for developing hypothermia. A warming pad can help to overcome this eventuality.

Equipment storage

Most established endoscopic suites use a single self-contained unit to store all basic equipment, including the video setup (Fig. 3-1). This reduces the incidence of damage and ensures easy access. Some of these self-contained units can be locked.

The large pieces of apparatus (electrosurgical generator, lasers, argon beam coagulator, and suction-irrigation devices) are usually free standing. Central sterile supply units usually provide standardized prepackaged instrument sets for the routine simple and more complex laparoscopic procedures. Special instruments, which are used for defined procedures as discussed below, will be sterilized and packaged individually.

These storage facilities will vary from unit to unit, but one fundamental principle must be observed: all equipment must be in proper working order and instantly available.

Suction

The ability to carry out suction and lavage is integral to laparoscopy. Suction capability is provided in all modern operating rooms and can be attached to the simple suction or combined suction irrigation cannula.

INSTRUMENTATION SPECIFIC TO LAPAROSCOPY

Insufflators

Insufflation may be achieved by means of any one of a number of pneumoperitoneum machines designed specifically for this purpose. Some are combined in modular fashion with light sources and/or electrosurgical generators. We prefer the use of single-purpose systems. They permit removal of any one of the components for repair and, therefore, loss of availability of the entire system does not occur in case of malfunction of one specific component.

Older insufflators can be set to provide gas flow rates of 1 L/minute or 3 L/minute (rapid flow). Although these insufflators are adequate for diagnostic and simple operative laparoscopy, they are inadequate for use during prolonged operations. Such procedures are inevitably accompanied by loss of intraperitoneal gas either through leakage from the numerous portals or by aspiration during removal of blood, lavage fluid, or the smoke or plume generated by electrical or laser energy. To compensate for this, a new generation of electronically controlled and fully automatic insufflators is available (Fig. 3-2). Once the surgeon sets the maximum intra-abdominal pressure and flow rate, the insufflator will deliver gas at rates up to the maximum set, every time it senses that the intra-abdominal pressure has fallen below the required level. When this preset intra-abdominal pressure has been reestablished the insufflator stops delivering gas.

Some such insufflators also have an integrated warmer to maintain the gas at body temperature to prevent body core cooling, which is a recognized effect of prolonged operative laparoscopy.

Light sources and cables

Most instrument manufacturers produce simple light sources that contain a single examining light of 150 watts or high-powered mercury vapour or xenon bulbs for video monitoring. Some units possess multiple functions, which may include a spare 150-watt bulb or a flash bulb or strobe light that can be connected by a synchronizing cable to a 35 mm camera. Newer models automatically vary the in-

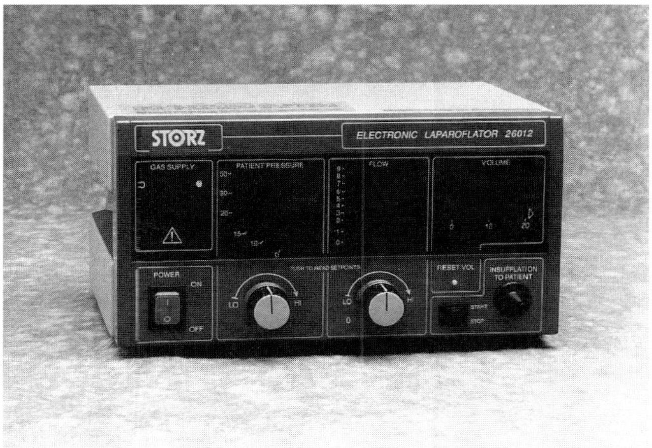

Fig. 3-2. Electronic rapid-flow insufflator. (Courtesy Storz Instruments.)

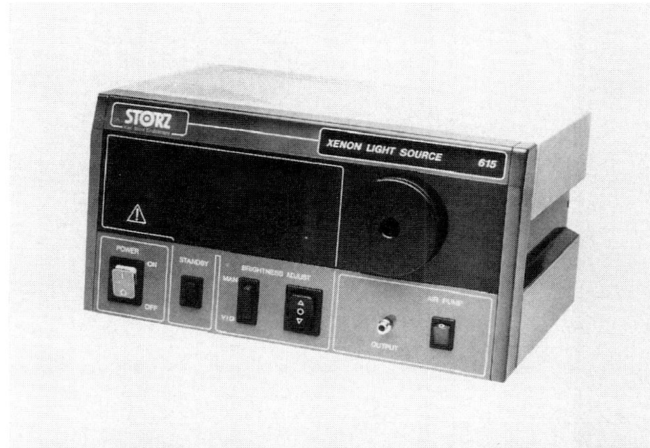

Fig. 3-3. Xenon light source. (Courtesy Storz Instruments.)

tensity of the light in response to signals from the video or still camera (Fig. 3-3). Bulbs should be replaced regularly in accordance with the manufacturer's instructions because a great deal of light intensity and efficiency is lost with repeated use.

The ability to transmit light from high-intensity external sources through the laparoscope and into the abdominal cavity has been accomplished by the application of fiberoptic technology. The intensity of the light delivered to the laparoscope is a function both of the power of the external light source and of the diameter of the cable. The larger the cable, the greater the number of fibers it can carry. Light transmission is improved as the number of fibers increases. Illumination power is reduced at each junction point in the system. This occurs particularly at the site where the cable joins the laparoscope. Light can be transmitted only from fiber to fiber and, if there is any degree of overlap, some light will be lost. Since overlapping is inevitable at the junction between the laparoscope and the fiberoptic cable, one manufacturer has placed a condensing lens at the end of the cable where it attaches to the laparoscope. This lens concentrates the light directly over the laparoscope connector post and thus increases the intensity of the illumination of the field of vision.

Other manufacturers have produced alcohol-filled cables that contain no fibers, thus negating the overlap effect. The fluid-filled cables also eliminate cracking and breaking of fiber bundles, which can occur if the cables are coiled too tightly. Such breaks in the optic fibers result in loss of their light-transmitting capabilities.

It is unfortunate that each manufacturer has developed its own specifications for coupling of the fiberoptic cables to the light source and to the laparoscope. This variation can be overcome by the use of special adaptors, but this results in some loss of light intensity.

External manipulators

It is advantageous in almost all cases of laparoscopy to be able to manipulate the uterus by a transcervical route. In those situations in which operative procedures are required in the vicinity of the lower large intestine, a blunt rectal probe can be of value. The uterine cannula is used unless the uterus is absent, where anomalies exist that prevent exposure of or access to the cervix, in the prepubescent female, and when an intrauterine pregnancy is suspected.

There are numerous uterine cannulas and manipulators. They all are used to manipulate or mobilize the uterus and facilitate the visualization of and access to all aspects of the pelvic structures. Most permit insufflation of a dilute dye solution (chromopertubation) to assess tubal patency.

For diagnostic procedures we prefer to use a rigid cannula such as the Cohen (Fig. 3-4). Manipulation of the postabortal or postpartum uterus may be more difficult due to its increased size and softness. The Hulka postpartum manipulator was designed specifically to mobilize such an enlarged, recently gravid uterus but does not possess chromopertubation capability. The Majoli manipulator is similar to the Hulka but does allow for chromopertubation (Fig. 3-5). The Valtchev has obturators of varying sizes to accommodate variations in the depth and position of the uterus (Fig. 3-6). The uterine end (into which the appropriate obturator is attached) is hinged and connected to a sliding rod mechanism that allows it to be placed at any angle to the shaft. There is a locking mechanism that, when tightened, fixes the obturator in the desired angle, thus maintaining the uterus in the desired position.

The rectal probe has a large-bore blunt obturator and a long shaft. If this specific piece of equipment is not available, two or three gauze swabs mounted on a sponge holder can be used instead.

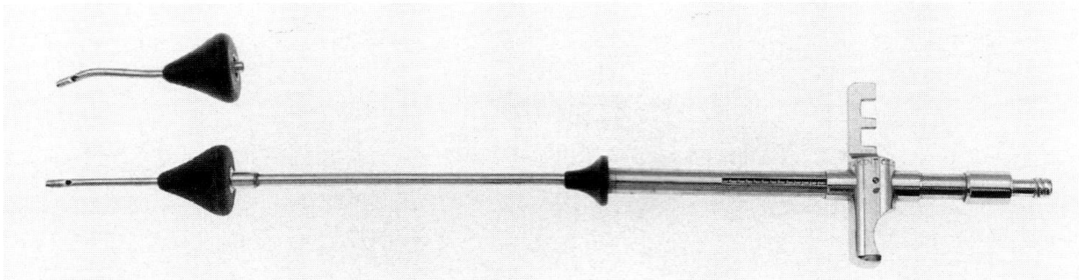

Fig. 3-4. The Cohen uterine cannula.

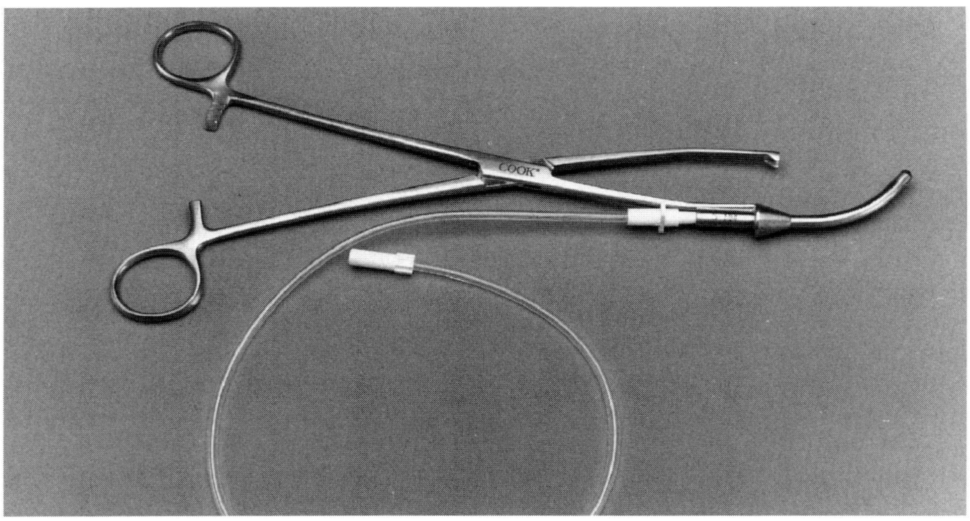

Fig. 3-5. The Majoli uterine manipulator. (Courtesy Cook Instruments.)

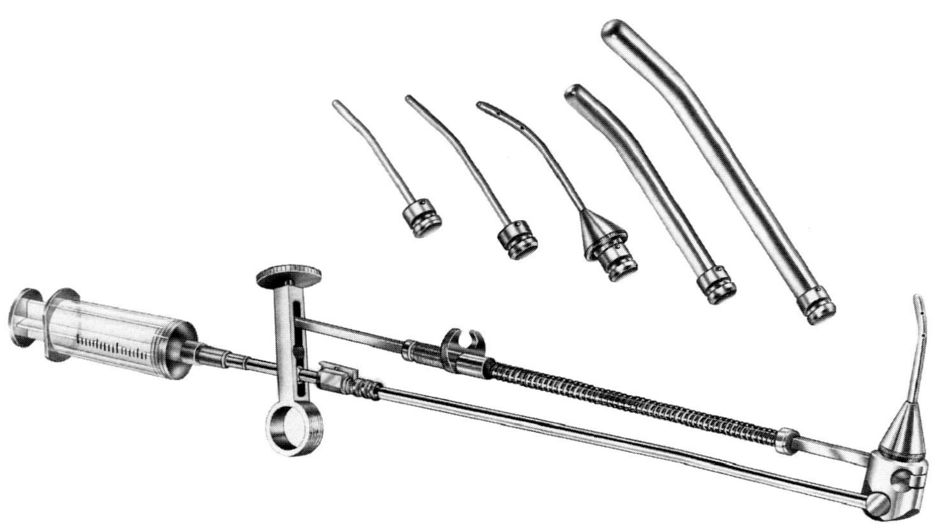

Fig. 3-6. The Valtchev uterine manipulator. (Courtesy Conkin Surgical).

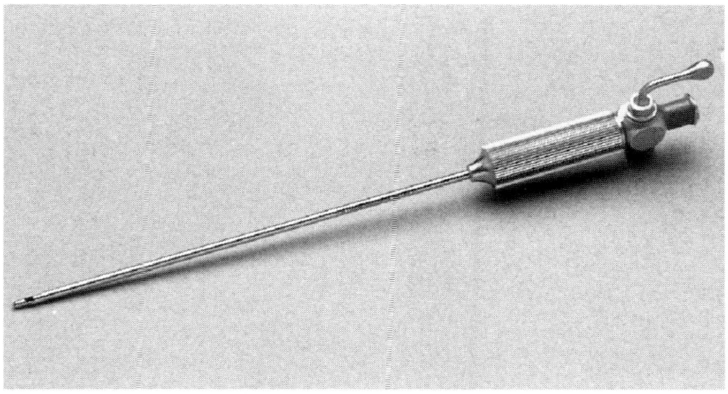

Fig. 3-7. The Verres needle.

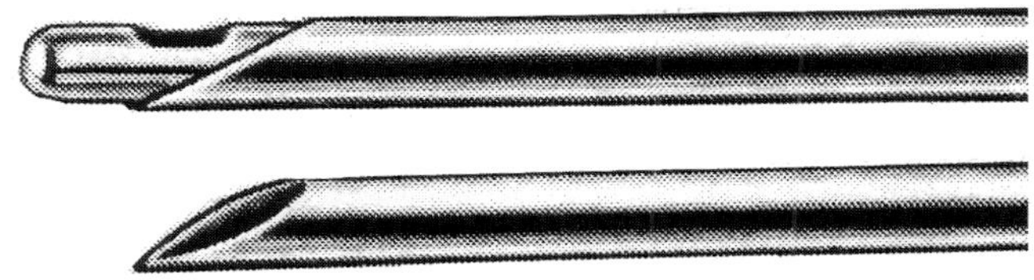

Fig. 3-8. The tip of the Verres needle.

Pneumoperitoneum needles

The Verres needle is the most frequently used (Fig. 3-7). It permits the creation of pneumoperitoneum but does not permit the simultaneous recording of intra-abdominal pressure during insufflation. A double-barrelled insufflating needle (Verres-Frangenheim) was developed to achieve this goal. Simultaneous recording of the intraperitoneal pressure is more important in pediatric laparoscopy in which the addition of very small volumes of gas may create significant increments in pressure.

The Verres needle was designed to prevent perforation of intra-abdominal viscera by the sharp tip. There are two working parts. An outer needle with a sharp bevelled edge is combined with an inner, spring-loaded, retractable blunt shaft that extends beyond the end of the needle point. When introduced through the abdominal wall, the sharp bevelled edge of the needle penetrates the tissue while the inner, spring-loaded blunt shaft is retracted due to tissue resistance. As soon as the peritoneum is penetrated, the blunt shaft is propelled forward by the spring-loaded mechanism beyond the sharp tip, thus converting the needle to a blunt tipped instrument (Fig. 3-8). To maintain this factor of safety, the Verres needle must be in proper working order and must be introduced slowly through the various tissue layers. If the needle is passed too rapidly into the abdominal cavity, the sharp point may still be exposed long enough to perforate viscera. A longer Verres needle equipped with a metallic stop, 3 cm from its tip, is available for transvaginal introduction.

A wider bore Verres needle can be used through which a needle scope can be inserted (see Chapter 5).

Telescopes

When selecting laparoscopy equipment, considerable importance must be placed on the after-sales service provided by the supplier. Aside from this service aspect, optical quality, optical distortion (especially at the periphery), the degree of magnification, and illumination of the field of vision are essential factors to be considered in telescope selection.

Diagnostic laparoscopes generally range from 5 to 10 mm in diameter, although smaller, specialized telescopes are also available. It should be remembered that as the diameter of cannula to accommodate a telescope increases, so does the size of the incision required to accommodate it and the force required to penetrate the abdominal wall. Of additional importance is the fact that the larger the diameter of trocar, the longer will be its tip and, hence, the greater the depth of penetration.

Diagnostic telescopes are available with different angles of view that are either straight-forward, 0 degrees, or fore-oblique, 30 to 45 degrees (Fig. 3-9). The selection of the viewing angle is the surgeon's choice; it has been our experience that the novice laparoscopist does better to gain early experience with the straight-forward view telescope. The angulated telescope has the advantage of permitting visualization of relatively inaccessible areas.

Small-diameter telescopes (5 to 7 mm) are more than adequate for diagnostic laparoscopy. Large-diameter telescopes (8 to 10 mm) are preferable to use with video equipment because greater light transmission is possible.

The operating laparoscope is by necessity of greater caliber than the simple diagnostic telescope, because the operating channel through which various types of instruments can be inserted varies in diameter from 3 to 5 mm. The angle of view through the operating laparoscope is always straight-forward (0 or 180 degrees), because any operating instrument inserted through the operating channel must always be in direct view of the operator.

Three major types of operating laparoscopes are available: (1) The Jacob-Palmer instrument has two right angles in the viewing system so that the eyepiece is offset but parallel to the telescope (Fig. 3-10). This is the simplest telescope to use because the impression that the operator obtains when looking through the eyepiece is identical to that obtained when looking down a simple diagnostic telescope. (2) The 45-degree angulated eyepiece increases the surgeon's operating field compared with the Jacob-Palmer telescope but otherwise offers very little, if any, advantage. (3) The 90-degree angle eyepiece telescope requires more experience for the operator to feel comfortable because the field of view is at right angles to the operative field. Operative laparoscopy is not synonymous with single-puncture laparoscopy techniques. Operating equipment can be in-

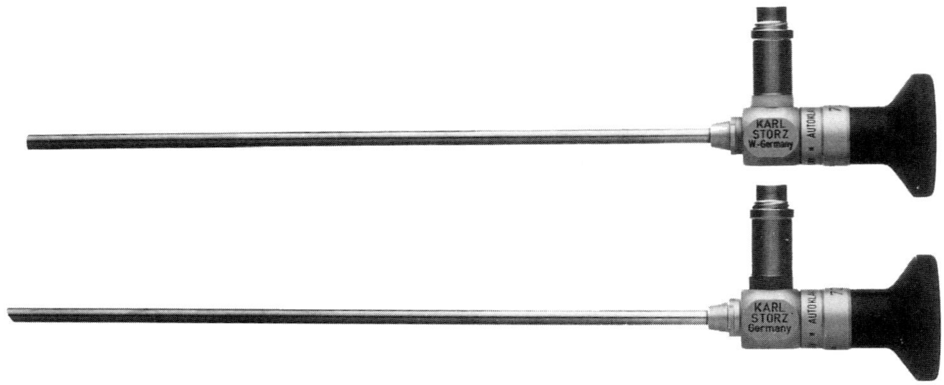

Fig. 3-9. Laparoscopes: straight-forward and fore-oblique *(bottom)*.

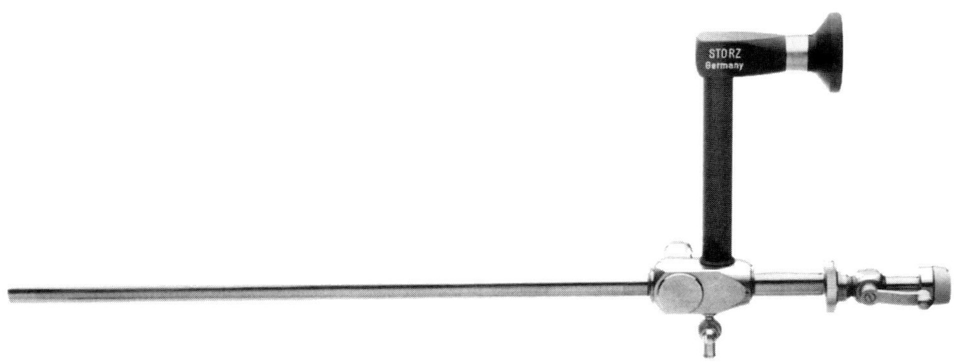

Fig. 3-10. Laparoscope with operating channel.

serted through ancillary punctures, even if an operating laparoscope is employed.

Although some attempt has been made to standardize the size of the eyepiece among different telescope manufacturers, this has not yet been fully accomplished. Until this goal is achieved, various camera lens adaptors will still be necessary.

In addition to the standard operating and diagnostic telescopes, specialized laparoscopes are available, which include the integrated bundle telescope (for photography referred to earlier in this chapter), telescopes with double posts for additional fiberoptic cable attachments, and telescopes combined with specialized operating instruments such as clip applicators.

The most recent developments are lenseless telescopes that transmit light in the usual manner but relay a video image by means of distally sited imaging chips. This telescope has an integral steel reinforced cable that carries the fiberoptic bundle and wires for picture transmission. The cable connects to a combined image processor and light source (Fig. 3-11).

Some telescopes are marketed as "steam autoclavable." However, the longevity of these telescopes will be decreased if autoclaved with steam rather than with gas or sterilized chemically.

Telescopes have a tendency to fog when first inserted into the abdominal cavity. This clouding of the lens can be overcome by touching the tip of the laparoscope to the fundus of the uterus, a loop of bowel, or the parietal peritoneum. This may cause a slight coating of the lens with serous peritoneal fluid and some loss of sharpness of the image when videography is being performed. Lens antifog material is available.

Principal cannulas and trocars

Cannulas are available in all the necessary diameters ranging from 3.5 to 11 mm to accommodate laparoscopes of varying calibers (Fig. 3-12). Cannulas made of metal are preferable to those made from an insulated material such as glass fiber (Fiberglas).

Cannulas may be equipped with one of three types of valves to prevent gas loss. The *trumpet valve* must be

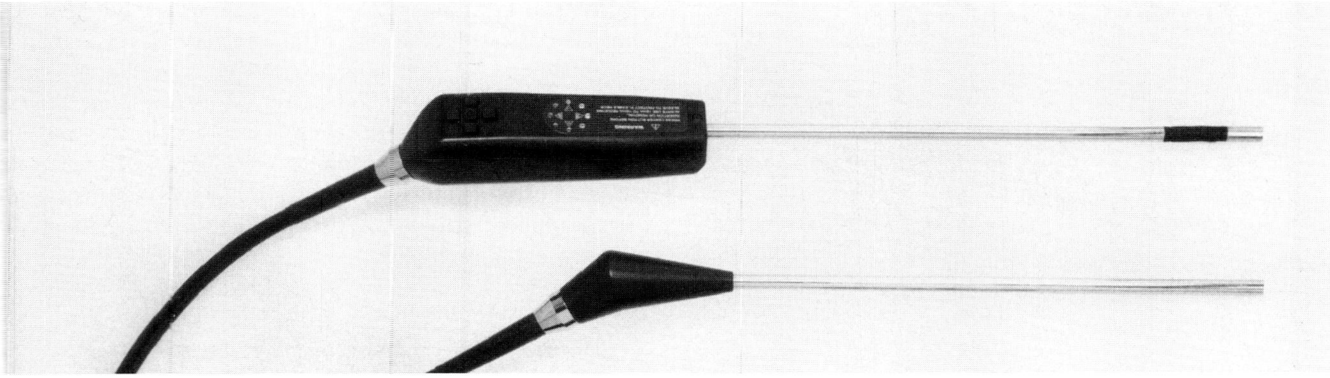

Fig. 3-11. Lensless laparoscopes with distally placed chips: with a rotating tip *(above)*.

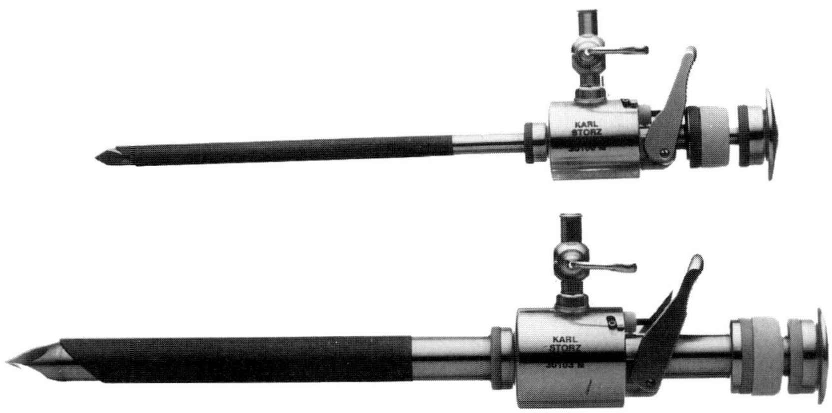

Fig. 3-12. Principal and ancillary trocars and cannulas. The lever controls the trap valve and the Luer-lock is used to connect the gas line.

opened by pushing the external plunger to permit the laparoscope to traverse the cannula. The *"trap-door"* or *"flapper" valve* automatically opens when the laparoscope is pushed against it. The pneumoperitoneum must be evacuated once the procedure has been completed. This is usually effected through the principal cannula. With trumpet-type cannulas, the piston is depressed. A metal key is used to open flap valves, unless the cannula is equipped with a lever that can be depressed to open the valve. Both of these valves work equally well but require regular maintenance in order to keep them moving freely and smoothly. Virtually all principal cannulas are fitted with a side Luer lock connector that will accommodate the gas tubing from the insufflator. Additional gas is insufflated directly through the cannula during the procedure in order to maintain appropriate abdominal distention.

The principal cannula, because of its larger diameter, is often used as a route for removal of tissue. Both types of mechanical valves complicate this process. The third valve mechanism relies upon a distally placed *malleable diaphragm,* the opening of which has the same configuration as a tricuspid valve. This valve fits snugly over the distal end of the cannula like a cup. It maintains gas-tight integrity during the procedure but can easily be removed to allow passage of specimens (Fig. 3-13).

If a cannula is damaged, the laparoscope will not pass smoothly through this sheath. A damaged cannula should be repaired or replaced immediately because very minor distortions in the shape of the cannula may result in scratching and damage to the laparoscope.

Trocars that fit the cannulas may have either pyramidal or conical tips. There is debate, even among experience laparoscopists, as to which tip is better. Trocar tips must be kept sharp. Dull trocars as well as conical tip trocars require greater force to penetrate the abdominal wall. The greater the force, the greater the risk of sudden, uncontrolled entry and damage to the viscera.

Most trocars are also fitted with a hollow channel with

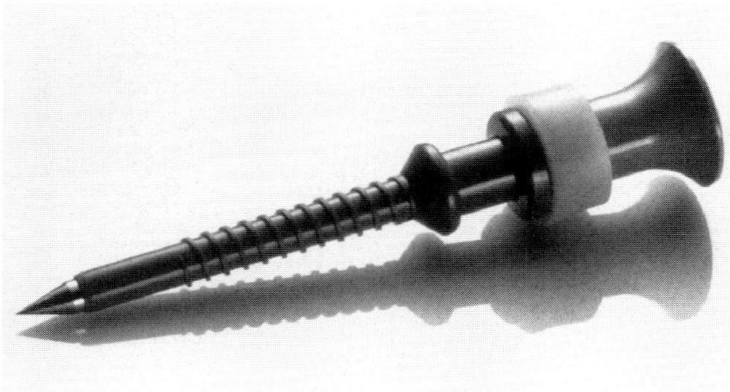

Fig. 3-13. Trocar and cannula with an integral molded spiral flange and a simple tricuspid-shaped valve. (Courtesy Apple Medical.)

openings at the tip as well as at the top of the instrument. This permits a rush of gas to occur when the peritoneal cavity is penetrated by the trocar. At this point, the surgeon need not pass the instrument any more deeply, thus reducing the risk of visceral damage (see Chapter 5).

Disposable primary and ancillary trocars and cannulas are available. Although they have the advantage of invariably having a sharp tip, they are expensive. They have been in vogue, but concerns about health care cost containment may preclude the universal use. In addition, there is a considerable environmental impact of all disposable medical equipment.

Ancillary cannulas and trocars

Ancillary instruments differ in diameters, which may range from 3 to 12 mm depending on their function. Appropriately sized cannulas accommodate these instruments. Giant 20 to 30 mm cannulas are available for tissue removal.

The smooth-sided cannulas are ideal for diagnostic purposes. During operative procedures there will be constant movement and interchange of the ancillary instruments. Frequently the cannula will slip out of the abdomen. This difficulty can be overcome by using special second puncture cannulas that are equipped with an external spiral flange. The cannula is screwed into the incision and becomes self-retaining. Most ancillary cannulas have been simple adaptations of earlier diagnostic models. Many are too long and equipped with unnecessary gas line connectors. Their valve systems are unnecessarily complicated. The best ancillary trocars and cannulas are relatively short and have an integral modeled spiral flange and simple valve (Fig. 3-13).

It is frequently necessary to use cannulas of differing sizes to accommodate ancillary instruments of larger or smaller bore than those first inserted. Larger cannulas are equipped with blunt obturators to dilate the secondary incision atraumatically, or the Heinkel-Semm dilator can be used. This is an ingenious arrangement of a solid guide rod that is passed through the 5 mm cannula. The cannula is removed and the skin incision enlarged. The dilator assembly is placed over the rod and used to screw an 11 mm sheath into the abdominal cavity (see Chapter 7). Adaptors are available that will permit the introduction of smaller instruments, without loss of gas tight integrity, unless cannulas equipped with the diaphragm valve arrangement described earlier are used.

Ancillary instruments

Virtually every manufacturer produces a complete line of ancillary instruments that can be used either through a second-puncture site (ancillary puncture) or through the operating channel of an operating laparoscope. The latter are, by necessity, much longer since their tip must extend well beyond the end of the laparoscope for adequate visual control of their function. Many instruments produced by a particular company are often the result of collaboration in design between a specific physician and the manufacturer and, as a result, will often bear the physician's name.

It is impossible and unnecessary to list here all of the available ancillary instruments. They range in size from 3 to 12 mm in diameter and fall into several broad categories that include:

Probes and retractors
Aspirating needles and suction/irrigation cannulas
Grasping forceps
Scissors
Biopsy forceps
Electrosurgery, laser, and the argon beam coagulator
Endocoagulation
Ligating and suturing equipment
Special function instruments

Each of these types will be described.

Manipulation probes and retractors. Probes are essential for displacing and retracting the intraperitoneal structures. They must be blunt to reduce the possibility of causing trauma during manipulation. The majority of these probes are marked with centimeter graduations so that structures can be measured (Fig. 3-14). The magnification properties of many telescopes make accurate estimation of size by visual methods alone difficult. To enhance the surgeon's ability to retract tissue, a variety of instruments have been produced that are introduced through the cannula in a closed position. Once in the abdominal cavity the distal end is expanded to form a series of tines or a triangular flat surface. The angle of the distal end with respect to the shaft may be able to be changed. Both opening and angling are effected by using proximally sited controls.

Aspiration needles and suction/irrigation cannulas. Some aspiration cannulas (puncture needle) have a narrowed, short front piece with a bevelled sharp tip, permitting penetration of cystic structures (Fig. 3-14). Simple

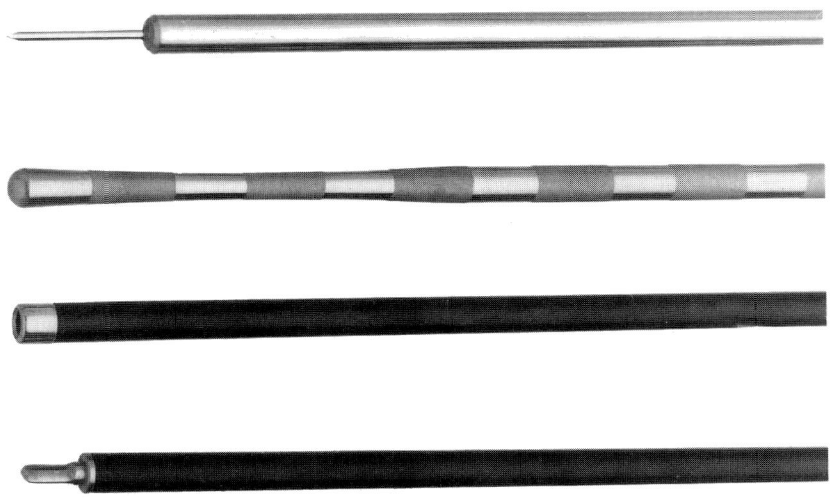

Fig. 3-14. Ancillary instruments *(from top)* aspiration needle, calibrated probe, insulated unipolar suction aspiration cannula, and insulated unipolar blade shaped electrode. (Courtesy Storz Instruments.)

blunt aspiration cannulas are extremely helpful for obtaining peritoneal fluid for culture or cytology, for aspirating blood that has accumulated in the peritoneal cavity, and to effect peritoneal lavage (Fig. 3-14). Some are equipped with a valve mechanism to prevent loss of pneumoperitoneum.

Suction irrigation cannulas designed for operative laparoscopy must have the capability to deliver irrigation fluid and suction as required. Thus they must have distal attachments for both inflow and outflow lines that are controlled by a finger-activated valve mechanism. This mechanism has three functions. When closed it permits neither inflow of fluid nor escape of pneumoperitoneum. When opened in one direction irrigation occurs; opening in the other direction converts the cannula into an aspirator. Irrigation solutions should be instilled under pressure. If low pressure is all that is required, a warmed bag of the irrigation solution can be suspended from an intravenous pole. Greater pressures up to 300 mm Hg can be provided by wrapping the IV bag in an inflatable cuff or by using specially designed pumps (Fig. 3-15).

Most irrigation suction cannulas will accommodate a unipolar needle electrode or laser fibre through a centrally placed channel (Fig. 3-16). Thus the same cannula can be used for cutting, coagulation, irrigation, aquadissection, (see Chapter 7), and aspiration.

Grasping forceps. Grasping forceps are used to steady tissue. If the tissue is to remain it is imperative the grasping forceps hold the structure firmly yet atraumatically. For fixing tissue that is to be removed, various patterns of toothed or ridged grasping forceps are available (Figs. 3-17 to 3-22). Many of these can be locked by an external mechanism. The most frequently used are 5 mm in size. Grasping forceps may be rigid or it may be possible to rotate either the jaws or the shaft and jaws independently of the handle. Others are designed so that the angle of the jaws with respect to the shaft can be altered up to 90 degrees (Fig. 3-23). These refinements have also been incorporated in some models of scissors and needle holders.

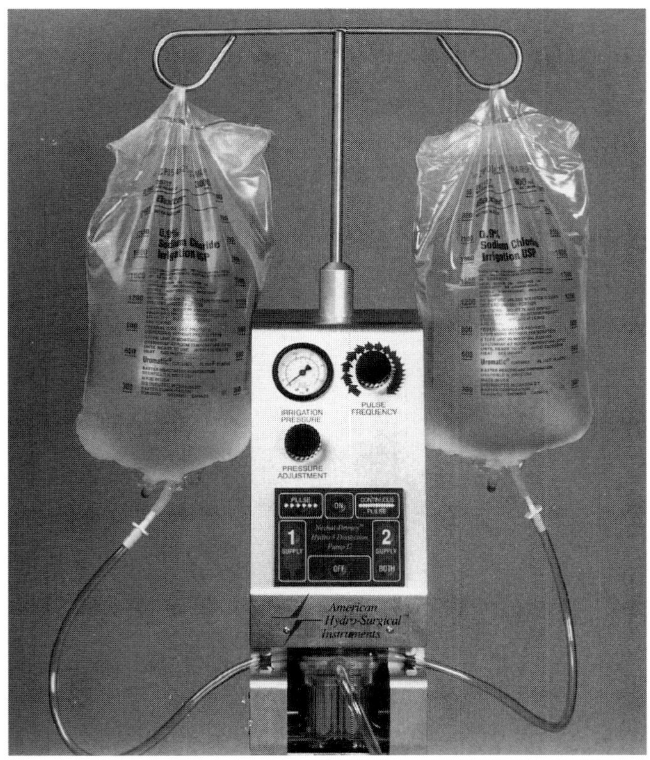

Fig. 3-15. The Nezhat-Dorsey pump. (Courtesy American Hydro-Surgical Instruments.)

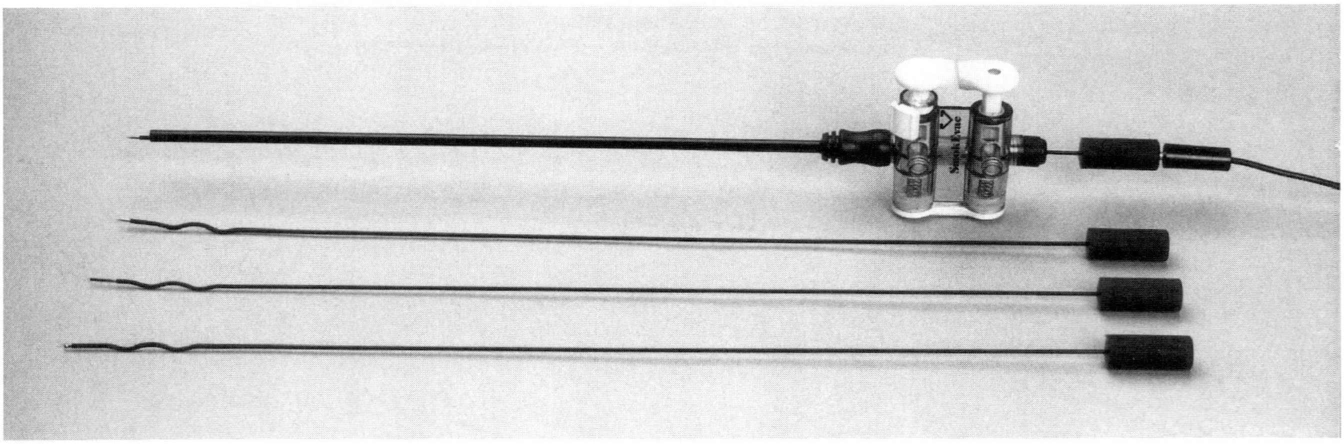

Fig. 3-16. The Nezhat-Dorsey suction-irrigation cannula and electrodes that can be introduced through the same cannula. (Courtesy American Hydro-Surgical Instruments.)

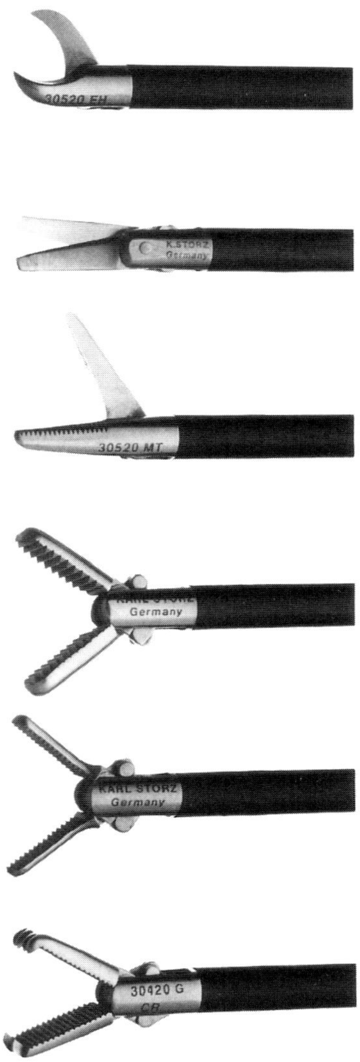

Fig. 3-17. Ancillary instruments, insulated: *(from top)* hook scissors, straight scissors, serrated straight scissors, grasping forceps, grasping and dissecting forceps, toothed grasping forceps. (Courtesy Storz Instruments.)

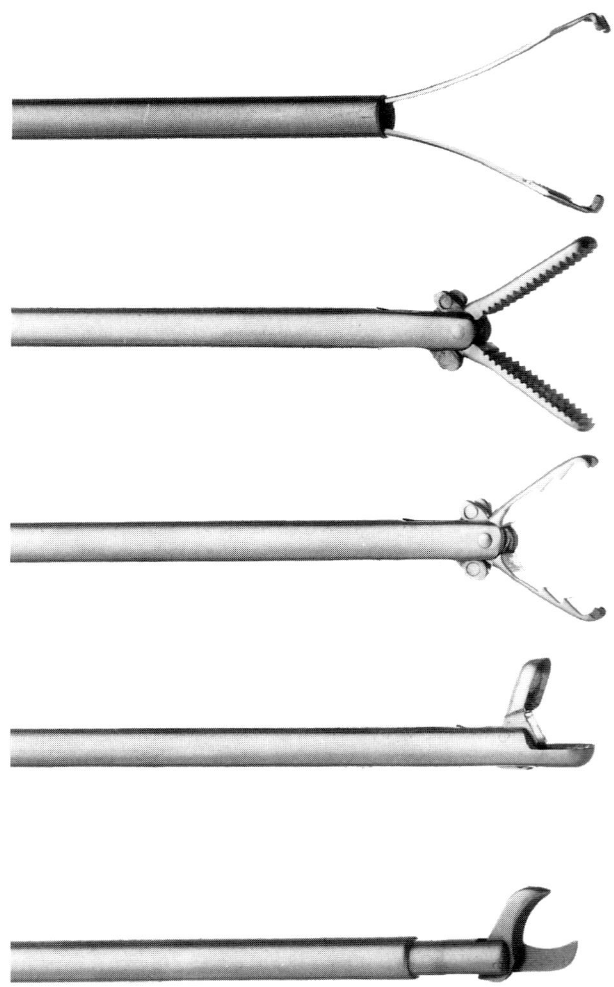

Fig. 3-18. Ancillary instruments: *(from top)* toothed grasping forceps, grasping and dissecting forceps, strong grasping forceps, biopsy forceps, hook scissors. (Courtesy Storz Instruments.)

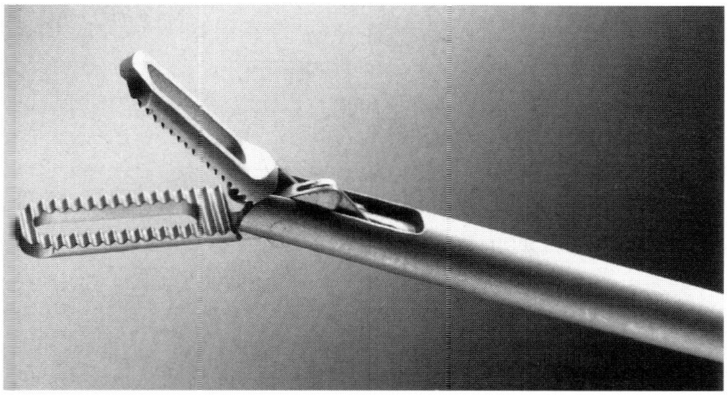

Fig. 3-19. Paddle forceps. (Courtesy Marlow Surgical.)

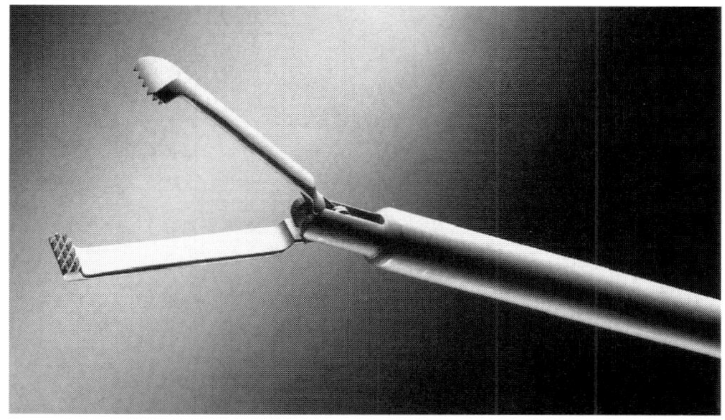

Fig. 3-20. Allis forceps. (Courtesy Marlow Surgical.)

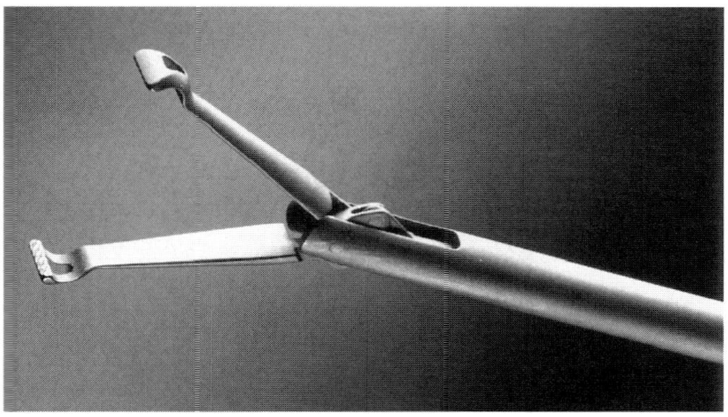

Fig. 3-21. Babcock forceps. (Courtesy Marlow Surgical.)

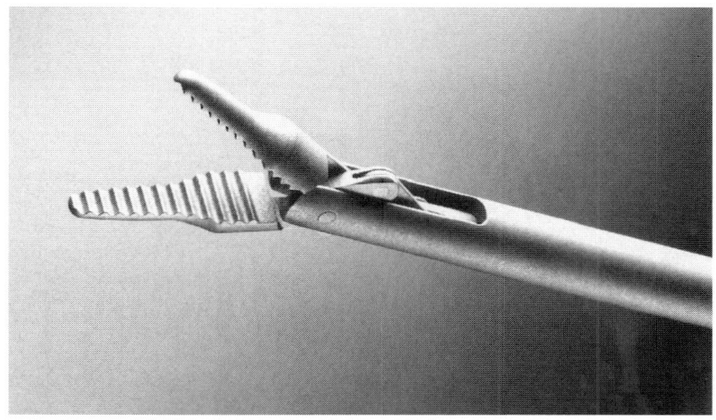

Fig. 3-22. Dolphin nose dissector. (Courtesy Marlow Surgical.)

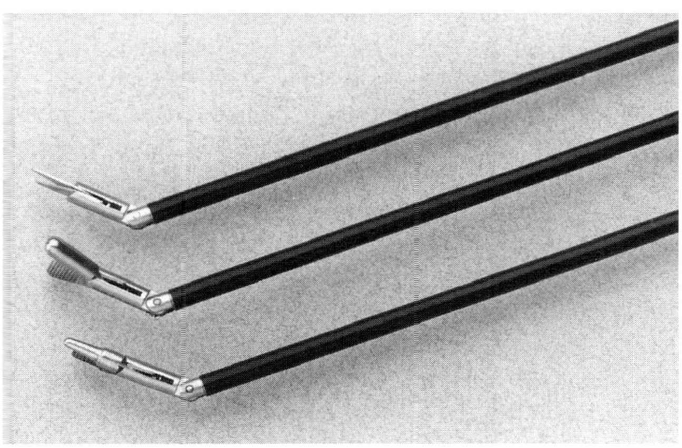

Fig. 3-23. Articulating forceps and scissors: *(from top)* scissors, grasping forceps, dolphin nose dissector. (Courtesy Microsurge.)

Grasping forceps may have electrosurgical capability (Figs. 3-17 and 3-23). Those that use unipolar current have insulated shafts, those that use bipolar do not. Two instruments at opposite ends of the size range may be particularly valuable. The 3 mm alligator forceps is used during delicate dissection of the fallopian tube, and may be used to advantage to tease open agglutinated fimbria. Large claw forceps (10 mm diameter) are used during myomectomy. Care must be taken when they are used as their teeth can inadvertently damage intrapelvic structures.

Scissors. Scissors of various designs are available (Figs. 3-17, 3-18, 3-23, and 3-24). They may combine unipolar or bipolar electrosurgical capability with the mechanical cutting action of the scissors (Fig. 3-25).

Hook scissors that have sharp tips that overlap are dangerous because they may inadvertently cause intraperitoneal trauma. We do not recommend the use of such scissors. When closed, scissors must have a smooth, rounded tip even if the blades are curved or hooked. This feature permits manipulation with the closed instrument while avoiding the risk of inadvertent trauma.

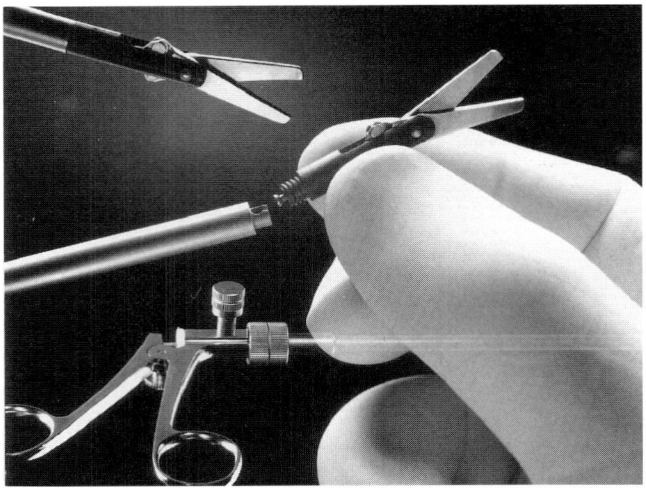

Fig. 3-24. Scissors with reusable, disposable tips. (Courtesy Marlow Surgical.)

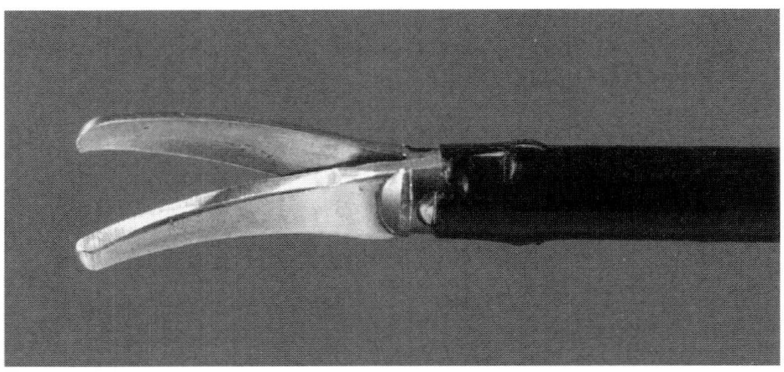

Fig. 3-25. Scissors with bipolar electrosurgical capability. (Courtesy Everest Medical.)

Just as with open abdominal surgery, it is advisable to retain one pair of scissors solely for cutting sutures or ligatures. These tend to become blunted even more quickly than scissors that are used for dividing tissue. This blunting is accelerated if the scissors are used as electrosurgical instruments. Scissors are difficult to maintain and sharpen. Because of the critical value of sharp scissors, we believe that a strong argument can be made for the use of fully disposable scissors (Fig. 3-25) or those models with reusable handles and sharp but interchangeable disposable/reusable blades (Fig. 3-24).

Biopsy forceps. The design of biopsy forceps is variable. The differences lie primarily in the function and shape of the jaws. Some of these are equipped with one fixed and one movable jaw, whereas others have two movable jaws. The jaw size and configuration determine the size of the eventual biopsy. Biopsy forceps with jaws that cross and with sharp cutting edges, are safer and provide better biopsies. Instruments that do not cut cleanly tear the tissue, with bleeding often resulting. Almost all biopsy forceps are insulated and thus have electrosurgical potential so that biopsy sites may be desiccated. The surgeon should remember that the biopsy specimen must be removed from the instrument before electrodesiccation is carried out, otherwise the biopsied tissue will also be destroyed. The "Palmer" biopsy drill forceps is capable of obtaining a large cylindrical core of material from the ovary and is the best instrument for this purpose.

All-purpose, good, biopsy punch forceps possess a mobile, hollow, upper jaw that when closed fits snugly within the sharp cutting edges of the fixed, hollow, lower jaw. A biopsy is obtained readily by the effective scissor-like cutting action of the edges as they cross.

Electrosurgery laser and the argon beam coagulator. A complete discussion of these energy sources will be found in Chapter 4. The fact that many of the other instruments have electrosurgical capabilities has already been mentioned. It will be sufficient to remark at this stage that no laparoscopy should be undertaken without instant access to bipolar and unipolar grasping forceps and electrodes. Laser energy may be delivered either through a specially adapted operating laparoscope, (for CO_2), or through laser-bearing fibers that can be inserted through ancillary cannulas (for Argon, KTP, Yag:Nd). The argon beam coagulator probe is inserted through an ancillary portal.

Endocoagulation. To avoid the risks associated with the use of electrical current the endocoagulator was introduced by Semm. It works on the electrical soldering bolt principle. The active part of the instrument is heated by an electrical current and used literally to cook the tissue to which it is applied. Heat is generated in a range of from 90 to 120 degrees Celsius. The generator produces an acoustic tone that waxes and wanes as the temperature rises and falls. The two most widely used endocoagulation instruments, the crocodile forceps and the point coagulator, are both 5 mm in diameter.

Ligating and suturing equipment. It may be necessary to ligate or suture tissues. The Endoloop is used to perform the former function. It is a modification of the Roeder loop, which was originally designed for tonsillectomies. A ligature is pretied in a fisherman's knot, the free end of which is mounted in a hollow plastic guide and embedded in the detachable proximal tip of the guide (Fig. 3-26). Unless the diaphragm cannula is available, an adaptor is used so that the Endoloop can be passed through a 5 mm cannula without loss of gas-tight integrity. Once the tissue to be ligated has been encircled by the loop, the proximal tip is snapped from the guide and used to pull on the free end of the loop while at the same time the distal end of the guide is used as a knot pusher. A full description of the techniques of extra- and intracorporeal knot tying will be found in Chapter 7. To place sutures laparoscopically, needle drivers and needle-holding forceps of both 3 and 5 mm sizes are available (Figs. 3-27 and 3-28). Straight, ski, and curved needles

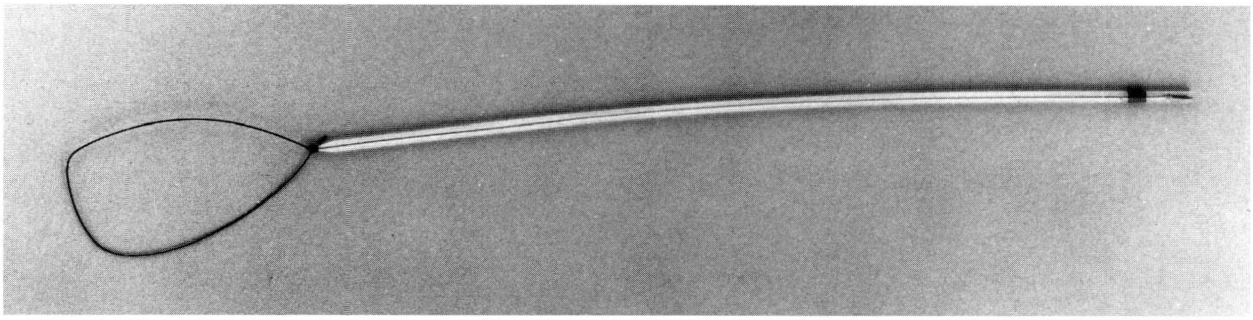

Fig. 3-26. Roeder's Loop. (Endoloop Courtesy Ethicon.)

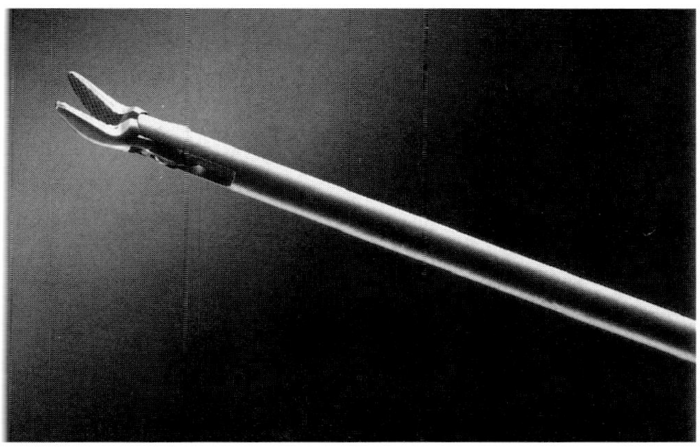

Fig. 3-27. Needle driver. (Courtesy Marlow Surgical.)

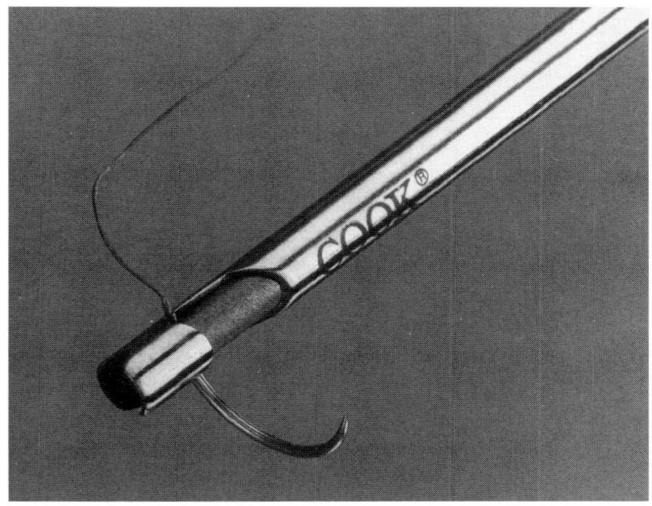

Fig. 3-28. Needle driver for curved needles. (Courtesy Cook.)

that are swaged to the sutures are used in laparoscopic surgery.

Special instruments. Special heavy duty scissors and a tissue morcellator are available. Both are introduced through 11 mm cannulas. The morcellator has a distal cutting blade that can be manually operated or mechanically driven. The cylindrical pieces of tissue are forced into the hollow shaft of the instrument. Tissue morcellation is described in Chapter 7.

Staples can be applied from preloaded delivery systems. Such instruments, when fired, will automatically place two sets of staples and divide the contained tissue with an integrally sited knife, leaving three rows of staples on each side of the incision. The equipment is of 12 mm diameter, and the staple cartridges are expensive.

The Endopouch (Ethicon) is an impermeable, flexible, plastic bag equipped with a drawstring. It can be passed through a cannula and opened within the abdominal cavity. Tissue can be placed within the sac and aspirated or morcellated without risk of spillage and removed in the bag without touching the parietes.

CONCLUSIONS

It should be apparent from this chapter that diagnostic laparoscopy can be carried out effectively with a set of simple instruments. Most laparoscopic surgery can be performed with a limited number of well-chosen instruments. Even as this chapter is being written the rapidity with which the instrument manufacturers are producing new equipment will no doubt ensure that by the time of publication some of the information given here will be out of date.

Chapter 4

ENERGY SOURCES FOR OPERATIVE LAPAROSCOPY

Malcolm G. Munro

Several energy sources are important to the performance of endoscopic surgery. Electrical, laser, or the mechanical energy from an oscillating probe may be harnessed to incise, resect, ablate, morcellate, or desiccate tissue. Appropriately applied, all of the energy sources are safe and effective. However, in untrained hands, imprudent use may result in injury. Consequently, it is mandatory for the endoscopic surgeon to become intimately familiar with the principles, applications, and safety aspects of the energy sources to be used during surgery. The purpose of this chapter is to acquaint the reader with the biophysical and surgical principles of each energy source.

ELECTROSURGERY

Electrosurgery is the use of electrical radiofrequency alternating current to raise cellular temperature in order to vaporize or coagulate tissue. In addition to providing hemostasis, these effects can be used to incise or ablate tissue. Electrosurgery must be distinguished clearly from the process of cautery, derived from the Greek *kauterion* (hot iron), in which the destruction or denaturation of tissue is caused by the passive transfer of heat or the application of a caustic substance.

Electrical energy has long been a critical and often criticized component of the armamentarium of the operative endoscopist. In the 1980s, the advent and promise of surgical lasers, combined with perceived dangers associated with electrosurgery, caused many to change the energy source used for their operative procedures. However, a reanalysis of data criticizing electrosurgery, together with improved equipment and a better understanding of electrosurgical instruments, has led to a renewal of interest and increased use of this important tool.

History of electrosurgery

The use of heat for the treatment of wounds dates to neolithic times.[1] The ancient Egyptians (c. 3000 B.C.) employed thermal cautery for ulcers and tumors of the breast. Hippocrates (469 to 370 B.C.) employed heat to destroy a neck tumor and Albucasis (*c.* 980) used a hot iron to control bleeding.[2,3] In the mid-eighteenth century, scientists, including Benjamin Franklin and John Wesley, began to investigate the effects of electrical energy on body tissue, with therapeutic applications relying on the use of *direct current* to heat an electrode. All these methods employed passive heat transfer, which resulted in coagulation and/or desiccation of the tissue, a form of cautery.[4]

In the latter part of the 19th century, investigators in Europe and the United States began experimenting with the biological effects of *alternating current* on tissue. Arsené D'Arsonval, a French inventor and physiologist, was one of these investigators and, in 1893, was the first to exploit these effects in a clinical fashion.[5] He designed capacitors, later modified by Oudlin, that developed a high-voltage discharge in the form of sparks with the ability superficially to destroy tissue, a process termed *fulguration* (from the latin noun *fulgur* for lightening and the verb *fulgurare,* to flash).

In 1907, Rivière, a student of D'Arsonval, demonstrated that if high-frequency alternating current was applied directly to tissue without sparking another electrosurgical process called "white coagulation" occurred.[6] Doyen was the first to apply therapeutic *bipolar* alternating current to tissue.[7] In the next 10 to 20 years, more powerful generators allowed these techniques to be employed in humans to treat nevi, granulation tissue, and bladder tumors.

The next important step in the development of electrosurgery was the invention of the vacuum tube by de Forest. With this device it became possible to produce the type of high-frequency, low-voltage alternating current necessary for the production of a third electrosurgical effect, *cutting*. The first reported use of a vacuum tube–generated, continuous sinewave current to cut tissue in humans was by Wyeth in 1924.[8] Bovie, a physicist, and Cushing a neurosurgeon, whom together are often given credit for the invention of electrosurgery, actually were only its most effective promoters. In 1926, Cushing used Bovie's side-by-side electrosurgical generators—one, a vacuum tube–based design for cutting, the other a spark gap version for coagulation—to perform neurosurgery on a patient with an otherwise inoperable vascular myeloma. The results of this and other procedures were published in 1928 and the machine served as the model for virtually all subsequent generators until the 1970s.[9]

The most recent significant development was the production of solid-state generators in the early 1970s. These devices provided the template for all currently available generators. Their principal advantage is that they can produce the complex waveforms useful for providing a combination of cutting and coagulation effects on tissue. These generators generally have isolated circuitry and may be fitted with other features that combine to add an improved margin of safety.

Endoscopically directed electrosurgery was first performed by Beer in about 1910 when he used an electrosurgical electrode to fulgurate bladder tumors under cystoscopic guidance.[6] One of the first attempts at using laparoscopically directed electrosurgery for adhesiolysis was by Fervers in 1933.[10] While Boesch in 1936 and Anderson in 1937 were the first to propose the use of unipolar electrosurgery under laparoscopic direction for human female sterilization [11,12] the first reported human cases were by Power and Barnes in 1941.[13] Electrosurgical ablation of the endometrium was first described in 1937 by Bardenheuer of Germany.[14] Popularization of laparoscopic electrosurgical sterilization in the mid-1970s is credited to Palmer.[15] In 1976 Neuwirth was the first to describe the use of electrosurgical resection in the uterus to deal with submucus myomata.[16]

In the 1970s and early 1980s there was widespread belief that unipolar electrical current could unpredictably arc long distances from the active electrode to other viscera causing significant thermal injury. Indeed, these concerns contributed to the further development and popularization of the bipolar techniques that were described by Frangenheim in 1972.[17] In addition, in 1981, because of purported significant morbidity and death secondary to electrically induced bowel injury, this perception led to the 1981 recommendations that severely limited the use of unipolar electrosurgery for laparoscopically directed sterilization.[18,19] However, in 1985, Levy and Soderstrom demonstrated that under reasonable conditions such injuries were infrequent and that almost all the purported bowel injuries were indeed secondary to physical, not electrical trauma.[20] In addition, there developed a better understanding of the risks presented by the use of high-power outputs (up to 600 watts) and the factors, such as "capacitive coupling," that contribute to electrosurgical complications. Subsequent reduction of the output potential of electrosurgical generators and modification of the guidelines for cannula use allowed the 1981 recommendation to be rescinded in 1985.[21] Safety has been further enhanced by newer generators with isolated circuits and monitoring systems for the early detection of separation of the dispersive or return electrode from the patient.

Unipolar electrosurgery has now become widely recognized as a highly acceptable method of cutting and obtaining hemostasis. Bipolar instruments offer some safety advantages when used for desiccation but are of limited use for cutting or vaporization. Safe and effective application of either requires the use of well-designed equipment and a sound understanding of electrosurgical principles.

Principles of electrosurgery

With the advent of surgical lasers, institutional credentialling committees ensured that surgeons clearly demonstrated a knowledge of laser physics prior to allowing them to use the equipment in their facilities. Unfortunately, such rigorous requirements had not been applied to electrosurgery. Consequently, generations of physicians had extensive experience with an instrument most did not understand. As a result, it should not be surprising that when endoscopic complications arose in association with the use of electrosurgery, there was apprehension regarding its continued use. We now know that these concerns were largely unfounded. Like all energy sources, electrosurgery should be respected, not feared. However, the surgeon must possess a clear understanding of the principles of electrosurgery for safe and effective use.

Principles of electrical energy

In modern electrosurgery, electrical energy is converted in the tissue to thermal energy. The desired effect in the tissue is determined by a number of electrical properties as well as factors such as tissue exposure time and the size and shape of the electrode.

Electrosurgery requires the formation of a circuit for passage of electrons that includes the electrodes, the patient, the electrosurgical generator (ESU), and the connecting wires (Fig. 4-1). In the bipolar mode, only the tissue interposed between the two electrodes is included in the circuit. However, in the unipolar mode, the entire patient is interposed between the active electrode and the large dispersive electrode. The small active electrode concentrates the current at the designated site, elevating the intracellular temperature, while the large dispersive electrode acts as the other pole, "collecting" the same number of electrons but in a diffuse fashion, preventing the occurrence of a thermal effect.

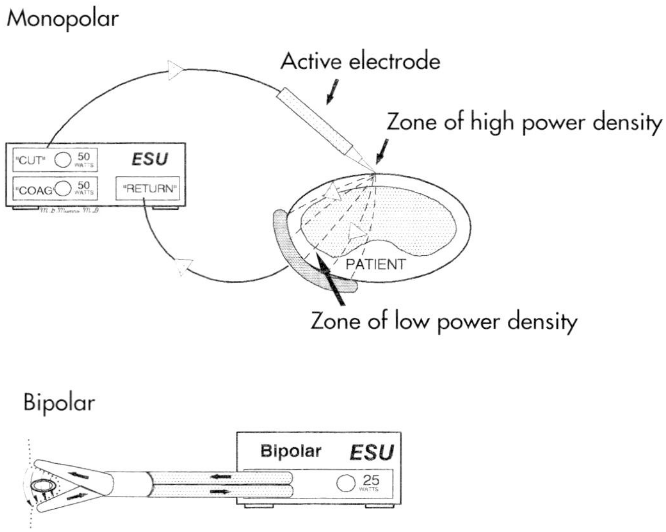

Fig. 4-1. Electrosurgical circuits. Each consists of an electrosurgical unit (ESU), two electrodes, and live tissue. Only a relatively discrete portion of the patient is included in bipolar systems while in monopolar, or unipolar, circuits the entire patient is interposed between the two electrodes.

Properties of electricity. The three interacting properties of electricity that effect the temperature rise in tissue are: current (I), voltage (V), and impedance or resistance (R). Current is a measure of the electron movement past a given point in the circuit in a given period of time. It is measured in *amperes*. Voltage describes the pressure with which the electrons are pushed through the tissue. It is measured in *volts*. Resistance is measured in *ohms* and is a reflection of the difficulty a given substance (e.g., tissue) presents to the passage of electrons. The term resistance is generally reserved for direct current while for alternating current the term impedance (I) is used.

In a given circuit, these properties are related by *Ohm's law:*

$$I = V/R$$

An effective hydraulic analogy explaining these properties has been designed by Roger Odell (Fig. 4-2). The height of the water tower creates the pressure (voltage) exerted upon the water in the outflow pipe. The water passes through the pipe (flow of current) which, if widened, would increase flow (decreased resistance) and, if narrowed, would restrict flow (higher resistance).

Power (W), the capacity to do work per unit time, is a product of current and voltage and is measured in watts:

$$(W = V \times I)$$

If Ohm's law is used to substitute for current $[W = V \times (V/R)]$, then wattage can be expressed in another way:

$$W = V^2/R$$

These relationships (Fig. 4-3) are helpful in explaining a number of features of electrosurgery. For example, the ratio of voltage to current is largely responsible for the differing effects on tissue, given similar electrode size and shape as well as tissue exposure time. In general, the "pressure" of increased voltage enhances the ability of the current to arc from the electrode to tissue. In addition, this pressure forces more energy into the tissue, a circumstance that fosters a greater degree of thermal injury. Equation 3 shows how, at a given ESU output in watts, the voltage in the circuit will diminish if the tissue resistance increases. This helps to explain how the cutting or coagulating characteristics of an electrode may change as tissues with different resistance are encountered.

Electrosurgical generator output. The ESU converts a 60 cycle/second diagonal (60 Hertz or Hz) low voltage alternating current into higher voltage radiofrequency (500 kHz to 3.0 MHz) current. The generator is also capable of producing current with a number of waveforms that allow for differing effects on tissue. Features of the output are identifiable on an oscilloscope (Fig. 4-4). The wave is generally symmetrical above and below "0" volts reflecting the nature of an alternating current. The peak voltage generated is depicted by the distance from the baseline to the apex of the wave.

All modern generators have ports for active and "return," or dispersive electrodes, and controls determining power output for each of the waveforms. While most ESUs have two outputs labeled "cut" and "coag," these terms do not accurately reflect the appropriate use of the energy, a feature that tends to add to confusion regarding the properties and purpose of the different waveforms.

The output labeled "cut" provides a continuous low-voltage waveform (Fig. 4-4). As it is seen on the oscilloscope, the waveform is in the form of a sinewave, reflecting the alternating polarity of an alternating current. Incidentally, this should help the reader understand that the current in radiofrequency electrosurgery does not flow in one direction via the active and dispersive electrodes but instead rapidly moves back and forth across the tissue.

The so-called *"coagulation"* mode is actually designed for fulguration only. It is an interrupted, dampened, and relatively high-voltage waveform (Fig. 4-4). Typically, the current is on only 6% of the time, referred to as a 6% *duty cycle*. The high-peak voltage allows the current to leave the electrode, striking the tissue with multiple visible arcs. This fosters the creation of the superficial coagulative and carbonization process called fulguration.

Blended currents were formerly created by combining

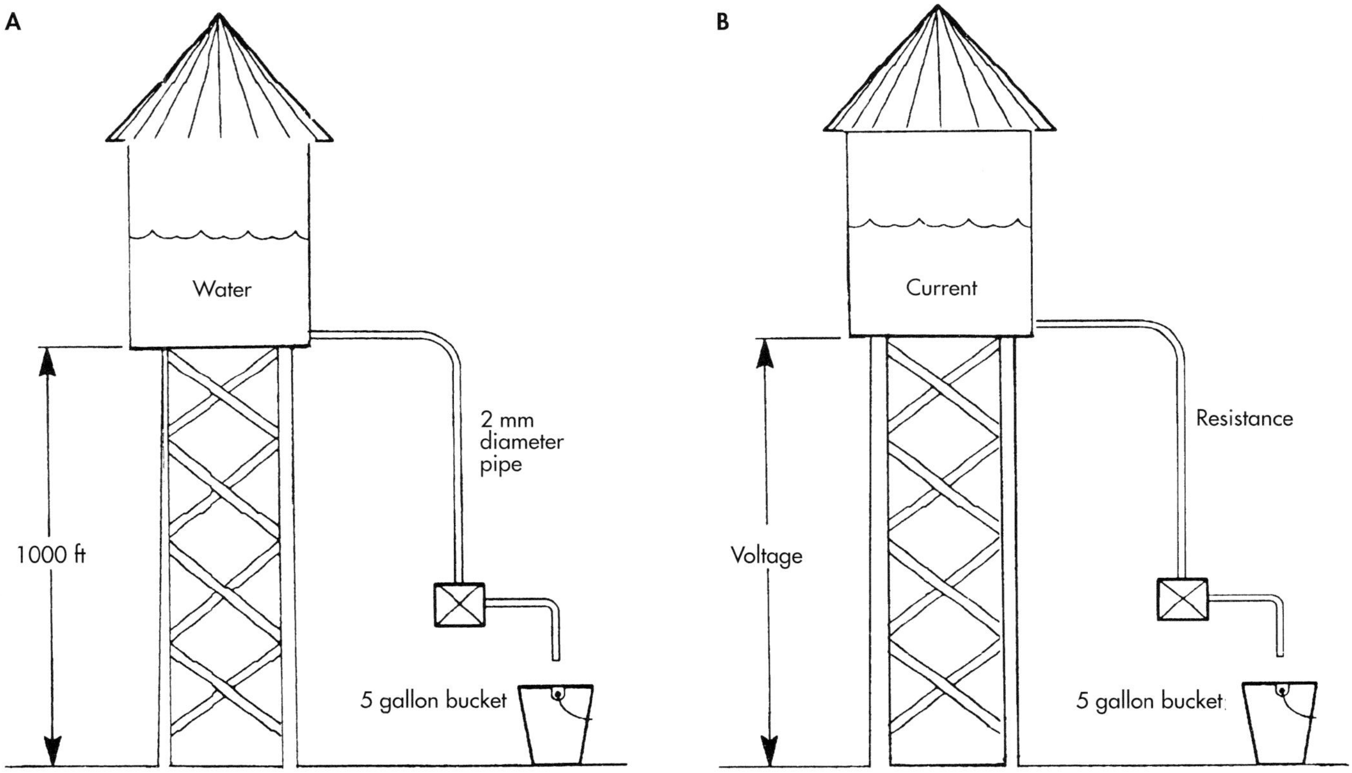

Fig. 4-2. **A,** The Odell water tower analogy explains Ohm's law (I = V/R). Voltage *(V)* is essentially electrical pressure and is represented by the height of the water tower. Current *(I)* is equated to the water flowing through the pipe—greater flow is the same as increased current. Electrical resistance or impedance *(R)* is depicted by the width of the outflow pipe. Flow *(I)* will be proportional to the height of the tower *(V)* and the diameter of the pipe *(R)*. **B,** The electrical terms corresponding to the water analogy in **A.** (From Odell R: Electrosurgery. In Sutton C, Diamond M, editors: Endoscopic surgery for gynaecologists, London, 1993, WB Saunders.)

the two types of waveforms described above. However, all modern ESUs create their "blended" currents by producing interrupted versions of the "cut" waveforms. When the current is interrupted and wattage is held constant, the generator increases the voltage of the output (W = V × I). In the water tower analogy (see Fig. 4-2), this is equivalent to elevating the level of the tower while intermittently turning the water flow on and off at the tap The increased pressure afforded by the height of the tower allows a greater amount of water to flow along the pipe per unit time. Typically it is possible for the operator to vary the effect by selecting from a number of blend modes that vary the duty cycle from, for example, 80% (Blend 1) to 50% (Blend 3). As the duty cycle diminishes, the peak voltage increases, a factor that allows more collateral thermal damage and a consequently greater hemostatic effect (see Figs. 4-4 and 4-8).

It is important to realize that all generators are not created equal. The duty cycles of the various "blend" modes vary from machine to machine. The peak voltages generated in any of the modes may vary significantly, depend-

Ohm's Law $I = \frac{V}{R}$

Power (W) $= V \times I$

$$W = V \times \frac{V}{R} = \frac{V^2}{R} \text{ watts}$$

Fig. 4-3. Substitution of the Ohm's law current *(I)* equation into the power equation demonstrates that power varies according to the square of the voltage and inversely with the impedance *(R)* of the circuit.

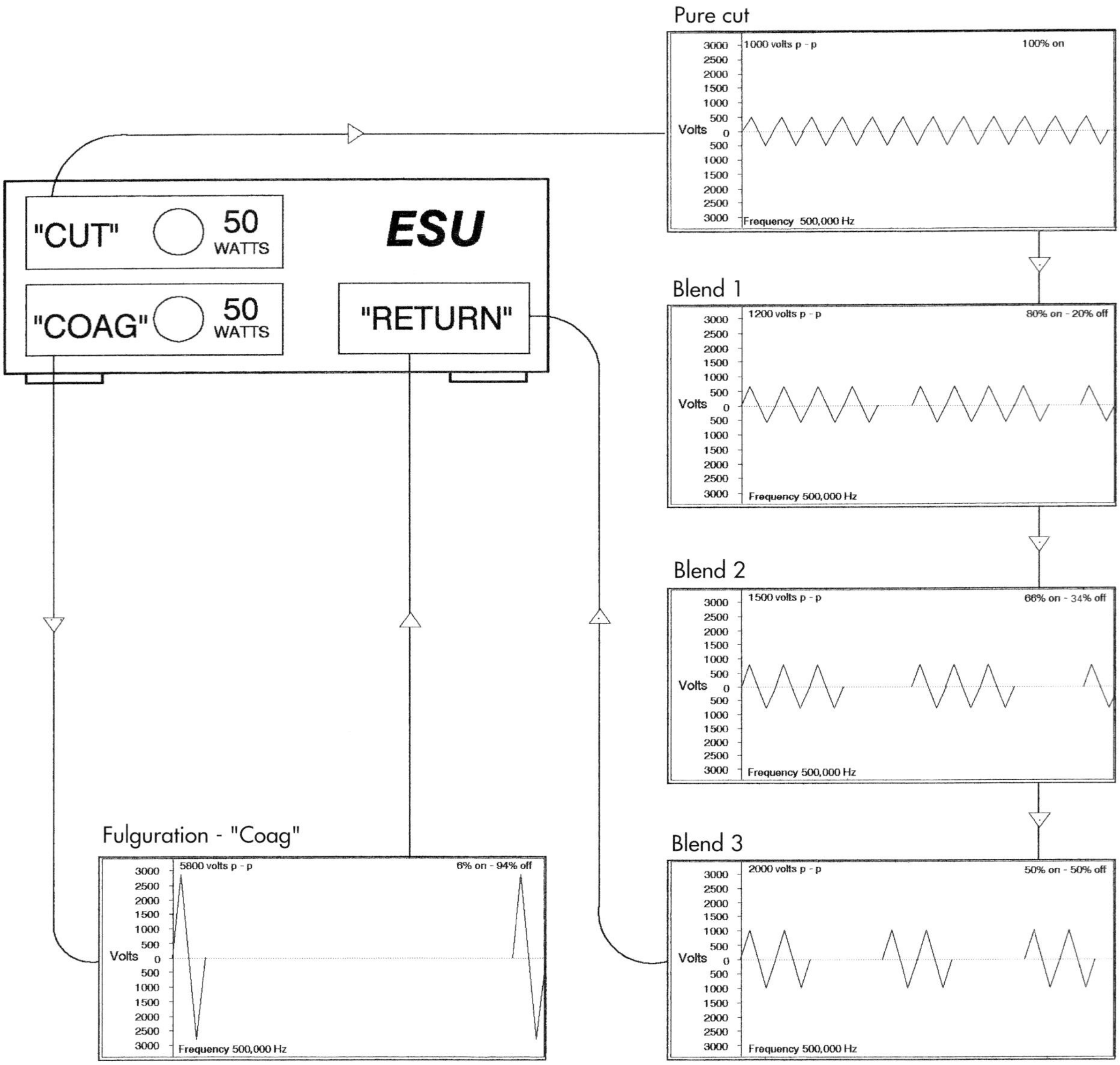

Fig. 4-4. Stylized representations of electrosurgical generator *(ESU)* outputs as they appear on the oscilloscope. Blended outputs are actually variations of the "cutting" current. Note that as the duty cycle (amount of time that the current is on) diminishes, the voltage must correspondingly increase, provided the power remains constant. The highest voltage is found in the fulguration output in which the duty cycle is only 6%.

ing, in part, on the purpose for which the machine was designed. For example, machines designed for operating room use generally provide peak voltages for the continuous and blended waveforms significantly higher than those provided by machines designed for outpatient loop electrosurgical excision of the cervix. This is largely because the operating room machines are designed to deal with tissue that has high impedance. The trade-off is that thermal injury will be greater with the increased voltage.

Most ESUs designed for operating room use can provide bipolar current. Modern generators provide only a continuous waveform, identical to the "cut" waveform, even though bipolar devices are not really capable of a cutting effect. The reasons for this will be explained in subsequent sections.

Effect of alternating current on cells. The first biophysical principles essential for the understanding of electrosurgery are those that describe the effect of radiofrequency alternating current on cells.

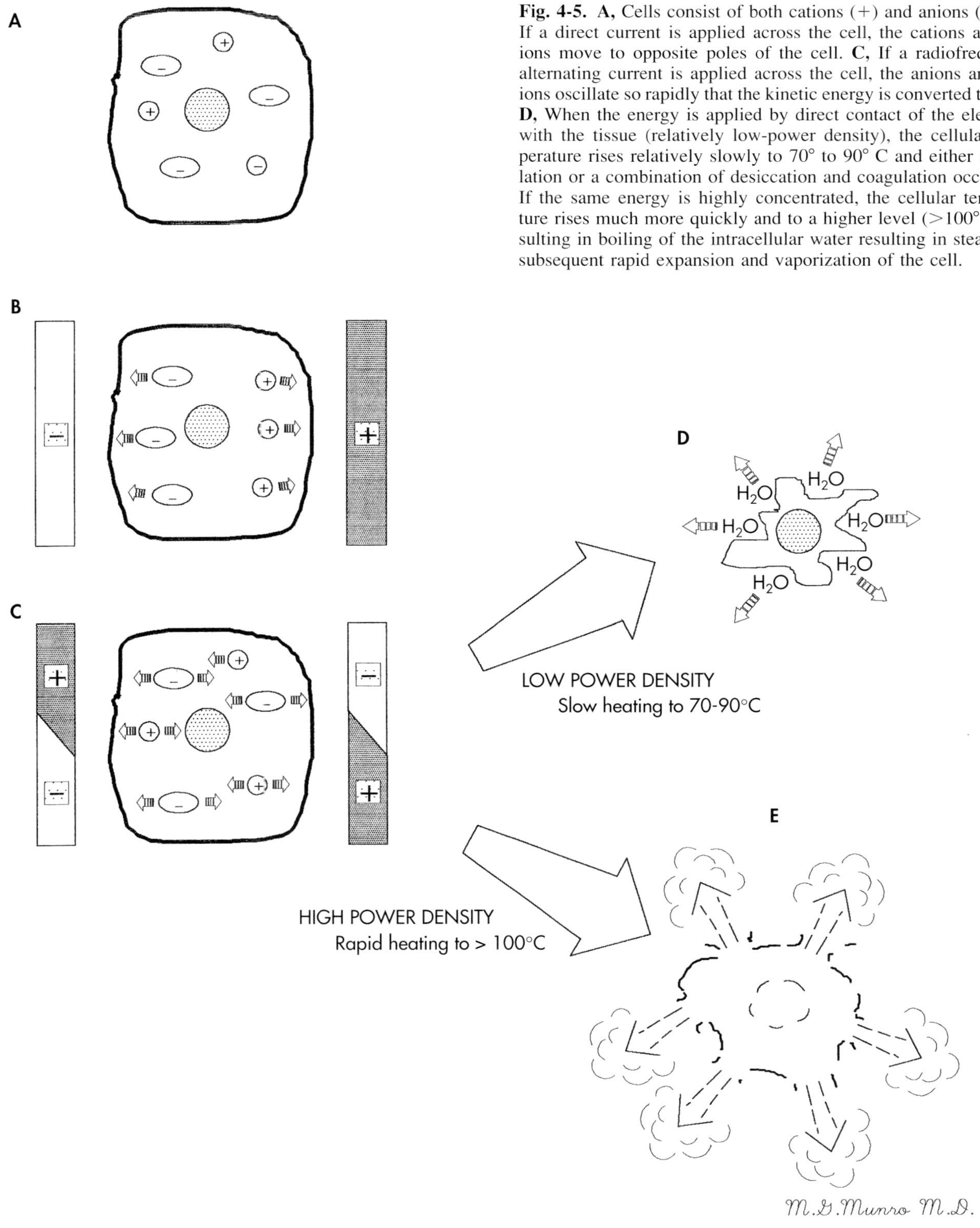

Fig. 4-5. A, Cells consist of both cations (+) and anions (−). **B,** If a direct current is applied across the cell, the cations and anions move to opposite poles of the cell. **C,** If a radiofrequency alternating current is applied across the cell, the anions and cations oscillate so rapidly that the kinetic energy is converted to heat. **D,** When the energy is applied by direct contact of the electrode with the tissue (relatively low-power density), the cellular temperature rises relatively slowly to 70° to 90° C and either coagulation or a combination of desiccation and coagulation occurs. **E,** If the same energy is highly concentrated, the cellular temperature rises much more quickly and to a higher level (>100° C) resulting in boiling of the intracellular water resulting in steam and subsequent rapid expansion and vaporization of the cell.

Cells contain both cations and anions. The former are small, positively charged particles like sodium and potassium, while the latter include large, negatively charged protein molecules. Alternating currents of different frequency will have different effects on the cell. When a radiofrequency (500 kHz to 3.0 MHz) alternating current is applied across the cell, these cations and anions rapidly oscillate within the cytoplasm, elevating the temperature within the cell (Fig. 4-5). If the intracellular temperature reaches about 70° to 80° C, protein denaturation occurs, initiating the process of "white coagulation." If the temperature rises more quickly to 90° C the cells lose water content *(dehydration)* but preserve architecture in the process termed *desiccation.* When the temperature quickly reaches 100° C and beyond, the intracellular water boils, and the subsequent formation of steam and intracellular expansion results in explosive vaporization of the cell. It is suspected that the explosive force results in acoustical vibrations that contribute to the cutting effect through the tissue. Finally, if the cellular temperature reaches 200° C the process of *carbonization* occurs.

If the frequency is below 30 kHz but above 20 Hz, the alternating current will predictably cause a *Faradic* effect—the depolarization of muscles and nerves resulting in fasciculation and pain. As described above, with radiofrequency current the cell's positive and negative ions oscillate so rapidly that depolarization does not occur. Despite these theoretical considerations, radiofrequency alternating current up to 1 MHz can cause neuromuscular stimulation [22] The exact reasons for such stimulation are not known but could include the influence of stray lower frequency arcs to tissue or *rectification,* the conversion of alternating current to direct current.

Tissue effects of electrosurgery

Electrosurgery may be used to either vaporize or coagulate tissue. If vaporization is extended in a linear fashion, cutting occurs. To a greater or lesser extent, a zone of coagulation will be created adjacent to any electrosurgical incision or other zone of vaporization.

The tissue effects depend upon a number of factors including the power, tissue impedance, the waveform, the shape and size of the electrode, and its proximity to tissue (i.e., contact or noncontact). Another factor is the peritoneal distension medium, if any, utilized for the procedure. (See the box below.) The basic principles will be discussed under the appropriate headings. Then a discussion of the factors that modify the tissue effect will follow.

Cutting. Vaporization of tissue is best achieved with a continuous, unipolar, low-voltage current, using a pointed or a thin loop-shaped electrode held near to but not in contact with the tissue (Fig. 4-6). The generator is activated, allowing the thin electrode to concentrate the current at its tip. The current then arcs to the tissue, rapidly elevating the local intracellular temperature and causing vaporization. As the electrode is advanced, an incision is fashioned as the process is maintained by continued arcing to and vaporization of the underlying tissue. Because the voltage is low and the current dissipates rapidly toward the return electrode, the thermal damage beside the cut is minimal, provided appropriate equipment and surgical technique are used.

The actual depth of coagulation injury incurred when electrodes are used for cutting is dependant upon a number of factors, including power output, electrode size and shape, waveform and peak voltage, and the speed and skill of the surgeon. Consequently, descriptions of the depth of coagulation injury should take the existence of such variables into consideration. While the minimum depth of thermal injury has been described as low as 100 μ or less,[23] more typical reported peritoneal injury studies suggest from less than 200 μ for pure cutting waveforms[24] to 300 μ for blended waveforms.[25] Such injury depths no doubt in part reflect the rather high-peak voltage outputs of the majority of the generators currently in general use. The use of lower voltage units will result in a correspondingly reduced depth of thermal injury.

Bipolar electrodes cannot be used effectively for cutting because it is difficult for the two electrodes to be oriented in a way that allows efficient vaporization to occur.

Desiccation and Coagulation. Coagulation is generally used to describe one or more of a number of related processes in which the cell is dehydrated and the protein is denatured but not destroyed by the thermal energy.

When an electrode is placed in contact with the tissue, all the energy is available for conversion to heat (Fig. 4-6). Furthermore, the relatively large contact area (particularly if it is from a flat electrode) reduces the power density, preventing elevation of the intracellular temperature to 100° C and allowing the intracellular water content to evaporate and desiccation and/or coagulation to occur.

Desiccation is the process in which temperature reaches about 90° C, resulting in cellular dehydration without protein denaturation. From a gross and microscopic perspective, coagulation is the result of a process similar to boiling the white of an egg—a white, homogenous coagulum. Microscopically it has been demonstrated that protein bonds are formed, creating the homogenous, gelatinous structure. Such a tissue effect is useful for occluding tubular structures such as fallopian tubes or blood vessels for the purpose of hemostasis. Because in practice it is difficult to distinguish clinically between these two processes, both will be referred to as coagulation.

Although any waveform may be used to create tissue coagulation, the cutting and blended outputs are preferred to the labeled "coagulation" mode. There are a number of potential reasons for this apparent paradox. First, the inter-

Factors influencing effects of electrosurgery on tissue

- Power output of electrical source
- Tissue impedance
- Waveform of alternating current
- Shape of electrode
- Size of electrode
- Proximity of electrode to tissue
- Peritoneal distension medium
- Speed of procedure
- Skill of the surgeon

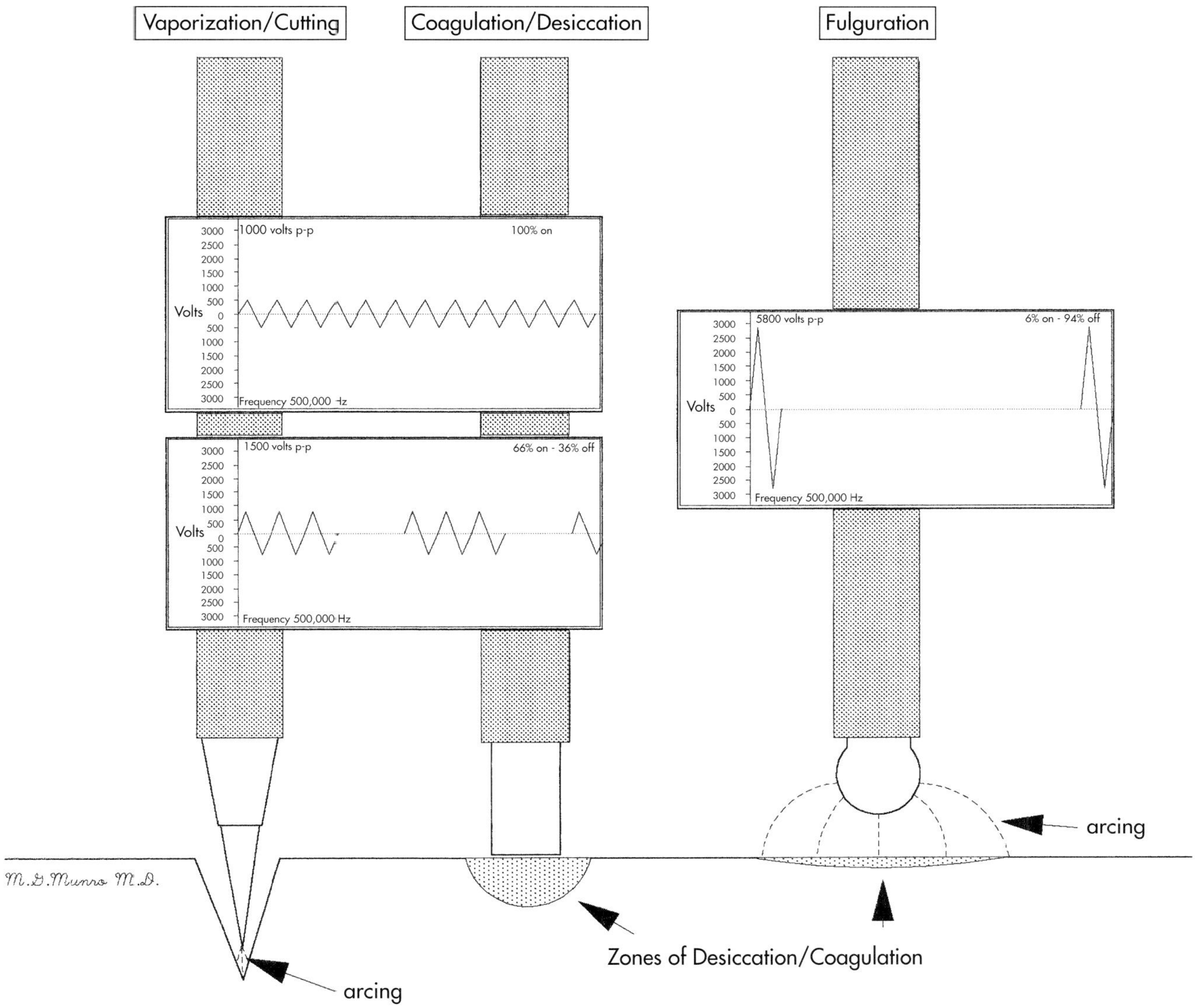

Fig. 4-6. Tissue effects. Vaporization or cutting, and coagulation or desiccation are each achieved using continuous or "blended" currents. Fulguration is performed with the relatively high voltage, modulated current with a short duty cycle. Vaporization and fulguration are noncontact procedures while coagulation and desiccation require tissue contact.

rupted nature of the "coagulation," or fulguration, current may cause an uneven amount of protein bonding, preventing, for example, complete occlusion of a blood vessel. In addition, such current may cause the more superficial layers of the tissue to become rapidly coagulated, increasing impedance, thereby inhibiting further transmission of current to the deeper layers. Finally, the fulguration effect near the electrode causes rapid heating and adherence of tissue, allowing the eschar to be pulled off with removal of the electrode, a process that often causes a recurrence of bleeding.

As a result of these considerations, coagulation should be performed with an electrode having a relatively large surface area, using the "cutting" or "blended" waveforms. If a blood vessel is to be coagulated, it should be first coapted by compressing it against adjacent tissue or by grasping it with a forceps. Either of these maneuvers reduces the effective volume to be coagulated and facilitates the thermal effect by preventing the flow of blood from removing heat from the site.

Fulguration. Fulguration, also known as spray coagulation or black coagulation, is a process in which the tissue is superficially carbonized by repeated high-voltage electrosurgical arcs that quickly elevate the temperature to 200° C or more.

The spraying of this energy onto tissue is accomplished using an interrupted, or modulated, high voltage with a very short duty cycle waveform (Fig. 4-6). The active electrode is held a few millimeters away from the tissue at a distance sufficient to allow the discharge to traverse the gap. Unlike the case with low-voltage continuous current, the interrupted high-voltage discharges seek variable paths to the tissue creating a spraying effect, thereby reducing the power density. The result is a relatively diffuse, but superficial, elevation of the tissue temperature so that coagulation and carbonization occur. The rapid superficial nature of this type of coagulation raises tissue impedance, preventing the current from continuing to heat the deeper layers of the tissue. Consequently, this type of coagulation is most preferred for the arrest of capillary or small arteriolar bleeding over a large surface area.

Variables affecting the tissue effects of electrosurgery

After the basic principles of electrosurgery are understood, the next step is to learn how to modify the tissue effects (see the box on p. 32). Familiarity with these variables is essential for safe and effective application of electrosurgical technique.

Generator Output. Understanding of the output characteristics of the ESU will enable the surgeon to vary the tissue effects. It is important to know that different generator brands have different output characteristics with varying peak voltages and variable duty cycles at the blend settings. These variables will, in many instances, affect subtleties of technique and tissue bioeffect. Virtually all ESUs have a means by which the output in watts may be controlled or set. Most of the newer varieties have a light emitting diode screen that reveals the exact wattage, while others have a logarithmic scale from 1 (lowest) to 10 (highest), making exact settings and adjustments more difficult.

For most generators the power output is proportional to both the voltage and current and inversely proportional to tissue impedance. Some machines will automatically adjust the voltage or current as impedance varies to maintain the desired output in watts. Others do not have this capability, allowing the power output to tissue to fall below the setting when impedance increases.

The appropriate power output for cutting will be the minimum amount necessary to create the desired combination of vaporization and coagulation. More power means more voltage and increased adjacent coagulation (Fig. 4-7). For fulguration, increasing the voltage by increasing the power output will generally allow more superficial coagulation within a given time interval. However, when deep coagulation is desired, higher power outputs may be counterproductive. This is because the higher energy levels may disproportionately heat the tissue adjacent to the electrode, causing premature superficial coagulation, resulting in-

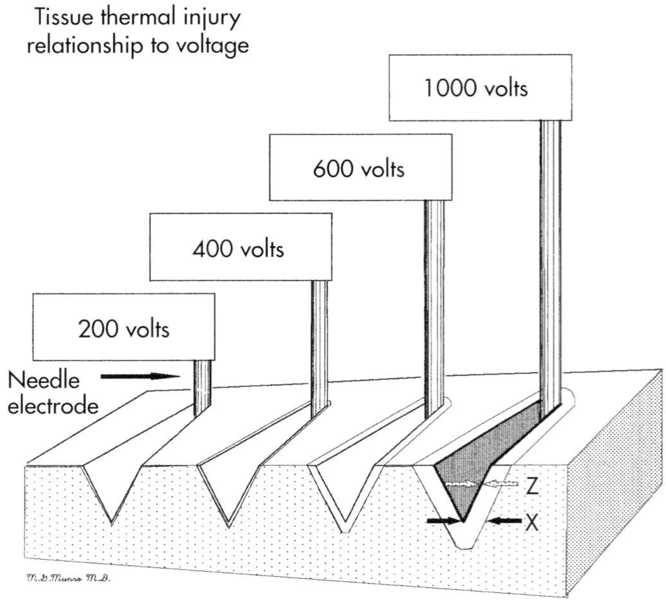

Fig. 4-7. Collateral thermal injury increases with increasing voltage.

creased tissue impedance and a tendency for the current to spark intermittently through tissue, resulting in deeper carbonization. In addition the increased impedance results in a decreased output of voltage by the generator ($W = V^2/R$). These effects prevent deeper coagulation of tissue. If sparking is seen when deep coagulation is described, the process should be interrupted and the power decreased. This concept is very important to the gynecologic surgeon using electrosurgery for occlusion of structures such as the fallopian tubes or blood vessels.

The voltage may be increased without changing the power settings by using *"blended waveforms"* with their increased peak voltage.* Blended waveforms result in greater thermal injury around an incision because the higher voltage pushes more current into tissue and because the interrupted nature of the current dictates a slower cutting speed (Fig. 4-8). This effect may be exploited when hemostasis is necessary along an incision line or when the surgery requires cutting or coagulating of tissue with relatively high impedance.

Power density. The power or current density is the total wattage striking the tissue per unit area of the electrode or current in contact with that tissue. This variable is of paramount importance in the performance of electrosurgery (Fig. 4-9). Given equal power outputs, power density is largely determined by the shape and size of the electrode. A very small electrode, such as a needle-shaped device, will

*"Blended waveforms" are, in modern generators, pure but modulated sinusoidal outputs. Older generators actually blended high-voltage modulated waveforms from the spark-gap side with continuous sinewave outputs from the "cutting" side.

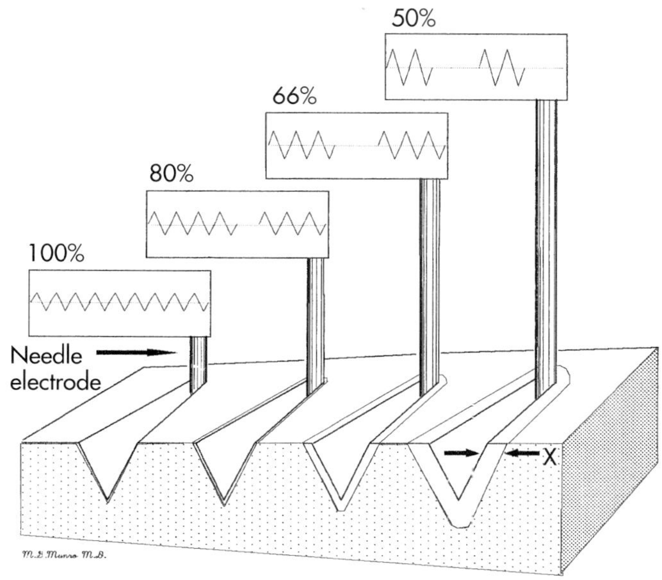

Fig. 4-8. As the duty cycle is reduced, the voltage increases if power remains constant. Collateral thermal injury increases because of the increased voltage and the reduced cutting speed secondary to the interrupted current.

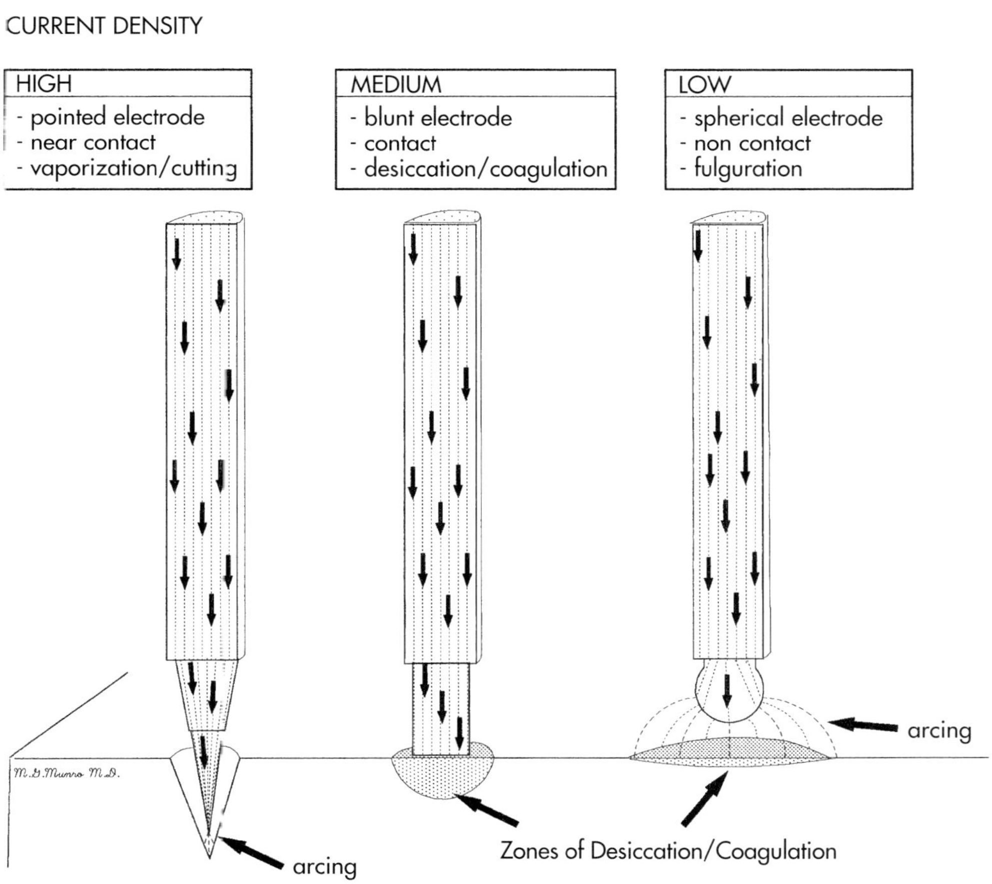

Fig. 4-9. Current density, or power density, is largely determined at equal power outputs by the shape of the electrode and its relationship to tissue. The same power and current type is passed through each of the stylized electrodes, but the shape of the electrode and its relationship to tissue determines the tissue effect. **A,** Concentrated noncontact with arcing results in vaporization. **B,** Dispersed contact electrosurgery causes deep desiccation and/or coagulation. **C,** Dispersion with arcing requires high voltage current and results in superficial coagulation or fulguration.

concentrate current so that the point of impact on tissue is very narrow and the power density high, allowing for the rapid elevation of cellular temperature and the creation of a narrow zone of vaporization. Given the same power, a wider, larger electrode, in contact with tissue, will dilute the power density, preventing rapid elevation of intracellular temperature. Instead, the temperature rises more slowly, causing protein coagulation and/or desiccation.

Fulgurating electrodes are preferably shaped in the form of a ball. This reduces the power density and facilitates the spraying effect, allowing a greater area of tissue to be fulgurated in a given pass.

Some electrodes are designed to serve a dual purpose. For example, a blade-shaped electrode may be employed as a cutting device holding the blade's narrow edge near the tissue, creating a high-current density. Alternatively, by placing the breadth of the blade in contact with the tissue, the resultant low-current density can be used for coagulation. Note that if the leading edge of the blade is used for cutting purposes, the flat sides may contact the edge of the incision as the electrode is passed through tissue, creating an additional degree of adjacent tissue coagulation (Fig. 4-10). Depending upon the clinical situation, this effect may be either an advantage or disadvantage.

An electrode at the other end of the power density spectrum is the "return" or *dispersive electrode*.* Given the same power output, this electrode has a very large area and dissipates the current so much as to allow essentially no significant tissue effect. This is why the dispersive electrode placed on a patient's body allows the flow of monopolar current without causing injury to the skin.

Electrode tissue proximity. An important factor in the performance of electrosurgery is the relationship of the active electrode with the target tissue (see Figs. 4-6 and 4-9).

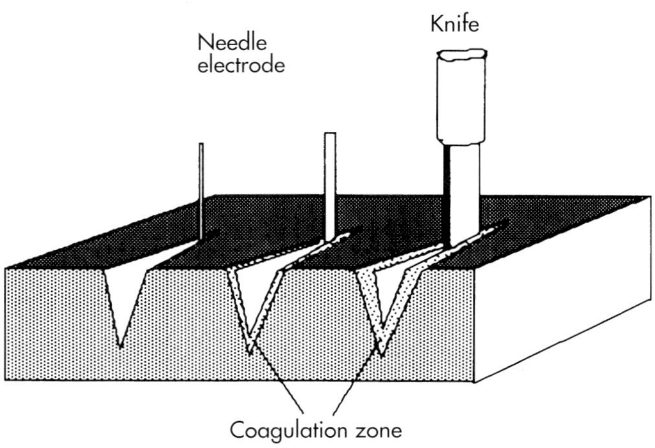

Fig. 4-10. The shape of the electrode also affects the amount of thermal injury—thick blades result in coagulation as the side of the instrument contacts the edge of the incision. (From Keckstein J: Tissue effects of different lasers and electrodiathermy. In Sutton C, Diamond M, editors: Endoscopic surgery for gynaecologists, London, 1993, WB Saunders.)

Cutting, a form of vaporization, is ideally a *near-contact* event where the current arcs from the active electrode to the tissue where the bioeffect is manifested. Vaporization is facilitated by the formation of a steam envelope between the electrode and the zone of destruction. This steam is generated by the vaporized intracellular water. If the electrode is held too far from the tissue, no arcing and, therefore, no vaporization will occur On the other hand, if the electrode touches the tissue, the power density diminishes and coagulation will occur, creating a greater degree of thermal injury to the tissue adjacent to the incision line.

Fulguration is also a noncontact electrosurgical activity employing higher voltage, interrupted current, usually with a short (e.g., 6%) duty cycle. Because of the higher voltage, the electrode can be held millimeters from the target, while the current is "sprayed" onto the tissue. The distance that the electrode is held from the tissue is dependent in part upon the design of the generator. As previously mentioned, different generators can, at a given wattage, have varying output voltages in the fulguration mode. Higher voltages will allow the electrode to send longer arcs to the tissue.

The deeper effect of white coagulation is best achieved with contact between a flat electrode and the tissue, creating the necessary lower current density. This activity, properly employed, causes sealing of blood vessels of up to several millimeters in diameter.

Tissue impedance or resistance. Impedance, or resistance, is offered by each aspect of the electrical circuit. Highly conductive tissues have a high water content and offer little resistance to the passage of current and the creation of electrosurgical effects. However, it is the tissue itself that provides the greatest degree of variability. Tissue that offers high impedance is generally relatively low in fluid content and therefore relatively non-conductive. Tissue such as bone, calloused skin, fat, or any previously desiccated tissue will impede passage of current and therefore will inhibit the creation of an electrosurgical effect.

If it is necessary to cut through tissue with relatively high impedance, increasing the voltage by either raising the power output or decreasing the duty cycle is usually effective. In such cases, the current is pushed through the relatively resistant tissue with greater force.

The rest of the circuit has variable impedance related to factors that include its length, its composition, and its cross-sectional area. While an important factor is the type of material used for the construction of the electrode, most manufacturers use similar substances. Consequently, the most relevant variable parameter is the environment in which the procedure is being performed, an issue discussed below under "Distension media."

*The term *return electrode* is technically incorrect with alternating currents as, with the alternating polarity, there is no constant directionality to the "flow" of current.

Time on or near tissue. The amount of energy imparted to a given volume of tissue is directly related to the time during which the electrode is near or in contact with that tissue. If, when used for cutting, the electrode is moved very slowly through tissue, there will occur a greater degree of collateral thermal injury. However, moving the electrode too quickly will also result in increased thermal injury (Fig 4-11). This may occur if arcing is prevented by the electrode coming in contact with the tissue. Such contact allows for much more energy transfer to adjacent tissue, more coagulation and ultimate slowing of the cutting process.

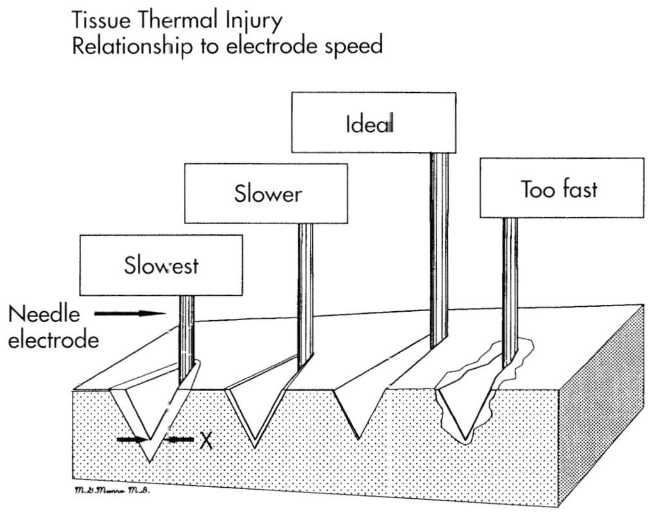

Fig. 4-11. The speed or cutting rate will affect the amount of thermal injury. If the rate is very slow, increasing thermal injury will occur. However, if the electrode is moved too quickly, contact will be made with the tissue, power density decreases, vaporization is impeded, and coagulation results.

In circumstances where coagulation is a desired effect, the time of contact will directly affect the extent and degree of tissue injury. Indeed, a more homogenous and deep effect will occur if the voltage is kept relatively low and the contact time is prolonged.

Distension media. The distension medium should be considered as a part of the electrical circuit. For procedures that require an arc, this concept is quite easy to understand. The arc only occurs when the electrical field between the active electrode and the tissue becomes strong enough to ionize the intervening medium. These ions collide with other molecules until the charge crosses the gap between electrode and tissue, completing the circuit (Fig. 4-12).

Different media possess varying ionizing capabilities. For example, the CO_2 medium employed for most laparoscopy cases is only 70% as effective as room air at transmitting a charge. Argon gas promotes conductivity of electrical current, a feature that is exploited by the argon beam coagulator (Fig. 4-13), which is essentially an instrument that allows fulguration to occur from a distance of one to two centimeters.

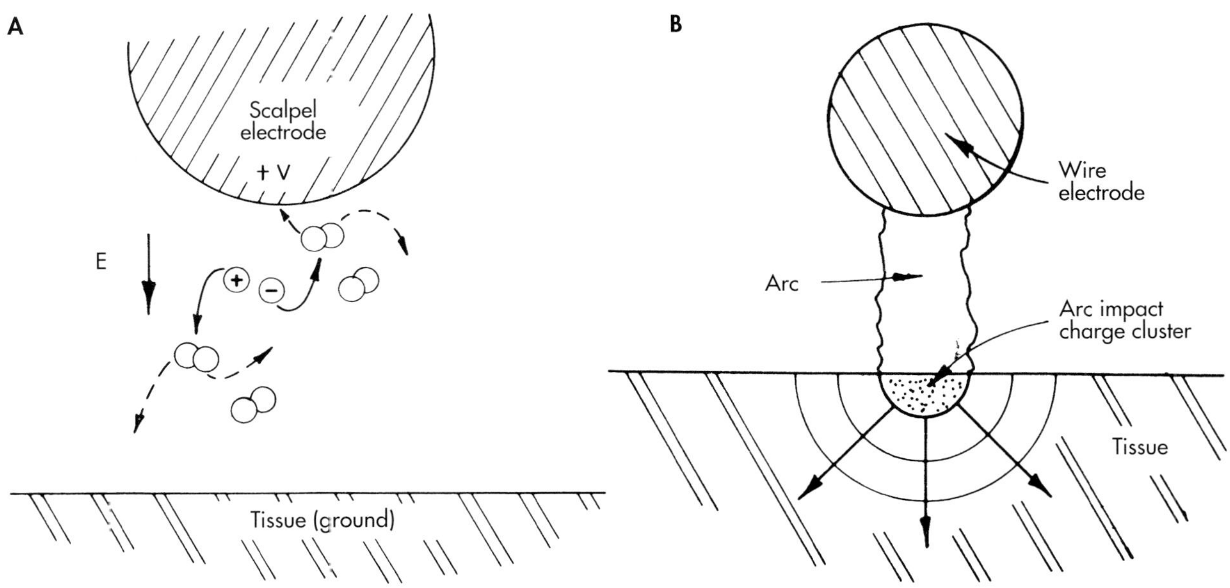

Fig. 4-12. Arcing. **A,** With sufficiently high voltage, the intervening medium is ionized and the resulting charged particles are accelerated by the electrical field to strike other molecules, forming more ions until the tissue is struck. **B,** The power density rapidly diminishes with distance from the point of the arc's impact. (From Pearce JA: Electrosurgery. New York: 1986, John Wiley & Sons.)

A 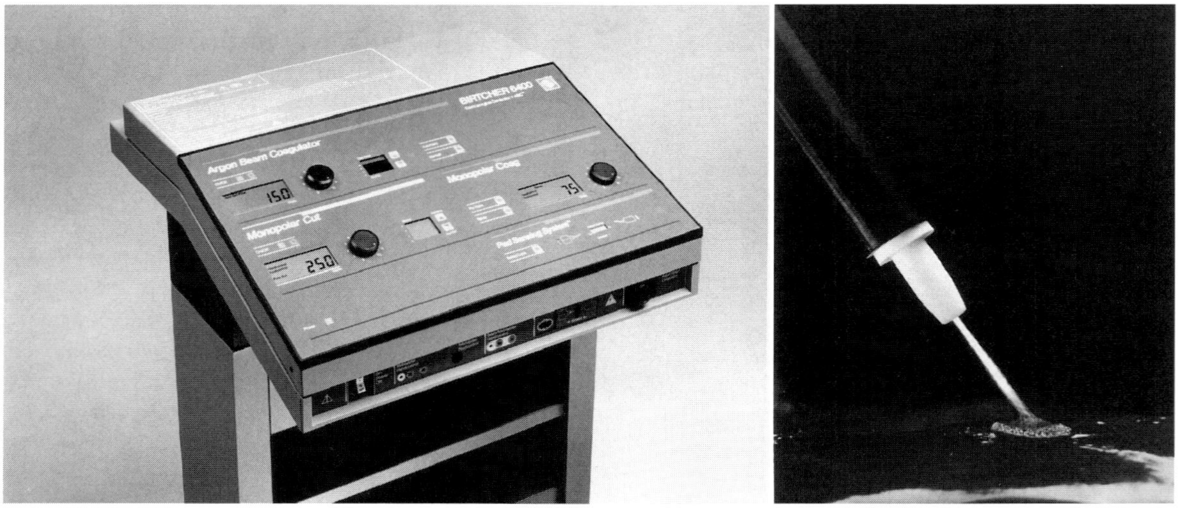 B

Fig. 4-13. **A,** The argon beam coagulator. **B,** It is actually a fulgurating device that uses a stream of argon gas to focus and direct the charge.

Other important variables. There are other concepts important for the effective use of electrosurgery. For example, active electrodes must be kept shiny and free of carbon that acts as an insulator, impeding the flow of current. In addition, a moist electrode and tissue will facilitate the formation of the steam envelope necessary for effective vaporization and cutting, a principle especially important in electromicrosurgery.

Laparoscopic applications of electrosurgery

Electrosurgery is the most flexible and cost effective method by which energy can be used during laparoscopy. For many reasons it is generally preferable to perform operative electrosurgical laparoscopic procedures using a multipuncture technique. These reasons include increased maneuverability of the electrode and the safety issues discussed later in this chapter. It is useful to have unipolar or bipolar attachments to most grasping forceps as this increases their flexibility and decreases the need for frequent instrument exchanges. In such cases, the encountered bleeding vessel may be grasped and coagulated with the same instrument.

For unipolar procedures a dispersive electrode must be applied to normal tissue as close as possible to the operative site. The foot or hand controls for the generator are controlled only by the operator. The combination of a smoke evacuation system attached to a hollow probe and a high flow insufflator will decrease operating time by quickly evacuating and replenishing the evacuated pneumoperitoneum.

Cutting. Cutting is most efficiently achieved through the use of the continuous low-voltage waveform from the "cut" side of the generator, utilizing a shiny, pointed, and moistened unipolar electrode. While the ideal output varies, with a pointed electrode about 1 mm in maximal diameter with a 100% duty cycle ("pure cut" output), it is usually in the range of 30 to 60 watts. The tip of the electrode is brought near to the tissue and the generator activated. The cutting action is created with a light, brushing or stroking action without actually touching the tissue. To remain effective at deeper levels, the edges of the incision should be retracted to avoid their contact with the sides of the electrode. If a greater degree of hemostasis is desired, it may be obtained at some loss of vaporization efficiency by using the slightly higher voltage *"blended currents"* that create a deeper layer of coagulation (see Fig. 4-8).

Large vessel hemostasis. Occlusion of the fallopian tube or other large vessel hemostasis is achieved by the process of white coagulation, best performed with the same continuous or blended currents used for cutting. The vessel or tissue should be grasped in the smooth jaws of either a unipolar or bipolar forceps attached to the electrosurgical generator. As previously noted, newer bipolar generators are available only with a continuous, low-voltage waveform. However, if the generator is an older model, with cutting, blended, and fulguration options, the dial should be set to "cut" or "blend." The simultaneous use of irrigation with the application of bipolar current may reduce the lateral spread of thermal injury. If bipolar current is employed, an ammeter may be used to aid in determining when complete desiccation or coagulation has occurred. When the interposed tissue is totally dehydrated it can no longer conduct current (Fig. 4-14). The ammeter will detect the loss of conductivity and then provide the surgeon with a visible or au-

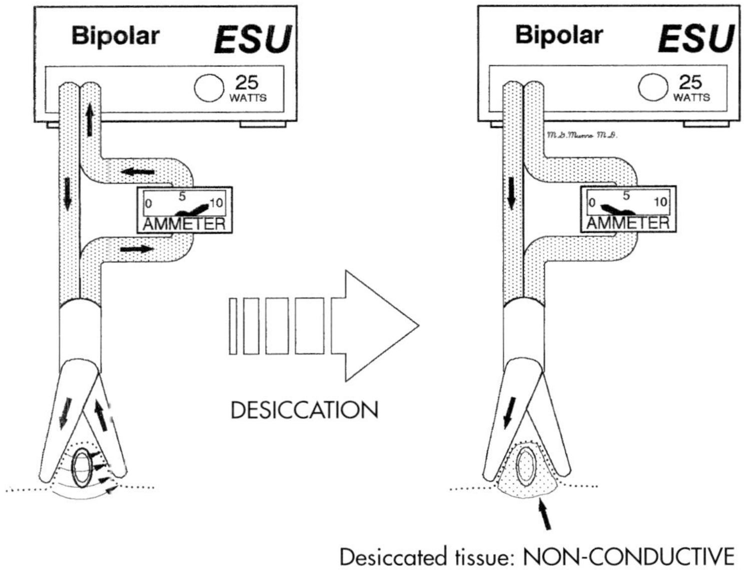

Fig. 4-14. Bipolar electrodesiccation—use of an ammeter to determine the end point of bipolar desiccation or coagulation. When the target tissue is completely desiccated, no more current flows and the ammeter drops to "0."

dible signal. Ammeters may be purchased separately (Electroscope Inc, Denver, Colo.) or they may be integrated into the ESU (Richard Wolf, Medical Instruments Corp., Rosemont, Ill.; Elmed Corp., Addison, Ill.). Flat or forceps style unipolar electrodes may also be used to coagulate, taking care not to injure vital structures such as bowel, bladder, or ureter.

Small vessel hemostasis. Small vessel hemostasis may be achieved by pinpoint desiccation. However, if large areas of small oozing vessels are encountered, control may require laparoscopically directed fulguration. This effect is in some ways more difficult to perform and associated with slightly greater risks of inadvertent injury because of the higher voltages in use. Consequently, fulguration should be used with care within the peritoneal cavity and only as a method of hemostasis for capillary or small arteriolar ooze. The electrode is preferably ball shaped and the current selected is the interrupted, dampened high-voltage waveform that comes from the "coag" output of most generators. The site should be made as free of blood as possible, the generator activated, and the electrode brought into proximity with the tissue until the arcing effect is seen. Another approach is to touch lightly or bounce the electrode off the site, allowing the arcing to occur. The latter approach, while more practical, is also more prone to allowing debris and carbonization to coat the electrode. In such instances arcing will be inhibited. The electrode should be removed and cleaned with an appropriate brush or pad.

Another way that laparoscopic fulguration may be achieved is with the argon beam coagulator shown in Fig. 4-13. This device employs a high-voltage, modulated, and dampened current with power outputs suitable for fulguration. A jet of argon gas is passed around the electrode, propagating the current to the target tissue in a relatively wide, low-power density "beam" 3 to 6 mm in diameter about 1 cm from the tip of the probe. The forced flow of the argon gas helps to keep the oozing site free of blood, allowing an improved fulgurating effect.[26] Problems with the device include the need for venting of the large volumes of argon gas and the current need for a 10 mm port for the device. The latter issue has been recently solved with the introduction of a 5 mm diameter probe.

Complications of electrosurgery

The complications of electrosurgery occur secondary to thermal trauma and can be classified into three basic types (Table 4-1). The first relates to unintended thermal injury through use of the active electrode(s). The second occurs when the current is diverted to another path, causing injury distant from the principal operative field. The final cause is injury at the site of the dispersive electrode. Injury associated with the active electrode(s) can occur with either unipolar or bipolar technique while trauma secondary to current diversion or dispersive electrode accidents only occurs with unipolar electrosurgery. The incidence of any of the complications of electrosurgery is reduced by adherence to safety protocols and a sound understanding of the circumstances that dictate when current can undesirably affect other tissue.

Active electrode trauma. One of the more common

Table 4-1. Management of complications

Mechanism	Prevention and management
Active electrode trauma	
Unintended activation	Surgeon must be in direct control of electrode activation Remove all electrosurgical instruments from peritoneal cavity when not in use Detach instruments not in use from the ESU
Increased zone of effect	Isolate vessels prior to coagulation Maintain adequate tissue margin
Unintended arcing to adjacent structures	Use ESU with lower voltage output
Diversion of current	
Grounding at site other than dispersive electrode	Use ESU with isolated circuits Use return electrode imipedance monitoring system
Direct coupling to adjacent tissue	Thorough examination of insulation on all instruments Keep shaft free of vital structures Maintain shaft visible in the operative field Remove all electrosurgical instruments from field when not in use Confirm electrode is not in inappropriate contact with other instruments before use
Capacitative coupling	Use only all plastic or all metal systems
Dispersive electrode burns	Use a return electrode impedance monitoring device

mechanisms by which the active electrode causes complications is by unintended activation. Typically, such a complication occurs when an electrode is left untended within the peritoneal cavity to be activated by accidental compression of the handswitch or depression of the foot pedal.[27,28] Control of the generator by someone other than the operating surgeon may be another source of accidental activation of the electrode. To prevent these kinds of injury, the surgeon should always be in direct control of electrode activation and all electrosurgical instruments should be removed from the peritoneal cavity when not in use. When removed from the peritoneal cavity, the instruments should be detached from the ESU or they should be stored in an insulated pouch. These measures will prevent damage to the patient's skin should the foot pedal be accidentally depressed.

Another mechanism by which the active electrode(s) directly cause complications is when the zone of vaporization or coagulation extends to involve large blood vessels or vital structures such as the bladder, ureter, or bowel. In laparoscopy, the use of bipolar current may reduce, but does not eliminate, the occurrence of thermal injury to adjacent tissue.[28,29] Consequently, care must be taken to isolate blood vessels prior to coagulation, especially when near vital structures, and to apply appropriate amounts of energy in a fashion that allows an adequate tissue margin.

Unintended arcing of current to nearby structures was a possibility when high-voltage (30,000 volts peak to peak) currents were used. Such mechanisms of injury are all but eliminated with the adoption of ESUs with lower voltage outputs.[29,30]

Thermal injury to bowel, bladder, or ureter, recognized at the time of laparoscopy, should be treated immediately (See Chapter 26), considering the potential extent of the coagulative necrosis when repairing the structure. The extent of thermal trauma will depend upon the characteristics of the energy transferred to tissue. A thermal incision made with a pointed electrode may be repaired in a fashion identical to one created mechanically. However, if a coagulative injury is generated, the thermal necrosis may extend for several centimeters from the point of contact. In such instances, wide excision or resection will be necessary.

Frequently, the diagnosis of visceral thermal injury is delayed. In such instances the trauma is diagnosed only after the signs and symptoms of fistula or peritonitis present. Because these complications may not present until 2 to at least 10 days following surgery, the diagnosis may be delayed unless both the patient and the physician are aware of the possible consequences. Consequently, patients should be advised to report any fever or increasing abdominal pain experienced in the postoperative period.

Current diversion. Current diversion can take a number of forms. One type occurs when an electrical current finds a direct path out of the patient's body via grounded sites other than the dispersive electrode. Alternatively, current may be diverted directly to other sites in the patient's body before it reaches the tip of the active electrode. In either instance, if the power density becomes high enough, unintended and severe thermal injury can result.

Alternate ground site burns. These injuries can only occur with ground referenced ESUs. In such generators, if the dispersive electrode becomes detached, unplugged, or otherwise ineffective, the current will seek any grounded conductor. If such a conductor is of a sufficiently small surface area, the current density may become high enough to cause thermal injury (Fig. 4-15). Examples include electrocardiograph patch electrodes or the conductive metal components of the operating table.

Modern ESUs function with isolated circuits. This allows them to be designed so that if any part of the circuit is broken, an alarm sounds, and/or the machine "shuts down," thereby preventing electrode activation. Since the widespread introduction of such generators, the incidence of burns to alternate sites has been reduced significantly. However, maximum safety is achieved only with the use of return electrode impedance monitoring systems discussed later in this chapter. Consequently, it is incumbent on sur-

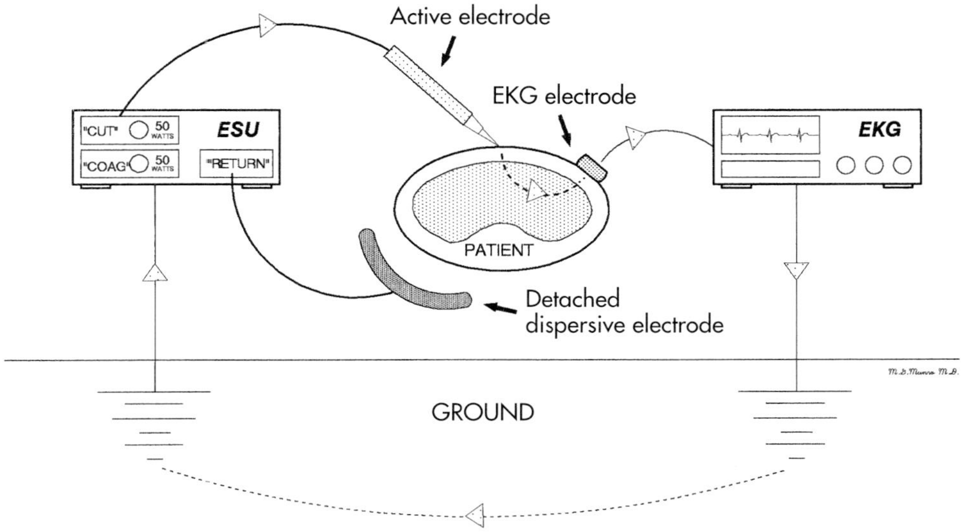

Fig. 4-15. Current diversion is a risk of ground referenced ESUs, particularly if the dispersive electrode is detached.

geons to establish the type of machine(s) available in their operating rooms prior to proceeding with surgery.

Direct coupling. Breaks in the insulation coating the shaft of an electrosurgical electrode allow for the possibility of current diversion to adjacent tissue. In laparoscopic procedures, bowel is the most commonly injured organ. The high-power density resulting from such small points of contact makes significant injury a real possibility (Fig. 4-16, *A*). The fact that the laparoscopic visual field frequently does not include the whole shaft of the active electrode makes it possible that such direct coupling can occur without the knowledge of the operator.

Prevention of such complications starts with the selection and care of hand instruments. Loose instrument bins should be replaced with containers designed to keep the instruments from damaging each other. Electrosurgical instruments should be examined prior to each case, searching for worn or obviously defective insulation. When found, the instrument should be removed and repaired or replaced. Despite all efforts, unobserved breaks in insulation may rarely occur. While the use of disposable instruments is often claimed as a way of reducing the incidence of insulation failure, there is no guarantee that this is the case, as invisible defects may occur in the manufacturing process. Consequently, when applying unipolar electrical energy, the shaft of the instrument should be kept free of vital structures and, if possible, totally visible in the operative field.

Direct coupling can also occur when an activated electrode touches and energizes a laparoscope, cannula, or other conductive instrument that is, in turn, near to or in contact with other tissue (Fig. 4-16, *B*). Such accidents usually happen following unintentional activation of an electrode or when it is energized when in contact with another conductive instrument. Prevention of direct coupling is facilitated by removal of the electrodes when not in use and visually confirming that the electrode is not in inappropriate contact with other conductive instruments prior to activation.

Capacitive coupling. *Capacitance* is the ability of a conductor to establish an electrical current in an unconnected parallel circuit. In any activated laparoscopic unipolar electrode, an electrical field is established around the shaft, a circumstance that makes the electrode a potential capacitor. This field does not pose a danger if the circuit is completed via a dispersive, low-power density pathway (Fig. 4-17, *A*). For example, if the electrode is passed through a metal cannula and capacitive coupling occurs (electrode to cannula), the current harmlessly "returns" via the metal cannula to the abdominal wall where it traverses to the dispersive electrode (Fig. 4-17, *B*). However, if the metal cannula is anchored to the skin by a nonconductive plastic retaining sleeve, the current will not return to the abdominal wall because the sleeve acts as an insulator. Instead, the capacitor will have to "look" elsewhere to complete the circuit. Consequently, bowel, often the nearest conductor, can become the target of a relatively high-power density discharge (Fig. 4-17, *C*). This problem also occurs with operating laparoscopes passed through plastic cannulae. The electrode could capacitively couple with the metal laparoscope, which, in turn, could be near to or in contact with bowel causing significant enteric thermal injury.

Prevention of capacitative coupling can largely be accomplished by avoiding the use of "hybrid" laparoscopic cannula systems containing a mixture of conductive and nonconductive elements. Instead all plastic or all metal cannula systems should be used. When and if operating laparoscopes are employed, all metal cannula systems should

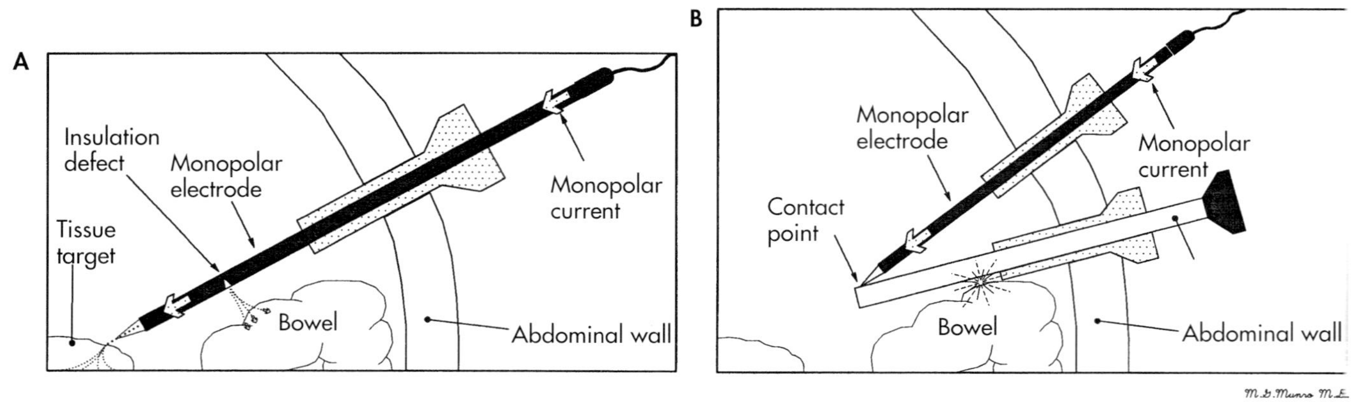

Fig. 4-16. Direct coupling may occur secondary to defective insulation of an activated electrode **(A).** Another cause is contact of the electrode with a conductor like a laparoscope **(B)** that is, in turn, in contact with or near other tissue.

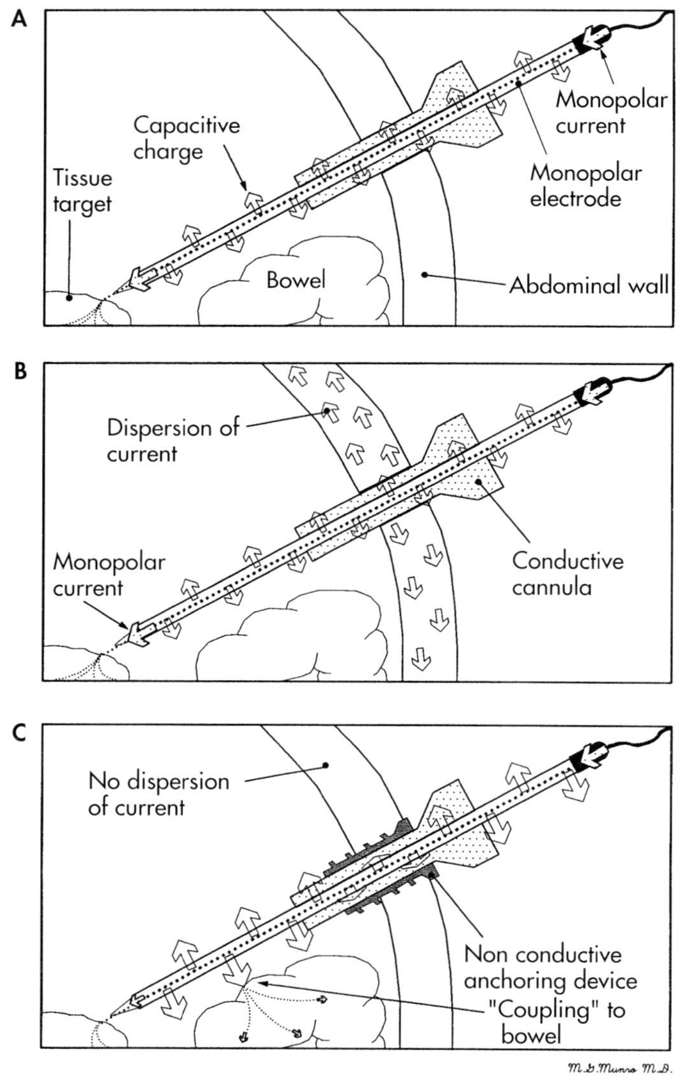

Fig. 4-17. Capacitive coupling. **A,** All activated monopolar electrodes possess a surrounding charge. **B,** As long as the current is conducted back to the abdominal wall no capacitative coupling occurs. **C,** Coupling will occur when current is not allowed to disperse via the abdominal wall.

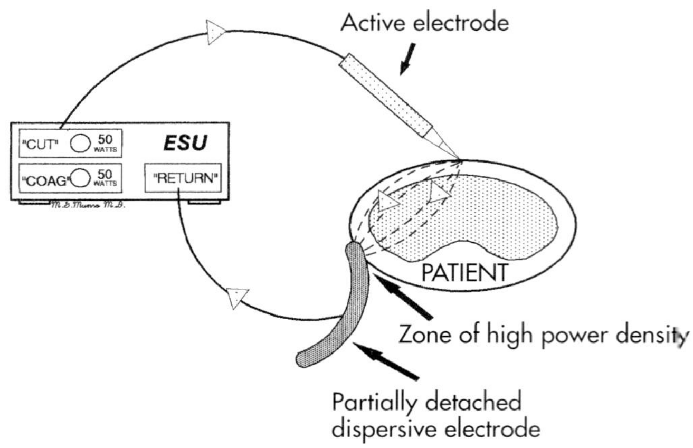

Fig. 4-18. Dispersive electrode burns. If the dispersive electrode is partially detached from the patient, the power density increases and a burn may result.

be the rule unless there is no intent to perform unipolar electrosurgical procedures through the operating channel.

Dispersive electrode burns. Thermal injury at the site of the dispersive electrode is rare with the use of isolated circuit generators with return electrode monitors. Most return electrode monitors are constructed as a dual electrode where the generator compares the impedance from the two sides of the pad. Without such devices, partial detachment of the "patient pad" could result in a burn. The thermal injuries occur because reducing the surface area of the electrode raises the current density (Fig. 4-18). With a return electrode monitor (REM), if significant dispersive electrode detachment occurs, the increased pad impedance is detected, an alarm sounds and the unit shuts off.

It is important for the surgeon to establish what type of ESU is being used in each case. Absence of a REM system is a reason for increased scrutiny of the positioning of the dispersive electrode before the surgery begins.

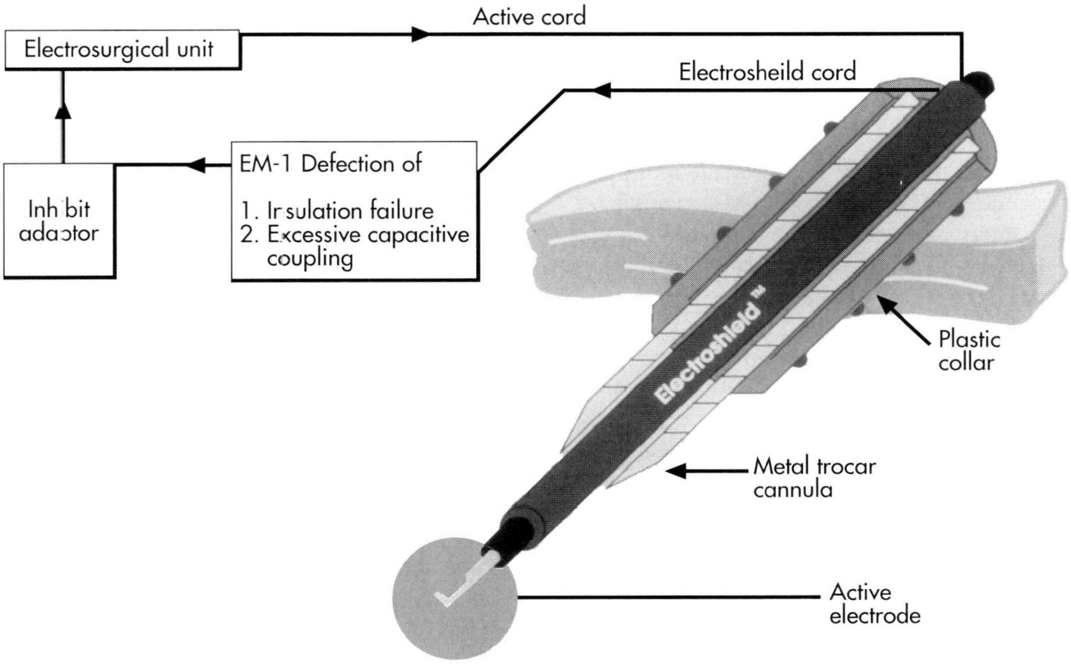

Fig. 4-19. The electroscope system. The shield provides protection from defective insulation and monitors for the presence of significant capacitance. If the latter occurs, the ESU is automatically turned off. (Courtesy Electroscope, Inc. Boulder, Colo.)

Electrode shields and monitors

A United States–based company (Electroscope Inc. Boulder, Colo.), has developed and released a system that helps to reduce further the chance of direct or capacitive coupling (Fig. 4-19). The reusable shield is passed over the shaft of the laparoscopic electrode prior to insertion into the peritoneal cavity. This shield protects against insulation failure and detects the presence of significant capacitance. Should an insulation break occur or when capacitance becomes threatening, the attached monitor automatically shuts down the generator. Unfortunately the shield enlarges the effective diameter of the electrode, making it necessary to use larger laparoscopic ports.

Safety considerations in electrosurgery

Electrosurgery has been rendered safe for use in surgical procedures provided there is adequate understanding and implementation of its principles, availability of modern electrosurgical generators, and appropriate education of medical and support staff. Nevertheless, to maintain this record of safety, a number of principles must be observed.

The equipment must meet acceptable standards. ESUs are ideally those with isolated circuits and return electrode monitors. Digital displays allow for more precise calculation of power output but are not essential for safety. The operating instruments should be in good working condition with intact insulation. The risk of capacitative coupling may be reduced if unipolar electrosurgery through the operative channel of an operating laparoscope is minimized or avoided. For bipolar coagulation, the use of a serial ammeter to aid in the determination of the end point of coagulation may reduce problems associated with inadequate treatment of the fallopian tube (pregnancy) or of severed blood vessels (bleeding).

Proper application of the dispersive electrode to an appropriate location is essential. Attachment over large body scars may hinder even transmission of the electrical current and consequently foster the development of thermal injury. The electrode should be applied as closely as possible to the operative site, without intervening potential sources of grounding such as ECG electrodes. For most gynecologic procedures an ideal site is the medial aspect of the thigh. To avoid accidental injury to either intra- or extraperitoneal structures from inadvertent activation of the active electrode, instruments not in use should be carefully placed in plastic holsters or detached from the electrosurgical generator.

Finally, care and prudence should be exercised when using electrosurgical instruments within the peritoneal cavity. The zone of significant thermal injury usually extends beyond the zone of visible injury and this must be kept in mind when operating in close proximity to vital structures such as bowel, bladder, ureter, and large and important blood vessels. It is equally important to impart the minimal amount of thermal injury (if any) necessary to accomplish the task at hand, even around nonvital structures, by using the ideal power output and the appropriate active electrodes.

LASER SURGERY

The term *laser* is an acronym for *l*ight *a*mplification by the *s*timulated *e*mission of *r*adiation. Lasers are sources of intense beams of radiant energy. The properties of this energy may be exploited in surgery, where the laser energy, or light, is directed to tissue. Here the light is converted to thermal and/or acoustic energy, resulting in vaporization and/or coagulation of tissue.

Lasers have been used with unique and spectacular effects in disciplines such as ophthalmology and dermatologic surgery. However, in the past few years many have come to question the value of laser assisted surgery within the pelvis and abdomen compared with similar procedures performed using mechanical means and/or other energy sources. This concern is largely related to the explosion in the cost of medical care combined with better understanding of electrical and other energy sources.

Despite these reservations, lasers do possess their own unique properties and, in well trained and experienced hands, are safe and effective surgical tools. Consequently, it behooves the aspiring endoscopist to become familiar with the principles of laser physics and applications in gynecologic surgery. The actual exposure the trainee will have to laser endoscopy will be dependent in part on the experience and bias of the teachers and in part on the available resources of the educational institution.

History of laser surgery

The history of lasers starts with Albert Einstein who, in 1917,[31] first proposed the theory of stimulated emission. This theory stated that a photon of energy could stimulate the emission of another identical photon from a suitably energized atom. Years later, V. A. Fabricant proposed that if the majority of a population of atoms was to be stimulated into a higher energy state *(population inversion),* a chain reaction would occur resulting in enhanced emission of identical photons. These seminal ideas were further developed over the ensuing two decades. The next significant development was the invention, reported in 1954, of a device that amplified microwave energy, the *maser* (microwave amplification by the stimulated emission of radiation), created by J. P. Gordon, H. J. Zeiger, and Charles H. Townes.[32] Over the next several years, maser principles were further developed by Townes, Arthur L. Schawlow, Nikolai G. Basov, and Aleksandr M. Prohhorov. However, it was Theodore H. Maiman who, in 1960, produced the first optical laser, a ruby laser.[33] Interestingly, for their efforts, Townes, Basov, and Prokhorov received the 1961 Nobel prize for physics. While Schawlow received a Nobel prize in 1981 (for laser spectroscopy), the inventor of the laser, Maiman, was never so honored.

The next few years saw the creation of a number of lasers that ultimately became useful for surgery. In 1964 both the CO_2 laser and the neodymium:yttrium-aluminum-garnet (Nd:YAG) lasers were reported.[34,35] Shortly after, in 1965, Bridges and colleagues developed the argon laser.[36] The first reported use of the CO_2 laser for reproductive surgery during laparotomy was by Bellina in 1974.[37] In 1979, Bruhat et al. described CO_2 laser applications under laparoscopic direction.[38] The KTP laser, essentially a modified Nd:YAG laser, was relatively recently reported in 1984 by Liu et al.[39] Other lasers, such as the tunable dye lasers,[40] are used in other specialties. It is quite possible that the future will present us with new devices with unique properties that may have value to the gynecologic surgeon.

Principles of laser physics

The laser's amplified beam of monochromatic light can be focused to deliver highly concentrated energy to the tissue that is then converted in the cell to thermal energy. It is through this thermal energy and its effect on the cell that the laser is able to vaporize or coagulate tissue. Understanding how the laser generates its beam of light is essential to effective and safe use of this energy source.

What is light? To understand the physics of a laser it is first necessary to understand light. To most people, light is a seemingly dichotomous entity, sometimes perceived as streams of energy and sometimes seen as color. In fact, light results from changes in the electronic structure of atoms or molecules as they absorb and emit energy. Consequently, light should be considered as the emission of packets of energy (photons) propagated in the form of electromagnetic waves, each of which has four variables; wavelength, amplitude, frequency, and velocity. In addition, the relationship of these waves to each other is described by the term *coherence*. For this discussion we will consider all such waves as light waves, regardless of their visibility or invisibility to the human eye.

The color of light is determined by the *wavelength* (λ), usually measured in nanometers (nm), which is the distance between two successive crests of the wave. Since lasers generally produce waves of only one wavelength, their light emissions are said to be *monochromatic*. Some lasers function in the visible spectrum while others produce waves in the near infrared or near ultraviolet spectrums and are therefore invisible to the human eye. *Amplitude* is a measure of the height of a wave and is an indication of its strength or power. *Frequency* (η) is the number of waves produced per second and is measured in Hertz. This property reflects the amount of energy in the wave. The *velocity* (c) of light is

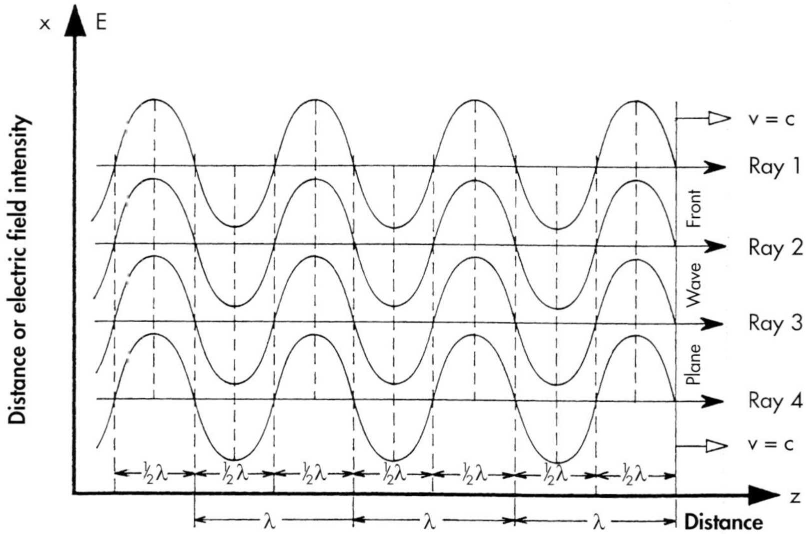

Fig. 4-20. Schematic representation of laser light. The four collimated, or parallel, rays emitting from a laser on the left (not shown) are also spatially coherent given the parallel peaks and valleys. Temporal coherence is evident in that all rays are similar in frequency, wavelength, and speed of propagation. Monochromacity is reflected by the fact that all the rays have the same wavelength. (From Fisher JC: In Shapshay SM, editor: Endoscopic laser surgery handbook. New York, 1987, Marcel Dekker.

essentially constant at 300,000 km (186,000 miles) per second. Because velocity is constant, any change in the frequency of the light results in an associated change in the wavelength. These properties are related by the equation

$$\lambda = c/\eta$$

When the waves of a beam of light are aligned so that their peaks and troughs match, they are said to be *spatially coherent.* This process has the effect of augmenting the amplitude of the beam, thereby increasing its brightness. If the waves are, in addition, of the same frequency, wavelength, and speed, they are *temporally coherent* (Fig. 4-20). Lasers produce coherent waves of light in the visible, near infrared or near ultraviolet spectrums.

Stimulated emission of light. Atoms and/or molecules may be manipulated to release monochromatic, coherent waves of light. An atom is a particle composed of a nucleus, made up of relatively large protons and neutrons, surrounded by a number of tiny orbiting electrons in discrete orbits of varying heights. The atom is said to be in its *ground state* if all its electrons are in their lowest possible orbits. Those electrons that are in higher orbits maintain that state because of their relatively higher level of energy (Fig. 4-21). An atom absorbs energy only in quantum, incremental amounts, by shifting some of its circulating electrons from lower to higher orbits. Such an atom is said to be in an excited state. When the electrons of such an excited atom inevitably drop back into their original orbits, an equal amount of energy is released. This discharge may occur spontaneously or it can be incited by collision with a photon of energy released by another atom, a process termed *stimulated emission.* In stimulated emission there result two photons of energy, each with the same frequency and directional characteristics of the stimulating photon (Fig. 4-21). If there are enough upper state or excited atoms or molecules in a given substance there can be a multiplying effect or chain reaction as each collision produces two identical photons of light.

Creating and maintaining an adequate number of excited atoms or molecules is critical to laser light production. What happens when energy is added to a population of atoms or molecules? Certainly, spontaneous emission of photons occurs. However, if the population is dominated by lower state atoms there will be more atoms available for absorption of spontaneously emitted photons than for stimulated release of energy. To achieve the amplification of light necessary for sustained stimulated emission, there must be a surplus of upper state atoms. The condition that occurs when the number of upper state atoms or molecules exceeds those in the lower state is referred to as *population inversion.* Successful achievement of population inversion depends upon careful selection of both the lasing medium and an appropriate supply of energy.

Various types of substances, including solids, liquids, and gases, can be used to create laser light. The medium that

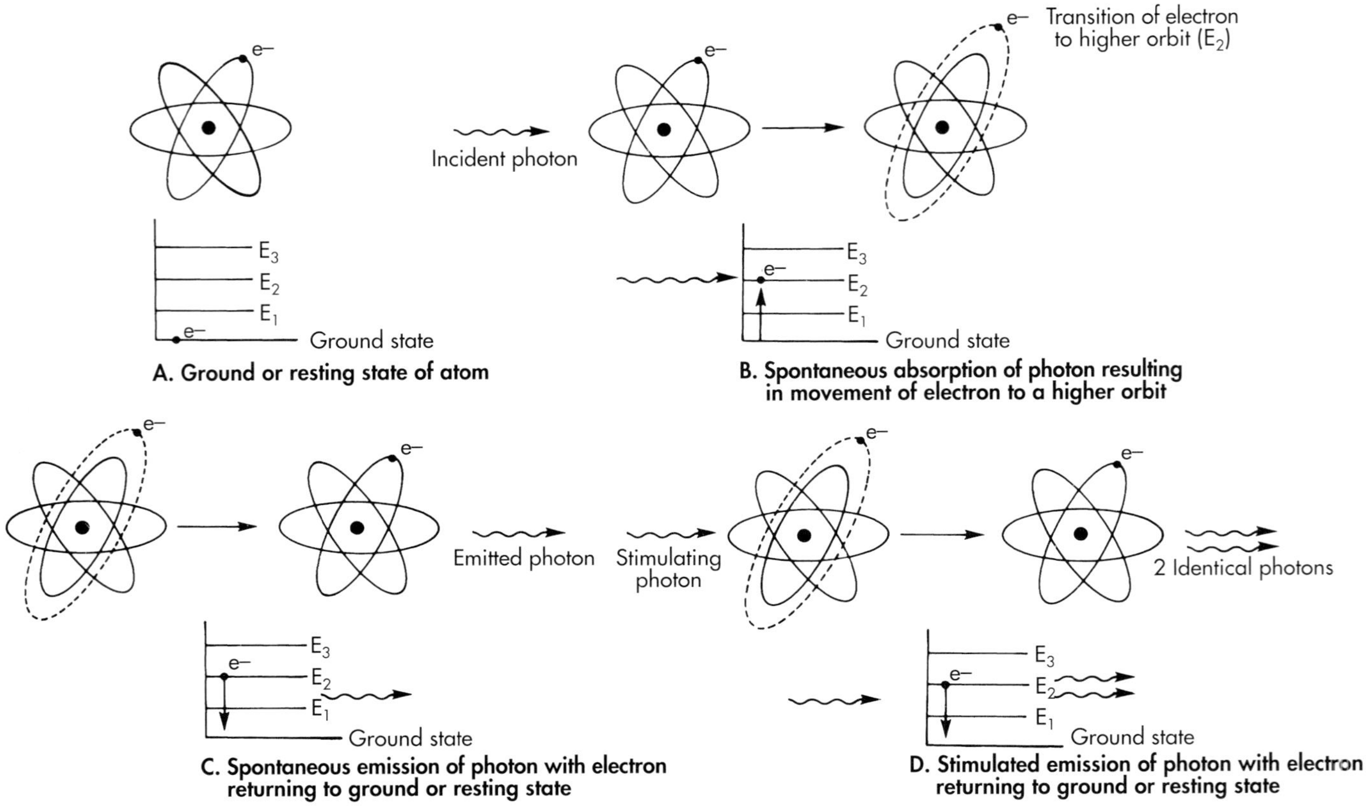

Fig. 4-21. Absorption and spontaneous and stimulated emission of radiation. (From Keye WR Jr: Laser surgery in gynecology and obstetrics. St Louis, 1990, Mosby–Year Book.)

is to be stimulated is placed into an long, cylindrical, resonant optical cavity with slightly concave mirrors perfectly aligned with each other at either end. Then the medium is energized by electrical or optical sources during a process called *pumping* that continues until population inversion occurs. The excited atoms spontaneously begin to emit photons of energy in random directions within the optical cavity. Those that are launched in parallel with the axis of the resonator are subsequently reflected back and forth by the mirrors. This allows photons moving parallel to the long axis of the cavity to dominate progressively as the chain reaction adds more and more photons of equal wavelength and frequency, all propagated along the same axis. This process serves to amplify the light. Eventually, sustained stimulated emission is attained, and a stream of photons is allowed to exit the optical cavity from one of the partially (from 1% to 20%) transmissive mirrors (Fig. 4-22).

Energy considerations. Energy is the capacity to do work. It is measured in Joules and may be expressed as a product of the frequency of the wave and a number called Planck's constant:

$$E = h \times \eta$$

where η = frequency and h = Planck's constant [6.63×10^{-34} joule seconds]. The energy (E) emitted by an excited atom during spontaneous or stimulated emission depends upon the difference between the energy in the upper state, or initial energy [E_1], and the ground state [E_2] of that atom ($\lambda = c/\eta$). In turn, these values will depend upon the particular atomic substance and its various electron orbits. The energy is emitted in multiples of the minimal difference between orbits or energy levels.

Other relationships can be deduced by substituting for frequency from the frequency, velocity, wavelength equation (Fig. 4-23). When this is done, energy can be reexpressed as follows:

$$E = h \times 1/\lambda$$

Consequently, energy can be seen to be inversely proportional to the wavelength and directly proportional to the frequency of the electromagnetic or light waves generated. Hence, the shorter the wavelength of laser light, the greater the amount of energy contained in the beam.

Power is measured in watts and is the amount of energy transferred or transformed per unit time. It may be expressed as follows:

$$1 \text{ W} = 1 \text{ joule/sec}$$

Properties of a laser beam. Laser light, by its nature, possesses a number of unique properties (see box on p. 47).

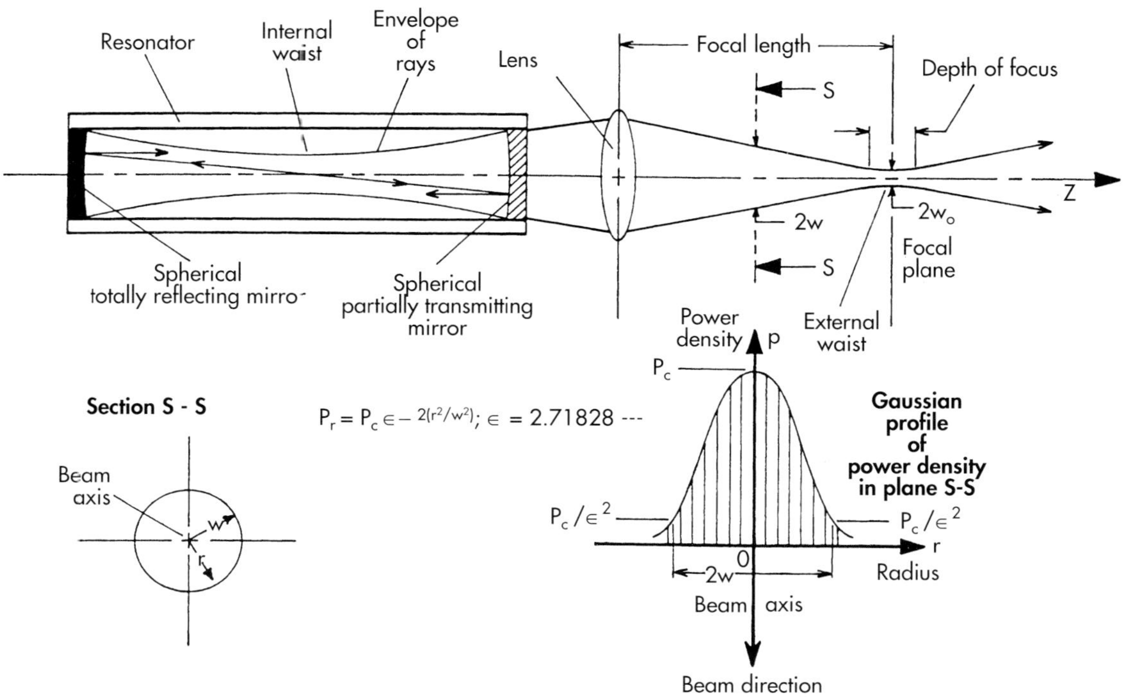

Fig. 4-22. Schematic representation of a laser with a focusing lens emitting a gaussian beam. The actual ratio between length and diameter of the resonator is much greater that depicted in this representation. (From Fisher JC. In Shapshay SM, editor: Endoscopic laser surgery handbook. New York, 1987, Marcel Dekker.)

$$\text{Wavelength } (\lambda) = \frac{\text{Velocity of light (c)}}{\text{Frequency } (\eta)}$$

$$\eta = c/\lambda$$

$$\text{Energy (E)} = h \times \eta \quad \text{(h = Planck's constant } 6.63 \times 10^{-34} \text{ Joule seconds)}$$

$$\text{Power density} = \frac{\text{Power (P watts)}}{\text{Area (A cm}^2\text{)}}$$

$$= \frac{110\text{ P}}{\text{d (mm)}^2} \quad \text{watts/cm}^2$$

Fig. 4-23. Summary of laser energy equations.

Properties of the laser beam

Coherence of light beam (peaks and troughs match)
Waves are parallel to each other (collimated)
Monochromatic
High degree of luminosity (brightness)
Intensity is easily varied (power density and TEM)
Rate of energy delivery to tissue (fluence) easily varied

The light must be spatially and temporally *coherent.* The waves are also *collimated* or parallel to each other. This property is what gives laser light its unique directionality, allowing for transmission over relatively long distances with little loss of energy. Because the laser beam is *monochromatic* the energy from a particular laser beam has a uniform effect on the target tissue. Finally, laser light waves have a high amplitude, giving the beam a high degree of *luminosity.* It is the brightest existing source of light (see Fig. 4-20).

The maximal power (P) setting for most surgical lasers ranges from 20 to 100 watts at the exit point of the optical cavity. Using an interposed lens, the beam may be focused or defocused at a given spot, thereby varying its intensity. The magnitude of power concentration at the tissue is referred to as the power density (PD), analogous to that found in electrosurgery but conceptually more easy to measure. It may be expressed as the power of the incident beam in watts

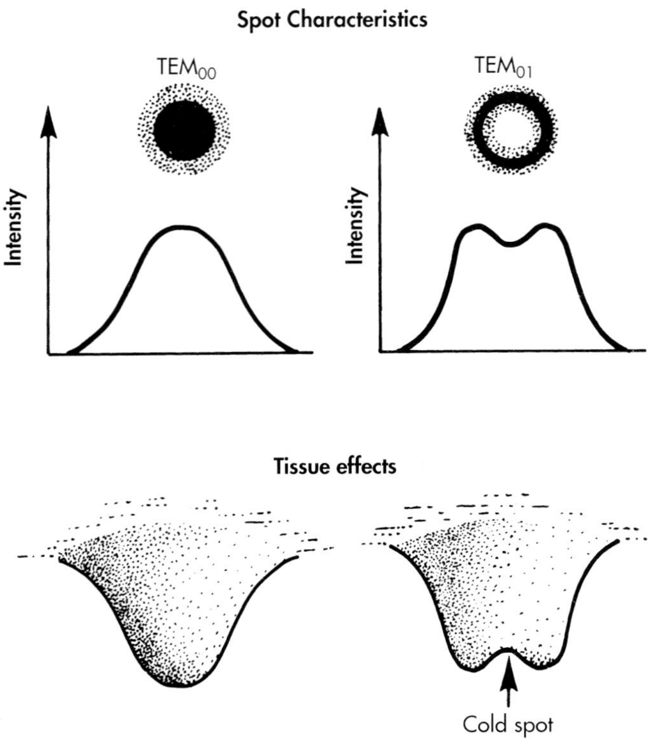

Fig. 4-24. Transverse electromagnetic mode *(TEM)*—its effect on the crater shape in tissue. (From Keye WR Jr: Laser surgery in gynecology and obstetrics. St Louis, 1990, Mosby-Year Book.)

divided by its area (A) in square centimeters or spot size (PD = P/A).

Another important property of the beam is the *transverse electromagnetic mode* (TEM) which reflects the variance in power density as perceived by cross-sectional analysis of the laser spot (Fig. 4-24). This property helps to determine the interaction of the beam with the target tissue and is usually denoted by two numeric subscripts—TEM_{mm}. The most common variety is the TEM_{00}, or gaussian mode, where the power density is greatest at the center, decreasing toward the periphery. This mode allows for the greatest concentration of energy within the smallest spot size. The TEM_{01} mode is the inverse—a "doughnut" shape with a ring of high-power density surrounded by less intense zones in the center and at the perimeter.

The last feature of laser beams to discuss is the capability of varying the rate at which energy is delivered to tissue, a property known as *fluence*. Laser beams with high fluence deliver an equal amount of energy to tissue in a shorter time than do those with low fluence (Fig. 4-25). A given beam can have its fluence significantly raised if the beam is interrupted while simultaneously raising the power delivered with each pulse of light. Because of the more rapid delivery of energy with highly fluent beams, there is less opportunity for heat conduction and consequent collateral thermal damage to adjacent tissue. The processes of superpulsing and ultrapulsing create examples of highly fluent laser beams.

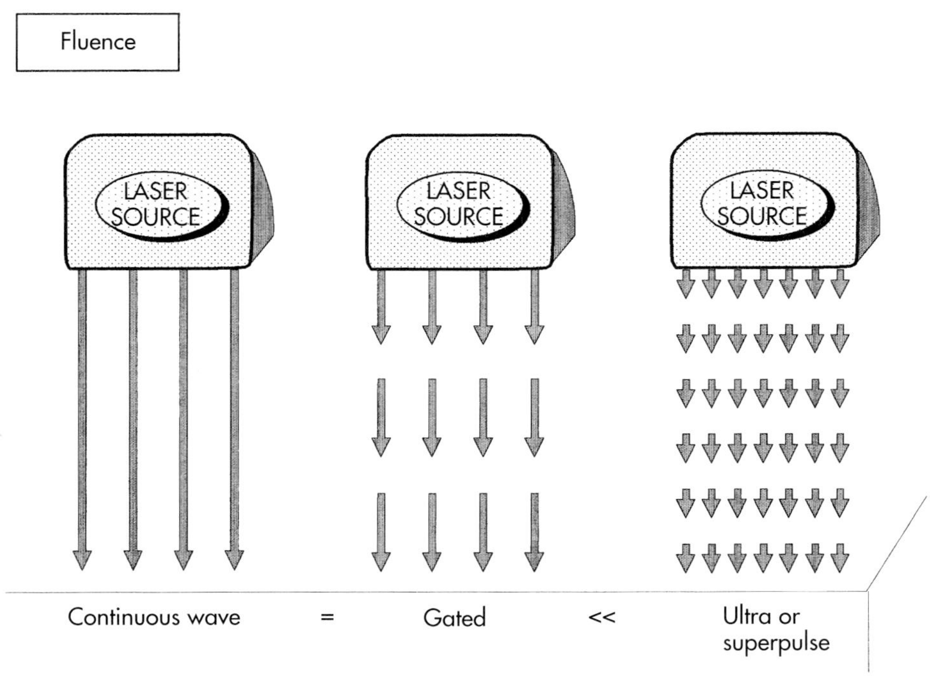

Fig. 4-25. Highly fluent outputs result in equal or greater amounts of energy delivery to tissue in a lesser period of time.

Tissue effects of laser surgery

When an incident laser beam strikes tissue, one or a combination of four interactions may occur: (1) reflection, (2) transmission, (3) scatter, and (4) absorption. When total reflection or transmission occur, there is no thermal effect on tissue. To create one or both of the desired tissue effects of vaporization and coagulation, absorption must occur, with subsequent conversion of the light energy into thermal energy. When scatter occurs, there may be an attenuated thermal effect dependent upon the amount of tissue absorption of the fragmented beam.

Effect on cells and tissue. When there is sufficient absorption of large amounts of the energy, there is rapid elevation of the intracellular temperature to more than 100° C. For example, in a cell with a high water content, capable of absorbing CO_2 laser light, the application of adequate power causes the water to turn instantly to steam, resulting in rapid cellular expansion and subsequent explosive vaporization. This is an event that is identical to electrosurgical vaporization except that a different source of electromagnetic energy is converted to heat. In either event, moving the energy source in a linear fashion results in linear vaporization, or cutting.

When the amount of light energy absorbed by the cell in a given period is reduced, dehydration of the cellular water and coagulation of the contained protein results. The deep coagulation achieved with laser energy is, at the cellular and tissue level, identical to the desiccation and white coagulation created by electrosurgical technique. The superficial coagulation and char formation created by the electrosurgical process of fulguration can also be replicated by prolonged exposure to low-power density laser beams.

Unlike electrosurgical energy, some laser wavelengths may be used to cut following coagulation of the tissue. Nd:YAG laser light propagated through a sapphire-tipped quartz fiber is an example. This system exerts at least some of its cutting action through the passive but focused application of heat from the sapphire tip. Paradoxically, unlike radiofrequency electrosurgery, this is a form of cautery.

Control of tissue effects. While there are a number of factors that affect tissue absorbance of laser light, the most important include (1) the power density and TEM of the beam, (2) the wavelength of the light, (3) the absorbance characteristics of the tissue, (4) the time of tissue exposure, and (5) the incident angle of the beam (see box above right). The importance and/or control of each of these variables will be discussed.

Power density and TEM. Safe and effective laser surgery can be performed only when the clinician has a sound understanding of the concept of power density and its control. The concepts of energy, power, and power density (PD) were briefly discussed above.

For purposes of this discussion PD may be defined as the average amount of radiant power striking the tissue per unit area of the tissue "illuminated" by the laser light. The amount of energy made available to a given volume of tissue for conversion to thermal energy is largely determined by the power density (PD).

Factors influencing effects of laser surgery on tissue

Power density and TEM of beam
Wavelength of light
Absorbance characteristics of tissue
Exposure time of tissue
Incident angle of beam

We previously learned that the PD of a laser beam in watts/cm^2 is theoretically calculated as the P in watts divided by the area (A) of the beam in square centimeters:

$$\text{PD watts/cm}^2 = \text{P watts / cm}^2$$

This equation expresses the fact that at a constant power, the power density is reduced exponentially as the diameter of the beam is increased. Conversely, a smaller beam area allows the creation of significantly higher power density. However, a number of factors complicate the calculation of the exact power density of the beam as it strikes the tissue. One of these is the TEM. Initially, we will consider a beam with a TEM_{00} or gaussian type distribution.

Classically, calculation of the area of a circular spot would be use the formula $A = \pi r^2$. However, clinically, spot sizes are set and measured according to their diameter, making the use of radius impractical. In addition, the diameters are measured in millimeters, not centimeters. Consequently the equation should be rewritten, first considering that the radius is half the diameter [$r = d/2$]. Therefore the area of the spot may be re-expressed:

$$\pi r^2 = \pi(d/2)^2 = \pi\ d^2/2^2 = \pi d^2/4$$

Substitution into the equation would result in:

$$\text{PD in watts/cm}^2 = \text{P watts}/\pi d_{cm}{}^2/4 \text{ or } 4P/\pi d \text{ watts/cm}^2$$

Now, the equation must be rewritten to allow the calculation of PD to be made in watts/cm^2 using the spot diameter in millimeters. Since 1 mm is 0.1 centimeter, 1 mm^2 is 0.01 or 1/100 cm^2. Consequently if the equation is to be expressed in watts/cm^2 but the diameter is expressed in millimeters, the equation must be divided by 0.01, or more easily, multiplied by 100. Now the equation may be expressed as follows:

$$\begin{aligned} PD = 100 \times 4P/\pi d^2 &= 400P/\pi d^2 \\ &= 127.3241\ (\text{P watts})/(d_{mm})^2 \text{ watts/cm}^2 \end{aligned}$$

The final modification of the calculation relates to the amount of power within the spot in a TEM_{00} beam. The power is maximal on the axis of the beam but falls gradually to zero at an infinite distance from that axis (Fig. 4-26).

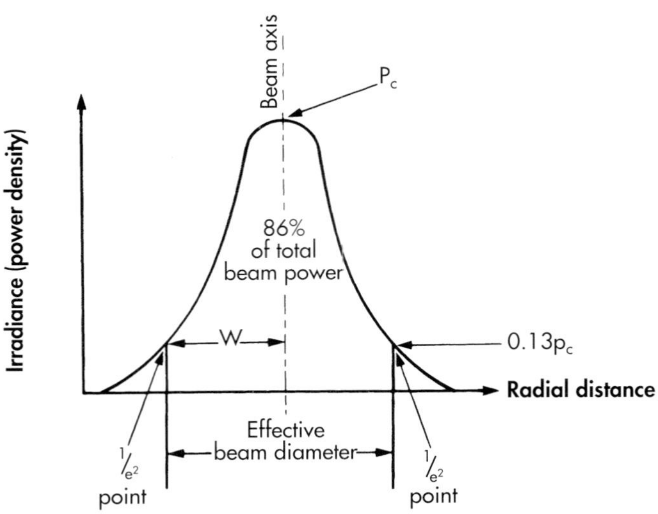

Fig. 4-26. Effective diameter of a gaussian beam. (From Wright VC, Riopelle MA: Gynecologic laser surgery: a practical handbook. Houston, 1982, Biomedical Communications.)

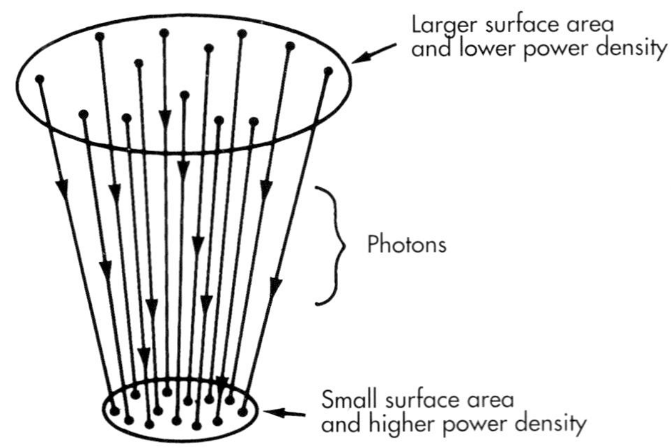

Fig. 4-27. Power density—schematic representation. (From Keye WR Jr: Laser surgery in gynecology and obstetrics. St Louis, 1990, Mosby-Year Book.)

This means that less than 100% of the beam's power is transferred to tissue within a fixed diameter. Consequently we refer to an effective diameter (d_e) of the beam within which 86.35% of the beam's power is concentrated in the gaussian mode. Calculating 86.35% of 127.3241 results in 109.944, or approximately 110. The final equation may be expressed as follows:

$$\text{PD watts/cm}^2 = \frac{110\ (\text{P watts})}{(d_e \text{ in millimeters})^2}$$

The power density is the most important calculation for the surgeons as they will frequently wish to make alterations during the performance of a case. The power density may be controlled by adjusting either the spot size or the power output of the laser. Doubling the beam diameter reduces the power density by ¼ while halving the spot diameter will increase the power density by a factor of four (Fig. 4-27).

By pulsing the energy source while simultaneously elevating the power per pulse (superpulse, ultrapulse), power density will also increase. The resulting increased fluence will correspondingly decrease the amount of residual thermal injury.

Remember that all of the calculations and relationships derived above were based on a beam with the gaussian distribution found in virtually all CO_2 laser systems. When any laser light is propagated down most fiber or hollow waveguides the Gaussian distribution is lost, a factor that will be discussed under endoscopic applications.

Wavelength and tissue absorbance. The optimal laser choice depends upon the characteristics of the tissue and the desired surgical effect—vaporization or coagulation. In most instances, laser energy must be absorbed by molecules and converted to thermal energy in order to create the desired surgical result. Because each laser has a unique wavelength, the ideal target substance will vary. Since water is the predominant molecule found in the tissues encountered by gynecologists, wavelengths readily absorbed by water are most efficiently and quickly converted to thermal energy. Carbon dioxide laser wavelengths (10,600 nm) are optimally absorbed by cells that contain 80% to 90% water, making them effective at cutting most of the tissues encountered in gynecology. However, if CO_2 laser energy is applied to already desiccated tissue the effect is attenuated resulting in diffuse, rather than localized, heating of the tissue.

The 1064 nm Nd:YAG laser light is rather poorly absorbed by water, a feature that fosters a deeper coagulating effect in tissue with high water content. On the other hand, light from Nd:YAG devices is selectively absorbed by proteins and red or black pigmented molecules. The 532 nm potassium-titanyl-phosphate (KTP) laser is, interestingly, a better cutting tool. The visible green KTP laser light is developed by using KTP crystals to double the frequency of the invisible near infrared Nd:YAG laser beam. Consequently, both these lasers may be contained within one machine, allowing the surgeon to change from one to the other with a switch.

The wavelength-dependent site-specific absorption of lasers operating in the visible and near infrared electromagnetic spectrum is most effectively exploited in ophthalmologic surgery. For example, the blue-green argon beam is easily transmitted through the cornea, lens, and vitreous but is absorbed by the retina, a feature useful for photocoagulation. Other lasers use similar properties for the removal of tattoos and birthmarks. Such properties may well have future importance in the treatment of gynecologic and other tumors utilizing the selective uptake of laser light activated dye. However, currently, in gynecology most lasers in the visible category are used to manifest a thermal effect.

Tissue exposure time. If the laser's wavelength and power density are kept constant, the zone of vaporization and/or coagulation of a given tissue varies directly with exposure time. This is because more laser energy will be available for transformation to thermal energy.

Controlling exposure time is an important concept in laser surgery. Because thermal conduction to adjacent tissue is reduced with shortened exposure time, there will be less coagulation. This will be desirable if a pure cutting effect is required but counterproductive if hemostasis is necessary. Therefore, the appropriate balance between hemostasis and vaporization must be considered.

In gynecology, vaporization and cutting are most efficiently accomplished with the CO_2 laser held away from the tissue, focusing the beam to the smallest possible diameter, usually about 0.1 mm. By using superpulsed or ultrapulsed modes, thereby making the beam more fluent, residual thermal tissue injury is held to a minimum. Conversely, a relatively defocused beam directed at tissue for a longer time will create superficial coagulation.

Incident angle of the beam. With any laser, the maximal absorption and power density occurs with the beam incident at right angles to the plane of the tissue. As the incident angle becomes more obtuse, there is more reflection of the light and a decreased power density secondary to the increased spot size. Consequently, for maximal absorption with the smallest spot size, the surgeon must keep the incident laser beam as close as possible to a 90-degree angle with the tissue.

Types of surgical lasers

Because much of the nature of the beam created by a laser is unique to the substance contained in the resonant optical cavity, there are a number of devices available to the surgeon, each with their own special properties, risks, applications, and cost of acquisition.

CO_2 laser. The CO_2 laser is the one most commonly used for gynecologic procedures. This is because of its ability to vaporize precisely or cut with limited thermal injury provided the tissue has 80% to 90% water content. The depth of the injury depends upon many of the variables described above but, with small spot size, adequate power, and limited time on tissue it is usually below 100 μ.[41-43] With the use of superpulsed and ultrapulsed modes the depth of thermal coagulation is even less.[41,44,45] Defocusing of the instrument allows for a superficial coagulating/carbonization effect similar to electrosurgical fulguration.

For most modern CO_2 lasers, the gas is contained in a sealed tube and excited by a radiofrequency electrical discharge. Because the wavelength of a CO_2 laser cannot be propagated via conventional quartz fibers, an articulated arm is generally used to deliver the beam to the operative site (Fig. 4-28). Each articulated joint contains a mirror that must maintain the beam centered, allowing it to be directed to the center of the next mirror in the series. Once the beam has been delivered to the end of the articulating arm, it may be focused by the interposition of a suitable system of lenses. The light is finally delivered to tissue by a hand-held probe, a mirrored micromanipulator, or, in laparoscopy, by a rigid or flexible hollow waveguide.* The surgery is performed in a noncontact fashion.

All lasers are capable of providing a continuous wave (CW) of light. For most CO_2 lasers, the beam can be modulated by "gating" or interrupting the output, allowing the energy to strike the tissue repeatedly for varying durations of time, usually measured in hundredths to tenths of a second. In this format, the wattage of the output does not vary. In the *superpulse* and *ultrapulse* modes, the duration of the pulses is extremely short but the pulse wattage is very high (see Fig. 4-25). For example, superpulsed lasers may provide pulses of 250 to 500 watts from 300 to 1000 times per second. Lasers equipped to provide ultrapulse may deliver up to 100,000 or more watts/cm^2 per pulse. While this may seem like a large amount of energy, the pulse duration is so short that the total tissue exposure in Joules remains very low. Consequently, these technologies, by creating high fluence, allow for tissue vaporization with reduced thermal trauma to the residual tissue.

Nd:YAG, KTP and argon lasers. The shorter wavelength of these lasers allows them to be propagated along flexible optical fibers. This property allows the laser light to be directed into locations otherwise unreachable with the CO_2 laser. The site-specific absorption characteristics of these lasers has been discussed above.

KTP laser light is created via crystals that are used to double the frequency of the 1064 nm Neodymium:Yttrium-Aluminum-Garnet (Nd:YAG) beam resulting in the 532 nm wavelength green-colored KTP output. Consequently these types of laser output are usually found in the same machine. KTP lasers are relatively efficient cutting tools, particularly in a pulsed mode and provided that there is adequate power. Nd-YAG lasers are intrinsically crude vaporization tools but good deep coagulating instruments because the wavelength is poorly absorbed by water. These tissue effects are generated with a noncontact technique, for touching the tissue with a bare fiber can result in so much temperature elevation that melting of the fiber's tip can occur. However, if the fiber is fitted with a sapphire tip, the laser energy, focused and converted to heat, can be used to create a relatively good cutting effect. Tips that allow greater contact with tissue result in lower temperatures and a greater coagulative effect. Paradoxically, these effects are classical examples of cautery, the passive transfer of thermal energy.

Argon lasers are composed of light beams with a com-

*More recently, specially designed, narrow and flexible conducting tubes have been developed, capable of conduction of CO_2 laser energy without significant loss of power.

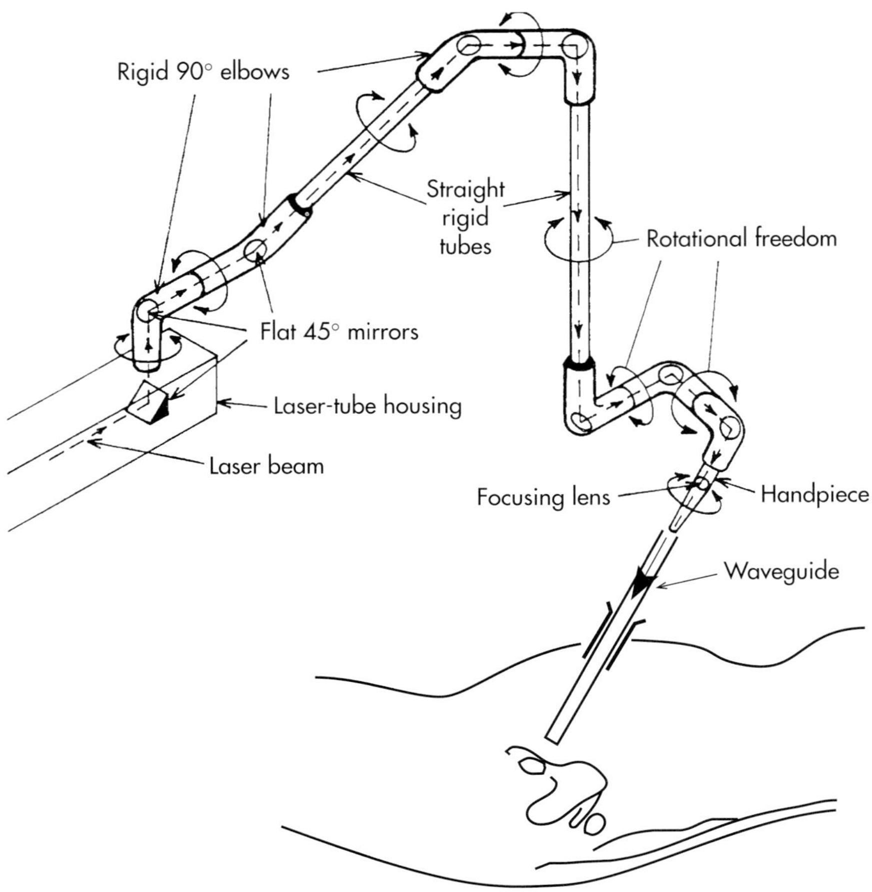

Fig. 4-28. Delivery of CO_2 energy. Typical articulated arm used to bring the laser energy to the operative field. For laparoscopy, the beam is directed into the peritoneal cavity via a wave guide. (From Fisher JC. In Shapshay SM, editor: Endoscopic laser surgery handbook. New York, 1987, Marcel Dekker.)

bination of wavelengths (488 to 514 nm). This type of laser energy seems to be more effective when used as an ablation tool directed at darkly pigmented targets.

Other laser and fiber types. A number of other laser types have surgical applications, however none of these have been widely introduced to gynecology. The "Fibertome" laser, produced by Dornier Medical Systems, utilizes Nd:YAG light and a fiber that contains an optoelectronic control system that allows temperature-controlled cutting with a bare fiber. The temperature-sensitive sensor in the fiber tip reduces the power to a level below that which causes melting of the fiber. Other fibers have been developed that may have potential in coagulating preset volumes of tissue based upon on-line monitoring of NADH concentrations.[46] Other new instruments include the Holmium:YAG laser, the Erbium:YAG device, and the CO laser, all with different tissue effects, advantages, and disadvantages. Their potential for use in clinical medicine is currently under evaluation.

Laparoscopic applications of lasers

During the 1980s, promise afforded by new technology, combined with the fear and ignorance of electrical energy, drove many to the near exclusive use of laser energy for endoscopic surgery. In the 1990s the high acquisition and operations costs associated with surgical lasers began to temper the enthusiasm. This situation, combined with a greater understanding of the surgical applications of electricity and data suggesting that laser energy was no more effective than electrical energy, has caused many surgeons to return to the less costly energy source. Nevertheless, many continue to use lasers effectively, and future developments may further exploit their unique properties. What follows is only a brief introduction to the laparoscopic applications of laser energy. Procedure-specific applications are detailed elsewhere in this text.

The laparoscope may be used to direct lasers in the performance of vaporization, cutting, excision, or coagulation of tissue. As described above, different lasers, used in differing ways in various environments, will be more or less suited to the task at hand.

One of the common problems encountered when either electrical or laser energy is applied laparoscopically is the evacuation of smoke. A number of methods may be used alone or in combination to achieve this task. The most common is the use of a smoke evacuation system in combination with the high-flow insufflation of CO_2 gas. The simplest method is to use periodic venting, although suction probes placed near the site are more effective and, perhaps, safer. There also exist closed systems that contain an in-line smoke filtration device (Richard Wolf Medical Instruments Corp, Rosemont, Ill.).

CO_2 laser. The CO_2 laser is most effective when used as a cutting tool, by vaporizing tissue with a relatively small amount of thermal injury. If defocused and used with a relatively low-power density, the laser can be used to obtain hemostasis of capillary ooze and bleeding from small arterioles. However, since the water content of blood absorbs the CO_2 laser energy this effect is limited in the face of significant bleeding.

Using a coupling lens, CO_2 laser energy can be focused into the peritoneal cavity through a hollow probe passed through the instrument channel of an operating laparoscope or an ancillary puncture site. As the energy is invisible, it is directed using an aligned helium-neon laser aiming beam. Because the beam must traverse the relatively long length of the probe (approximately 30 cm), the focal length is necessarily long. This feature limits the ability to focus the beam to around 1 mm and lengthens the depth of focus. A long depth of focus creates a situation in which tissue beyond the site of surgery is at risk for injury, a circumstance that requires care, concentration, and, on occasion, the use of an absorptive or dispersive backstop. Older coupling devices required that the surgeon manipulate the direction of the beam with a joystick. However, the newer couplers produce an aligned beam without such a device.

The coupled systems deliver a coherent laser beam with a TEM_{00} or gaussian mode. This allows precise cutting at a distance, but the long focal length limits the ability to reduce power density by defocussing with simple back and forth movement of the probe.

Another method of delivering CO_2 laser energy is through rigid hollow waveguides. These instruments bounce the beam down the narrow inner channel (<1 mm diameter) of the guide. The nature of such a method of propagation is that energy and coherence are, to some extent, lost. Consequently the spot lacks the gaussian mode of the spot, a factor that limits the cutting effectiveness of the beam at given power outputs. In addition, because of the relative lack of coherence, the greatest power density for a given output exists very near the tip of the probe. Defocusing may therefore be achieved by pulling the device back from the target.

Flexible, hollow waveguides have historically delivered more promise than performance, since their ability to transmit CO_2 laser light is generally increasingly limited as the guide is progressively flexed. However, the guides continue to improve and may soon find clinical applicability.[47]

Nd:YAG, KTP, and argon lasers. As previously described, the laser light created by these devices can be propagated along optical fibers, usually made of quartz. In gynecologic endoscopy, the most commonly employed fibers are 600 μm in diameter, although 200 μm and 100 μm fibers are also available. The fibers may be passed through narrow channels in either operating laparoscopes or ancillary cannulas, and the lack of coupling devices and articulated arms generally makes them more easy to use than CO_2 lasers. The divergent nature of the beams precludes the need for a backstop. In addition, the colored lasers may be used through irrigation solutions. However, the thermal injury associated with these lasers is greater than that for either properly applied CO_2 laser or monopolar electrosurgical energy, making their use on vital structures inadvisable. The use of sapphire-tipped fibers as contact cutting devices may make for effective cutting action with relatively reduced collateral thermal effect.

KTP and argon lasers have similar wavelengths but somewhat different effects on tissue. The KTP laser is more effective as a cutting instrument while the argon laser is limited in this role, being more effective at tissue coagulation. With each, the blue-green beam is easily seen, obviating the need for an aiming beam. There is no need for flowing gases or focusing devices. The best tissue targets are vascular lesions or those rich in hemoglobin or hemosiderin.

There are a number of disadvantages to the argon and KTP lasers. Eye filters are needed, there is possible breakage of the fibers, and special water cooling and electrical connections are required. In addition, the cost of each of these lasers is high relative to the CO_2 laser and, especially, electrosurgery.

Nd:YAG laser light is less readily absorbed by hemoglobin and hemosiderin-rich tissue than is that from the argon or KTP laser. With the advent of sapphire tips, the YAG laser can be used safely in the peritoneal cavity. However, because most of these devices are air cooled, they present at least a theoretical risk of air embolization. Additionally, the tips of the YAG laser remain hot for several seconds after turning the laser off. Care must be exercised to avoid inadvertent contact with tissue when the laser is initially disengaged to allow for sufficient cooling of the sapphire tip.

Safety considerations and complications in laser surgery

The safety of the patient and the operating team is of paramount importance. If the laser is in the visible or near infrared spectrum the windows in the operating room must be covered. Operating rooms must be labelled on the out-ide door(s) indicating that a laser procedure is in progress. Protective eye wear should be available outside the door of the operating theater for use by individuals entering the room. All personnel participating in, or watching, the procedure must wear safety goggles or appropriate protective eye wear. The patient's eyes must also be properly protected. The optical density for protective eye wear must be appropriate for the wavelength of laser employed.

The production of laser plume has been associated with respiratory complications and has been implicated as a possible source of mutagenicity. While approximately 75% of the solid particulate matter in laser plume has a diameter less than 1μ, virtually all is larger than 0.1μ. When inhaled, this small particulate matter is capable of traveling directly to the furthest reaches of the tracheopulmonary system and being deposited in individual alveoli. To eliminate this plume, a suction device is necessary, preferably with a filter capable of extracting particles as small as 0.1μ. Although CO_2 laser laparoscopy is associated with more particulate formation than that resulting from the use of argon, Nd:YAG, or KTP lasers, plume is generated by the latter three wavelengths and adequate smoke evacuation systems are necessary.

There are a number of complications that are uniquely associated with the use of laser energy, some of which have been previously alluded to.

As is the case with other energy sources, inadvertent operation of the laser may result in injury to the patient or operating room personnel. Unique to lasers is the ability of the coherent and collimated light to reflect from the shiny surfaces of polished instruments and equipment, causing injury within or remote from the surgical field. For example, within the peritoneal cavity, the use of such instruments may reflect CO_2 laser light, causing intestinal burns. If fired extraperitoneally, the same laser can cause injury to the water-containing cells of the cornea or sclera. KTP, argon, and Nd:YAG lasers, because of their ability to be propagated along glass, can, even at laparoscopy, cause injury to the retina of the operating surgeon, necessitating the use of special filters and/or safety glasses. Because such light has the potential to scatter elsewhere in the room, the tinted safety goggles should be worn by the patient and staff.

Fire or explosion may result from the heating of flammable materials or gas. Consequently, sponges and drapes used in or near the operative field should either be fire resistant or be kept moist. It is also important to avoid the use of alcohol-based antiseptic solutions.

The fact that the laser is utilized within the peritoneal cavity reduces the opportunity for some of these complications but does not eliminate their occurrence. Most can be minimized or eliminated with appropriate training, care, and the establishment of laser safety protocols.

OTHER ENERGY SOURCES

While electrical and laser energy are the most commonly employed energy sources used in endoscopically directed gynecologic procedures, inventors and investigators are evaluating the use of other energy sources. No doubt, some of these will be found valuable for at least some applications.

Harmonic scalpel

The energy produced by ultrasonic transducers may be exploited for the purposes of cutting, coagulation, or emulsification of tissue. One of the devices that has been developed and marketed for laparoscopically directed use is the harmonic scalpel (Ultracision Inc., Smithfield, RI). The hand-held device is a probe activated by ultrasonic transducers in the handle that longitudinally vibrate the shaft at 55 kHz (Fig. 4-29, *A*). This back and forth motion, with an excursion of up to 80 μ, creates localized tissue effects that may result in cutting and/or coagulation, depending upon the configuration and/or orientation of the probe tip.

Coagulation apparently results from mechanical denaturation of protein. It is thought that the mechanical energy from the vibrating probe breaks protein hydrogen bonds, resulting in a sticky coagulum. While some of the mechanical energy is converted to heat, there seems to be less than that associated with other energy sources.

Cutting probably results from at least two mechanisms. The first is the actual cutting action that results when a relatively sharp blade vibrates on tissue at 55,000 times/second. This is the mechanism dominant when cutting tissue with high-protein density such as fascia, skin, and muscle. The second mechanism is postulated to be a process of fragmentation where cells are disrupted following the creation of a low-pressure zone at the tip of the vibrating probe via a process termed *cavitation*. The reduced local atmospheric pressure caused by the vibrating tip of the probe may be compared with that created in front of a propellor in water or air. The drop in pressure causes intracellular water to turn from liquid to gas at 37° C, resulting in the same cellular explosion that occurs secondary to electrosurgical or laser energy. This mechanism of cutting is thought to be dominant when cutting low-protein density tissue such as liver parenchyma and fat.

Unfortunately there is a paucity of published studies evaluating the characteristics of tissue incisions created by the harmonic scalpel. One study from the dermatology literature demonstrated thermal injury in skin lesions to be less than that incurred by electrosurgery and the CO_2 laser. In this study tissue healing was slower than with a conventional scalpel.[48]

For laparoscopic surgery the harmonic scalpel is manufactured as a 30 cm probe in both 5 and 10 mm diameters. A variety of tips may be used to vary the tissue effect (Fig 4-29, *B* and *C*). The blunt tip provides superfi-

A 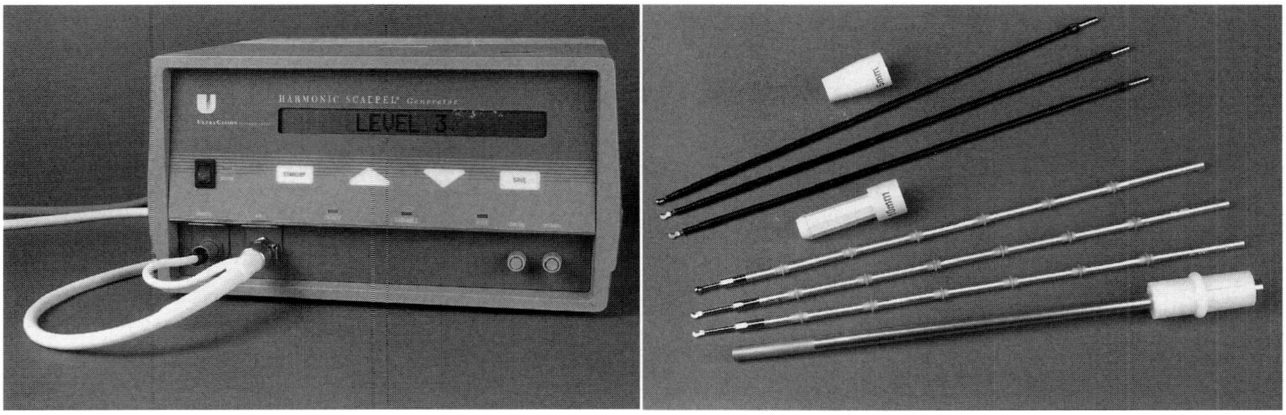 B

Fig. 4-29. A, The harmonic scalpel. **B,** laparoscopic probes.

cial coagulation of large bleeding areas that otherwise would be the target of electrosurgical fulguration. The knife-tipped probes are used for cutting or, if turned on their side, may be employed for coaptive coagulation of blood vessels up to 3 mm in diameter. More recently the company has applied the same energy to a set of shears, designed to simultaneously cut and coagulate tissue. All of the probes are connected to an ultrasonic handle that, in turn, is linked to the base unit. The base unit is plugged into a standard wall 110 volt output. A pedal footswitch is used to activate the transducers contained in the handle.

A number of aspects of operating with the harmonic scalpel require adjustment of surgical technique. The tissue must be stabilized to allow the vibrating probe to manifest its localized affect. A good example is the case of filmy adhesions which vibrate like a loose guitar string unless stabilized by retractors. On the other hand, more inherently stabile tissue like the uterus or peritoneum may be readily incised with the harmonic scalpel. Blood vessels must be coapted prior to coagulation by either compressing them against adjacent tissue or lifting them with the probe tip. Early experience with the ultrasonic shears suggests that problems with tissue stabilization may be largely solved.

Clearly the devices have a number of advantages over electrosurgery. There is no smoke or plume produced, and the energy seems to remain localized to the site of application. However there is currently much more flexibility with laser and electrosurgical techniques. Further study of thermal injury following laparoscopically directed application of the device will be necessary. Consequently, it remains to be seen if surgeons and the manufacturer can overcome some of the inherent drawbacks encountered in this intriguing method of delivering energy to tissue.

Endocoagulation

In 1966, Professor Kurt Semm, from Kiel, Germany, reported his development of a new method of applying thermal energy to tissue.[49] This technique, called endocoagulation, passes electrical current through a teflon-coated probe, heating the tip to temperatures that reach up to 120° C. Coagulation of the tissue is by the direct application of the heat to tissue—a form of cautery. It differs from electrosurgery because there is no current actually traversing the patient's tissue. Endocoagulation is limited because of its inability to cut tissue and because the depth of thermal injury is limited to only the superficial layers.

The Kiel group has reported on the applications of *cautery* when used under laparoscopic guidance.[50,51] However this information does not reflect relative efficacy of the method.

Laparoscopic endocoagulation probes and endocoagulation generators are available from a number of manufacturers (Karl Storz, America Inc., Culver City, Calif.; Wisap, Munchen, Germany).

REFERENCES

1. Major, RH: History of medicine, vol I and II, Springfield, Ill., 1954, Charles C Thomas.
2. Licht SH: The history of therapeutic heat. In Licht SH, editor: Therapeutic heat and cold, ed 2, New Haven, Conn., 1965, Elizabeth Licht publications.
3. Geddes LA, Silva LF, DeWitt DP, Pearce JA: What's new in electrosurgical instrumentation? Medical Instrumentation, 1977.
4. Stillings D: John Wesley: electrotherapist. *Medical Instrument* 8:66-7, 1974.
5. Bettman RB, Crohn NN. Diathermy in the production of deep temperature. *JAMA* 88:532-7, 1927.
6. Kelly HA, Ward GE: Electrosurgery, Philadelphia, 1932, W.B. Saunders.
7. Doyen E: Sur la destruction des tumeurs cancereuses accessibles: par la methode de la voltaisation bipolaire et de l'electro-coagulation thermique. *Arch d'Elect Physiother Cancer* 17:791-5, 1909.
8. Pearce JA: Electrosurgery, New York, 1986, John Wiley & Sons.
9. Cushing H, Bovie WT: Electrosurgery as an aid to the removal of intracranial tumors. *Surg Gynecol Obstet* 47:751-84, 1928.
10. Fervers C. Die laparoskopie mit dem Cystoskope. Ein beitrag zur vereinfachung der Technik und zur endoskopischen Strangdurchtrennung in der bauchole. *Med Klin* 29:1042-5, 1933.

11. Boesch PF: Laparoskopische sterilization. Swchweizerische Zeitschrift für Krankenhaus und Anstaltswesen, 1936.
12. Anderson ET: Peritoneoscopy. *A J Surg* 35:135-9, 1937.
13. Power FH, Barnes AC: Sterilization by means of peritoneoscopic fulguration: a preliminary report. *Am J Obstet Gynecol* 41:1038-43, 1941.
14. Bardenheuer R: Elektrokoagulation der uterusschleimhaut zur behandlung klimakterischer blutungen. *Zentralb Gynäkol* 209:1937.
15. Palmer R, de Brux J. Essais de sterilization tubaire celcoscopique par electrocoagulation *Bull Fed Soc Gynecol Obstet Lang Fr* 14:298, 1962.
16. Neuwirth RS, Amin HK: Excision of submucus fibroids with hysteroscopic control. *Am J Obstet Gynecol* 126:95-9, 1976.
17. Frangenheim H: Laparoscopy and culdoscopy in gynaecology. London, 1972, Butterworth.
18. Deaths following female sterilization with unipolar electrocoagulating devices. *MMWR* 30:149, 1981.
19. AAGL 1981 Board of Trustees Recommendations, June 11, 1981.
20. Levy BS, Soderstrom RM, Dail DH: Bowel injuries during laparoscopy: gross anatomy and histology. *J Reprod Med* 30:168-72, 1985.
21. American Association of Gynecologic Laparoscopists News Scope, 4:1-13, 1985.
22. LaCourse JR, Miller WT, Vogt M, Selikowitz SM: Effect of high frequency current on nerve and muscle tissue. *IEEE Transs Biomed Eng BME* 32:82-86, 1985.
23. Oringer MJ, Ed Kelly WJ, Harrison JD: Laboratory experimental evaluation of efficacy of clinical electrosurgical techniques in electrosurgery in density, Philadelphia, 1975, W.B. Saunders.
24. Munro MG, Fu YS: Loop electrosurgical excision in the peritoneal cavity: preliminary experience in the rat model. In press.
25. Filmar S, Jetha N, McComb P, Gomel V: A comparative histologic study on the healing process after tissue transection: I. Carbon dioxide laser and electromicrosurgery. *Am J Obstet Gynecol* 160:1062-1067, 1989.
26. Daniell J, Fisher B, Alexander W: Laparoscopic evaluation of the argon beam coagulator: initial report. *J Reprod Med* 38:121-125, 1993.
27. Gomel V, James C: Intraoperative management of ureteral injury during operative laparoscopy. *Fertil Steril* 55:416-419, 1991.
28. Grainger, RA, Soderstrom RM, Schiff SF, et al: Ureteral injuries al laparoscopy: insights into diagnosis, management and prevention. *Obstet Gynecol* 75:839-843, 1990.
29. Corson SL. Electrical considerations of laparoscopic sterilization. *J Reprod Med* 11:159-164, 1973.
30. Engel T. The electrical dynamics of laparoscopic sterilization. *J Reprod Med* 15:33, 1975.
31. Einstein A. Zur quantentheorie der stralung. *Physio Z* 18:121-128, 1917.
32. Schawlow AL, Townes CH: Infared and optical masers. *Physiol Rev* 112:1940, 1958.
33. Maiman Th: Stimulated optical radiation in ruby masers. *Nature* 187:493-494, 1960.
34. Patel CKN, McFarlane RA, Faust WL: Selective excitation through energy transfer and optical maser action in N_2-CO_2. *Physical Rev* 8:470-473, 1964.
35. Geusic JE, Marios HM, Van Vitert CG: Laser oscillations in Nd-doped yttrium-aluminum, gallium and gaddinium garnets. *Appl Phys Lett* 4:182, 1964.
36. Bridges WB, Chest AN: Visible and UV laser oscillation at 119 wavelength in ionized Ne, Ar, Kr, Xe, O and other gases. *Appl Opt* 4:573, 1965.
37. Bellina JH: Gynecology and the laser. *Contemp Obstet Gynecol* 4:24-29, 1974.
38. Bruhat M, Mage C, Manhes M: Use of the CO_2 laser via laparoscopy. In Kaplan I, editor: Laser surgery III, Proceedings of the third international society for laser surgery. Tel-Aviv, 1979, Ot-Paz.
39. Liu YS, Denz D, Belt R: High average power intracavitary second harmonic using KT:OPO_4 in an acouto optically switched Nd:YAG laser oscillation at 5 kHz. *Opt Lett* 9:76, 1984.
40. Sorokin PD, Lan JR: Stimulated emission from an organic dye, chloroaluminum-phythalocyanine. *IBM J Res Dev* 10:162, 1966.
41. Luciano AA, Whitman G, Maier DB, et al: A comparison of thermal injury, healing patterns, and postoperative adhesion formation following CO_2 laser and electromicrosurgery. *Fertil Steril* 48:1025-1029, 1987.
42. Filmar S, Jetha N, McComb P, Gomel V: A comparative histologic study on the healing process after tissue transection: I. Carbon dioxide laser and electromicrosurgery. *Am J Obstet Gynecol* 160:1062-1067, 1989.
43. Bellina JH, Hemmings R, Voros J, Ross LF: Carbon dioxide laser and electrosurgical wound study with an animal model: a comparison of damage and healing patterns in peritoneal tissue. *Am J Obstet Gynecol* 148:327-34, 1984.
44. Badaway SZA, El Bakry MM, Baggish MS, Choe JK: Pulsed CO_2 laser versus conventional microsurgical anastomosis of the rat uterine horn. *Fertil Steril* 46:127-31, 1986.
45. Baggish MS, El Bakry MM: Comparison of electronically superpulsed and continuous-wave CO_2 laser on the rat uterine horn. *Fertil Steril* 45:120-127, 1986.
46. Bethuan J, Muller G, Schaldach B, Zur C: Fiber design for interstitial laser treatment. The international society for optical engineering 1420:234-241, 1991.
47. Kaplan I, Giler S, Dror R, Gannot I: Preliminary expirements of possible uses in medicine of novel plastic hollow fibers for transmission of CO_2 radiation. *Lasers Surg Med.* 10:291-294, 1990.
48. Hambley R et al: Wound healing of skin incisions produced by ultrasonically vibrating knife, scalpel, electrosurgery and carbon dioxide laser. *J Dermatol Surg Oncol* 14:1213-1217, 1988.
49. Semm K: New apparatus for 'cold-coagulation' of benign cervical lesions. *Am J Obstet Gynecol* 95:963-967, 1966.
50. Semm K, Mettler L: Technical progress in pelvic surgery via operative laparoscopy. *Am J Obstet Gynecol* 138:212-217, 1980.
51. Semm K, O'Neil-Freys I: Conventional operative laparoscopy. In Sutton CJG, editor: Baillières clinical obstetrics and gynecology. *Laparoscop Surg* 3.3:451-486, 1989.

Chapter 5

PRINCIPLES OF DIAGNOSTIC LAPAROSCOPY

"It is only by meticulous attention to detail, complete familiarity with the instruments, and extensive knowledge of the intrapelvic structures and through experience, that laparoscopy can be performed safely, accurately and to the maximum benefit of the patient."[1] It is the purpose of this chapter to take the reader, step by step, through those aspects of the laparoscopic techniques that have proved to be effective.

PREOPERATIVE INVESTIGATION

Prior to performing gynecologic laparoscopy, a complete history should be taken and a physical examination performed (box at right). Any laboratory testing indicated by the patient's presenting complaints should be completed before the procedure. If general anesthesia is to be used, the patient's fitness must be evaluated. The hemoglobin level should be ascertained and, where indicated, a urinalysis performed and cervical and vaginal cultures taken to identify both the common infective organisms and *Chlamydia* and *Mycoplasma*. If a recent Papanicolaou smear has not been performed, one should be carried out. Informed consent must be obtained in a manner that clearly demonstrates that the patient has understood the nature of the procedures to be performed and the benefits and risks.

Components of the preoperative investigation for diagnostic laparoscopy

Complete history
Thorough physical examination
Laboratory tests as indicated
Evaluation regarding route of anesthesia
Hemoglobin level measurement
Cervical and vaginal cultures and treatment as necessary
Informed consent

PREOPERATIVE EQUIPMENT CHECK

It is the responsibility of the surgeon to ensure that all the equipment is available and is in perfect working order before the patient enters the operating room. The light source is switched on to confirm that the bulbs are working.

The insufflator system is tested. The surgeon must be satisfied that there is an adequate supply of carbon dioxide (CO_2). Standard low flow rate insufflators, which are suited only for diagnostic purposes, are checked as follows. The internal tank is filled, and the flow of gas turned on. If a finger is placed over the outflow nozzle, the pressure manometer should record a steep rise in pressure. Even though 3 to 5 L will be adequate for diagnostic laparoscopy, if more prolonged procedures are to be performed, it may be necessary to refill the internal tank. To overcome this cumbersome step and permit a more rapid rate of insufflation, high-flow insufflators have been developed. The flow rate is automatically regulated based upon pressure and flow settings that the surgeon must establish. Flow rates may be variable but the pressure setting should not exceed 15 mm of mercury.

On many occasions it may be necessary to proceed directly from diagnostic to operative laparoscopy. All other potentially needed equipment, including a rapid flow insufflator, should be available and in working order. Pretesting of the instruments is discussed below.

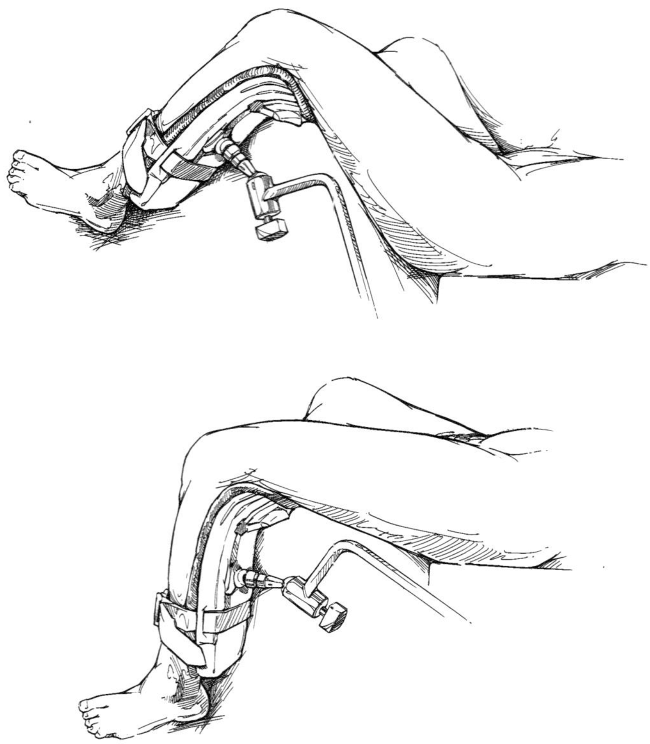

Fig. 5-1. Positioning of the patient.

ANESTHESIA AND PATIENT POSITIONING

Although local anesthesia can be used, we prefer to carry out laparoscopy with the patient under general anesthesia. It offers greater comfort to patient and surgeon alike, especially if extensive diagnostic manipulations are required within the peritoneal cavity and increases safety during operative laparoscopic procedures. While the nature of the general anesthetic agents used is in the province of the anesthetist, certain basic principles should be stressed. Because of a risk of hypercarbia, patients should be intubated and receive assisted ventilation. If the surgeon is right handed and hence will stand to the patient's left side, any intravenous lines should enter through the patient's right arm. The presence of an intravenous system in an extended arm can interfere with the mobility and comfort of the surgeon or assistant and increases the risk of an injury to the nerves of the brachial plexus. If the arm is placed by the patient's side rather than on an extended arm support, this inconvenience is avoided. Care must be taken that any arm so placed is protected when the table is moved to facilitate laparoscopic manipulations.

Before the induction of anesthesia, the patient should void. Anesthesia is induced with the patient horizontally supine on the table, which remains horizontal. Although some physicians will perform laparoscopy in this position, our preference is to place the patient in lithotomy stirrups (Fig. 5-1). Such positioning offers several advantages. There is easy access to the vagina. Hysteroscopy can be performed concurrently, if it is indicated. Unless there is reason to suspect the presence of an intrauterine pregnancy, it is important that the surgeon be able to manipulate the uterus during gynecologic laparoscopy (unless, of course, the patient does not possess a uterus). This is critical with most operative procedures. The dorsal lithotomy position allows the insertion of a uterine manipulator.

Although the dorsal lithotomy position is of great value, incorrect positioning of the flexed knees in the stirrups can be a hindrance to the manipulation of ancillary instruments. To facilitate laparoscopic evaluation and surgery, low lithotomy of Lloyd-Davis stirrups should be used; they should be angled as necessary toward the patient's feed (Fig. 5-1). The surgeon must ensure that the nerves and blood vessels of the legs are protected from pressure.

Once the patient is in the lithotomy position, the table is broken so that there is easy access to the perineum. A common mistake is to permit the patient's buttocks to remain too far up from the edge of the table. Frequently, uterine manipulation will require depressing the angle of any manipulator nearly 90 degrees to the horizontal plane, and this can be achieved only if the patient's buttocks protrude for 1 or 2 inches from the distal end of the table. If there is any reason to anticipate the need for unipolar electrosurgical capability, the ground plate is affixed to the patient's thigh.

TECHNIQUE OF LAPAROSCOPY

Laparoscopy must be performed in a logical sequence of steps, which include:

- Pretesting of the instruments
- Perineal and bladder care
- Induction of the pneumoperitoneum
- Introduction of the principal trocar and cannula
- Introduction of the telescope
- Introduction of ancillary instruments
- Laparoscopic survey
- Removal of the instruments and abdominal closure

Pretesting of the instruments

After being gowned and gloved the surgeon must pretest the sterile equipment.

The Veress needle should be examined to ensure that it is working perfectly. It should be assembled correctly with the outer sheath screwed snugly against the hub. The blunt tip must be freely mobile within the external sharp pointed sheath, and the hole in the blunt tip should be free and pointing in a direction diametrically opposed to the back of the sharp needle. Cracks can occur around this opening, and cases have been reported in which the tip of a Veress needle has fractured and fallen into the peritoneal cavity. The integrity of the tip should be checked. The needle should be connected with the polyethylene line to the insufflator and pressures within the system tested with the flow rate set at

1 L/minute. Pressures within such a system will rarely exceed 10 mm Hg but can vary between 5 and 10 mm Hg. An accurate knowledge of the baseline pressures within the system is imperative if accurate placement of the needle tip within the peritoneal cavity is to be confirmed (as will be described later).

The telescope should be examined to confirm that the lenses are clean and are not loose. When video equipment is to be used, the camera is draped, attached to the telescope, and the system adjusted so that the best picture is obtained.

A particularly troublesome problem can be encountered if valves in the cannulas jam during the performance of laparoscopy. These should be tested to ensure proper assembly, free mobility, and gas tight integrity. Endoscopic operative instruments are miniaturized and many have distal hinges. If such instruments have not been properly cleaned they can jam. They should be tested prior to their use.

Perineal and bladder care

It is the trivia of medicine that causes the most discomfort to our patients. The long tradition of pubic and perineal shaving is of no advantage in reducing infection and causes the patient a great deal of discomfort as the hair grows back. However, second punctures are frequently made below the pubic hair line and may be closed with adhesive tape. To permit entry below the pubic hair line and appropriate closure of this incision, we encourage our patients to remove a small square of the suprapubic hair (in the midline) at home. Otherwise a small area, in the operative site, is removed with scissors once the patient has been anesthetized.

The patient's abdomen, perineum, and vagina are washed with antiseptic solution. She is draped and a bimanual pelvic examination performed to assess the size, mobility, and, particularly the position of the uterus. The presence of any other pelvic anomalies is noted. The status of the bladder is noted. The patient should have been asked to void immediately before anesthesia was induced. If, however, any doubt exists it is safer to catheterize the patient. An dwelling catheter should be necessary only if prolonged operating time is anticipated.

The uterine manipulator of choice is inserted through the cervix and locked in place. (This step is omitted if an intrauterine pregnancy is suspected.) In order to effect proper uterine manipulation, which will permit the best laparoscopic visualization, any uterine manipulator used must be of rigid construction.

Induction of the pneumoperitoneum

"It is this step above all that is critical in the avoidance of major complications and in ensuring proper visualization and room to perform any necessary intraperitoneal manipulations."[1] Traditionally the distending gas is introduced through a needle and the principal trocar and cannula are introduced only after the establishment of the pneumoperotoneum. Direct insertion of the primary trocar and cannula with subsequent induction of pneumopertoneum has been advocated.[2] This approach may reduce operating time by a minute or two but is more hazardous in the patient with a scarred abdomen, those who are very thin, or in whom a mass is present. We prefer the use of the Veress needle to induce pneumopertoneum in the following fashion.

Inspection, palpation, and percussion of the abdomen. The presence of abdominal scars from previous surgery will influence the placement of the Veress needle. Their position(s) should be noted. The abdomen should be palpated to detect any evidence of organomegaly or unsuspected intra-abdominal tumors that might be damaged by the introduction of the Veress needle or the larger trocar and cannula.

Although rare, on occasion the stomach may have been inadvertently inflated during induction of anesthesia. Any difficulties in intubation should have been communicated by the anesthetist to alert the surgeon to this possibility. If such is the case, the stomach is at risk of perforation. If the upper abdomen is gently percussed, any areas of undue resonance will be noted. If indeed the stomach does appear to have been inflated, a nasogastric tube should be introduced by the anesthetist and the gas aspirated.

Introduction of the Veress needle. The Veress needle is usually introduced intraumbilically where the peritoneum is adherent to the abdominal wall. The needle may also be introduced in the midline anywhere between 5 cm above the pubic symphysis and the umbilicus or the lateral border of the rectus at either the left or right McBurney's point. The principal inconvenience of these insufflation sites is due to the lack of adherence of the peritoneum to the parietes. The Veress needle may tent the peritoneum without penetrating it, leading to a preperitoneal insufflation. Confirmation of proper needle placement (described later) is essential prior to the insufflation of the peritoneal cavity. Another important site of needle insertion is the left upper quadrant at the lateral border of the rectus two fingerbreadths below the left costal margin (Fig. 5-2). Pneumoperitoneum may be effected transvaginally by introducing the Veress needle (or preferably a modified one with a metallic stop 3 cm from the tip) into the pouch of Douglas. The most common site for introduction of the Veress needle (and the principal trocar and cannula) is intraumbilically. This technique of needle placement will be described first, and indications for the alternate techniques will be described later.

To insert the Veress needle, the skin below the umbilicus is stretched toward the pubic symphysis by placement of the thumb and forefinger of the nondominant hand on either side of the umbilical margin. This stretching will expose a natural fold within the umbilicus. Insertion of closed tissue forceps, which are then permitted to spring open, will provide similar exposure. An incision sufficiently large to

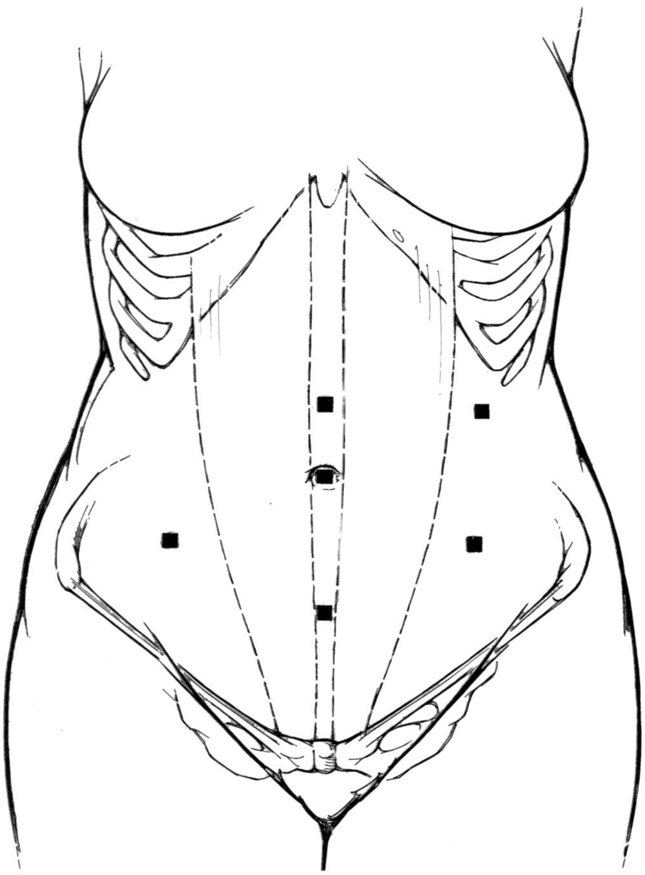

Fig. 5-2. Sites of introduction of the Veress needle.

accommodate not only the Veress needle but also the principal trocar and cannula is made through one of the umbilical folds and should divide the skin only. A pointed no. 11 blade is adequate for this purpose and is also of value in making second or subsequent punctures. The Veress needle, which has been disconnected from the gasline, is grasped between the finger and thumb of the dominant hand. In order to ensure maximum safety, the inner blunt cannula should be able to travel freely. In addition, the surgeon should have estimated the length of needle necessary to reach the peritoneal cavity. If the shaft of the needle is grasped at this point, any sudden advance will be prevented by the grasping fingers (Fig. 5-3).

The tip of the needle is inserted through the skin incision. The nondominant hand grasps the hypogastrium and elevates the parietes. The Veress needle is advanced at a 45 degree angle toward the hollow of the sacrum. As it penetrates the peritoneum, the displaced distal hub will click against the tap, indicating that penetration of the peritoneum has occurred. With experience, the surgeon recognizes each layer of the abdomen as it is traversed and the sudden sharp advance as the tip of the needle enters the peritoneal cavity. The abdominal wall is released by the nondominant hand and proper placement of the needle tip is confirmed.

Confirmation of needle placement and insufflation. To confirm proper placement of the needle tip, a syringe test is performed. A 10 cc syringe containing 5 cc of normal saline is connected to the needle. Gentle withdrawal on the plunger should not produce any gas bubbles or blood; 4 cc are injected into the peritoneal cavity and aspiration once again performed. If the needle is correctly positioned, there will be no recovery of saline. If, however, the needle has inadvertently entered the bowel, stained saline will be returned; on those occasions in which the needle has entered the preperitoneal space, clear saline may be obtained.

Further confirmation of correct placement is obtained by connecting the gas line to the Veress needle, turning the gas on, and noting the pressure displayed by the insufflator. In a well-anesthetized patient, the difference between the pressure when the system was originally tested and that now obtained should not be greater than 5 mm Hg. If higher pressures are recorded, the surgeon should suspect that the needle is either in the preperitoneal space or has entered an intra-abdominal viscus or omentum. If insufflation pressures are high, the lower abdominal wall should be grasped with both hands and gently shaken. This is frequently sufficient to dislodge omentum from the tip of the needle. If such a maneuver fails to relieve the increased pressures, the angle of the needle should be increased as on occasion the distal hole will simply be impinging against the anterior abdominal wall. If these maneuvers fail to relieve increased pressure, the Veress needle should be removed and a second insertion made.

If gas pressures are normal with flow set at 1 L/minute, percussion over the right costal margin should demonstrate loss of liver dullness within 45 to 60 seconds. This is the most convincing demonstration that the Veress cannula is indeed within the peritoneal cavity. If, however, after passage of 1 L of gas liver dullness does not disappear, it is almost certain that the tip of the Veress needle is in the preperitoneal space or in a viscus. Under these circumstances, the needle should be withdrawn and repositioned. If this simple precaution is neglected and gas is permitted to continue to flow, once sufficient gas has entered the preperitoneal space liver dullness will disappear.

Once the surgeon is satisfied that the gas is flowing into the peritoneal space, flow should continue until between 2 to 5 L have been insufflated. The volume required will be dependent on the depth of anesthesia, the size of the patient, and the size of the trocar and cannula to be inserted. The optimum amount of gas for the individual patient is assessed more by the distended feel of the abdomen than by the numbers shown on the dials of the insufflator.

Insufflators are equipped with a rapid insufflation system that will deliver 3 to 10 L/minute. Increasing the flow rate above 1 L/minute is absolutely contraindicated until the surgeon is completely satisfied that the Veress needle is accurately placed freely within the peritoneal cavity. Once a

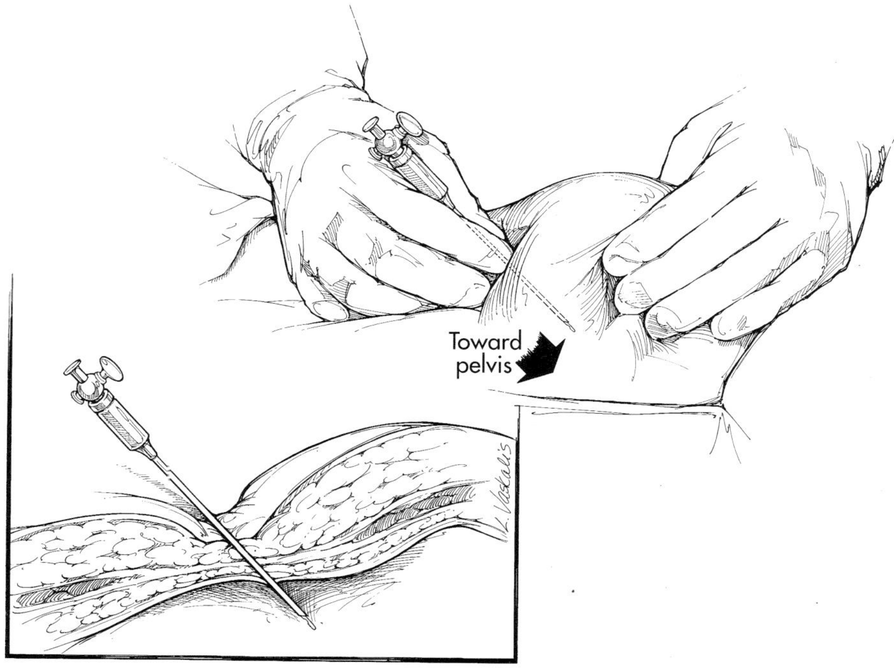

Fig. 5-3. Insertion of the Veress needle.

satisfactory pneumoperitoneum has been established, the Veress needle is removed.

Alternate sites for a Veress needle insertion. Introduction of the Veress needle in the intraumbilical position in patients with previous abdominal surgical scars may put intra-abdominal contents at risk if they are adherent to the abdominal wall. In a small group of patients, tumors or enlarged organs may be in jeopardy. It is under these circumstances that alternate sites in the abdomen must be selected, their location being dictated by the area at risk.

If the Veress needle is introduced in the lower abdomen, it should be angled toward the center of the hollow of the sacrum. If introduced in the midline above the umbilicus, the angle of approach should be similar to that used at the intraumbilical site. If inserted beneath the left costal margin, the needle must be introduced in a direction that does not place the intrathoracic structures at risk.

The vaginal approach should only be undertaken: (1) in a patient who has a uterus, (2) in whom there is no reason to suspect that the cul-de-sac is obliterated and (3) if the bimanual pelvic examination reveals no evidence of thickening or masses within the cul-de-sac.

If the original attempt to produce pneumoperitoneum leads to preperitoneal emphysema, the gas line is disconnected from the Veress needle and the preperitoneal space emptied of as much gas as possible. While second attempts can be made through the same site, an alternate site may also be employed.

Introduction of the principal trocar and cannula

Once an adequate pneumoperitoneum has been established, the next step is to introduce the principal trocar and cannula through which the telescope will be passed. The risks associated with this step are to a large extent related to the force that must be exerted and the control that can be applied to the instrument. Three factors influence the degree of force required: (1) If the skin incision is too small, passage through the skin will be impeded and greater force must be applied. (2) The diameter of the trocar and cannula will directly influence the force required to effect parietal penetration. Since the early days of laparoscopy, the evolution of laparoscopes of narrower bore but yet effective optical resolution have greatly reduced the force required to introduce the principal trocar and cannula. (3) Sharp trocars can be inserted more readily than blunt ones.

The trocar and cannula appropriate to the size of the telescope to be used are grasped in the dominant hand. The trocar should fit snugly against the upper border of the cannula and is fixed in that position during introduction by the ball of the thumb. The trocar and cannula are introduced subcutaneously for a distance of about 2 cm. The angle of introduction is increased to 45 degrees toward the hollow of the sacrum. The ulnar border of the nondominant hand is placed on the abdominal wall and encircles the cannula to act as a stop should a sudden thrust force the cannula through the abdominal wall (Fig. 5-4, *A*). There is no need

A

B

C

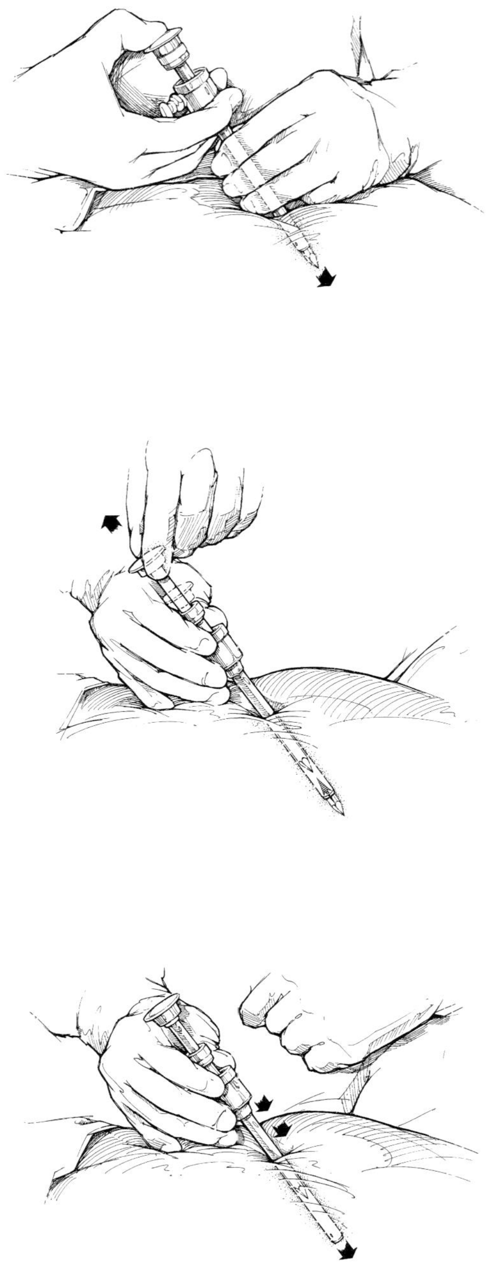

Fig. 5-4. Insertion of the principal trocar and cannula. **A,** The nondominant hand encircles the cannula to act as a stop. **B,** Once the tip of the trocar is in the peritoneal cavity and evidence of gas escape is noted, the trocar is retracted within the cannula. **C,** The cannula is further advanced.

to elevate the parietes provided the abdomen has been distended sufficiently.

The trocar should be hollow with a hole at its distal tip that connects with a hole at its proximal end. As the trocar and cannula are advanced, gas will be heard to escape as the trocar tip enters the peritoneal cavity. At this point, the trocar should be retracted within the cannula and the cannula further advanced for 1 or 2 cm, to ensure that it is adequately placed within the peritoneal cavity (Fig. 5-4, *B* and *C*). This retraction of the sharp trocar tip into the cannula is designed to prevent trauma to the intraperitoneal organs. The trocar is removed and excess gas is allowed to escape, leaving in the peritoneal cavity the optimal amount required for the procedure.

Introduction of the telescope

Next, the telescope, which previously has been connected to the light source, is introduced. Although the video camera and monitor are integral to modern operative laparoscopic technique, initial observation with the naked eye offers certain advantages. The unaided eye is able to discriminate between subtle shades of color, which is particularly important in the detection of early stages of endometriosis.

Viewing commences as the telescope traverses the cannula to ensure that if any organ has been impaled upon the sheath it will be visualized and not dislodged by passage of the telescope. If direct visualization confirms accurate placement, the gas line is attached to the tap on the side of the cannula and the insufflator set to the desired automatic flow rate.

Once the telescope has been inserted and the surgeon is assured that no intraperitoneal damage has been occasioned by either the Veress needle or the large trocar and cannula, a systematic diagnostic evaluation should be performed. Since at this point the table is still in the horizontal position, it is appropriate to inspect the upper abdomen. If a clear view cannot be obtained, the table should be placed in Fowler's position.

Once the abdomen has been inspected, the table is placed in sufficient Trendelenburg position to allow access to the pelvic organs. The appendix is seen best in this position. If a uterine manipulator is in place, it can be used in a fashion that enables the fundus of the uterus to perform like a piston and dislodge much of the loose bowel from the pelvic cavity. This preliminary dislodgement of bowel will permit an initial pelvic inspection so that appropriate ancillary portals can be selected.

Introduction of ancillary instruments

A thorough pelvic assessment cannot be performed unless, as a minimum, a calibrated probe is inserted. In addition, it may be necessary to introduce grasping forceps, scissors, or instruments with electrosurgical and/or laser capability. Such ancillary instruments are introduced through second and, when necessary, third and fourth portals. It is most usual to introduce probes and instruments for diagnostic laparoscopy and tubal sterilization supraumbically in the midline. Additional portals may be made as necessary

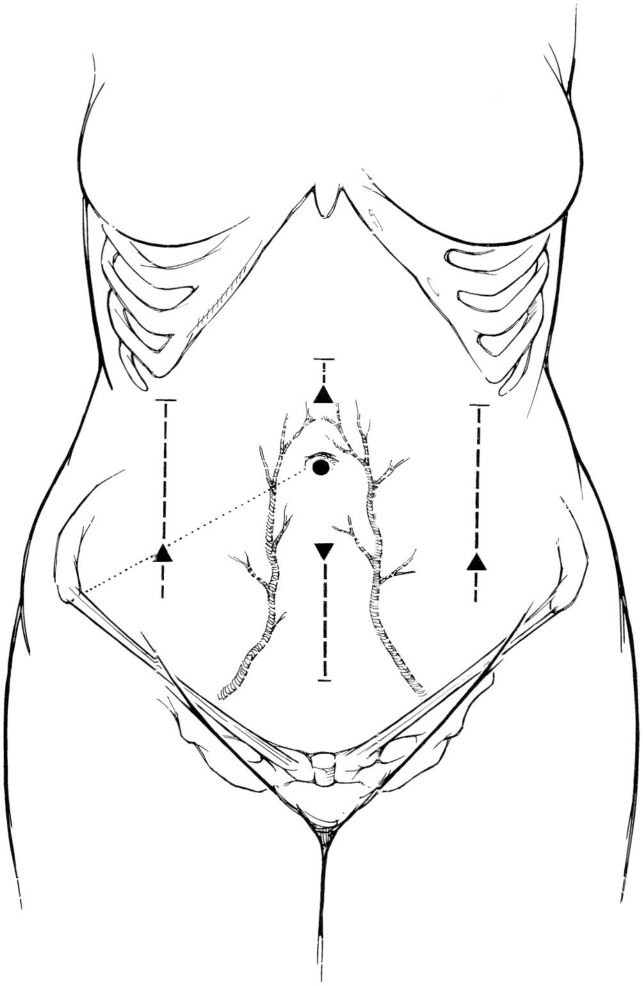

Fig. 5-5. Site of ancillary portals. ●, Principal; ▲, ancillary.

laterally at the outer borders of the rectus sheath. These punctures are placed at a higher level than the suprapubic midline portal to provide the optimal angle of approach for operative instruments. While in most instances this can be achieved at McBurney's points, it may be necessary to site them even more cephalad (Fig. 5-5).

In order to avoid trauma to the structures of the abdominal wall, the site of secondary puncture should be indented with the index finger and observed with the laparoscope in the abdomen. The site of indentation will be readily seen and can be confirmed to be free of both bladder and parietal blood vessels. The obliterated umbilical arteries are useful landmarks for avoiding major parietal blood vessels. When the site has been chosen, it is transilluminated with the laparoscope, further confirming the absence of vessels. Secondary incisions of sufficient size to accommodate the trocar and cannula are made at selected points. The trocar and cannula are inserted through the skin and fascia. To avoid causing intraperitoneal trauma, further advance of the trocar and cannula is controlled by direct laparoscopic observation (Fig. 5-6). The finer points of surgical laparoscopy will be discussed in the appropriate chapters.

Laparoscopic survey

The laparoscopic survey encompasses the thorough visualization of the entire peritoneal cavity. The survey includes successive observation and assessment of the parietal peritoneum, the visceral surfaces, and specific abdominal and pelvic organs. The surgeon begins by gaining a general impression about the peritoneal cavity with the assessment of the upper abdomen, liver, gallbladder, stomach, and diaphragm while the patient is still in the horizontal position. A normal spleen is usually not visible; in addition to steep Fowler's a right lateral decubitus position is required to display this region. The Fowler's position also facilitates the visualization of the other upper abdominal organs. Successively, the transverse, descending, and ascending colon and the small bowel are inspected.

The patient is now placed in the Trendelenburg position and the cecum and appendix are assessed. Manipulation with a blunt probe will expose the appendix and allow assessment of ileal loops for the presence of a Meckel's diverticulum or other lesions. The bowel is displaced from the pelvis by the manipulation of the uterus with the uterine cannula, if one is in place, and/or with the blunt probe. A general panoramic inspection of the pelvis is first performed with the laparoscope kept at some distance from the pelvic contents. The laparoscope is then advanced and pelvic organs are scrutinized systematically as described under "The Endoscopic Survey" in Chapter 9. Manipulation of the uterus in both the anteroposterior and side-to-side directions along with the use of a probe greatly facilitates the inspection.

It is beyond the scope of this chapter to describe the appearance of the various pathologic entities that may be encountered in the pelvis. We do discuss, below, the challenges certain patients and procedures present.

Removal of the instruments and abdominal closure

Once any laparoscopic procedure is finished a final survey is made to ensure that there is no unsuspected trauma or bleeding. The ancillary instruments and, thereafter, their cannulas are removed. The internal aspects of the secondary puncture sites are inspected with the laparoscope. If there is no internal bleeding, the telescope is removed. With the patient still in the Trendelenburg position, the valve of the principal cannula is opened and the gas expelled from the peritoneal cavity. Keeping the abdominal wall compressed with the nondominant hand, this cannula is removed with the valve in the open position. Pressure from the hand will prevent introduction of room air that will cause subsequent shoulder pain. Keeping the valve open will also prevent negative pressure sucking bowel or omentum into the puncture wound.

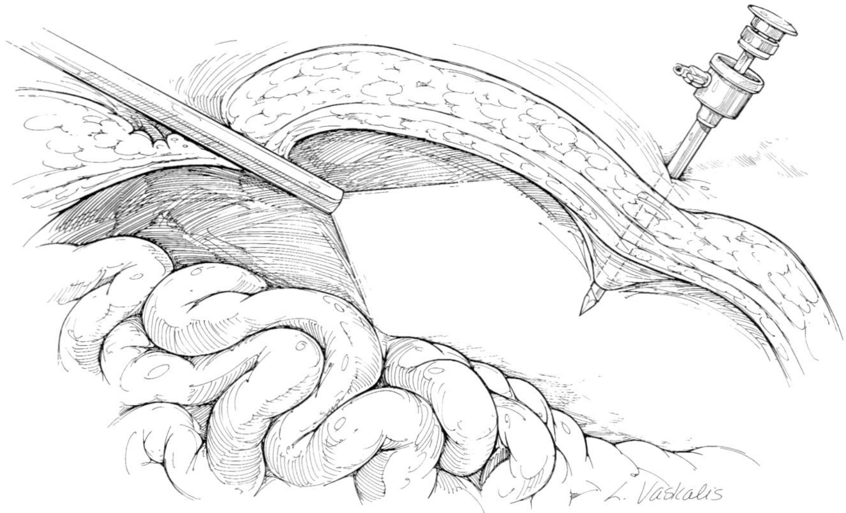

Fig. 5-6. Introduction of ancillary trocar and cannula under direct laparoscopic vision.

When the instruments are removed, the incisions are closed. Incisions of less than 5 mm can be closed with simple cutaneous sutures or, preferably, with steristrips. Larger incisions should be closed in two layers. Repairing the fascial defect will prevent hernia formation.

ALTERNATE APPROACHES

Open laparoscopy

The preceding sections have alluded to the damage that may be occasioned by the Veress needle and the principal trocar and cannula. In order to avoid these risks the technique of open laparoscopy was introduced.[3] It is based on the principle that direct opening of the abdominal cavity carries less risk than the blind introduction of sharp instruments. A small subumbilical incision is made through the outer parietes and the peritoneum identified and incised under direct vision. The open laparoscopy trocar and cannula are the key to this procedure. The trocar has a blunt rounded end. The trocar and cannula are introduced through the small peritoneal incision. Four hooks are provided on the cannula that are sutured to the peritoneal edges to ensure gas tight integrity. With the trocar and cannula in place, the gas line is connected and the pneumoperitoneum established. The blunt trocar is removed and the telescope inserted. Open laparoscopy now proceeds in the same manner as standard laparoscopy.

While this technique should at least theoretically carry less risk than that with traditional laparoscopy, bowel damage has been reported to occur at the time of peritoneal entry. Open laparoscopy takes longer to perform. Because we have not been convinced of the reputed advantages of this technique, we have not introduced it into our practices.

Gasless laparoscopy

The pneumoperitoneum serves the purpose of elevating the anterior abdominal wall to provide space in which the surgeon can work. Loss of this working space, caused either by aspiration or loss of gas tight integrity of the cannulae, slows the procedure. Significant loss of gas will also occur when the vagina is opened or an abdominal incision is extended. "Gasless laparoscopy" has been introduced in an attempt to provide space in which to operate without the need for continuous gas replacement. The anterior abdominal wall is elevated mechanically with a special device (Fig. 5-7).

An umbilical incision is made and the peritoneum entered. In this respect gasless laparoscopy is similar to open laparoscopy. The incision must be of sufficient size to accommodate the abdominal wall elevator and a laparoscope, which are inserted. The lifting device is adjusted to raise the anterior abdominal wall. Ancillary portals are placed. These cannulae are large, do not have valves, and will accommodate conventional instruments. Indeed, more than one instrument at a time can be inserted through the same cannula. The flexible construction of these cannulas allows them to adapt to the configuration of the instruments and also permits a wider range of movement.

This approach is still in the developmental stage. It does offer the surgeon the advantage of being able to use conventional instruments and techniques. Suturing is easier and faster. Larger ancillary cannulas will accommodate the removal of larger tissue specimens. In addition, when a combined laparoscopic and vaginal operation is undertaken, two surgeons can work simultaneously, since opening the vaginal wall does not hamper the work of the abdominal surgeon.

There are disadvantages. While pneumoperitoneum provides a domelike elevation of the whole abdominal wall, the currently available elevation devices lift the midline but not the flanks. Access to the upper abdomen and the pouch of Douglas is restricted. There is no increase in intra-abdominal pressure to inhibit excursion of the bowel with

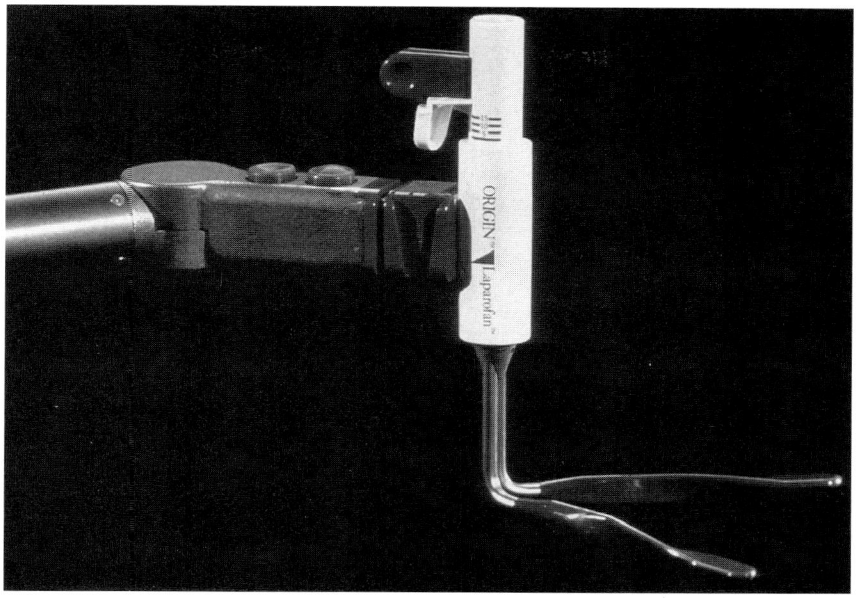

Fig. 5-7. Mechanical elevating device for gasless laparoscopy.

respiratory movements. The hemostatic effect of the pneumoperitoneum is also absent.

LAPAROSCOPY IN SPECIAL SITUATIONS

Obese and very thin patients

In cases of extreme obesity, laparoscopy may present rather more difficulty. A longer Veress needle may be required. The intraumbilical approach is valuable because it is the thinnest point of the abdominal wall. Whereas in the average patient the Veress needle is angled at 45 degrees, an approach closer to the vertical may be used in the obese patient. Positioning is important. Any degree of flexion of the thighs will result in the abdominal panniculus doubling its thickness and folding in such a way as to make the procedure almost impossible. To avoid this, the Veress needle may be introduced prior to putting the patient's legs in the lithotomy position, or, preferably, the lithotomy stirrups should be positioned in such a way that the patient's legs are not unduly flexed. In some of these patients, if no contraindications exist, transvaginal insufflation via the cul-de-sac may be the method of choice. A special needle is available for this purpose.

Whereas it is obvious that the obese patient presents certain mechanical problems, the very thin patient is at greater risk. The distance between the anterior abdominal wall and the abdominal aorta is often very small. Further, the force required to introduce the Veress needle is often less than anticipated because the fascia is thin and offers little resistance. To avoid this risk, the Veress needle must be grasped close to its tip, the abdominal wall must be completely elevated by the nondominant hand and the angle of induction modified so that the Veress needle is at about 25 to 30 degrees to the upper abdominal wall.

In all potentially difficult laparoscopies, it is a wise precaution to overinflate the abdomen through the Veress needle. Gas should be run in to achieve overdistention but should not exceed a pressure of 15 mm Hg, which would impede venous return through the vena cava. This added distention provides more room for entry of the large trocar and cannula. Once it is established that the large trocar and cannula are correctly positioned, some of the gas can be allowed to escape to reduce overdistention and laparoscopy performed safely.

Pediatric patients

Pediatric laparoscopy requires special instruments (see Chapter 3). It carries risks similar to those encountered in the very thin patient. The distance between the anterior abdominal wall and the aorta is very short. Due to the thin fascia, which offers little resistance, the force required to introduce the Veress needle is significantly less than that in the adult. For these reasons, the Veress needle must be grasped close to its tip; the abdominal wall must be completely elevated; and the angle of the needle pointed toward the pelvis is modified so that it is almost parallel with the upper abdominal wall.

The pneumoperitoneum will be established quickly because of the small overall volume of the peritoneal cavity. In addition, small increments of gas cause dramatic changes in the intraperitoneal pressure. Therefore extreme vigilance is necessary. The double-barrelled Veress-Frangenheim needle, which permits simultaneous recording of the intraperitoneal pressure during the induction of pneumoperitoneum, is especially useful in these cases.

From the foregoing, it is clearly evident that, in children, extreme care must be exercised in the insertion of the Veress needle, the principal trocar, and cannula and in all of the successive steps of the procedure. Once the laparoscope has been introduced into the peritoneal cavity, the gas line is connected to the tap on the side of the principal cannula, but the tap is kept closed. The tap is reopened only if additional gas is required during the procedure and only for as long as it takes to top up the pneumoperitoneum.

High-risk patients

Contraindications to laparoscopy are discussed in Chapter 6. Introduction of the Veress needle, the principal trocar and cannula, and ancillary cannulas carries greater risk if the patient is pregnant, has organomegaly, or has intra-abdominal adhesions. There are techniques to minimize the risks in such patients, which will now be described.

Intrauterine pregnancy. The larger the gravid uterus the greater the probability that it may be traumatized or that it will obscure the areas the surgeon wishes to examine. These risks and limitations must be taken into account when considering laparoscopy in a pregnant woman, especially once the uterus has attained the size of 16 weeks or greater. The use of an intrauterine cannula is contraindicated. The site of introduction of the Veress needle must be carefully selected.

If the uterus is still within the pelvis an intraumbilical insertion is possible, provided the needle tip is not permitted to penetrate the parietes any further than is absolutely necessary. If the uterus is larger, the Veress needle can be introduced supraumbilically in the midline or in the left upper quadrant. The former approach places the transverse colon and stomach in jeopardy, so the needle must not be introduced too far into the peritoneal cavity. The latter approach is more likely to avoid the transverse colon and the stomach. The Veress needle is usually introduced vertically to avoid inadvertent penetration of the diaphram and pleura. This approach is particularly valuable in patients with severe adhesive disease and will be discussed in more detail shortly.

Once an effective pneumoperitoneum has been established, the principal trocar and cannula can be introduced supraumbilically in the midline. The depth of penetration of the principal trocar and cannula is a function of its diameter; the narrower the gauge the shallower the penetration. As such the smallest suitable laparoscope should be used in the pregnant patient.

The site of induction of any ancillary trocar and cannulas will be more cephalad than usual. The insertion of these instruments must take into account the obliteration of the pelvis by the uterus and decreased space due to the upper displacement of the bowel. Insertion is made under constant laparoscopic observation. A sharp trocar will penetrate the parietes efficiently and can be withdrawn into the cannula as soon as the cannula has entered the peritoneal cavity. A blunt trocar may cause peritoneal tenting and reduce the clearance between its tip and vital organs. If this occurs the angle of entry can be directed toward the tip of the laparoscope, which is withdrawn into its cannula. Further insertion of the ancillary trocar-cannula will proceed into the safety of the principal cannula. Every endeavor should be made to disturb the pregnant uterus as little as possible.

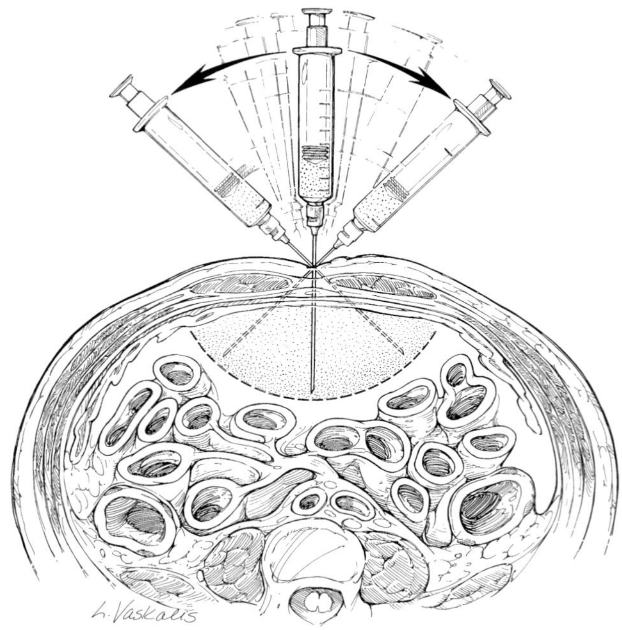

Fig. 5-8. Testing for free space under the umbilicus.

Organomegaly or abdominal mass. Laparoscopy may be performed in the presence of hepatomegaly or splenomegaly, which are rare occurrences, or in the patient with an abdominal mass. To prevent traumatizing the enlarged organ or the mass, the borders of the organ or mass must be carefully delineated by palpation and percussion of the abdomen of the anesthetized patient. Furthermore, alternate sites of entry for the Veress needle and principal and auxiliary trocar and cannulas should be selected.

Intra-abdominal adhesions. The presence of intra-abdominal adhesions must be suspected in patients who have had prior abdominal surgery, especially bowel surgery. Evidence of adhesions may be obtained from the previous operative reports. In such cases, an umbilical entry carries the risk of traumatizing a bowel loop, especially if adherent to the parietes. In the majority of such cases it is possible to induce the pneumoperitoneum by inserting the Veress needle in the left upper quadrant as described earlier.

Once a satisfactory pneumoperitoneum has been created it may be still possible to introduce the principal trocar and cannula intraumbilically. Prior to the umbilical introduction of the trocar and cannula, a simple test should be performed to ensure the safety of this approach. A 10 cc or 20 cc glass syringe containing 5 cc of normal saline is connected to an

18 gauge needle. The needle is inserted through the intraumbilical site and advanced 1 cm at a time. At each one of these steps the presence of gas is elicited. Gas bubbles will appear in the saline and will elevate the plunger of the glass syringe. The goal is to establish whether or not there is adequate free space to introduce the principal trocar and cannula safely. The limits of the potential space can be defined by gradually advancing the needle vertically and in various directions (Fig. 5-8).

If, however, it proves impossible to insert the principal trocar and cannula in the umbilical area, it may still be possible to gain access to the peritoneal cavity through another abdominal site. Once again, insertion of the trocar and cannula must be preceded by carrying out the above-described safety test.

A better approach is to insert the new needle-scope that fits through the outer sheath of a special Veress needle. Alternatively a narrow-gauge telescope (e.g., cytoscope) can be introduced through a 3 mm cannula through the same upper quadrant insufflation site. This permits determination of the extent and nature of the adhesive process and assessment of umbilical and other sites for insertion of the principal and ancillary trocar and cannulas.

REFERENCES

1. Gomel V, Taylor PJ, Yuzpe AA, Rioux JE: Laparoscopy and hysteroscopy in gynecologic practice. Chicago, 1986, Year Book Medical Publishers.
2. Jarret II JC: Laparoscopy: Direct trocar insection without pneumoperitoneum. *Obstet Gynecol* 75:725-727, 1990.
3. Hasson HM: Open laparoscopy: A report of 150 cases. *J Reprod Med* 12:234, 1974.

Chapter 6

INDICATIONS AND CONTRAINDICATIONS OF DIAGNOSTIC LAPAROSCOPY

INDICATIONS

Laparoscopy is an invasive method of diagnosis, assessment, and surgical access. Diagnostic laparoscopy is indicated when, following assessment of the history, physical examination, and the ancillary investigations appropriate to the presenting symptoms, direct visualization of the peritoneal cavity is required to substantiate the working diagnosis. (See box at right.)

Laparoscopy plays an important diagnostic role in patients who are suffering from infertility and pelvic pain. If imaging and laboratory investigation are unable to clarify the nature of the underlying disorder in the asymptomatic woman with abnormal pelvic findings, a diagnostic laparoscopy should be performed. The use of laparoscopy for these purposes is described in Chapters 9, 10, 11, and 12.

The second function is assessment of the severity of conditions so that effective management can be planned. This role is particularly relevant in cases of tubal infertility, endometriosis, acute pelvic inflammatory disease, and some cases of gynecologic malignancy. These first two functions have until recently constituted the primary indications for laparoscopy.

Because laparoscopy provides direct access to the peritoneal cavity, the last decade has seen enormous advances in our ability to use this property to enable us to perform many operative procedures without recourse to laparotomy. Within the next 10 years a chapter describing the indications for surgical laparoscopy will be succinct and didactic. At present, while it is possible to list those procedures that can be performed laparoscopically, clear understanding of those which should be performed laparoscopically is still evolving. Chapters 13 to 25 describe these laparoscopic operations and, using currently available data, attempt to evaluate their place.

Indications for diagnostic laparoscopy

Use

Direct visualization of the peritoneal cavity

Applications

Infertility
Pain (acute and chronic)
Endometriosis
Neoplasia

CONTRAINDICATIONS

There are contraindications to laparoscopy as a means of access (see box on p. 69). Once it is understood that laparoscopy is merely the means of access by which a number of specific procedures can be performed, then it becomes apparent that the contraindications to any specific procedure—proposed to be performed laparoscopically—are properties largely inherent to the procedure itself. A secondary consideration, once it has been decided that the procedure is indeed indicated, is whether or not it should be performed laparoscopically.

The decision not to perform an operation should be based upon simple medical facts. The decision not to perform the procedure laparoscopically will be made if such an approach is associated with greater relative risk. It is now be-

> **Contraindications to diagnostic laparoscopy**
>
> ***Procedural considerations***
>
> Laparoscopic approach in a given case may carry greater risk
> Increased operating time
> Increased cost
>
> ***Major contraindications***
>
> Severe cardiorespiratory disease
> Large abdominal and diaphragmatic hernia
> Generalized peritonitis
> Severe ileus-intestinal obstruction
> Inexperienced surgeon
>
> ***Relative contraindications***
>
> Prior abdominal surgery or inflammatory bowel disease
> Extremes in body weight
> Intrauterine pregnancy
> Large intra-abdominal mass
> Displaced or enlarged organs

coming apparent that increased operating time, cost of equipment, and cost of the procedure may also constitute contraindications to the laparoscopic approach. It is easy to justify laparoscopic tubal sterilization or management of tubal pregnancy. Justification becomes difficult if an operation takes twice as long if performed laparoscopically as opposed to traditional means. Just as the indications for laparoscopy are evolving so are the contraindications. These will be addressed in subsequent chapters. The general contraindications to laparoscopy will be described now.

When properly performed laparoscopy is a safe procedure. There are nonetheless circumstances in which it should either not be undertaken or performed with the greatest of caution.

Major contraindications

Under the following circumstances laparoscopy is extremely hazardous.

Severe cardiorespiratory disease. The patient who suffers from severe compromise of cardiopulmonary function is placed at risk by two mechanisms. The pressure exerted by the pneumoperitoneum may compress the vena cava and azygous system and hinder cardiac return, leading to cardiac decompensation. The diaphragm may be splinted, both by the pneumoperitoneum and by the weight of the intra-abdominal organs which fall cephalad when the patient is placed in the Trendelenberg position. This splinting will reduce respiratory tidal flow. The build up of carbon dioxide may be further aggravated by absorption of gas from the pneumoperitoneum. The resultant hypercarbia may cause cardiac arrhythmias.

The decision to operate on such patients will be influenced by the opinion of the anesthetist and by the anticipated length of the procedure.

Large abdominal and diaphragmatic hernia. In both cases the pressure exerted by the pneumoperitoneum may aggravate large hernias by forcing the contents through the hernial orifice. Strangulation of an abdominal hernia can then occur. The presence of abdominal contents in the thoracic cavity may further embarrass cardiorespiratory function. This advice obviously is not valid if the indication for the laparoscopy was to repair the hernia.

Generalized peritonitis. The ileus associated with severe generalized peritonitis places the distended bowel at risk of perforation by either the Veress needle or the primary trocar and cannula. In such gravely ill patients the underlying cause of the peritonitis will probably be amenable to treatment only by laparotomy.

Severe ileus-intestinal obstruction. In all such patients, except in those in whom the obstruction is believed to be due to bowel adhesions, the gynecologist is well advised to avoid laparoscopy because of the possibility of bowel perforation. Gynecologists of consummate surgical skills have been able to perform laparoscopic adhesiolysis but their patients have had to accept the risk of bowel trauma. Gastrointestinal surgeons are exploring the possibilities of laparoscopic bowel resection, but these techniques do not fall within the purview of the gynecologist.

Inexperienced surgeon. The days of "see one, do one, teach one" are long gone. No one who is incompletely trained should attempt to carry out a laparoscopy.

Relative contraindications

There are circumstances in which, although indicated, laparoscopy should be performed with more than usual caution.

Prior abdominal surgery or inflammatory bowel disease. Bowel can become adherent to any peritoneal scar, a risk that increases with the number of times that the abdomen has been opened. The techniques used to minimize risk have been described in Chapter 5. This risk is magnified if the previous laparotomy had been performed for peritonitis, bowel resection, or to create a neostomy. The patient in whom a diagnosis of regional ileitis or ulcerative colitis has been made should be approached with the same degree of caution. It is imperative that these patients are clearly informed of these additional risks.

Extremes of body weight. Particular hazards may be encountered in both the very obese and the very thin patient. The strategies to be used are described in Chapter 5.

Intrauterine pregnancy. Pain is the most common contraindication for the performance of laparoscopy in the pregnant patient. The larger the gravid uterus the greater the possibility that it might be traumatized or that it will obscure the areas that the surgeon wishes to examine. The value of laparoscopy must be questioned after the uterus has attained the size of 16 weeks.

Large intra-abdominal mass. It was previously stated, "Only under the most unusual circumstances would laparoscopy be the approach of choice in the patient with a large mass. The risks to the intra-abdominal contents, including the mass itself, are greatly increased and the value of the laparoscopic evaluation diminished."[1] This advice requires modification in light of recent developments. A useful concept is that it is no longer the size of the mass but the degree of skill of the surgeon that is the determining factor. If the surgeon is confident that the mass can be dealt with laparoscopically or the indication is purely diagnostic, laparoscopy is not contraindicated, although the patient should consent to laparotomy if it becomes necessary. Laparotomy is still the primary approach when it is apparent preoperatively that laparoscopic removal would not be feasible. The general principles of diagnostic laparoscopic technique in such patients have been described in Chapter 5. The specific details of management of ovarian tumours, uterine fibroids, and pelvic abscesses will be discussed later in this book.

Displaced or enlarged organs. Particular care must be taken in patients in whom it is recognized that intra-abdominal organs are misplaced or enlarged. A pelvic kidney will lie in the direct line of advance of the Veress needle, trocars, and cannulas. The spleen of a patient who suffers from malaria or hematogenous cancer may be sufficiently enlarged as to extend to the iliac fossa. Its borders must be delineated and the decision made as to whether or not laparoscopy can be performed safely.

REFERENCES

1. Gomel V, Taylor PJ, Yuzpe AA, Rioux JE: Laparscopy and hysteroscopy in gynecologic practice. Chicago, 1986, Year Book Medical Publishers.

Chapter 7

PRINCIPLES OF OPERATIVE LAPAROSCOPY

There are aspects of technique that are particular to each specific operative procedure and these will be described in succeeding chapters. The principles of operative laparoscopy are common to all surgical interventions and will be discussed in this chapter.

The general principles include:

- Patient selection
- Preoperative care
- Operating room setup
- Anesthesia and general preparation
- Prerequisites for safety
- Placement of secondary portals

The fundamentals of surgical technique include:

- Hemostasis
- Knotting techniques
- Dissection (to include adhesiolysis, which so often must be performed as a preparatory step)
- Removal of tissue
- Pelvic lavage and prevention of adhesion formation
- Wound closure
- General postoperative care

GENERAL PRINCIPLES

Patient selection

Operative laparoscopy should only be performed by a fully trained surgeon who is able not only to carry out the definite procedure but is skilled in the recognition and management of any complications that might arise. Patients should have given fully informed consent and should have indicated preoperatively whether or not they are willing to have the operation completed through a laparotomy incision if the laparoscopic approach proves to be inadequate or if complications warrant such intervention.

Only indicated procedures should be carried out, and clearly the contraindications described in Chapter 6 must be observed. If these conditions are satisfied, the decision must be taken about the suitability of any given patient for admission either to a day care or in-patient facility. In many institutions the in-patient function will be sited in a short stay unit. This decision will depend upon the nature of the operation to be performed and the patient's suitability for general anesthesia in a day care setting. The American Society of Anesthesiologists has introduced a classification system, the ASA system (see box on p. 72). In general only ASA 1 and 2 patients will be suitable candidates for laparoscopic surgery, most of which can be performed in a day care facility.

A general history should be taken and a physical examination performed. A minimum of routine laboratory testing is required, but the hemoglobin level should be measured and, in the case of an anemic patient who is to undergo elective surgery, the anemia should be corrected. Cross matching or banking of autologous blood will be required only for major procedures. Routine urinalysis provides little information except in those patients with a history of urinary tract symptoms. In such patients any urinary infection should be treated before surgery. Material is obtained, if indicated, from the cervix and vagina for microbiologic evaluation. Any infection so identified should be treated preoperatively. (See lower box on p. 72.)

Preoperative care

Very little preoperative preparation is required. Unless a Foley catheter is to be inserted, which should be done after the patient is anesthetized, she should void immediately preoperatively. Bowel preparation is rarely necessary but must

The American Society of Anesthesiologists' classification of physical status

Class 1

The patient has no organic, physiologic, biochemical, or psychiatric disturbance. The pathologic process for which surgery is to be performed is localized and does not entail a systemic disturbance.

Class 2

Mild to moderate systemic disturbance caused either by the condition or to be treated surgically or by other pathophysiologic processes

Class 3

Severe systemic disturbance or disease from whatever cause, even though it may not be possible to define the degree of disability with finality.

Class 4

Severe systemic disorders that are already life threatening and not always correctable by operation.

Class 5

The moribund patient who has little chance of survival but is submitted to operation in desperation.

Components of the preoperative investigation in surgical laparoscopy

Suitability for out-patient vs. in-patient surgery
Complete history
Thorough physical examination
Laboratory tests as indicated
Hemoglobin level measurements
Correction of anemia as necessary
Banking of autologous blood*
Cervical and vaginal cultures and treatment as necessary
Informed consent

*In major procedures only.

be undertaken whenever it is believed that the large bowel may be at risk. Antibiotic prophylaxis is not used routinely. In those patients who are at increased risk of infection, antibiotics (usually a cephalosporin) are administered preoperatively by the intravenous route.

Shaving is not required, but it is advisable to clip small areas of the pubic hair if it is anticipated that secondary portals might be established at these sites.

Operating room setup

Operative laparoscopy is performed most successfully by a team that is thoroughly familiar with the procedures to be performed and the instruments to be used. This familiarity is enhanced by the following clearly defined routines. One such routine is setting up the operating room.

There is no one way in which an operating room should be configured, as this will be the function of the limitations of the physical space and the preferences of individual surgeons. As a general principle, however, the physical space should be large enough to accommodate the surgical team and their equipment. If several senior surgeons use a laparoscopic facility, they should endeavour to agree upon a mutually acceptable standardized way of setting up.

The following description is meant to serve as a template, but is not to be considered a dictum. Consideration must be paid to the placement of the personnel, anesthesia equipment, imaging equipment, energy sources, insufflator, suction, and lavage equipment, table for vaginal instruments, table for basic laparoscopy set, and table for all potentially needed ancillary instruments.

Personnel. The operating team will vary from one composed of a surgeon, nurse, circulating nurse, and an anesthetist when minor surgical procedures are undertaken to a full team for major procedures of a surgeon, nurse, circulating nurse, one or two assistants, and anesthetist. For surgeons who use the laser, a laser technician will also be present within the operating room. It is important that all members of the surgical team have freedom of movement and do not hinder each other's actions.

If a minor procedure is being performed, a right-handed surgeon will generally stand on the patient's left and the nurse, who is assisting, on the patient's right or between the patient's thighs. The circulating nurse will act as required. When the full team is working, a right-handed surgeon again will usually stand on the left but may need to move to the patient's right or between the patient's legs. The scrub nurse will usually remain to the surgeon's left and the assistants will be positioned either between the patient's legs or to the right, depending on the needs of the surgery. Once again the circulating nurse will help and if a laser technician is in the operating room, the technician will be with the laser at all times. The anesthetist will always be at the top of the table (Fig. 7-1).

Anesthesia equipment. The anesthesia equipment, the anesthetic machine, drug trolley, and any necessary monitors should be at the head of the table. All suction and electrical leads should be positioned so that they do not become entangled with similar leads for the operative procedure. The equipment should be placed in such a way that the surgical team has freedom of movement through an arc of 240 degrees from the left-hand side of the anesthetist's screen to the right-hand side of the anesthetist's screen.

Imaging equipment. A single monitor is satisfactory for minor procedures. For more major procedures it is very helpful to have a primary monitor for the surgeon and a secondary monitor so that the nurse and assistant or assistants can follow the procedure. It is usual to have the primary monitor light source and video recording equipment

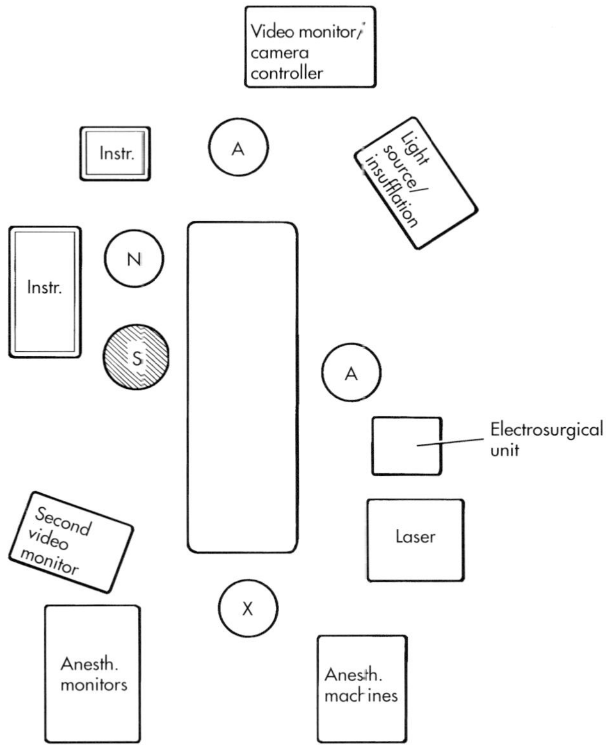

Fig. 7-1. Operating room set up.

mounted on a wheeled stand. The secondary monitor is also mounted on a wheeled stand or may be ceiling mounted. Once the surgical team has been positioned, the monitors are set up in such a way that the surgeon and assistants are looking at the screens *en face*. This would mean that for a minor procedure the primary monitor will be between the patient's legs and for a major procedure if an assistant is to work between the patient's legs this monitor must be moved to one or the other side of the assistant so that the surgeon's view is not interrupted. Usually the primary monitor is situated caudally and the secondary monitor cephalad so as to be easily seen by the assistant(s) and scrub nurse (Fig. 7-1).

Energy sources. Electrosurgical generators and, when indicated, lasers should be positioned close together so that either the circulating nurse or the laser technician can adjust the settings conveniently as required. They are usually placed to the patient's right and somewhat cephalad so that they are clear of the operating team and any necessary leads from the equipment to the patient are well out of the way. While it is quite possible to perform laparoscopic surgery with electrosurgical means alone, if a laser is being used the electrosurgical equipment must be available and the ground plate connected to the patient in case it is necessary to use electrosurgery to secure hemostasis.

Insufflator(s) suction and lavage equipment. Insufflators must be sufficiently close to the patient so that the gas line reaches the cannula without being under undue tension. While these insufflators can be stacked in the same trolley as either the electrosurgical equipment or the imaging equipment, lavage suction pumps should be kept separate from electrosurgical generators because of the risk of fluid spillage causing shorts.

Instrument tables. The table that carried the instruments for vaginal and on occasion rectal manipulation will be used early in the procedure and will then be pushed out of the operative area. If it is anticipated that vaginal operative procedures are to be performed, these sterile instruments should be on a separate table covered with a sterile towel which is kept out of the operative area until they are required. The nurse should have in close proximity a small table upon which are set up the basic pieces of laparoscopic equipment. In the standard setup this is usually to the nurse's left in close proximity to the patient's left leg. A larger table should be placed near both the surgeon and the scrub nurse so that both have easy access to any ancillary surgical instruments that may be required during the surgery (Fig. 7-1).

Because of the complexity of the equipment used, unless attention is paid at the start of the procedure to the arrangement of all gas insufflation lines, light cables, lavage tubing, suction tubing, and electrosurgical leads, a mare's nest of tubing and cables can occur, hindering the actions of surgeon, nurse, and assistant(s). It is very important that such cables and lines be set out in a logical, sequential fashion so that they do not become entangled.

An adhesive plastic pocket, designed rather like a carpenter's apron, is commercially available that can be affixed to the drapes of one or other thigh. It is very useful for receiving and holding frequently used and changed instruments so that they are more accessible to the surgeon and assistant than those on the rather more distantly placed table.

Anesthesia and general preparation

With the exception of tubal sterilization, which can be performed with the patient under local anesthesia, general anesthesia (usually with muscle relaxation, endotracheal intubation, and controlled positive pressure ventilation) will be used for operative cases.

If local anesthesia is used the patient is usually also given an intravenous narcoleptic agent. The sites of the primary cannula and secondary portal are injected with 0.25% of bupivacaine (Marcaine) or 0.5% lidocaine (Xylocaine). Each layer of the abdominal wall must be infiltrated. It is also usual to drip local anesthetic solution onto the segment of the tube to be occluded by inserting a spinal needle through the secondary portal. Because of the exquisite sensitivity of the parietal peritoneum all movements of the instruments must be deliberate and gentle.

The agents used to produce general anesthesia are within the purview of the anesthetist. Certain basic principles should be observed. While the anesthetist may wish to use an arm board to establish an intravenous line and induce anesthesia, use of these boards can place the brachial plexus at risk when the patient is placed in the Trendelenberg position. Once anesthesia has been established the arm should be placed at the side, taking care to ensure that the limb is not at risk from any moving parts of the table. The deep Trendelenberg position may also place pressure on the brachial plexus if shoulder restraints are used. As little as 15 minutes of such pressure can result in nerve damage. It is preferable to use nonslip mattresses or, if they are not available, to make certain that any shoulder restraints are properly positioned.

Once the patient is asleep the legs are placed in the stirrups. The abdomen, perineum, and vagina should be washed with an antiseptic solution and draped. The surgeon must be assured that the bladder is empty. If it is not, the patient should be catheterized. This is also the time when any necessary indwelling catheter is inserted. A thorough bimanual examination is performed. Any intrauterine or intrarectal manipulative instruments are fixed in place. The abdomen is palpated and percussed to identify any masses or evidence of organomegaly (see Chapter 5). The surgery may now proceed.

Safety prerequisites

The objective of laparoscopic surgery is to complete the procedure successfully with an absolute minimum of risk to the patient. To do so, certain safety precautions should be observed that are universal, no matter which specific operation is being performed. Some have already been mentioned but bear repeating. Only fully trained surgeons should operate on fully informed patients for a clearly appropriate indication in the absence of any contraindications. In addition:

The patient should be under general anesthesia with muscle relaxation and the bladder and, when necessary, the bowel should be empty.

Unless there is reason to the contrary, the surgeon must be able to manipulate the uterus with a rigid intrauterine mobilizer. In cases in which tubal patency is to be tested, the mobilizer should have chromopertubation capability.

All the instruments that will or potentially will be required should be present in the operating room, sterilized, and in perfect working order (see Chapter 3). All energy sources must be working and properly insulated and grounded. Safety precautions for the use of lasers must be observed.

Assistants and nursing staff should be skilled and familiar with their roles and the equipment.

A proper pneumoperitoneum must be achieved and maintained so that there is always adequate space in the peritoneal cavity in which to work.

The patient must be placed in deep Trendelenberg position for pelvic procedures and bowel manipulated away from the operative site.

Prior to beginning any operative procedure the surgeon must identify all the intrapelvic and intra-abdominal landmarks and the lesion which is to be removed or corrected.

Nothing should be cut, electrodessicated, lasered, ligated, or sutured until it has been identified and the surgeon is assured that there is sufficient distance between this tissue and the surrounding structures so that they are protected from injury.

Placement of secondary portals

Details of placement and positioning of secondary portals have been given in Chapter 5. In principle, blood vessels of the anterior abdominal wall, particularly the inferior epigastric vessels, must be avoided. Transillumination of the anterior abdominal wall may reveal the superficial vessels. It will be necessary to identify the obliterated umbilical arteries and to place secondary portals medial or well lateral to them to avoid damage to the inferior epigastric vessels. Self-retaining cannulas are used during prolonged procedures to prevent slippage and the development of subcutaneous emphysema. The ancillary portals are sited so that the ancillary instruments can be used to their best mechanical advantage and far enough from the operative site that the instruments' actions are not impeded. Furthermore they must be sited sufficiently distant from each other so that the instruments and telescope can be moved freely.

FUNDAMENTALS OF SURGICAL TECHNIQUE

There are certain basic steps that are integral to every surgical procedure. These steps include securing hemostasis, tissue dissection and division, removal of the specimen, pelvic lavage, and wound closure. Each will be described below; steps integral to specific procedures are discussed in Chapters 13 through 26.

Hemostasis

It is always preferable to prevent rather than stop bleeding. Smaller vessels may be induced to constrict by earlier injection of vasopressive substances. The surgeon must ensure that the solution is properly diluted. Vasopressin can be used in a concentration of 5 IU to 10 IU in 100 ml of normal saline. Concentrated solutions can have spectacular effects on the blood pressures of both patient and anesthetist. Epinephrine in a concentration of 1:200,000 is more likely to produce cardiac arrhythmias and be followed by reactionary hemorrhage when its results have worn off.

Laparoscopic surgery has the additional advantages that the intra-abdominal pressure is elevated to a level that is usually higher than the blood pressure in small vessels, and the warm irrigation solutions used also have a hemostatic effect.

Every endeavour should be made to occlude blood vessels prior to their division. To do so may require that an individual vessel be identified (e.g., the uterine artery or vein). Alternatively the pedicle which contains vascular structures can be secured (e.g., the infundibulo-pelvic ligament).

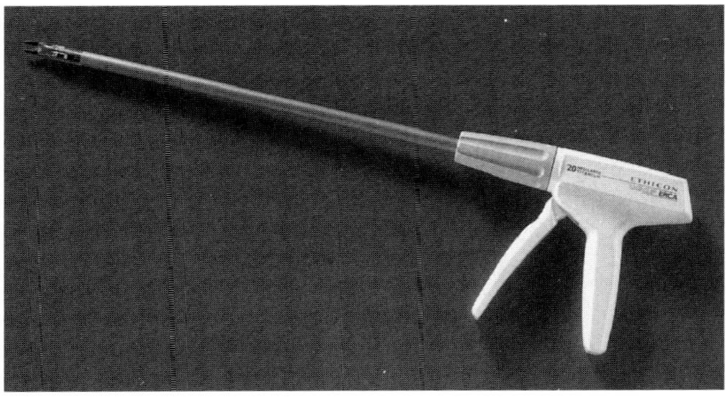

Fig. 7-2. Multiple clip applicator.

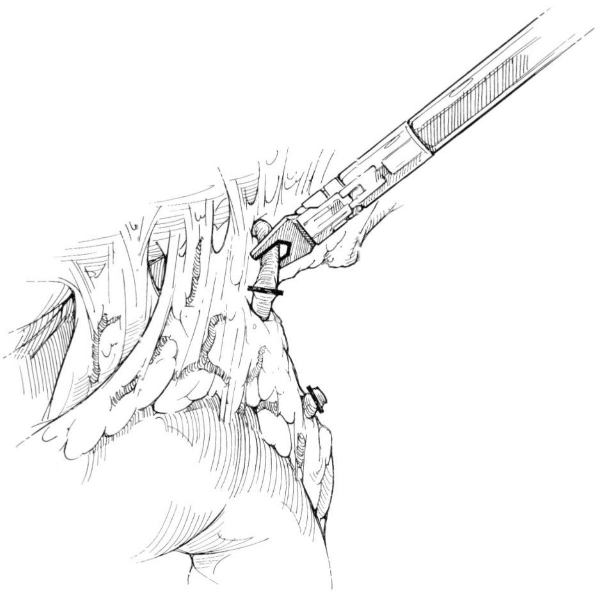

Fig. 7-3. Clip application prior to division of vessel.

Securing intact blood vessels. Occlusion of vessels can be effected with electrical energy, clips, ligatures, or suture ligatures.

The method chosen for occlusion will depend upon the location, caliber of the vessel, and the surgeon's preference. Vessels that are in close proximity to vital structures should not be electrodessicated. Use of clips, ligatures, or suture ligatures is preferable under these circumstances.

Electrodesiccation. Vessels up to the size of the uterine artery can be electrodessicated. If electrodesiccation is used to secure hemostasis the following principles apply:

All but small vessels must be skeletonized.

The flow of blood in the vessel must be interrupted, otherwise the energy will be dissipated. This interruption of flow can be achieved by compression of the vessel with forceps with either monopolar or bipolar capability.

No current should be passed until the surgeon is satisfied that only the vessels will be electrodessicated.

Current of sufficient intensity must be applied until complete desiccation has occurred.

Division should not be carried out until a sufficient length of the vessel has been occluded.

Clip application. Clip applicators are available for single or multiple applications (Fig. 7-2). The vessel is identified and space created around it to accommodate the clip. Application is effected by placing the open clip around the vessel and firing the applicator. The vessel is divided between two clips (Fig. 7-3).

Ligatures and sutures. Vessels, particularly larger ones, can be ligated or suture ligated. These techniques are also applicable to the securing of pedicles. A detailed description of these techniques will be described later to avoid repetition.

Securing already divided blood vessels. If bleeding is encountered it is dealt with as follows. The bleeding vessel is identified, usually with the help of irrigation. Small vessels can be spot desiccated. Larger vessels must be clamped either with electrical forceps for desiccation (Fig. 7-4, *A*), or with simple grasping forceps if the vessel is to be clipped (Fig. 7-4, *B*), ligatured, or suture ligatured. It must not be forgotten that laparoscopic surgery should be regarded as laparotomy avoided. If reasonable laparoscopic methods fail to control hemorrhage the surgeon should feel no inhibition to proceeding to laparotomy to deal with the bleeding.

Securing of pedicles. Pedicles can be electrodessicated, ligated, suture ligatured, or stapled.

Electrodesiccation. The principles of the use of electrodesiccation have been described above. Thickness is the limiting factor to the use of electrodesiccation for securing pedicles. While this approach is effective for thin pedicles like the mesosalpinx, meso-ovarium, and round ligament, it is less effective and time consuming if applied to major pedicles. These are better dealt with by ligatures, suture ligatures, or stapling devices.

Ligatures and sutures. Laparoscopic suturing and knot trying are new skills for many surgeons and do take some time to master. Time spent on the pelvic-trainer acquiring facility with these techniques is well repaid by shorter operating times.

A ligature is a fine piece of material that is not attached to a needle. It is used to occlude a blood vessel or pedicle by enclosing it in a loop of the material and compressing the vessel or pedicle by tying a knot. Two types of ligatures are used during laparoscopic surgery: those with pretied knots and those where the knot must be tied extracorporeally or intraperitoneally.

The Roeder loop (Endoloop) has a pretied slip knot (Fig. 7-5). The loop provided prepackaged in a plastic applicator with a distal end that snaps off. The applicator serves as a knot pusher. To prevent loss of gas during the application of such a loop, an adaptor is inserted through a

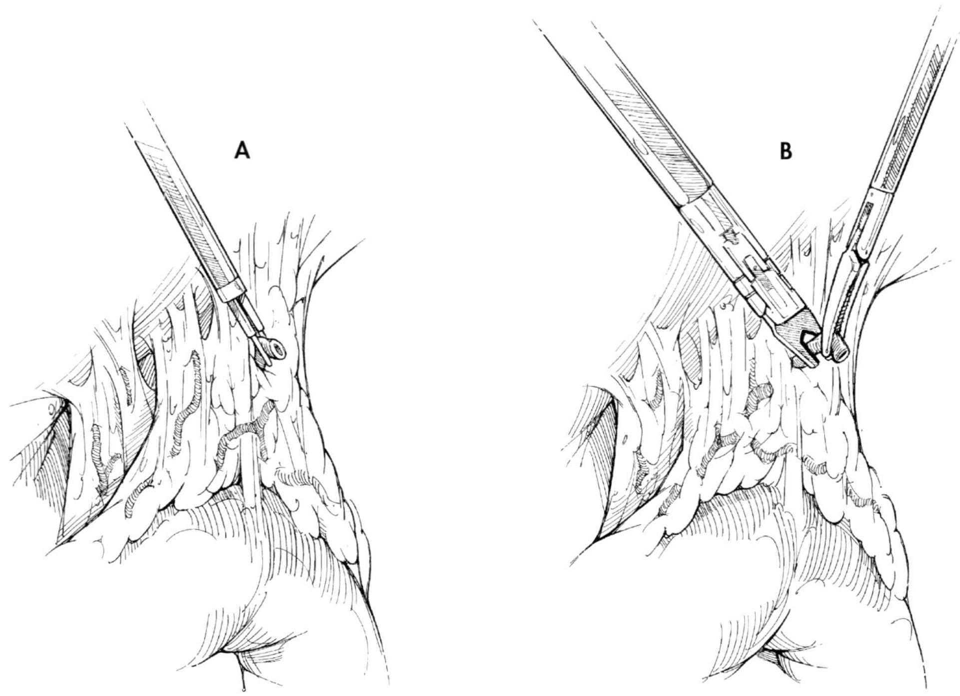

Fig. 7-4. Securing an already divided blood vessel. **A,** By bipolar electrodesiccation. **B,** By clip application.

5 mm cannula, unless special cannulas are used. The Endoloop fits through the adaptor (Fig. 7-5, *A*). The pedicle or vessel to be ligated is identified and the loop is placed over this structure. A grasping forceps is introduced through a contralateral portal, passed through the Roeder loop, and used to grasp the pedicle or vessel and elevate it through the loop (Fig. 7-5, *B*). The distal end of the applicator is then snapped off and the applicator is advanced to push the knot down onto the pedicle or vessel while tension is maintained with the grasping forceps to ensure that a sufficient piece of tissue is included in the tightening loop. The tip of the applicator is used to position the knot and tighten it (Fig. 7-5, *C*). After the knot has been tightened, the grasping forceps are replaced with scissors that are used to divide the ligature about 0.5 to 1 cm from the knot and to excise redundant tissue, if necessary (Fig. 7-5, *D* and *E*). The introducer and redundant ends of the ligature are now withdrawn. The pedicle or vessel is examined to ensure that it is dry. Second ligatures can be applied to larger pedicles.

A simple ligature is applied by carrying one of its ends into the peritoneal cavity with grasping forceps. These forceps are used to maneuver the ligature around the pedicle or vessel which are steadied by a second pair of grasping forceps. Once the ligature is satisfactorily placed, the end is withdrawn from the peritoneal cavity if an extraperitoneal knot is to be tied. Alternatively a shorter piece of material can be carried in its entirety within the peritoneal cavity, maneuvered into place, and knotted intracorporeally. These knotting techniques will be described later.

A suture is a piece of ligature material mounted on a needle. If the suture is used primarily to occlude a vessel or pedicle it is described as a suture-ligature. Sutures are also used for closing tissue defects. Suture ligatures and sutures can be inserted laparoscopically and the knot tied either extra- or intracorporeally. Sutures may be mounted on straight, ski type, or curved needles. The suture caliber can vary from 7-0 for delicate suturing to 1-0 to 3-0 for suturing and suture-ligating.

Straight and ski needles are introduced as follows. The suture is grasped by the needle holder close to its attachment to the needle. As the tip of the needle holder is placed in the cannula, the needle will hinge backward so that it lies parallel with the shaft of the needle holder and the point is directed away from the peritoneal cavity (Fig 7-6, *A*). The needle holder and needle are passed through the cannula until the needle can be seen. Grasping forceps that have been introduced through the contralateral cannula are used to steady the needle and position it so that it can be taken by the needle holder (Fig. 7-6, *B* and *C*).

Straight needles may be used for suture ligation. They are less satisfactory if the surgeon wishes to place a line of sutures. A ski needle is rather better for these purposes, but suturing is best carried out with a curved needle. Larger curve needles may simply be introduced through a 10 mm or 11 mm cannula. Such a needle can also be introduced easily through a 10mm cannula or through a 5 mm cannula by using the following approach:

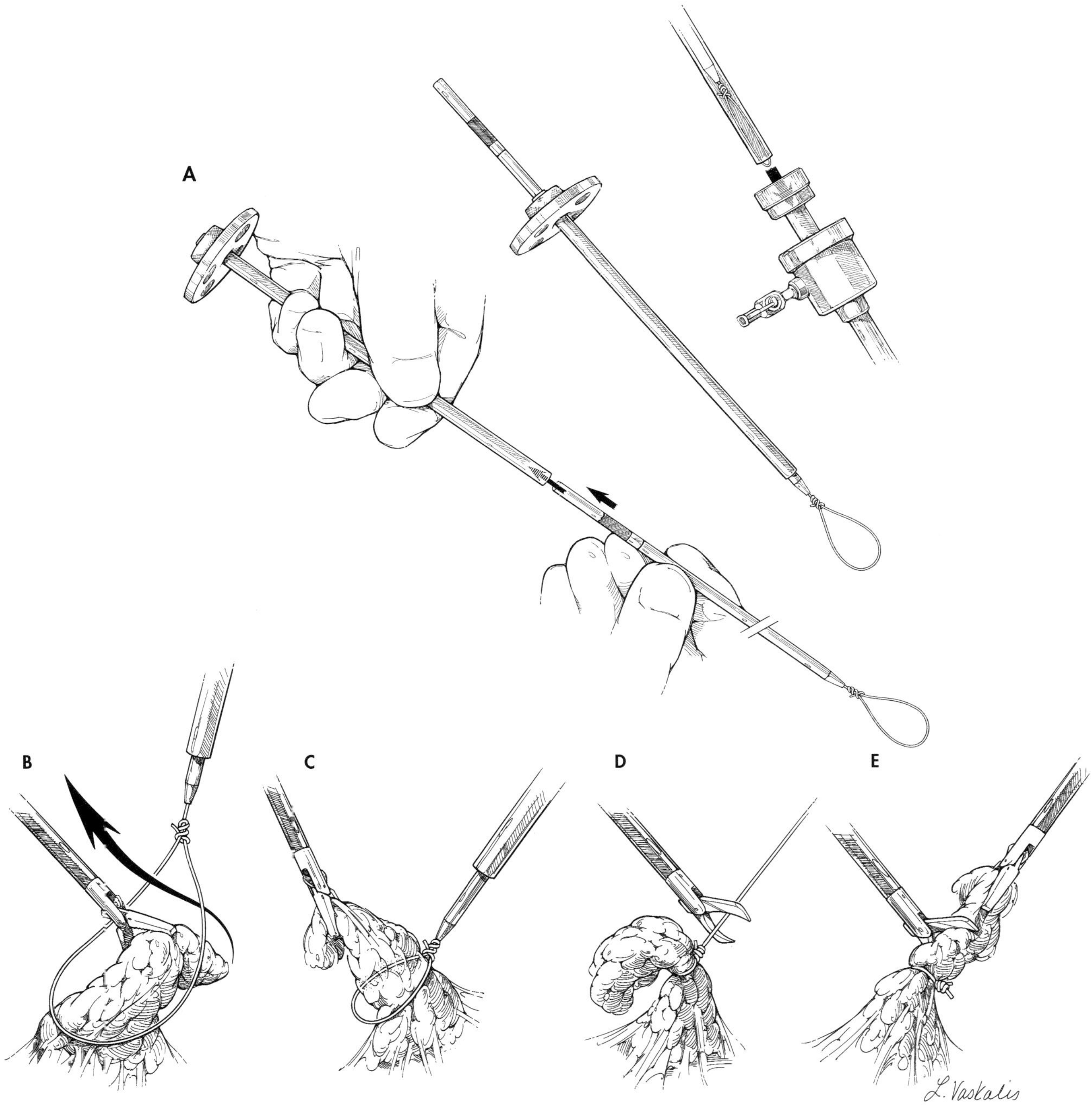

Fig. 7-5. Application of Roeder's loop. **A,** Loading the loop into the adaptor. **B,** Application of the loop. **C,** Tightening of the loop. **D,** Cutting ligature. **E,** Excision of redundant tissue.

The cannula is removed from the abdomen (Fig. 7-7, *A*) and the needle holder passed through the cannula.

The free end of the suture is grasped with the needle holder and pulled through the cannula (Fig. 7-7, *B*).

The needle holder is reinserted through the cannula and the suture grasped approximately 2 cm to 4 cm from the swage point (Fig. 7-7, *C*).

The cannula and the included needle holder are reintroduced, thus dragging the needle alongside through the cannula track into the peritoneal cavity (Fig 7-7, *D*).

The needle is regrasped with the holder (Fig. 7-7, *E*).

Alternatively, the suture can be grasped 10 cm or more from the swage point. The cannula is reintroduced, as before, dragging the suture alongside it. The suture, in the peritoneal cavity, is grasped with a pair of forceps or a second needle holder introduced through another portal (Fig. 7-7, *F*). The cannula is withdrawn once again and the needle is pulled through the cannula track into the peritoneal cavity (Fig. 7-7, *G*). Finally the cannula together with the enclosed needle holder are reinserted.

Suturing is effected by repositioning the grasping forceps to steady the tissue to be transfixed and passing the needle through the tissue until the tip of the needle can be seized by the grasping forceps. The needle is pulled through the tissue and passed back to the holder. To remove the needle from the peritoneal cavity (through a 5 mm cannula) the suture is grasped near the swage point, as before, with the needle holder within the auxillary cannula. The cannula, needle holder, and needle are withdrawn completely.

Knotting techniques

The knots of ligatures, suture ligatures, and sutures can be tied either intracorporeally or extracorporeally. The technique of knot tying of a suture ligature will be described. Essentially the same technique is used for simple ligatures although in this case there is no need to deal with the needle.

Extracorporeal knotting. The suture ligature has been introduced leaving one end extracorporeally. The needle has been passed through tissue and is safely held in the needle holder. The grasping forceps are used to pull more suture material into the peritoneal cavity and this loop is pulled through the tissue so that the needle has enough slack to be easily withdrawn to the surface. This is effected by holding straight or ski needles close to the swage point and withdrawing the needle holder into the cannula. Large curved needles are removed as previously described. Small curved ⅜ needles can be removed through the cannula.

Slip knot. The needle is cut from the suture and the two extracorporeal ends used to make a single throw knot which is held between the thumb and a finger (Fig. 7-8, *A*). A loop has now been formed between the single knot and the top of the introducer. One of the free ends is wrapped three times round this loop and brought between the sides of the loop and the bottom and middle of the three turns which have just been made (Fig. 7-8, *B*). Traction is now exerted on this end of the suture to tighten the knot and this short

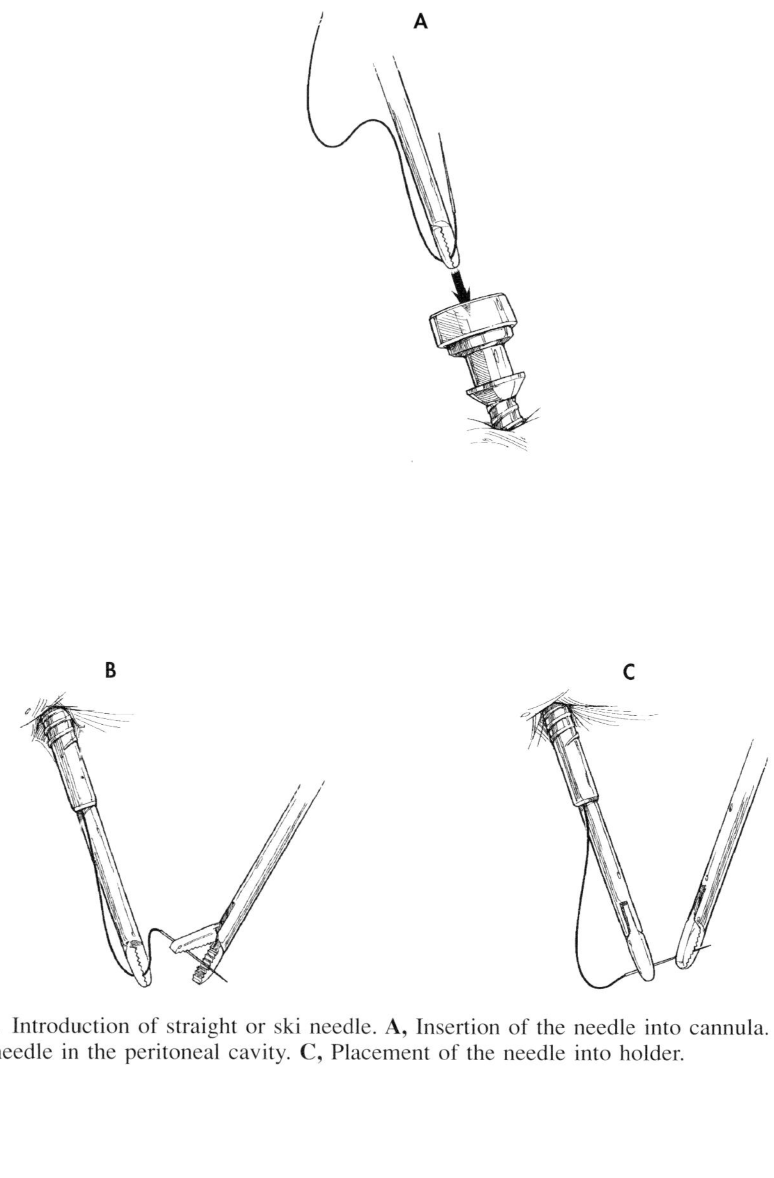

Fig. 7-6. Introduction of straight or ski needle. **A,** Insertion of the needle into cannula. **B,** Grasping the needle in the peritoneal cavity. **C,** Placement of the needle into holder.

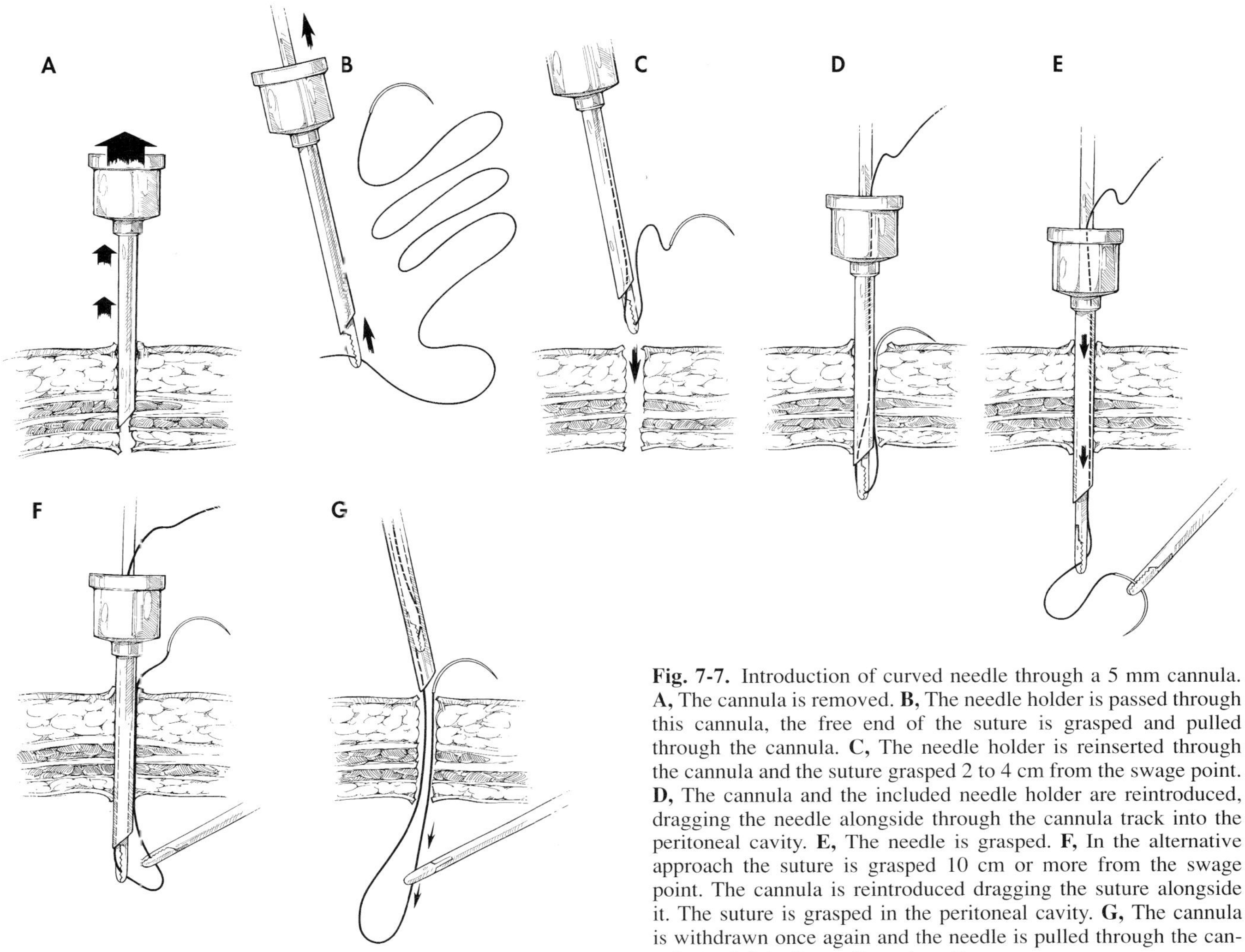

Fig. 7-7. Introduction of curved needle through a 5 mm cannula. **A,** The cannula is removed. **B,** The needle holder is passed through this cannula, the free end of the suture is grasped and pulled through the cannula. **C,** The needle holder is reinserted through the cannula and the suture grasped 2 to 4 cm from the swage point. **D,** The cannula and the included needle holder are reintroduced, dragging the needle alongside through the cannula track into the peritoneal cavity. **E,** The needle is grasped. **F,** In the alternative approach the suture is grasped 10 cm or more from the swage point. The cannula is reintroduced dragging the suture alongside it. The suture is grasped in the peritoneal cavity. **G,** The cannula is withdrawn once again and the needle is pulled through the cannula track into the peritoneal cavity.

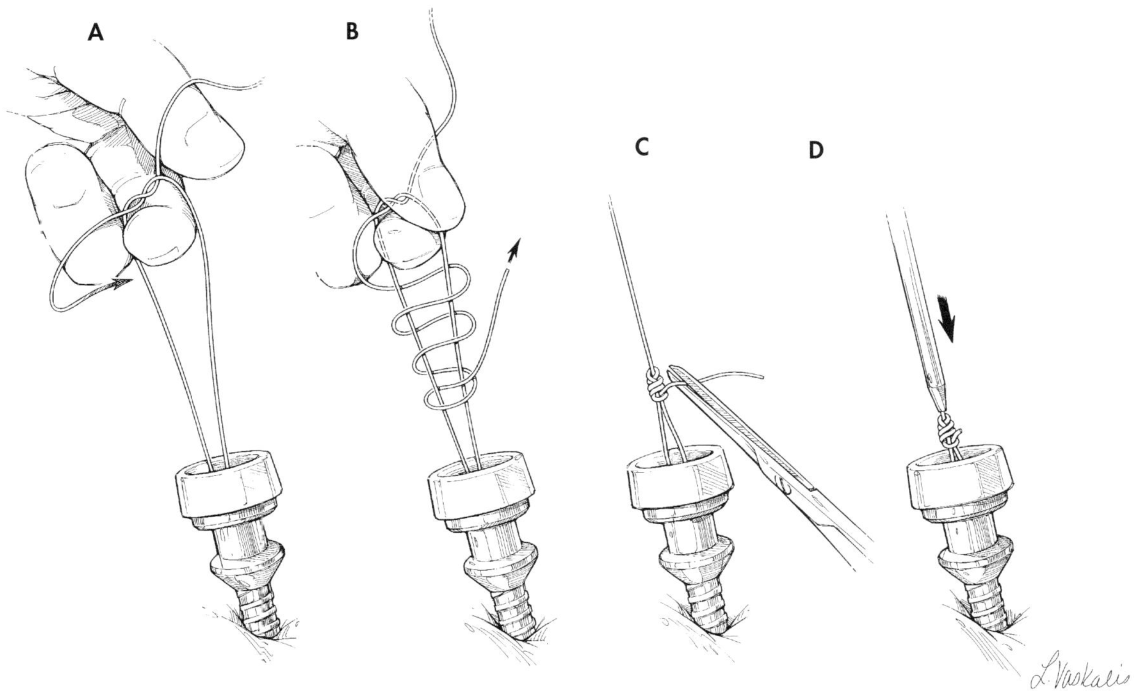

Fig. 7-8. Extracorporeal knotting: slipknot. **A,** The two extracorporeal ends of the suture are used to make a single throw knot. **B,** One of the free ends of the suture is used to form a slip knot. **C,** The slip knot is tightened and the short end is cut. **D,** The knot is pushed into place with the knot pusher.

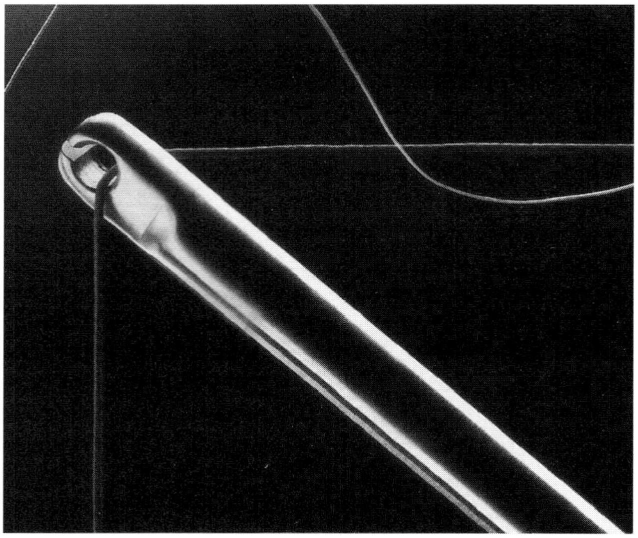

Fig. 7-9. The Clarke knot pusher. (Courtesy Marlow, Willoughby, Ohio.)

end is cut (Fig. 7-8, *C*). The long end of the suture is passed through a Roeder knot pusher, which is used to push the knot down into the abdomen and tighten it snugly in place (Fig. 7-8, *D*). Finally the long end is cut.

Surgical knot. An extracorporeal knot similar to the familiar surgical knot can be tied with the aid of a Clarke knot pusher (Fig. 7-9). This is a rigid instrument, the working end of which is a ring from which a small area has been removed. This allows the ring to be placed on the suture material. A single throw knot is tied and the Clarke knot pusher applied on the suture near the knot (Fig. 7-10, *A*). While maintaining tension on both ends of the suture the knot is maneuvered with the knot pusher through the cannula to its desired location (Fig. 7-10, *B*). This step is repeated to apply two or three more throws (Fig. 7-10, *C*). The suture is cut and redundant suture removed. When using this technique for knot tying the equipment should be introduced into the peritoneal cavity through an anciliary cannula without a trap valve.

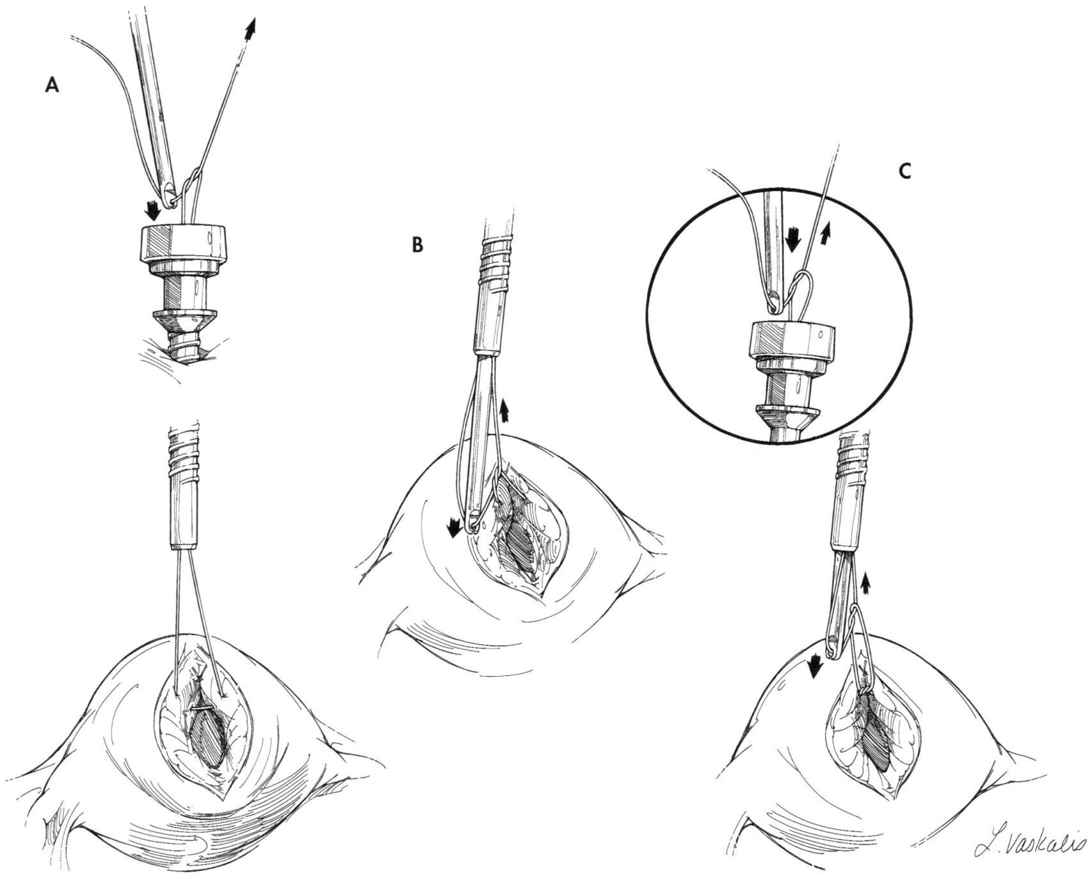

Fig. 7-10. Extracorporeal knotting: surgical knot. **A,** A single throw knot is tied and the Clarke knot pusher applied on the suture near the knot. **B,** The knot is maneuvered to its desired location. **C,** The above steps are repeated to apply two or three more throws.

Intracorpeal knotting. Intracorporeal knotting is performed in a manner similar to a routine instrument tie but is technically more difficult to master. If a suture has been placed, the suture is pulled through the tissue until a 4 to 5 cm tail is left. The needle is parked like a pin in a pin cushion in a convenient safe place. The needle holder is used to make a double loop of the long end of the suture around the head of the grasper. The grasper seizes the tail of the suture and pulls it through the double loop (Fig. 7-11, *A*). This first throw is pulled tight by traction and counter traction from grasper and holder (Fig. 7-11, *B*). A second double loop is made round the grasper (Fig. 7-11, *C*) and pulled tight to make a square flat knot (Fig. 7-11, *D*). The second double loop can be replaced by adding two or three additional single loops. Scissors are use to cut either both ends if a suture ligature has been inserted or the tail end if the surgeon wishes to place a continuous suture.

Once suturing or suture ligating has been completed, needles are removed as previously described.

Staples. Pedicles can be secured by using prepackaged commercially available automatic stapling devices (Fig. 7-12). The device is an applicator that contains a cartridge of staples and a cutting blade. The control mechanism is an external pistol grip. When the grip is compressed the tissue is enclosed within the jaws of the cartrige. The surgeon now is able to confirm that the application is satisfactory or release the jaws and reposition them. Once the instrument is properly positioned, the device is triggered. Six overlapping rows of staples transfix the tissue and the blade divides the tissue leaving three rows of staples on each side of the in-

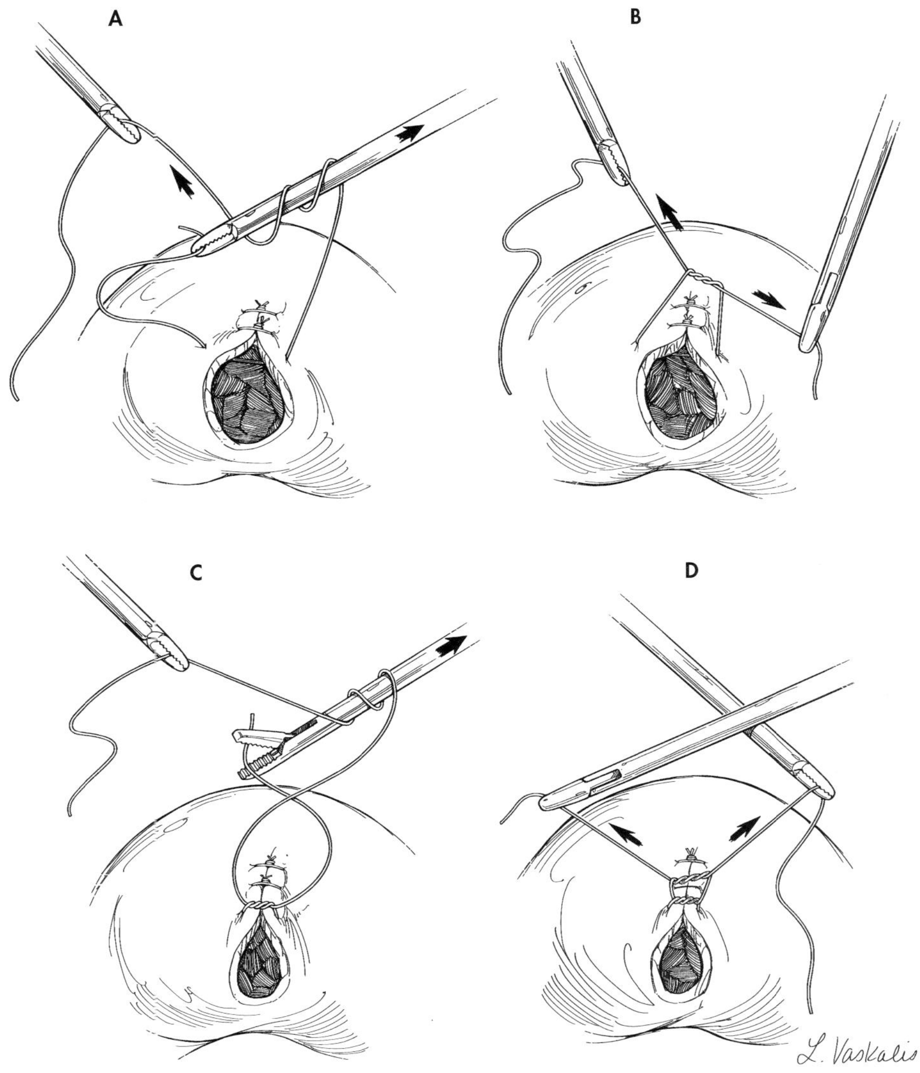

Fig. 7-11. Intracorporeal knotting. **A,** The needle holder is used to make a double loop of the long end of the suture around the head of the grasper. The grasper seizes the tail of the suture and pulls it through the double loop. **B,** This first throw is pulled tight. **C,** A second double loop is made around the grasper. **D,** Second double loop pulled tight to make a flat (square) knot.

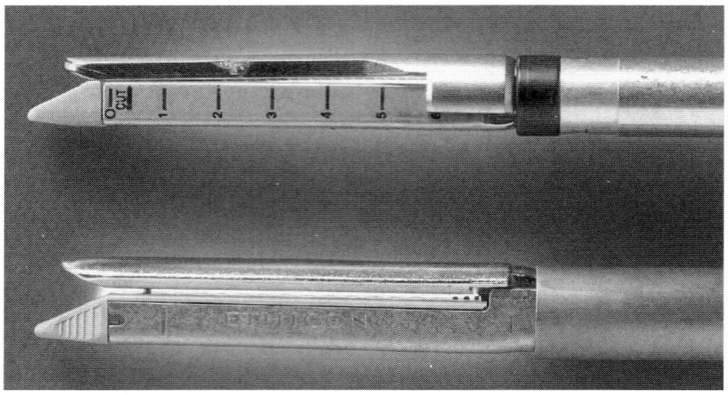

Fig. 7-12. Stapling device: Functional end. (Courtesy Ethicon Endo Surgical, Cincinnati, Ohio.)

cision. These six-row devices are of large caliber and include substantial widths of tissue. This means that a large ancillary cannula must be used and application of staples can be affected safely only where sufficient space exist. In addition, these devices, which are disposable, are very expensive. Smaller devices which will insert three overlapping rows of staples are well advanced in the developmental process.

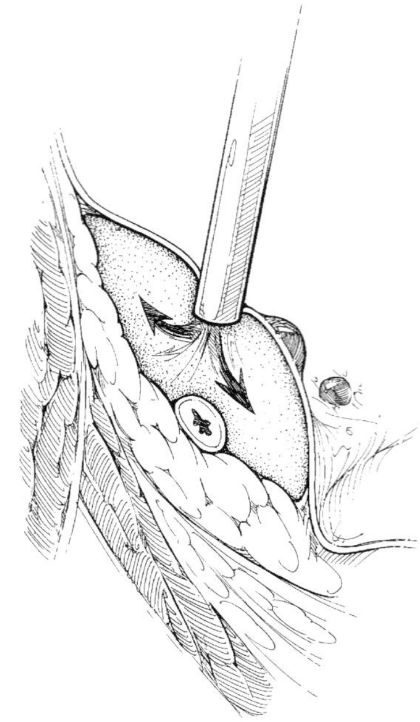

Fig. 7-13. Hydrodissection: The tip of the suction irrigation cannula is placed in the desired tissue plane and fluid is introduced under pressure.

Dissection

Tissue can be separated by either sharp or blunt dissection. Sharp dissection is performed with scissors, electrosurgical energy, or laser energy. The details have been described in Chapter 4.

Sharp dissection. The principles of sharp dissection include:

- Making every effort to occlude blood vessels prior to cutting
- Ensuring that the tissue to be divided has been properly identified and that everything in the path of the cutting instrument is under direct vision before, during, and after the cutting stroke is made
- Leaving enough tissue on a pedicle distal to any ligatures or staples to prevent slippage of the ligature or staples
- Dividing adhesions as close to healthy tissue as possible without putting the underlying tissue at risk
- Ensuring that vital structures are well away from the area to be divided
- Using countertraction to display the tissue to be cut

Blunt dissection. Blunt dissection is carried out by traction and countertraction with grasping forceps by opening the blades of scissors or grasping forceps between the tissue planes or by hydrodissection. The principles of mechanical blunt dissection will be enumerated. The technique of hydrodissection will be described in detail.

Blunt dissection should be performed in such a way to ensure that:

- No undue traction is ever placed on a vital structure
- Atraumatic forceps or blunt probes are used gently on tissues that are not to be divided or removed
- Blood vessels are skeletonised and occluded before they are disrupted
- Nothing that has not been identified is dissected

Hydrodissection. The use of copious lavage is an integral part of laparoscopic surgery. This lavage should be carried out with physiologic solutions (Ringer's lactate or saline to which heparin may be added when desirable) that are maintained at body temperature. Use of cold solutions during prolonged procedures can result in a significant lowering of the core temperature. The hydrostatic pressure of the lavage solution can be used to dissect tissue planes atraumatically.

The fluid can be introduced under pressure by simply wrapping a plastic bag of the solution in a pressure cuff. Automated pumps maintain a preset pressure. The suction-irrigation cannula is equipped with a two-way valve to control both functions.

The technique of hydrodissection is simple. The tip of the suction-irrigation cannula is placed in the desired tissue plane, either through a natural route of access or by creating a small aperture by sharp dissection. When the fluid is introduced under pressure, it will seek the path of least resistance, thus atraumatically creating a line of dissection and developing a tissue plane without putting adjacent organs at risk of perforation (Fig. 7-13). Once the planes have been displayed, they are more accessible to safe sharp division or blunt dissection with the tip of the irrigator. The fluid that accumulates behind the tissue planes can also be used as a backstop for the carbon dioxide laser.

Adhesiolysis. It is frequently necessary to perform a preliminary adhesiolysis to gain access to the operative site. To avoid repetition in subsequent chapters this technique will be described here.

All of the principles of securing hemostasis and dissection must be observed. As a general rule, filmy adhesions are usually avascular and are amenable to sharp or blunt dissection. Dense, fatty adhesions tend to be vascular but will often have avascular areas that can be used to gain access to the tissue layers to identify and occlude their major blood vessels. Lysis of cohesive adhesions will necessitate development of a dissection plane by sharp and blunt dissection and hydrodissection. Very fibrous and extremely cohesive adhesions, usually secondary to previous pelvic surgery or repeated severe infections, may not be amenable to laparoscopic dissection.

The performance of safe adhesiolysis requires the observation of the following measures:

Dissection should always commence in well exposed areas.
Each adhesive layer must be clearly identified, grasped, and retracted to achieve optimal exposure.
It is essential to recognize what lies behind the adhesion before dissection begins.
Transection must be carried out parallel to the organ of interest.
Adhesions must be divided one layer at a time.
Shallow adhesions are simply transected. Broad adhesions are excised by dividing them both along the organ of interest and at their distal attachments and removed from the peritoneal cavity.
Transection can be achieved mechanically using sharp scissors, electrosurgically, or with laser energy.
Scissor division can be effected close to vital structures but sufficient distance must be maintained if electrosurgery or laser is being used.
The instrument used for division must approach the tissue to be divided at a right angle.
Vessels encountered along the transection line should be electrodesiccated prior to division.

Adhesions may have to be removed from three sites: the anterior abdominal wall (to permit safe placement of secondary portals), loops of bowel, and the pelvic structures. Omental adhesions can be very vascular and, if they are adherent to the anterior abdominal wall, it may be difficult to establish a proper line of approach. This difficulty can often be overcome by introducing a 5 mm laparoscope through one of the secondary portals and effecting the dissection from a caudad start point. Such fatty vascular adhesions should be divided one layer at a time, skeletonizing and occluding blood vessels when possible. Broad vascular adhesions may be desiccated or ligated prior to division (Fig. 7-14).

Filmy shallow adhesions are simply divided, occluding the infrequent blood vessel that will be encountered prior to division (Fig. 7-15). Broad adhesions are divided at both ends and removed. When, as is often the case, these adhesions are multilayered, they should be divided one layer at a time. Hydrodissection is a simple way of developing these layers.

With cohesive adhesions it will be necessary to identify the proper dissection plane. This is achieved by placing a small incision between the two adherent structures (Fig. 7-16, *A*) and by developing a plane either by spreading the jaws of the scissors, by blunt dissection, or by hydrodissection (Fig. 7-16, *B*). No thermal energy should be used in such cases.

Adhesions between loops of bowel are tethered at both ends to a particularly vulnerable structure. The cleavage planes should be developed by using hydrodissection and the adhesions divided at their mid-points using scissors to avoid any potential spread of electrical or laser energy to the bowel wall.

Once the adhesiolysis has been completed, copious lavage is performed and, unless the returning fluid is clear, the areas of division are examined to identify and deal with any residual bleeding points.

Removal of excised tissue

The removal of excised tissue can present an interesting technical challenge.

Removal of small specimens. Small specimens can be pulled through one of the ancillary cannulae. Softer, readily dividable tissues, such as fallopian tube, normal ovary, or products from an ectopic gestation may be removed either intact or morcellated through an 11 mm cannula. If a 10 mm laparoscope has been used for the procedure and if a laparoscope with an operating channel (operating laparoscope, Jacob-Palmer) is available, this telescope is used. A strong grasping forceps is introduced through the operating channel of the laparoscope and the specimen is grasped and removed together with the laparoscope through the 11 mm cannula. Cannulas with automatic trap valves hinder removal of specimens.

If a laparoscope with an operating channel is not available, a 5 mm laparoscope is introduced through one of the auxiliary portals for viewing purposes. A strong grasping forceps is inserted through the principal (11 mm) cannula to retrieve the specimen. With certain cannulas it will be necessary to use a reducer if the grasping forceps is of 5 mm caliber.

The third option, if neither an operating laparoscope nor a 5 mm scope is available, is to extend the skin incision of the suprapubic midline portal and replace the 5 mm cannula with an 11 mm cannula. To change the cannulas, a 5 mm probe without a handle (the same diameter throughout) is introduced into the peritoneal cavity through the suprapubic cannula while it is still in place. The cannula is

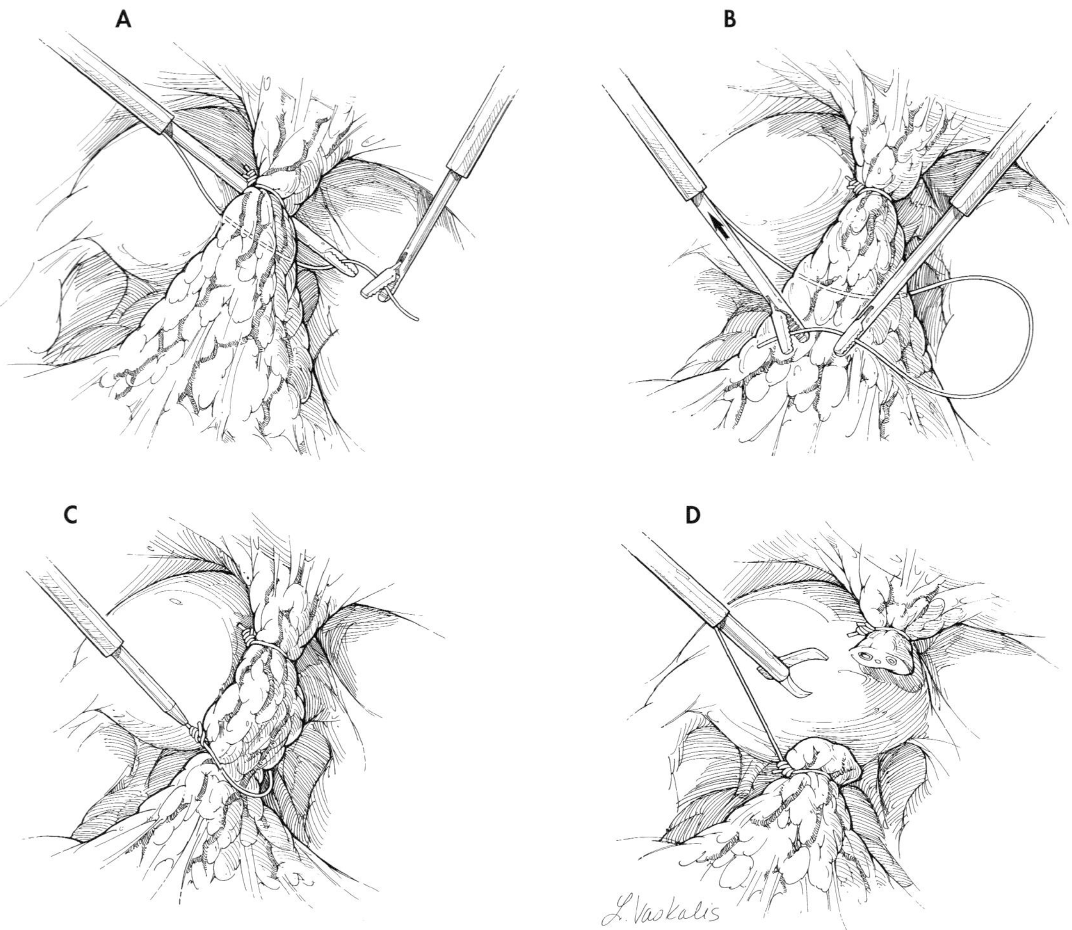

Fig. 7-14. Division of broad vascular adhesions. **A,** The adhesion has been ligated at one end. A second ligature is introduced. **B,** The second ligature is maneuvered around the vascular adhesion and the end pulled out through the cannula from which it had been introduced. **C,** A slip knot is tied extracorporeally. The long end of the suture is passed through a Roeder's knot pusher, which is used to push the knot down into the abdomen and to tighten it at the opposite end of the vascular adhesion. **D,** The adhesion is transected and the suture cut.

removed while the probe is left in its track. An 11 mm cannula is used together with a special trocar combination—a hollow trocar that has a grooved conical end and an opening both at the tip and at the top of the trocar—permitting the introduction of this trocar around the probe that remained in the track. The trocar cannula combination is passed over the probe and the grooved conical tip of the trocar is used to enlarge the track by rotating it in a clockwise manner. The larger cannula is thus introduced through the same but enlarged track into the peritoneal cavity. The specimen is retrieved through this cannula.

Removal of large specimens. Removal of large specimens continues to present a serious challenge for the surgeon. Specimens that are too large to be removed intact fall into one of two categories: either their intact removal is indicated or desirable or morcellation presents no inconvenience. Teratomas and benign neoplastic ovarian cysts fall into the former category. Fibroids and an excised uterine corpus (after subtotal hysterectomy) fall into the latter group.

A colpotomy incision, either horizontal or vertical, can be made either by laparoscopy or by the vaginal route.

An abdominal incision is usually made by enlarging the suprapubic midline site of entry. The skin can be incised transversely and the incision carried down to the facia. The adipose layer is dissected from the fascia in the midline which is incised in the midline. The recti muscles are separated and the peritoneal opening enlarged.

Transabdominal removal of larger specimens may also be accomplished with the use of giant (20 mm and 33 mm diameter) cannulas. The introduction of such cannulas will necessitate a sufficiently large incision to accommodate them but will either permit removal of the specimen intact and without touching the abdom-

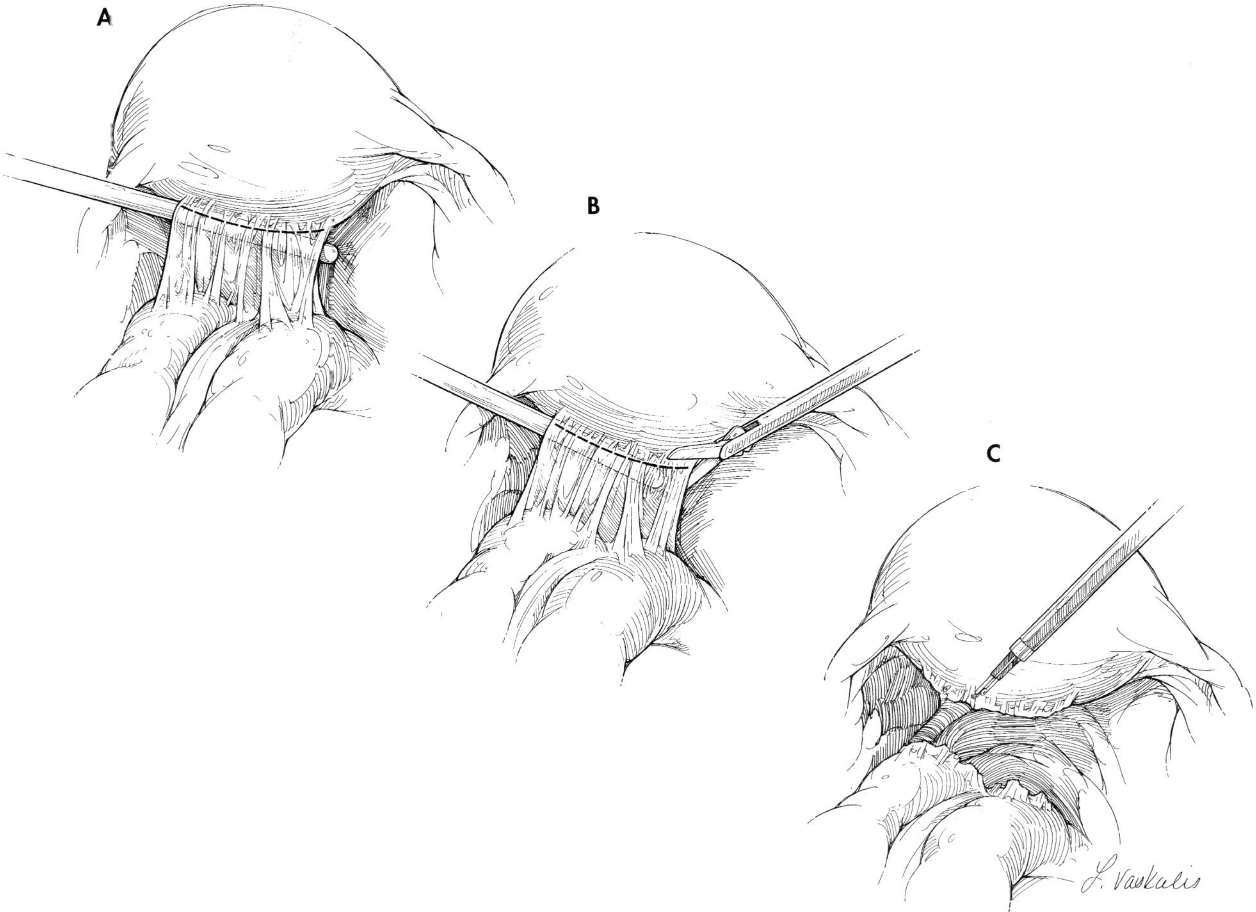

Fig. 7-15. Division of filmy adhesions. **A,** The adhesions are exposed. **B,** They are divided one layer at a time parallel to the organ of interest. **C,** Any bleeding vessels are visualized by irrigation and are electrodesiccated.

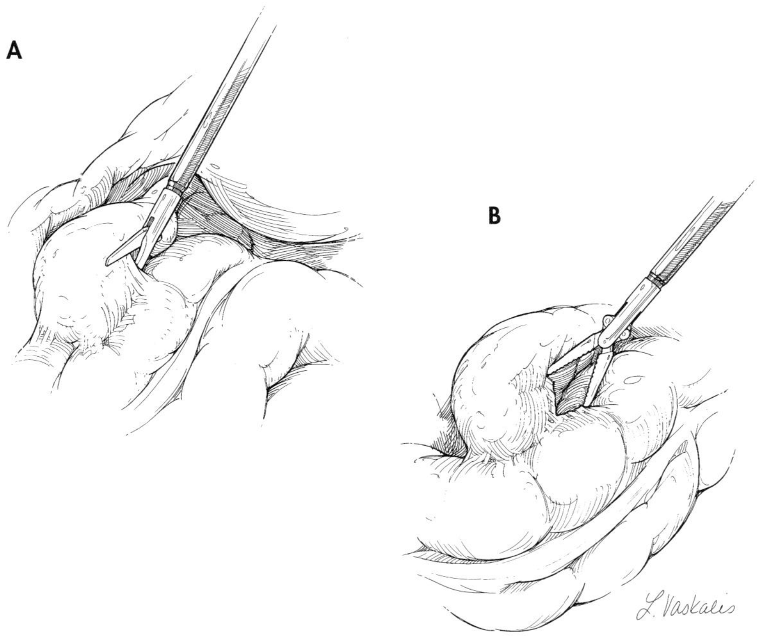

Fig. 7-16. Division of cohesive adhesions. **A,** A small incision is made between the two adherent structures. **B,** A dissection plane is developed by spreading the jaws of the scissors or dissecting forceps.

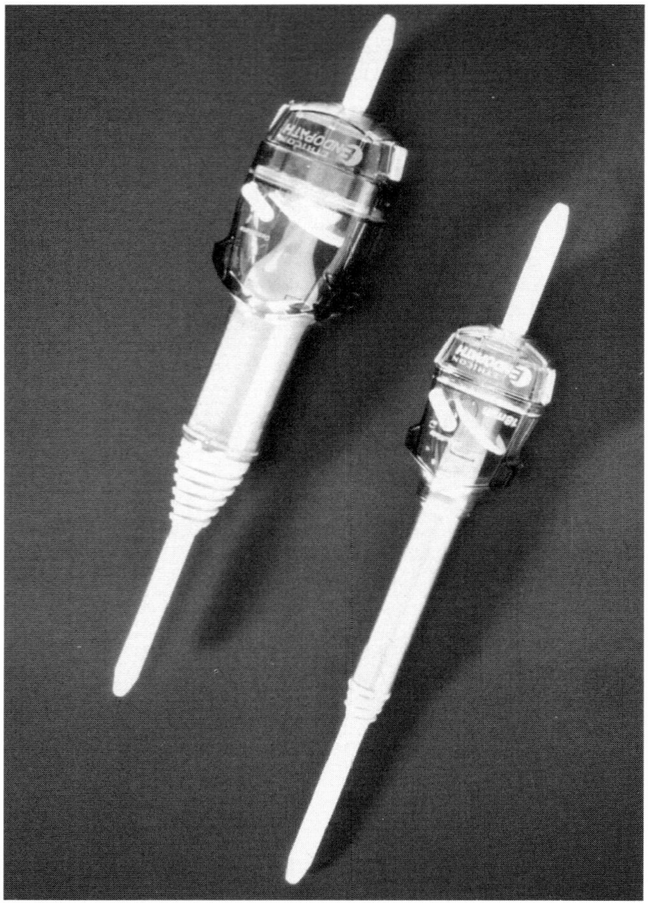

Fig. 7-17. Large cannula (up to 33 mm in diameter) allows removal of large specimen without contact of the parieties. (Courtesy Ethicon Endosurgery, Cincinnati, Ohio.)

inal wall or will reduce the number of pieces in which the specimen is to be subdivided (Fig. 7-17).

Morcellation. If morcellation of the specimen is not contraindicated and if removal through a colpotomy incision is desired, once the incision is made the specimen is pushed from above into the colpotomy. The surgeon or assistant working from below grasps the specimen with appropriate instruments such as single-toothed tennaculi. Morcellation is carried out under direct vision using a scalpel and the specimen is removed piecemeal.

Removal through the abdominal route is accomplished by making a minilaparotomy incision as described above. However it is useful to grasp the specimen with a strong-toothed forceps introduced through the cannula before the minilaparotomy incision is made and the cannula removed. Thus, once the incision is made, it will be possible to pull the specimen into the incision for intact removal or morcellation. Morcellation is carried out by using a scalpel on the partly exteriorized specimen (see Chapter 19).

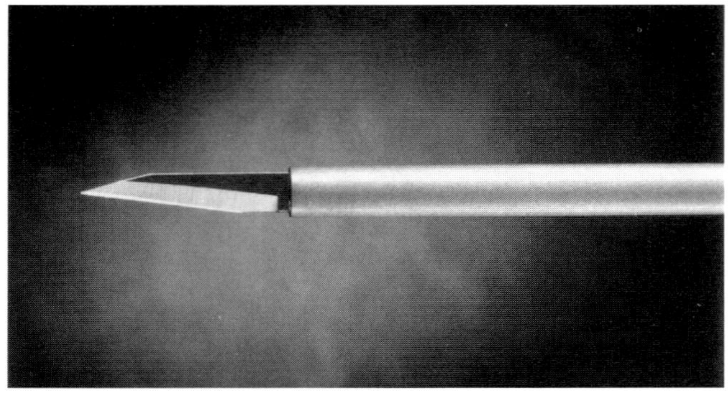

Fig. 7-18. Scalpel handle (5 mm) and retractable scalpel blade for laparoscopic use. (Courtesy Sharpe Endosurgical, Minneapolis, Minn.)

Intraperitoneal morcellation of the specimen into strips that can pass through an 11 mm cannula has been described. This is accomplished by introducing into the peritoneal cavity a number 11 scalpel blade attached to a scalpel handle modified for laparoscopic use (Fig. 7-18). The specimen is cut into longitudinal strips that will pass through the largest cannula in use. This technique is tedious and time consuming. Another approach is to morcellate the specimen with improved laparoscopic morcellators that are now available. Motorized versions of these are under development. The Semm serrated edged macromorcellator (Wisap, Tomball, Texas) is one of these manual devices. The instrument is available in 11 mm, 15 mm, and 20 mm shaft diameters and obviously requires preliminary insertion of an appropriately sized cannula to permit its introduction into the peritoneal cavity. The specimen is grasped either with a claw-shaped forceps or a myoma drill (that possesses a tip like a corkscrew) introduced through the morcellator. The latter has a cylindrical shaft with a serrated cutting edge. Rotation of this shaft while pulling on the forceps or the drill will excise a cylindrical piece of the specimen that remains within the morcellator (Fig. 7-19, *A*). This tissue is removed. By repeating the same step the whole specimen is removed piecemeal (Fig. 7-19, *B*). Morcellation of large specimens may be tedious and fairly time consuming. Improved motorized versions will facilitate this task in the future.

Use of an endopouch. When it is necessary or desirable to remove the specimen intact and when it is preferable to remove it without forcing it through an abdominal or colpotomy incision because of the risk of implantation of neoplastic or trophoblastic cells the following approach is used. An impermeable, strong, flexible plastic sac (Endopouch, Ethicon; Lapsac, Cook), sufficiently large to accommodate the excised specimen, is introduced into the peritoneal cavity through the largest portal. The specimen is dropped into the sac which is closed by pulling the drawstrings at the aperture of the sac. The drawstrings are delivered through

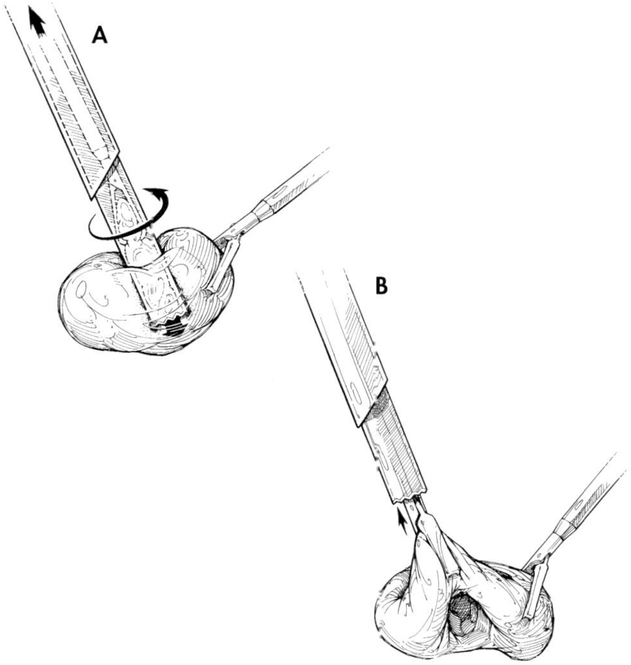

Fig. 7-19. Morcellation of tissue and removal from the abdomen with the use of the Semm macromorcellator. **A,** The specimen is grasped with forceps introduced through the morcellator shaft. Rotation of this shaft while pulling on the forceps excises a cylindrical core of tissue. **B,** By repeating the same step the whole specimen is removed piecemeal.

the incision (abdominal or colpotomy). Smaller specimens can be removed intact together with the closed sac. With specimens too large to be removed intact, such as teratomas or neoplastic cysts, the aperture of the partly delivered sac is opened and the specimen morcellated or the cyst drained within the sac under direct vision. This morcellation or decompression permits the removal of the sac including the specimen through a much smaller incision.

Pelvic lavage and prevention of adhesion formation

In order to reduce the risk of infection, the likelihood of adhesion formation, and the amount of postoperative discomfort it is important to remove all blood, fibrin, and any spilled fluids (e.g., from an endometrioma or other ovarian cyst) from the peritoneal cavity. This is effected by using copious amounts of lavage both during the operation and once the procedure has been completed. It is always easier to remove blood before it has had time to clot. Large clots can be difficult to remove, often being too large to fit through the aspiration cannula but yet too friable to be extracted with grasping forceps. The addition of heparin to the lavage solution decreases clotting of blood and facilitates the suction of such fluid from the peritoneal cavity.

Precautions against the formation of adhesions

- Leave fresh irrigation fluid in the peritoneal cavity at the end of the procedure
- Handle tissues gently
- Keep tissues moist
- Perform meticulous hemostasis
- Approximate tissues accurately
- Use fine and inert sutures

Once the operation has been concluded the pelvis is flooded with irrigation fluid, the pneumoperitoneum pressure is reduced, and the operative site inspected. Once the fluid is clear further inspection may be carried out with the lens of the laparoscope placed below the surface of the fluid. This underwater observation is remarkably effective for identifying any bleeding vessels by the smoky trail of blood that stains the fluid. If such vessels are seen they can be spot coagulated. Once this inspection has been completed, the fluid in the pelvis is aspirated, and the patient is placed in a foot-down position. This maneuver will cause any blood and/or irrigation fluid that may have pooled in the upper abdomen or paracolic gutters to drain into the pelvis from whence it can be easily aspirated. This maneuver will also permit inspection of the undersurface of the diagphram and lavage and suction of any upper abdominal collections under direct vision.

Some surgeons will leave up to 1 L of fresh irrigation fluid in the peritoneal cavity to create an artificial ascites in an attempt to reduce the formation of adhesions. Other precautions to achieve the same end are essentially those derived from sound microsurgical practice and include gentle tissue handling (keeping the tissues moist), meticulous hemostasis, accurate approximation of tissues (or at least as accurate as laparoscopic technology permits) and use of ligatures and sutures of inert and as fine materials as is possible. (See box above.)

During the development of microsurgery a large number of adjunctive agents were used in attempts to prevent adhesion formation. These were either instilled solutions or applications of biologic membranes. Despite early enthusiasm for high molecular weight dextran, subsequent studies failed to show that it was any better than normal saline in physiologic solution. The instillation of adrenal corticosteroids, while initially promising, was discontinued when it was noted that patients who had received such instillations frequently developed large plaques in the peritoneal cavity. It has subsequently been determined that these plaques occur when hydrocortisone acetate, an irritant suspension, is used. Hydrocortisone succinate does not produce these plaques. Presently there is intense interest in the use of various commercially available biologic membranes. At the moment they are expensive and remain to be of proven value.

Wound closure

Incisions of less than 5 mm can be closed with steristrips, clips, or subcuticular sutures. Larger incisions should be closed in two layers, ensuring that the defects in the fascia are repaired to prevent hernia formation. The skin can then be dealt with by any of the methods just described above.

GENERAL POSTOPERATIVE CARE

The principles of postoperative care include immediate observation to ensure that the airway remains clear and that the patient recovers from the anesthetic. Immediate observation is necessary to detect any signs of developing complications. Vaginal bleeding can occur from tenaculum punctures. These should have been inspected before the patient was taken from the lithotomy stirrups and sutured if necessary. Leakage usually occurs from the abdominal puncture sites if an artificial ascites has been created. It is of no consequence but both the patient and the recovery room staff should be warned that it might occur. Progressive elevation of the pulse rate, depression of the blood pressure, and signs of developing peritoneal irritation should alert the recovery staff and surgeon to the possibility that internal hemorrhage or peritonitis may be developing.

The amount of and specific medications required for analgesia will be predicated upon the complexity of the procedure that has just been performed. They may range from orally administered codeine medications to patient self-administered intravenous narcotics for those who have undergone the most major procedures. Along with the analgesic it may be necessary to provide an antiemetic. Finally, in the absence of complications, early ambulation and discharge are recommended for best results.

Chapter 8

DOCUMENTATION: TECHNICAL AND LEGAL CONSIDERATIONS

John M. Leventhal

"The historian, essentially, wants more documents than he can really use."

HENRY JAMES

In the sense that we must be the recorder of events, physicians are also historians. Whether it is the historian/physician or the litigious world in which we live that demands the documents, it is probable, as James predicted, that often there are indeed more than can be really used. No matter. Too much or too little, it is the universally accepted standard of medical care to document in some form every operative procedure. The documentation techniques may vary widely but, however recording is accomplished, it remains a legally mandated step in the appropriate care of the patient undergoing surgery.

Rapidly evolving electronic techniques for the recording of surgical procedures have begun to replace the more traditional forms of documentation in many centers throughout the world The dictated operative summary and written operative note remain, in most institutions, the minimum accepted standard for documentation. However, these paper documents by their nature are subjective and often not produced in a timely manner. Their accuracy with respect to what is actually seen or done is frequently as reflective of the surgeon as it is of the surgery. On the other hand, the video camera has no problem with objectivity. As imaging technology advances, it is increasingly probable that electronic imaging, in one form or another, will very soon become the new gold standard to which the surgeon will be held responsible. In no area is this more likely to occur than in the field of endoscopic surgery in which the documentation equipment itself has become an integral part of the equipment used to carry out the procedure. The advent of electronic microcircuitry has brought surgical documentation into the field of high technology and has made possible a whole variety of exciting forms of imaging. Real-time dynamic video imaging of any endoscopic operation has made the details of the procedure available to a wide range of secondary observers.

GENERAL AND LEGAL ASPECTS OF DOCUMENTATION

What is documentation?

A working definition, as well as the established objective of documentation, might be simply stated as *the recording of observed phenomena preserved in a format available to secondary observers.*

Why document?

Documentation of an endoscopic procedure serves a variety of purposes which include:

Patient information and education
Health professional education
Review by the surgical team
Communication with referring and other physicians
Documentation for the patient record
Follow-up review
Possible medico-legal documentation

Providing easily understood graphic information to the patient both before and after the operative procedure is of cardinal importance. The use of archive photographs or videotapes *before* the proposed surgery is an outstanding method of achieving truly informed consent. These materials serve to give the patient (and the family as well) a real

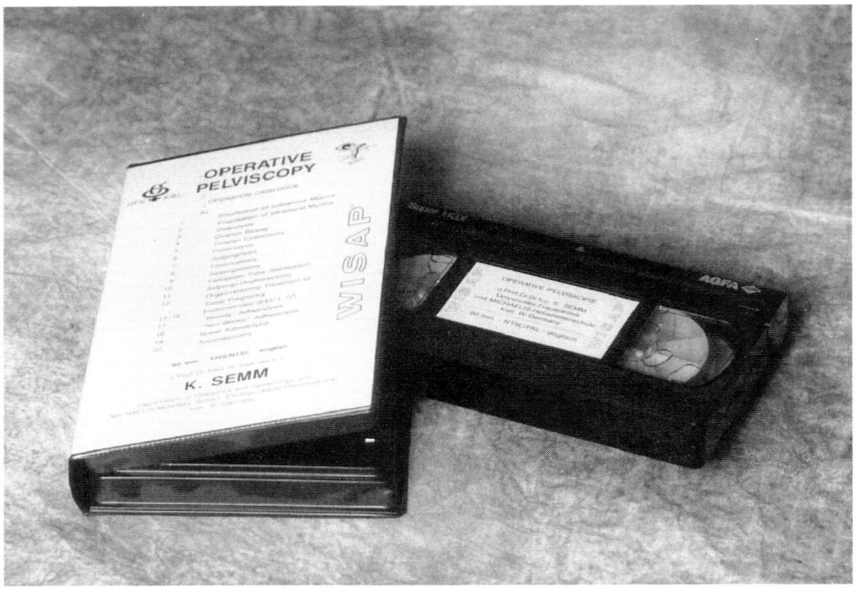

Fig. 8-1. Teaching videotape used for preoperative counseling.

basis for understanding the proposed surgery (Fig. 8-1). A videotape of the actual operation shown to the patient after the procedure can be compared with the preoperative visual briefing material and used to illustrate clearly the operative treatment. There is little question that enabling the patient to observe "first-hand" the surgical findings allows for the fullest understanding of the physician's observations and treatment. Not only is this important from the educational standpoint, but it can be argued that the patient's complete understanding of the problem often makes for both more effective treatment and a better outcome. When the problem is one of infertility, this understanding is frequently critical.

Videotapes or videodisks of endoscopic surgery are particularly valuable for the teaching of other physicians and members of the operating team. The availability of such material, even though unedited, often makes the use of professionally produced teaching tapes unnecessary. The unedited tape, used with the written permission of the patient (with the patient identification deleted), is often more valuable as a teaching aid than an extensively edited version and more importantly is usually immediately available within the office or institution.

In the important area of communication between the patients' physicians, video recordings and photographs are far more informative than the typed operative dictation for making known the findings of a procedure.

Why video documentation?

Most forms of traditional documentation are, by their nature, subjective. The fact that they comprise the initial observer's concept of what was viewed at the time of the operative procedure means that they often reflect as much the background and bias of the observer as they do the properties of the objects being observed. Therefore the written progress note or operative dictation is at best an interpretation and, in modern parlance, not "transportable" to others as objectively representative of the original observations. In its attempt to record accurately the findings of a surgical procedure, even the most detailed operative dictation falls short of being truly objective. It can never be more than a document created out of the mind of the surgeon (or, unfortunately, too often the less experienced junior assistant) and is therefore only a version of what was observed. The subsequent reader (the secondary observer) usually has no recourse to the original "data" and, for better or worse, must draw conclusions or base actions on subjective documentation. Modern video documentation, on the other hand, can provide each secondary observer with a fresh opportunity to draw conclusions based upon the original visual data. In the context of accuracy, video documentation is real-time recording and as such provides for more informed evaluation of the operative findings. From both the purely objective and legal standpoints, this increased accuracy may well serve in the near future to make the videotape the document of official reference.

Is the videotape a document?

The American Heritage Dictionary defines a document as "1. A written or printed paper bearing the original, official, or legal form of something, and which can be used to furnish decisive evidence or information. 2. Anything serving as evidence or proof, as a material substance bearing a revealing symbol or mark."[1] Certainly the videotape or disk is not a "written or printed paper," but it *is* a document "serving as evidence or proof." Therefore, we must accept, as has the legal profession, that the *videotape is a document.*[2] The video recording of operative procedures has become so commonplace and used in so many types of surgery that it represents in today's world as much of a document as any of the more traditional forms.

Legal status today

From the legal accountability standpoint, all of the reasons to document are important. However, the legal status of videotaping of procedures is vague in most jurisdictions both in the United States and abroad, and has been seldom addressed by legislative bodies creating the law. Critical questions remain largely unanswered by the laws or the courts at the present time. Is the videotape an official part of the medical record? Whose record? Where should it be maintained and for how long? Does the videotape belong to the patient, the doctor, or the hospital? Can the tape be edited during or after the procedure? Can surgeons tape only those portions of the procedure that they feel are significant?

Very few courts in the U.S. charged with interpreting statutes have rendered decisions relating to video documentation or attempted to answer these questions. In a New York case in 1986 a physician was supported by the court in refusing to comply with a patient's demand for a videotape of a procedure when the demand was made outside of the discovery procedures attendant to the malpractice action.[3] In Massachusetts in 1990, legal advice sought by a Boston hospital concerning the disposition of video documents held that declaring the videotape to be a part of the hospital record made the hospital responsible for its storage and preservation and made it discoverable in any action brought against the institution. It was therefore the opinion of the attorneys that any video record made by a physician should belong to, and be kept by, the physician. They further advised that copies (never the original) of the videotape be given to the patient *only* if requested and signed for. The result of this opinion was to shift the responsibility and liability for that record to the physician and away from the hospital. In this latter instance, of course, the legal advice was sought by and rendered in the interest of the hospital and would perhaps have been somewhat contrary to that given to an individual physician seeking similar information. These examples bring to light possible conflicts of interest between the physician and the hospital, and demonstrate the dilemma that stems from the inability of law-making bodies to keep pace with rapid advances in medical documentation technology.

One area that has been addressed by many jurisdictions in the U.S. is that of informed consent. It may well be that the consent laws offer a useful platform on which the patient and physician can reach prior agreement with respect to the various issues involved in graphic documentation.[4] These might include consent to record, ownership of the records and archiving. It is perhaps from the consent laws of the various states that a method for defining the legal status of video documentation can be derived. If it is true, as some experts contend, that the informed patient is less likely to be the litigious patient, then perhaps videotapes of various endoscopic procedures are especially valuable sources of preoperative and postoperative information and need to be regulated by the consent document itself. An understanding of the status of visual documentation serves both the patient and the physician. While it should never be forgotten that the video record of the actual procedure can be helpful to a defendant physician involved in litigation, it must also be remembered that it is a potential source of trouble as well. If we are going to use the video document as the preferred medium for recording endoscopic procedures, the eventual legal decisions will have to take into account the protection and interests of both the patient and the physician.

TECHNICAL ASPECTS OF DOCUMENTATION

A thorough understanding of the technical aspects of the recording medium and the methods of intraoperative recording is essential if the surgeon is going to be ultimately liable for the electronic documentation. Video imaging is a form of dynamic imaging, meaning that real-time motion is recorded. Static imaging is represented by the still photograph or frame-frozen video image that captures a single moment of the procedure. Both dynamic and static imaging have important roles to play in the documentation of endoscopic procedures.

Illumination

In order to produce usable and accurate documentation, all visual recording systems, whether dynamic or static, depend upon sufficient illumination of the observed subject matter. This illumination in turn can be thought of as being dependent upon four variable factors: (1) the sensitivity of the recording system, (2) the transmission efficiency of the lens system used with the recording equipment, (3) the illuminating power of the light source, and (4) the size of the image to be recorded.

Sensitivity of the recording system. Sensitivity of photographic film, such as used to obtain 35 mm slides, is a function of the chemical composition of the emulsion layer of the film. Color film emulsions are also made to compensate ("balanced") for various light temperatures, thus rendering accurate color under a wide variety of lighting conditions. While the sensitivity of photographic film varies with the chemical composition of the emulsion, video sensitivity is a function of the electronics of the camera and recording system (see below).

Transmission efficiency of the lens system. The efficiency of the transmission of light in any lens system is dependant on the design of the lens bundle, the diameter of the endoscope, the light-transmitting properties of the lens material itself, and the distance over which the light must

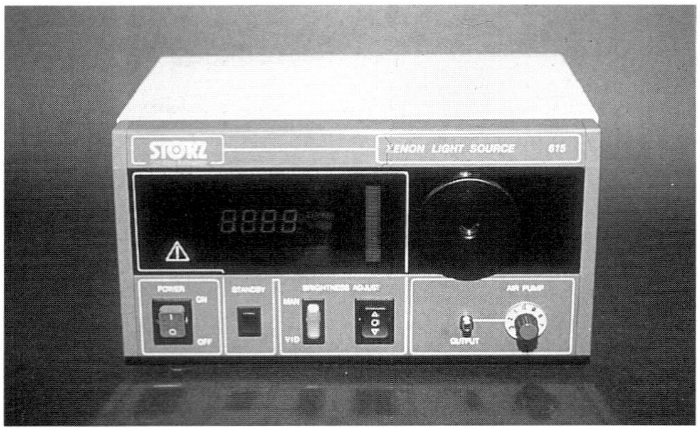

Fig. 8-2. A typical metallic arc light source used for endoscopic procedures. (Courtesy Karl Storz Endoscopy America.)

travel. Rigid endoscopes are made up of a series of glass lenses comprising a lens system. The design of the system is such as to provide for some predetermined degree of magnification and optimal light transmission.

This time-honored design, however, may be giving way to an entirely new concept. Recently, with the advent of high sensitivity, high-resolution microprocessor chips, the lens-filled endoscope has begun to share the stage with a whole generation of entirely new instruments that employ a solid state microchip camera mounted at the distal end of a solid "endoscope." When employed with these electronic systems, conventional lenses are used only for focus and magnification purposes and have little influence on the light transmission characteristics of the system.

The illuminating power of the light source. Since all visual documentation requires imaging onto light-sensitive material (silver halide emulsion in the case of film and light-sensitive pixels in the case of microprocessor chips), sufficient illumination of the recorded object is essential. Electronic recording usually requires less light intensity than photographic imaging; thus even very fast (high ASA rating) film is usually not as light sensitive as the electronic sensors of a microprocessor chip. The illumination of the object must therefore be matched to the sensitivity of the primary recording medium, rendering a recorded image that is an accurate reproduction of what is being observed.

Sufficient light depends on the source of illumination: the light generator (Fig. 8-2). Most modern light sources for endoscopy use a metallic arc bulb that produces light in the "daylight film" range of 5,000° K to 6,000° K and is capable of producing brighter illumination (more lumens) than incandescent sources. However, unlike an incandescent source, the intensity of which can be varied throughout its entire range of illumination, it is important to remember that the intensity of a metallic arc source can be varied only over a relatively small range. This property becomes an important consideration in the design of video cameras, which respond to the illumination intensity over a wide range depending on the amount of light reflected by the object being observed. This property of matching light intensity to the image requirement is generally addressed in the video camera by providing either an iris shutter driven by the light reflected from the field or by automatically dimming the illumination over the small range that is available with the metallic arc source.

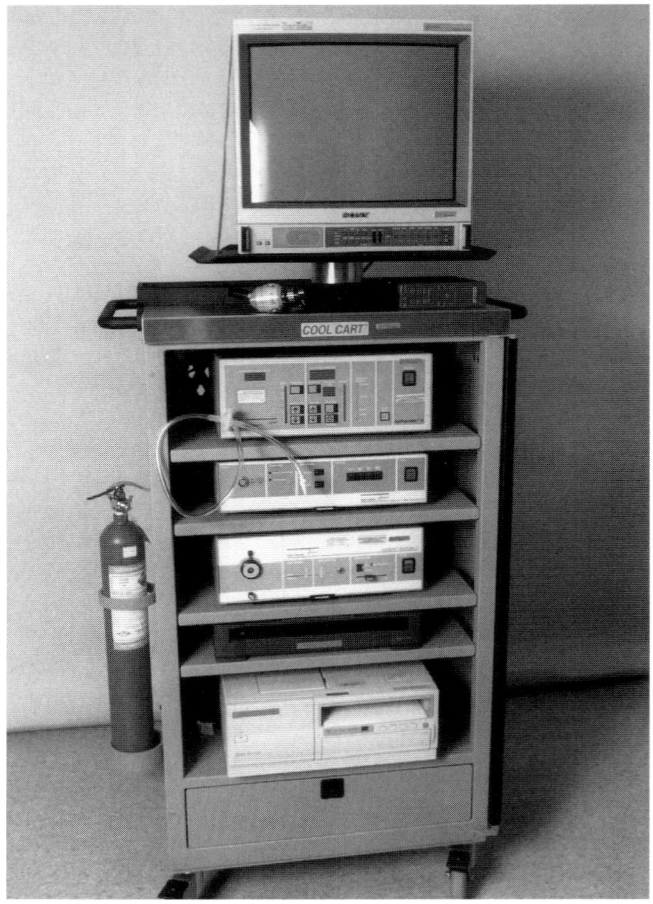

Fig. 8-3. An endoscopic video recording system consisting of videocamera, monitor, and video cassette recorder (VCR).

The size of the recorded image. The amount of light necessary for optimal imaging on film is inversely proportional to the size of the recorded image. It therefore requires more light for a 35 mm slide image than it does for a 16 mm frame of a movie film. This principle no longer applies in the case of electronic imaging in which the light gathering properties of the microprocessor chip are dependent upon the sensitivities of the individual units (pixels) and their density in the electronic chip array but not upon the size of the chip.

The video system

The basic video system consists of a video camera, monitor, videotape, and video cassette recorder (VCR) (Fig. 8-3). In the near future, optical laser disks and video frame grabbers will become additional routine components to most systems in medical use. The video system serves to record endoscopic procedures, but it also serves as the means by which the surgeon visualizes the operative field. Video monitor visualization has been used for years by orthopedic surgeons performing arthroscopy. The general surgeon, more recently introduced to laparoscopy, has learned to be totally dependent upon it. The surgeon's eye in effect has been moved from the endoscopic eyepiece to the color video monitor. The endoscopic observations, previously under the eye of the surgeon alone, can now be seen by the entire operating team as well. This has allowed much more efficient surgical teamwork and, not insignificantly, a more comfortable position for the surgeons.

Video formats

The video format refers to the electronic method by which the image is obtained and recorded onto videotape. Currently there is no world-wide agreement on the best electronic format for video recording equipment. The desire to have a single format, however, has given rise to numerous international meetings over many years, unfortunately without the emergence of a universal system. In North America, parts of South America, Japan, and parts of Asia, the **N**ational **T**elevision **S**tandards **C**ommittee (NTSC) format is in general use. In most of Europe and Australia the **P**hase **A**lternation **L**ine (PAL) format is the usual standard, although in France the **SE**quence de **C**ouleurs **A**vec **M**emoire (SECAM) format is used. Other standards exist and newer ones arise at an alarming rate. Each format has its enthusiastic proponents and has advantages and disadvantages with respect to image quality. Despite considerable consumer pressure, it is unfortunate that there will probably not be agreement on a universal format for a number of years to come. This disparity makes it difficult for physicians wishing to present videotapes at overseas lectures or meetings. Equipment exists for the conversion of videotapes from one format to another, but the process is expensive and not available everywhere.

EQUIPMENT FOR VIDEO DOCUMENTATION

In the past decade the endoscopic video camera has evolved from a two pound cylinder the size of a flashlight to a half-ounce unit little larger than the surgeon's finger. Concurrent with the reduction in size, advancing technology has made possible great improvements in light sensitivity and image resolution. The improvement in camera resolution has been accompanied by significant improvement in the quality of videotape media as well, allowing for considerable smaller and less bulky VCR equipment. The bulky expensive ¾ inch cassette recorder (Sony U-Matic) has been replaced almost universally by ½ inch VHS or Beta machines. These, in turn, are slowly giving way to high-resolution 8 mm recorders using very small 2-hour cassettes. The result of this miniaturization has been an ever increasing distribution and utilization of video systems, accompanied often by decreasing costs.

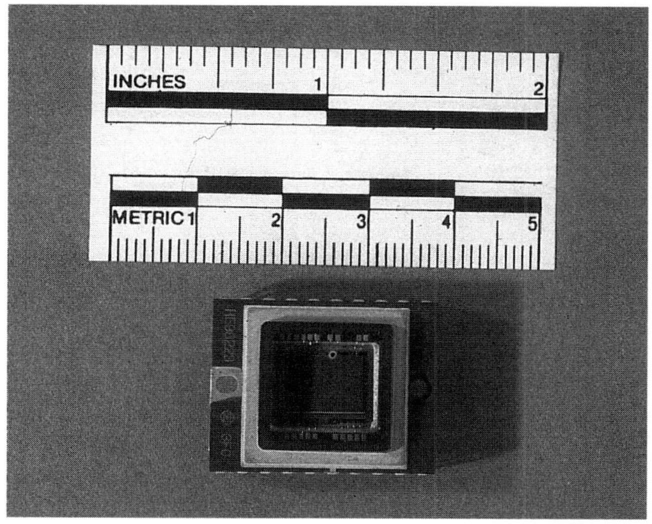

Fig. 8-4. A charged coupled device microprocessor chip.

In today's properly equipped operating room, the essential components of a basic video documentation system are five in number:

The video camera
The camera controller and video recorder (VCR)
The monitor
The light source
The endoscope

The video camera

Although possibly still in use in some operating rooms, the medical vacuum tube camera is almost an historic curiosity. Highly sophisticated vacuum tube cameras of much greater complexity are still used in most commercial television studio work and continue to provide (but only by the smallest of margins) the highest image resolution. Even this application is slowly giving way to a three-chip solid state camera with equivalent resolution. For medical and most other applications, however, the tube camera has been replaced by the solid state microprocessor or single chip camera. Advances in solid state camera technology have been extremely rapid, so that today these miniature units are capable of resolutions and light sensitivities almost indistinguishable from those of larger, bulky tube cameras.

There are currently two basic types of microprocessors used in solid state video cameras: (1) the **C**harge-**C**oupled **D**evice (CCD) chip and (2) the **M**etal **O**xide **S**emiconductor (MOS) diode chip (Fig. 8-4). As a general statement, the CCD chip has greater light sensitivity but, until very recently, somewhat less resolution capability than the MOS chip. Improvements in both types of chips, however, have occurred quickly. The addition of a negative charge to the MOS chip, creating the **N**egative **MOS** diode chip, has resulted in a marked increase in light sensitivity for this device. In its present form the MOS or NMOS diode chip camera strikes a state-of-the-art compromise between sensitivity, dynamic range, noise, and what is termed "lag" (the effect of light "contaminating" the image before it can be moved from the collecting diode to the storage register). Continuing improvements in CCD technology, such as the **H**ole **A**ccumulator **D**iode (HAD) sensor and the **F**rame **I**nterline **T**ransfer CCD (FIT CCD) by Sony, have served to advance this technology at a dazzling rate.

Both the CCD and MOS microprocessors are integrated circuit (IC) devices, which utilize the principle of changes in the electric resistance of a metallic or silicon oxide surface in response to varying intensities of light. The part of the chip facing the object being recorded is divided into an array of **PIC**ture **EL**ments called PIXELs, which are arranged along horizontal scanning lines. One of the major factors in determining the resolution of a chip is the number of horizontal lines. Therefore the greater the number of lines of pixels in a particular camera, the greater is its power of resolution. The NTSC format contains 700 pixels per line, whereas the PAL and SECAM formats contain 833 pixels per line. The latter formats therefore have inherently better resolution per line than the NTSC format used in the U.S.

Decisions regarding the purchase or updating of endoscopic video systems are especially difficult in the current climate of almost explosive technical change. The desired equipment specifications of today are often obsolete within a year. Economic probity, however, dictates that one must choose equipment on the basis of need and not of novelty. If the system in current use provides useful and accurate documentation, it should be retained. However, if a new video camera is being considered for purchase, it should have all or most of the following features:

- NTSC format (PAL or SECAM where appropriate)
- Horizontal resolution of at least 500 lines–preferably more
- Recorder on-off control at the camera head
- Simple one-hand focusing at the camera head
- Automatic and continuous white balancing
- Automatic light intensity control or controllable from camera head

The camera controller and video recorder (VCR)

The image information gathered by the camera chip is processed in the camera controller circuitry. Light striking a pixel in the chip induces changes in resistance that are stored in the controller in the "image register." The information stored in the image register is rapidly and sequentially "swept" or transferred to temporary storage in the "storage register," thus freeing the image elements (pixels) for the next fragment of light stimulation. The rate at which this transfer occurs is known as the "frame rate" and is measured in images per second. The frame rate varies with different electronic formats (see below). For NTSC format, used in the U.S., the frame rate is 30 per second, while for PAL and SECAM the rate is 25 frames per second.

Because of its relatively low cost and compatability with most video systems, magnetic videotape remains the most widely used medium today for recording. It is no longer necessary to employ ¾ inch (Sony U-Matic) tapes for top quality imaging. Half-inch VHS tapes (200 horizontal lines), Super VHS tapes (400 horizontal lines), and now 8 mm tapes of equal image quality are in increasingly common use and are perfectly satisfactory (Fig. 8-5). Image display on most television monitors and recording onto magnetic tape require the conversion of the digitally acquired image to an analog image (D-A conversion).

For over a decade, and probably for all future time, we have lived and will continue to live in a world of computers. Computers are digital machines and are not only extremely adept at image handling and display but also can add analysis and language (both audio and visual) to an acquired video recording. Medical video systems have already begun to move significantly into the digital age to accommodate the use of the computer. The laser videodisc, which is similar to the familiar compact disk or CD from our home entertainment systems, is a digital recording medium for archiving and fast retrieval of information. As an example, the Laser Videodisc Recording System, produced by Sony is capable of storing up to 24 minutes of video or 43,500 still color images and associated audio per side with random access of any image within 0.5 seconds or less.[5] This, and other similar systems beginning to appear on the market, is fully capable of communicating with an external computer for facilitation of computer-controlled recording and playback operation (Fig. 8-6).

The rapidly emerging concept of multimedia presentation is as fully available to the medical community as it is to the corporate world. Videotape has the inherent disadvantages of physical bulk and slow, inefficient access to specific images, while the videodisc can be instantly accessed, is small and rugged, and requires very little storage space. The videodisc (**W**rite **O**nce **R**ead **M**any or WORM) is recorded by laser-induced phase alteration of the reflectivity of the layered media material and is virtually not alterable. This characteristic of nonerasability may make this type of CD more acceptable than magnetic videotape as admissible evidence in litigation. Rewritable compact disks, however, are now available and may become the recording media of choice in the future. Computer compatability allows for detailed historic and diagrammatic data to be recorded along with operative findings, and may well be the precursor for the medical record of the future.

The monitor

At least two monitors should be available in the operating room for comfortable viewing by the surgeon and assistants (see Chapter 7). Two electronically different monitors are available in today's market: analog and digital. In

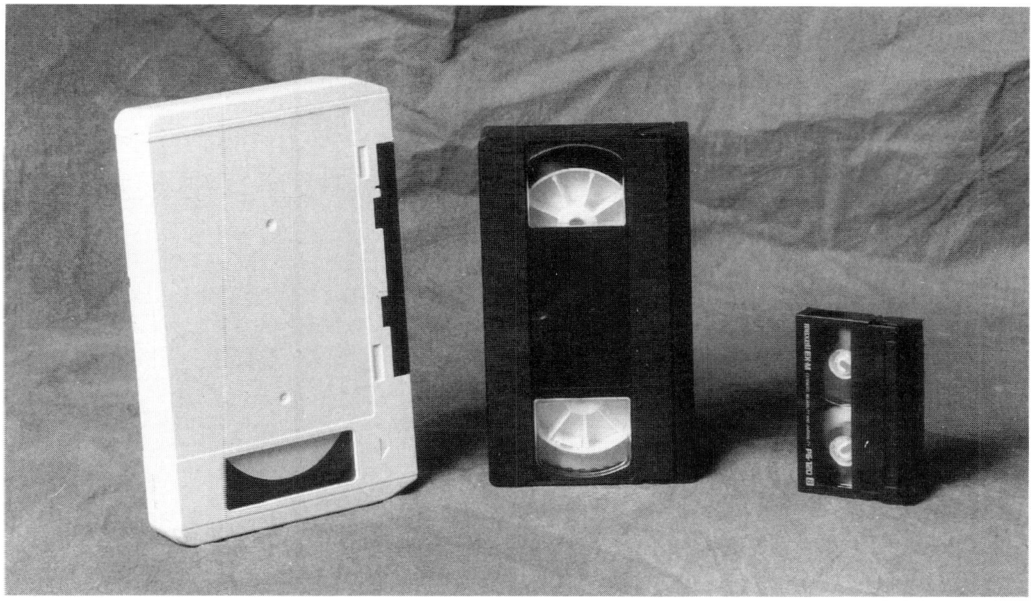

Fig. 8-5. Videotapes in current use for recording endoscopic procedures (¾ inch U-Matic, ½ inch VHS, and 8 mm).

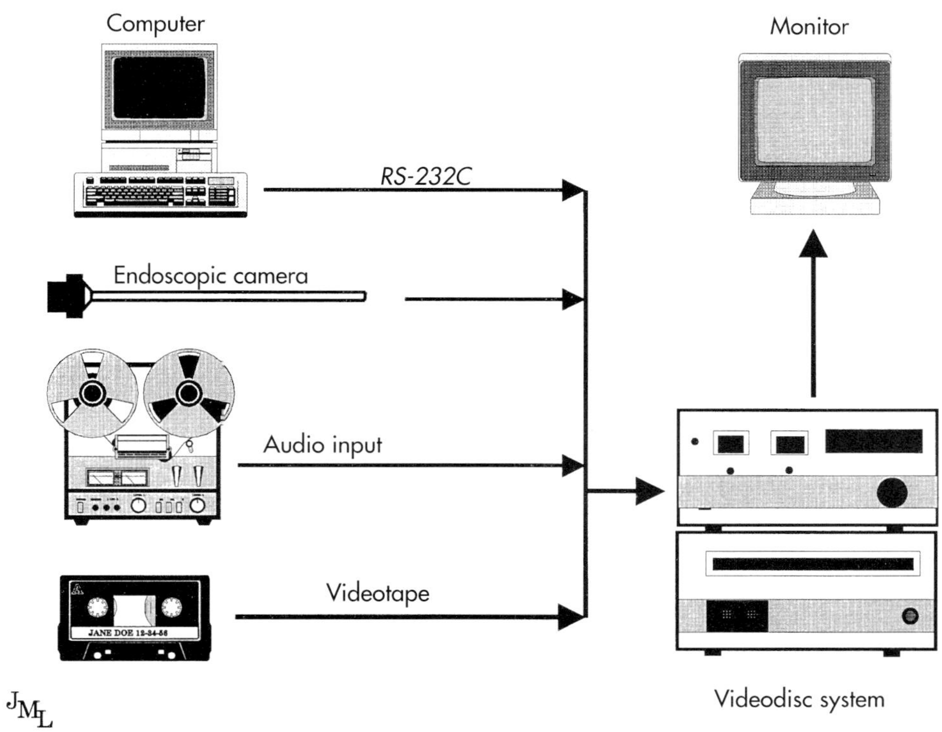

Fig. 8-6. Schematic representation of a laser videodisc system as may be utilized for endoscopic documentation.

widest use in operating rooms at the time of this writing are analog monitors. The home television set is a more familiar example of an analog monitor. Almost all monitors are capable of resolution higher than that of the camera used to acquire the image. This resolution gap is rapidly closing with advancing microchip technology, allowing the resolution of modern video images to approach that of color film. Because the original image is acquired as digital data with the solid state camera, a digital-analog converter is a necessary component of the camera controller when an analog monitor is used. Digital monitors, on the other hand, process the digital signal directly, are in increasing use, and will eventually replace their analog counterparts.

The light source

A wide variety of light sources for endoscopy are available. For the surgeon desiring both photographic and video capability, a metallic arc light with built-in synchronized electronic flash for still photography and automatic light control is essential (Fig. 8-2). As video frame grabbing (see below) becomes more widely used, silver halide (film) photography will slowly be replaced, and the electronic strobe flash will no longer be necessary.

The endoscope

Good endoscopic imaging requires ample light. Generally speaking, the larger the diameter of the endoscope the greater the light transmissability and therefore the better the video recording. The major determining factor is the diameter of the fiberoptic bundle within the endoscope itself. In the case of laparoscopy, the diameter of the laparoscope should be 10 mm and, 12 mm if equipped within an operating channel.

ADDITIONAL VIDEO IMAGING TECHNIQUES

Frame grabbing (still video)

The electronic answer to still imaging is called *"frame grabbing."* The process involves the capture, in digital form, of a single frame from the storage register of the camera and the subsequent printing out to hard copy material such as paper or transparency film. The process requires a computer for storage of the acquired frame and for output to a suitable printer to produce the "hard copy" or picture. A number of color printers are available, and depending on the system used, both prints and slides can be produced. Fig. 8-7 illustrates a typical modern system that allows for instantaneous frame grabbing at any moment during the operative procedure. The quality of the final image obtained with such equipment is equivalent to that of a still photograph.

This approach to static imaging (still pictures) has proved to be especially valuable for capturing illustrative segments of the operative procedure for insertion into the patient's hospital or office chart. It must be remembered, however, that, although informative, these pictures may raise some questions of admissability in a court of law because of having been taken out of context with respect to the whole operative procedure.

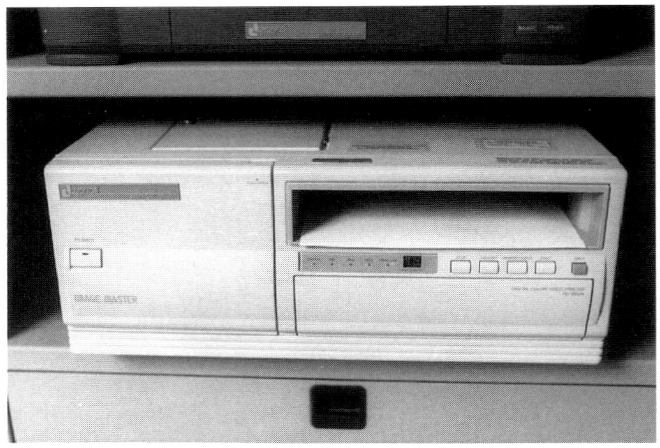

Fig. 8-7. A color printer is an integrated component of a video imaging system designed for use in the operating room.

3-D video

Three-dimensional medical video, although not at present a technology applicable to endoscopic procedures, bears mentioning because its development has involved innovations that will be important for endoscopic imaging in the future. The technology was developed for neuromicrosurgical use in the mid-1980s at the St. Louis University Medical Center with the encouragement and help of many international electronic corporations. Originally the idea of a young neurosurgical resident, Doctor Gregory J. Bailey, the concept has matured to the point at which 3-D prerecorded tapes have been available for teaching of open microsurgical procedures for a number of years.[6] The application of these methods to endoscopic imaging and the possibility of providing the surgeon with a three-dimensional view through the endoscope is exciting.

ARCHIVING

The storage of visual records is as important as it is difficult. Ideally, archiving of this material should require minimum space and should allow rapid and accurate retrieval of specific information. This ideal is rarely achieved. Most endoscopic surgeons who routinely document with videotape have cabinets and even rooms full of tapes that are usually not systematically catalogued and are therefore very difficult to find much less to use for viewing a specific segment of data. It is simply not possible even to approach the ideal with videotape, which over time, even in the 8 mm format, begins to occupy inconvenient amounts of physical space.

However, the answer is available. It is possible to transfer video images from videotape or directly from the camera controller at the time of surgery to laser videodiscs (see above). Capable of extremely large storage capacity measured in gigabytes, they allow almost instant retrieval of specific information. Whole segments of video imaging can be archived on a single disc, and, with data compression techniques now in use, entire operations or very many videotape segments can be stored on a single disc. Identification of interesting parts of a procedure, for instance, can be coded digitally on the videodisc and retrieved in milliseconds by barcode reader or database search on a computer. Color transparency slides can also be scanned, digitized, and stored in enormous quantity on a single disc, and can even be intermixed with video images. Since this visual documentation data is stored in digital form, it can be transmitted over long distances by telephone or satellite and thus can be available for viewing in widely separated geographic locations simultaneously and at any time.

The legal time requirements for the preservation of archived visual documents in any form remain to be established. This author suggests that archived video records be kept for the same length of time as the patient chart and then destroyed or overwritten.

THE FUTURE

The future of endoscopic imaging continues to parallel the development of digital imaging technology. There are few fields of information management changing more rapidly. The optical lens endoscope will probably be replaced by the electronic endoscope with the camera chip embedded into the distal end of the instrument. Looking through the endoscope will then cease to be an option. The surgeon will then be dependent upon the video system. Image quality will continue to improve tremendously, borrowing technology from other imaging fields. Today high-resolution scanners (2,000+ lines), which employ essentially the same technology as video cameras, are capable of resolutions finer than the grain in conventional films, and camera resolution improves with each passing month.

True three-dimensional recording and viewing is in its infancy, but is already being applied to endoscopy in some interesting ways. Virtual reality systems are under intense development at present and beginning to open possibilities almost impossible to imagine. A virtual reality trainer for laparoscopic cholecystectomy for instance, which allows the surgeon to manipulate the operative field in a way that is completely interactive and realistic, has already been introduced. The computer-generated organs displayed are, at this point, still largely diagrammatic, but their replacement with video images of live structures is under serious development and not far in the future. Seemingly the subject of science fiction, telesurgery, a procedure utilizing virtual reality techniques to allow the surgeon to operate upon a patient in an electronically linked, but geographically distant, operating room, is already in the experimental stage.

In the near term, however, the legal system must address the questions raised by visual imaging technology. Whether the resultant decisions will apply in any universal sense remains to be seen, but local and institutional regulations are already in place in some areas. In the interm, the suggestion by attorney Green to use the informed consent as the vehicle for agreement between patient and physician in matters concerning documentation deserves serious consideration.[4] With that in mind, a set of reasonable and practical guidelines for video documentation of endoscopic procedures is offered.

GUIDELINES FOR VIDEO DOCUMENTATION

The Consent Form should be the defining document for all agreements between the patient and physician (and/or hospital) concerning the employment and disposition of the video record. To that end it should:

1. State that a video recording of the procedure will be made and that the resultant tape or disk will be used to inform the patient of the operative findings and may be used (without identifying information) for instructional purposes as well.
2. Clearly state that the physician may edit the tape or be selective in choosing which parts of the procedure to record.
3. Confirm the patient's right to view the recorded material postoperatively and to obtain a copy if desired. It should further state that the original videotape is the property of the physician (or hospital).
4. Contain a provision confirming the patient's understanding that the physician may choose not to record the procedure.

Every video document should be identified at the beginning and end with the patient's name, hospital or office record number, date of the surgery, and surgeon.

The original of the recording, whether it be on videotape or compact disk, should be held in safekeeping by the physician or the hospital (if it is to be made a part of the official hospital record) for a period of time corresponding to the maximum statute of limitations applicable to the particular patient.

If the patient requests, an exact copy of the original may be given, the receipt of which should be acknowledged in writing and made a part of the patient record.

Under no circumstances should the surgeon erase or edit out a portion of the recording that contains material depicting a surgical mishap. Such action could subject the surgeon to charges of records alteration in any subsequent litigation.

CONCLUSIONS

Are we accountable when we use the video camera to record our endoscopic procedures? It seems likely, with the rapid increase in the number of video imaged operations, that this technology will ultimately replace the written or dictated operative record or at least be required to augment it. If that proves to be true, then the legal significance of the video record will parallel that of the written account. It is not likely, however, that the techniques and legal requirements for video imaging in surgery will be standardized at any early date. However, as the use of the video document becomes more and more widespread in medical litigation, it becomes increasingly important for every endoscopist utilizing the video camera to adhere to a minimal set of guidelines with respect to the obtaining of informed consent from the patient and the identification and recording of the endoscopic procedure.

The visual documentation of endoscopic procedures is presently the province of the video camera and its many peripheral devices. There is little question that some measure of accountability for what appears on the video record will rest with the surgeon. From the legal viewpoint, in the litigious atmosphere we find ourselves at present, it must never be forgotten that the video document presents not only an objective picture of what was performed correctly but also what may have gone wrong as well.

REFERENCES

1. Morris W editor: The American Heritage Dictionary of the English Language, New College Edition, Boston, 1978, Houghton Mifflin Co.
2. Miller, R.D.: The presentation of expert testimony via live audio-visual communication. *Bull Am Acad Psychiatry Law* 19:5-20, 1991.
3. Hill v. Springer, 132 N.Y.S. 2d 255, 1986.
4. Green HD Jr: Medical Technology vs. the Law, *Professional Medical Monitor* 1:7-9, 1991.
5. Sony Corporation: LVR-5000A/LVS-5000A Specifications EIA/NTSC, Publication V-9888-A, 1993.
6. Bailey GJ: Three-dimensional imaging in microsurgery. *Bull Am Coll Surg* 78:20-26, 1993.

Chapter 9

INFERTILITY

Radioimmunoassay and laparoscopy have been the two most significant advances in the investigation of the infertile couple in the last 20 years. The role of laparoscopy is primarily in the diagnosis and management of tubal and peritoneal causes of infertility. It is the purpose of this chapter to describe the applications of laparoscopy in the investigation of the infertile patient.

While laparoscopy plays an integral role in the investigation and management of the infertile female, it is an invasive procedure. Although no infertility investigation is complete without an endoscopic evaluation, abuses have occurred in the premature employment of this technique. This chapter will define those investigations that should be performed in the infertile couple prior to the laparoscopic evaluation.

"The investigation of the infertile couple should be concluded as rapidly, accurately, inexpensively, and as least invasively as possible. Based upon these criteria, in most instances endoscopic evaluation should be one of the later investigations. In addition, the emotional needs of the couple must be considered at all times."[1]

The investigation of the patient requesting reversal of a previously performed tubal sterilization, while not truly representing infertility, will be included in this chapter.

PRELIMINARY INVESTIGATION OF THE INFERTILE COUPLE

At the first visit of any infertile couple, a history is taken and a physical examination of both partners is performed. The fertility status of the male partner must be established first. The results of his history and physical examination are further clarified by the analysis of two and, where indicated, several properly collected semen samples. Further investigation of the male partner is dependent on these results. It is possible to triage the male partners into two groups; normozoospermic and oligo or azoospermic.

Initial clinical categorization of the female partner into either "infertile, apparently ovulatory," or "infertile, probably anovulatory or oligo-ovulatory" is made on the basis of the menstrual history. Absence of menses or disorganization of the menstrual cycle suggests anovulation or oligo-ovulation. The presence of regular vaginal bleeding accompanied by the molimina associated with ovulatory cycles is taken as presumptive evidence of ovulation. Supportive evidence of normal endocrine status is noted when stigmata of chromosomal or endocrine disorders are excluded by physical examination.

In addition, certain general laboratory tests may be ordered for both partners at the first visit. These should include, where appropriate, bacteriologic studies of the semen, urine, and female reproductive tract. The female partner's rubella titer is always measured.[2]

Further investigation of the female partner may be directed toward (1) assessment of ovulation; (2) assessment of sperm, cervical mucus interaction; (3) detection of intrauterine, tubal, peritubal, and peritoneal factors; and (4) evaluation of other potential causes of infertility.

Assessment of ovulation and of the luteal phase

A menstrual interval of 26 to 35 days has been shown to correlate with more sophisticated tests of ovulation in 97% of women.[3] If confirmation is required, evidence of ovulation may be obtained by assessment of the basal body temperature graph, luteal phase serum progesterone level, or endometrial biopsy.

Recent findings suggest that some women may elaborate progesterone without rupturing a follicle and releasing an egg, the so-called luteinized unruptured follicle (LUF) syndrome.[4-5] The laparoscopic diagnostic feature is the presence of a corpus luteum without evidence of an ovulation stigma. This enigmatic syndrome remains controversial since it has been detected in women who have borne children. It is doubtful whether the search for LUF syndrome constitutes a valid indication for laparoscopy, although incidental observations may be made if laparoscopy for other indications is performed at an appropriate time in the menstrual cycle.

In 1949[6] Jones postulated that some women might suffer from a relative defect in progesterone production—the luteal phase defect (LPD). Despite more than 40 years of intense interest in this syndrome its very existence is still unclear. A short luteal phase was said to be clinically indicative of the condition. Lenton et al.[7] have shown that in normal women the 95% confidence interval for lengths of luteal phase is 10 to 17 days. The elevation of basal body temperature lasts for less than 11 days in 18% of apparently normal women.[8] Endometrial dating is inaccurate. Errors can occur from biologic variability either within or between individuals or from observer inaccuracy. In a group of 13 parous volunteers, histologic changes were assessed by two observers. When the histologic findings were compared with the date of onset of the next menstrual period, the classic method of dating, only 16 of 26 samples (65%) were congruent.[9] Similar prevalences of delayed menstruation have been reported in both fertile and infertile groups of women.[10]

Mid-luteal serum progesterone values measured in 579 cycles in 159 women with unexplained infertility were compared with similar values in 267 cycles in 58 normal women. There was no difference in the prevalance of abnormal values detected in either group.[11] Taylor and Collins in an extensive review remarked "it must be concluded that the usefulness of histologic dating and measurement of serum progesterone values, as presently understood, contribute little to the understanding of the cause of otherwise unexplained infertility. This is particularly so when it is recognized that pregnancy occurs with similar frequency in women with normal endometrium and in women with delayed endometrial developments."[12]

Assessment of sperm-cervical mucus interaction

The assessment of sperm cervical mucus interaction is fraught with difficulty. While demonstrating evidence of sperm deposition and providing information about the quality of the cervical mucus and the behavior of the sperm, the traditional postcoital test "lacks validity as a test for infertility."[13] Other sperm-mucus interaction tests are currently under investigation; their exact role and significance are as yet unclear.[12] Such tests assess the transport of spermatozoa through the lower part of the genital tract. The ability of the sperm to traverse the female genital tract is better assessed by extended postcoital testing by which sperm are sought in the peritoneal washings.[15] At present, to perform this test, laparoscopy is required. Although the concept is simple, laparoscopy should not be undertaken for this purpose alone. Furthermore, the logistics of timing the laparoscopy in many operating rooms to accommodate a woman's menstrual cycle are difficult. Such a test should be performed immediately prior to ovulation and may be undertaken during an appropriately timed laparoscopy for other purposes.

Assessment of other causes of infertility

Although serum antisperm antibody testing is now readily available in most centers, the significance of such antibodies, especially in the female partner, has not been determined. It is possible that the detection of sperm antibodies in seminal plasma and/or cervical mucus may have more prognostic significance.

ASSESSMENT OF UTERINE, TUBAL, AND PERITONEAL CAUSES

The decision when to investigate uterine, tubal, and peritoneal factors will be dependent upon the apparent fertility status of the male partner and the ovulatory status of the woman. This section will address the methods of assessment. The timing of these tests in the overall investigation of the infertile couple will be discussed later.

Falloppius described the oviducts as "tubae" (Latin "trumpets") resembling as they did the straight trumpets of classical Rome. Modern transliteration to "tube" has led to the perception of a long, narrow, hollow structure requiring only patency to function. Translation to "trumpet," with its complex array of curves and valves, would have expressed the complexity of tubal function better.

Most major insults to the fallopian tubes follow either infective or traumatic events. The traumatic events might include intraabdominal surgical procedures and intrauterine manipulations.[16] Endometriosis is associated with infertility. As the investigation of the individual couples will progress at differing speeds, clinical indication of urgency in investigation of the tubal structure and pelvic peritoneum would be valuable. Procedures designed to assess function are being developed and will be discussed later. Early attempts to use radioactive microspheres as oocyte surrogates to evaluate oocyte transport were not clinically valuable.[17] Recently, Uher et al. have introduced biodegradable microspheres into the pouch of Douglas either by laparoscopy or cul-de-sac puncture.[18] These were collected in a cervical cap 24 hours later. The microspheres, which were recognizable by fluorescence, were demonstrable in the cap in 66% of 69 patients with unexplained infertility and 100% of 20 patients with male factor infertility. This report suggests a further avenue of investigation. Fimbrial microbiopsy has proved insufficiently representative of the total picture of the tubal mucosa to be of prognostic significance.[19]

The investigative procedures currently used routinely include hysterosalpingography and laparoscopy, which primarily assess tubal patency and tubal architecture. How well

Table 9-1. Clinical factors as predictors of pathological findings during laparoscopy among infertile couples

Clinical factor	Percentage with abnormal findings at laparoscopy (95% CI)		Kappa value
	Factor absent	Factor present	
Pelvic pain	37(25,49)	81(64,98)	0.32*
Appendectomy	37(25,49)	59(40,78)	0.19*
D&C	37(25,49)	65(44,86)	0.10*
History positive†	32(27,37)	69(61,77)	0.33*
Abnormal pelvic exam	40(35,45)	80(68,92)	0.15‡
Duration of infertility more than six years	40(35,45)	57(46,68)	0.11‡

*Cumming and Taylor, 1979.
†History positive for any: pelvic infection, intrauterine device, endometriosis, ovarian surgery, or tubal surgery.
‡Portuondo et al, 1984.

do laparoscopic findings correlate with clues detected in either the history or physical examination? Table 9-1 demonstrates the correlation between historic or physical findings and the presence or absence of an intra-pelvic abnormality. Although these clinical factors have some predictive value, it must not be forgotten that 60% to 75% of patients with hydrosalpinges will neither have a history of pelvic pain or pelvic infection nor positive physical findings.[20-21] The history and physical examination are indirect evidence only and a negative history and physical findings do not preclude the presence of intra-pelvic lesions. As fallopian tube obstruction will occur in 12% to 33% of infertile couples,[22-24] early investigation of tubal patency is indicated.

Contraindications to hysterosalpingography

Absolute

Possible pregnancy
Uterine bleeding
Lower genital tract infection
Pelvic inflammatory disease
Allergy to the contrast material used

Relative

Recurrent pelvic infection

HYSTEROSALPINGOGRAPHY

Hysterosalpingography (HSG) is a contrast study of the uterine cavity and fallopian tubes. It is a simple, inexpensive, safe, and rapid diagnostic procedure that provides valuable information about the uterine and tubal architecture.

Contraindications

Contraindications to HSG are possible pregnancy, uterine bleeding, lower genital tract infection, acute pelvic inflammatory disease (PID), and allergy to the contrast material (box at right). Hysterosalpingography in women with a history of repeated pelvic infections in the past or any suggestion of recent exacerbation should be approached with caution. In such women there is a significant risk of reactivation of quiescent pelvic inflammatory disease. This may occur in approximately 3% of patients.[25] This is a serious event, given that the risk of sterility rises from 13% after one episode of tubal infection to 36% after two.[26] To combat this risk some centers prophylactically administer antibiotics. Factors that would identify the woman at risk include a history of prior infection or surgery, adnexal tenderness or enlargement, and in whom secondary infertility has been identified. These factors would have predicted reinfection in 50% of the women who suffered this event.[25] Although the consequences of reinfection are serious, the 3% incidence is sufficiently low to suggest that routine treatment prophylaxis is not necessary for all women. Women in the high-risk group or with lower genital tract infection should be treated with antibiotics.

During the preliminary history and physical examination possible contraindications (see box) must be sought, and lower genital tract infection must be ruled out. The patient must be given the necessary information about the procedure. The success or failure of the procedure are entirely dependent on the thoroughness with which the HSG is performed. Details of technique will now be described.

Technique

Timing. Hysterosalpingography must be timed between the complete cessation of menses and ovulation (days 6 to 12 in most cycles). This will avoid the risk of disturbing a luteal phase pregnancy. Such timing also avoids radiation exposure to the oocyte that will resume meiosis following the LH surge. Injection of the medium can cause cramping. Administration of a prostaglandin synthetase inhibitor before the procedure will reduce the patient's discomfort.

Contrast medium. The radiopaque material for HSG may be oil or water soluble. Water-soluble media appear to be better tolerated by the patient, since the pain experienced during the procedure usually is less. Aqueous contrast medium coats the surfaces without sticking to them, produces sharp and finely shaded images and greater visual detail of the lesions, and enables better assessment of the intraluminal architecture and of the tubal mucosal folds. It is eliminated within 30 minutes.

Lipid-soluble medium is eliminated very slowly and may cause a granulomatous inflammatory reaction and, rarely, an embolism.[27] There may be a higher pregnancy rate in women with unexplained infertility when an oil-based medium is used.[28-29]

A recent study[30] demonstrated that exposure of macrophages to ethiodol oil-soluble contrast medium decreased their phagocytosis and adherence. This alteration in membrane function is caused by a reduction of membrane-negative surface charge and microviscosity. The authors hypothesized that the slow absorption of the oil medium may cause a long-term reduction in macrophage function, resulting in increased fertility.

When the hypothesis that use of an oil-soluble medium would improve the pregnancy rate as compared to use of an aqueous medium was tested in a prospective randomized fashion, no difference was detectable.[31] Furthermore, no comparison has ever been made between hysterosalpingography and a period of observation. The question of whether conceptions following HSG represent the passage of the contrast medium or simply the passage of time remains to be answered. As such we prefer to use water-soluble medium and advise our patients that the test is performed for diagnostic purposes only.

Procedure. After emptying her bladder the patient lies on the radiographic table with her hips flexed and the vulva exposed. A bivalve speculum is inserted into the vagina, and the cervix and upper vagina are washed with an antiseptic solution. Visible cervical mucus is removed. A modified Cohen cannula with a Teflon acorn tip is attached to a syringe containing contrast medium and the medium is injected through the cannula to ensure removal of air bubbles. The length of the acorn tip should be no more than 1 cm. The cervix is grasped with a tenaculum and traction is applied. If the patient is asked to cough and the tenaculum applied as she does so, it is remarkable how little she will notice its application. The cannula is inserted into the cervical canal under direct vision and countertraction is applied on the tenaculum to ensure a tight seal. The bivalve speculum is then removed and the patient's legs are extended. It is imperative to remove the speculum, especially if a metal variety is used, prior to the injection of the contrast material to avoid obscuring the cervical canal and vaginal fornices.

Preliminary films are of limited value as identification of areas of pelvic calcification or misplaced intrauterine contraceptive devices can be achieved by examination of the earliest film.

The contrast medium is injected slowly from the syringe attached to the cannula. It is essential that the cannula and syringe be free of air and completely filled with the contrast material prior to its introduction into the cervix in order to avoid injection of air, which may lead to misinterpretation of the findings.

Hysterosalpingography must be performed under fluoroscopic control using an image intensifier. The contrast material must be injected very slowly to avoid discomfort, contraction of the uterus, spasm of the uterotubal junction, and obscuring lesions with excessive contrast material.

Radiographs are not taken according to a fixed schedule but rather to record salient features as they appear on the monitor. On the average, five films are taken.

The endocervical canal, isthmus, and uterine cavity are visualized fluoroscopically initially as the contrast material is injected slowly and intermittently. Firm traction is maintained on the cervix to straighten the uterus. It is important to obtain films early during the procedure in order to record properly any intrauterine lesions and the intratubal architecture. Detail of such lesions is obscured by larger amounts of contrast material in the uterus, tubes, and/or the peritoneal cavity. Complete filling of a normal uterus requires 2 to 3 ml of contrast material. The fallopian tubes start filling at this stage. This is an optimal time to obtain a film (Fig. 9-1). The flow of the contrast through the tube and the initial passage into the peritoneal cavity is observed next. A film is taken at this point (Fig. 9-2). Injection of medium is continued slowly until tubal patency is unquestionably established. Care must be taken not to inject excessive amounts of contrast because this will obscure (flood) tubal images. Manipulation of the uterus with the cannula may be necessary to display specific tubal segments. A film is taken to confirm dispersal of medium within the peritoneal cavity (Fig. 9-3). After injection of a further 1 to 2 ml of contrast material, the cannula is removed and a film is quickly taken (evacuation film).

A true lateral film may be useful especially if there are abnormal findings. This exposure is taken after traction on the cervix is temporarily released. It will provide

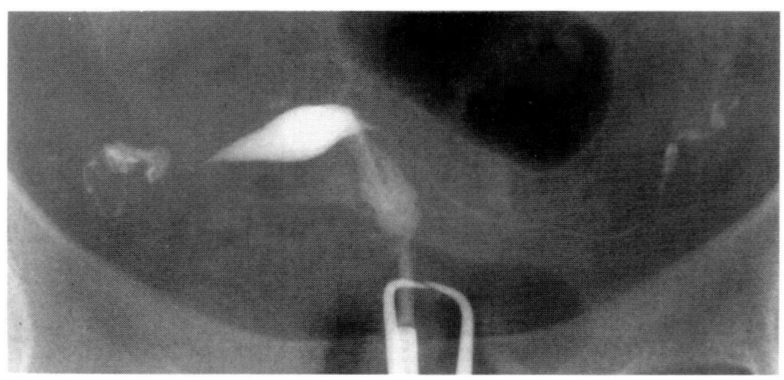

Fig. 9-1. HSG: Early film.

precise information regarding the position of the uterus, the status of the cervix and isthmus, location of intrauterine lesions (Fig. 9-4), and the course and configuration of the tubes.

The last, often neglected, phase of the procedure is a delayed fluoroscopic examination and film taken 10 to 20 minutes after the removal of the cannula if water-soluble contrast material is used. In the interim, the patient is encouraged to be up and about. This last film provides confirmation of tubal patency and more accurate diagnosis of fimbrial stenosis or occlusion. It may also yield useful information about periadnexal adhesions, the external contour of the internal genitalia, and the shape of the ovarian fossa. The contrast medium may outline the ovaries, the uterus, and the periphery of the tubes, producing a double contour image that enables the thickness of the tubal wall to be assessed (Fig. 9-5).

For the reader who wishes to explore the possibilities of hysterosalpingography further, Musset's classic test[32] is highly recommended.

Complications. With adherence to proper technique complications are rare. Major complications include:

1. Intolerance to iodine especially when intravasation of contrast medium occurs
2. Pelvic inflammatory disease, which can be avoided by proper adherence to measures mentioned earlier, including examination of the cervical mucus to rule out lower genital tract infection

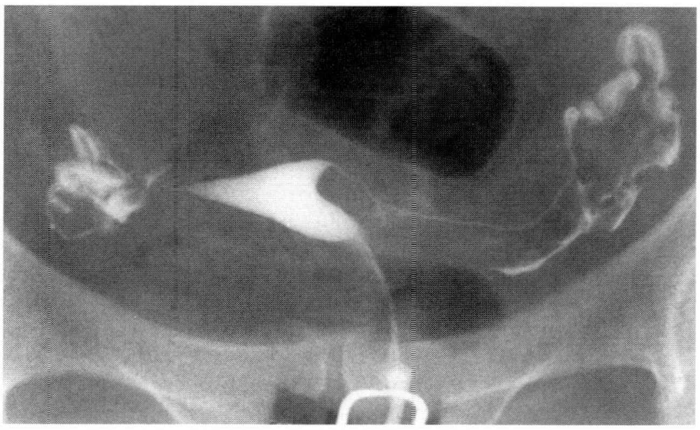

Fig. 9-2. HSG: Initial spill of contrast from the tube (same patient as in Fig. 9-1).

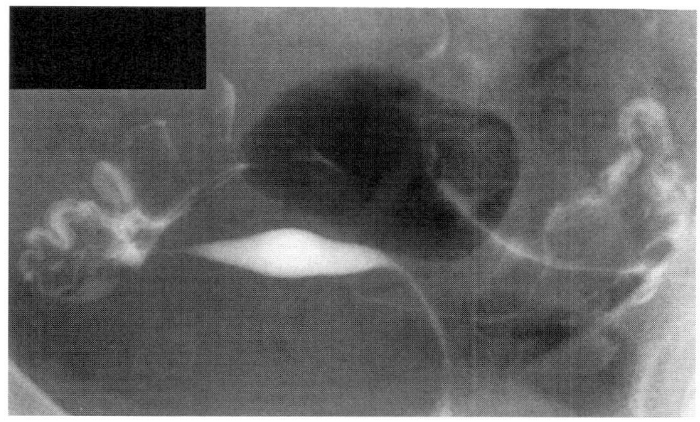

Fig. 9-3. HSG: Normal findings, with dispersal of contrast in the peritoneal cavity (same patient as in Fig. 9-1).

A

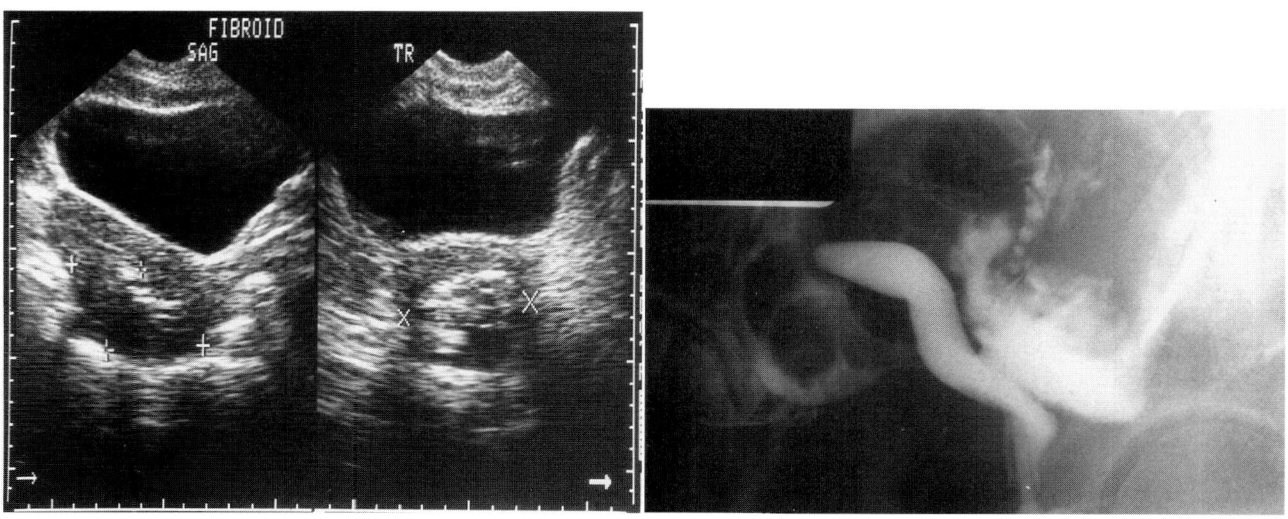

B

Fig. 9-4. **A,** Ultrasonography: The sagital view of the uterus demonstrates a posterior fibroid. **B,** HSG: Lateral view demonstrating the position of the uterus, uterine cavity, and cervical canal. Contrast has flowed into the cavity of a large fibroid (same patient as in **A**).

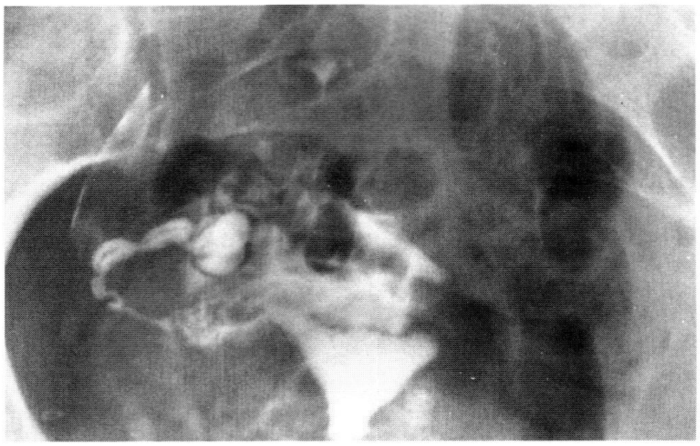

Fig. 9-5. HSG: Contrast material surrounds the opacified right tube and indicates the thickness of the tubal wall.

3. Perforation
4. Bleeding from the tenaculum site

Hysterosalpingographic findings

Hysterosalpingography provides valuable information about the uterus and oviducts.

Uterine abnormalities. Marked widening or funneling of the internal os may indicate cervical incompetence. Abnormal uterine findings include:

1. Fusion anomalies (Fig. 9-6)
2. A T-shape, secondary to in utero exposure to diethylstilbestrol (Fig. 9-7)
3. Submucous fibroids
4. Endometrial polyps (Fig. 9-8)
5. Intrauterine synechia (Fig. 9-9)

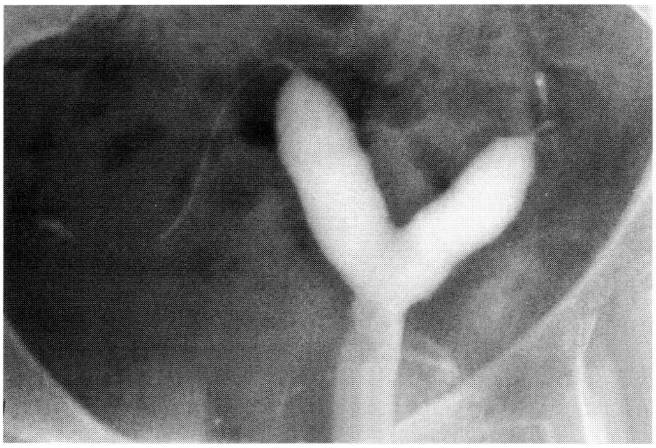

Fig. 9-6. HSG: Septate uterus.

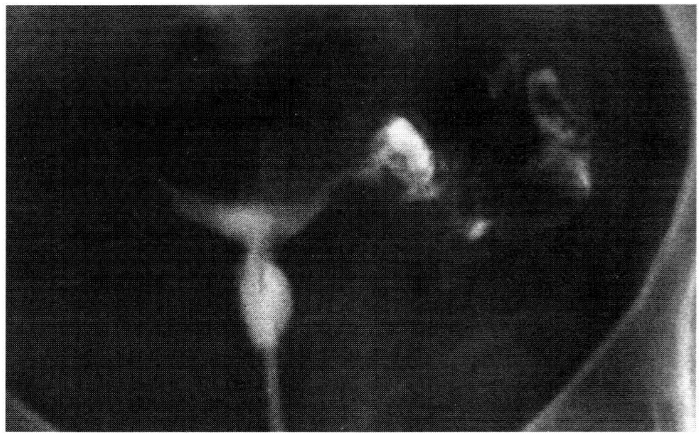

Fig. 9-7. HSG: T-shaped uterus.

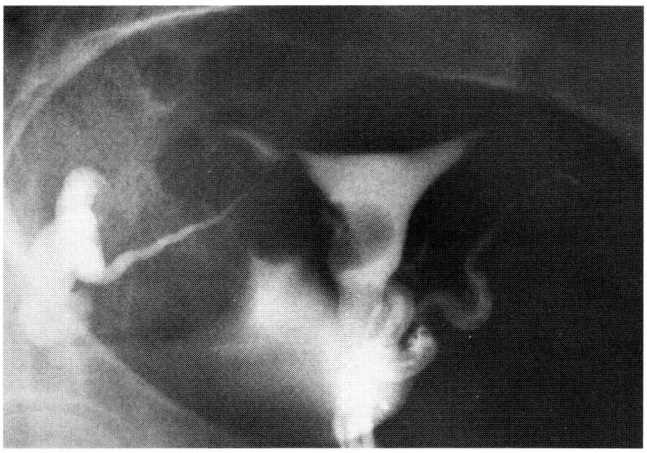

Fig. 9-8. HSG: Large filling defect in the uterine cavity and right hydrosalpinx.

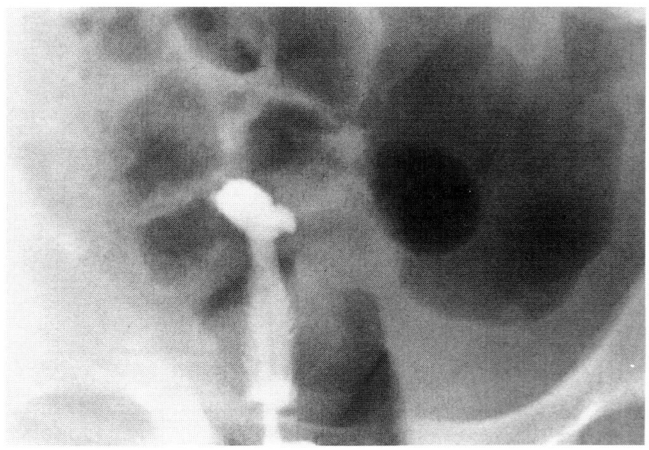

Fig. 9-9. HSG: Complete obliteration of the uterine cavity in a patient with Asherman syndrome.

6. Other less commonly identified lesions such as adenomyosis and polypoid endometrial hyperplasia.

Tubal abnormalities. The general configuration of the tubes may suggest the presence of a specific disease process. Exposure to diethylstilbestrol at the time of development of the genital tract may lead to shorter, hypoplastic oviducts with narrow abdominal ostia. Extremely tortuous oviducts that present no resistance to passage of the contrast medium have been associated with infertility in the absence of other specific anatomic abnormalities.[33] Tubes that appear fixed in the pelvis, especially when their position is abnormal suggest the presence of periadnexal adhesions. Sequelae of genital tuberculosis usually produce typical hysterosalpingographic images.

Abnormalities of the tubocornual region. Failure of contrast medium to enter the oviduct may be unilateral or bilateral. (See Table 9-2). This occurrence may be artifactual and due to tubal spasm. Spasm is more common in an anxious patient or if the HSG is poorly performed. If cornual spasm is suspected, administration of 1 mg intravenous glucagon, followed by a 5-minute delay before resuming injection of contrast material, results in relief of the condition in the majority of instances.

In the presence of a true cornual occlusion, hysterosalpingography permits the assessment of the intramural segment. This is important, since a patent and normal intramural segment allows a juxta-uterine tubocornual anastomosis to be performed. Images suggestive of salpingitis isthmica nodosa (SIN), endometreosis, or intramural polyps may be encountered with or without frank cornual occlusion. Salpingitis isthmica nodosa may produce a radiographic picture of simple obstruction to the passage of contrast medium, or there may be some evidence of interstitial spread of the fluid with small spicules of contrast apparently radiating from the tubal lumen, giving a bushy or berry-like appearance. In the earlier stages of the condition, this latter appearance will be associated with passage of contrast (Fig. 9-10). As the condition progresses, obstruction in the isthmus or intramural oviduct occurs. Endometriosis may also provide a similar image; frequently in this case the punctate pattern is more pronounced and larger.

Cornual polyps are not an uncommon finding in the in-

Table 9-2. Abnormalities of the oviduct

Abnormality	Signs	Comments
Tubocornual region		
Failure of contrast to enter tube	Simple obstruction	May be due to tubal spasm May be unilateral or bilateral
Salpingitis isthmica nodosa (SIN)	Appears as a simple obstruction or as spicules of contrast radiating from tubal lumen	May be unilateral or bilateral
Endometriosis	Similar to SIN, with more pronounced punctate pattern	
Polyps	Small globular or elongated vacuoles surrounded by contrast medium	
Isthmus		
Occlusion	Contrast outlines portion of the isthmic segment	Most commonly due to prior surgical sterilization or tubal pregnancy; less commonly to SIN; and uncommonly to tuberculosis and endometriosis
Ampulla		
Intraluminal adhesions	Patchy filling defects	Caused by endosalpingeal infection
Tubal pregnancy	Obstruction, calcifications	
Infundibulum		
Hydrosalpinx	Obstruction usually bilateral	Most common type of occlusion
Phimosis of distal tubal ostium	Intraluminal retention of contrast medium and slow intraperitoneal spill from stenosed tube	Both conditions are usually sequela of pelvic inflammatory disease
Intraperitoneal spread		
Adhesions	Localized pooling and loculation of contrast medium around distal end of oviducts	

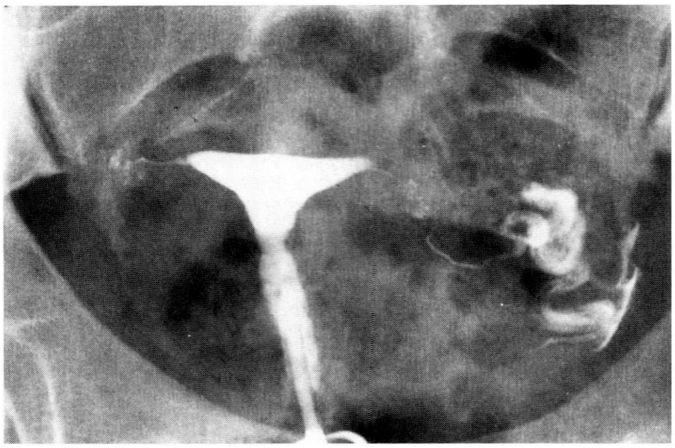

Fig. 9-10. HSG: Bilateral salpingitis isthmica nodosa with occlusion on the right but passage of contrast in the left tube.

tramural segment of the tube or proximal isthmus. They appear as small globular or elongated images (vacuoles) surrounded by contrast medium, and they may occupy the center of the lumen or may be clearly seen at the superior or inferior margin (Fig. 9-11). When seen in this fashion, they obviously do not completely obstruct the passage of contrast medium. Prospective studies have not shown their presence to affect the likelihood of conception,[34] nor has their removal improved the chances of pregnancy.[35] Infrequently, they may cause frank occlusion.

Abnormalities of the isthmus. Isthmic occlusion is most commonly due to prior surgical sterilization (Fig. 9-12). The other relatively common cause is segmental resection for tubal pregnancy. Less commonly, isthmic occlusion is associated with salpingitis isthmica nodosa; rarely, it may be due to pathologic entities such as tuberculosis or endometriosis. A previously unrecognized or expectantly treated ec-

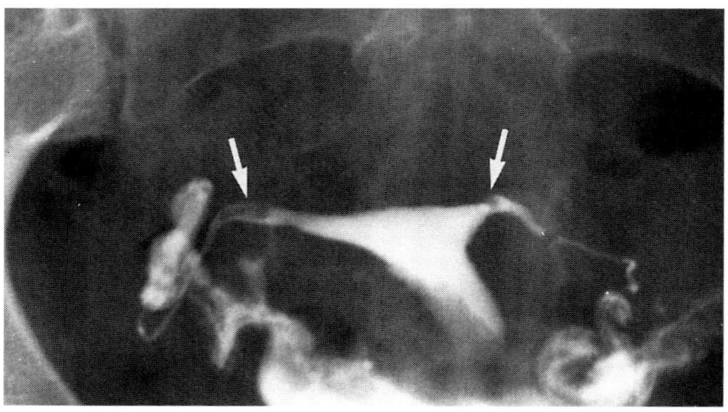

Fig. 9-11. HSG: Bilateral cornual polyps *(arrows)*.

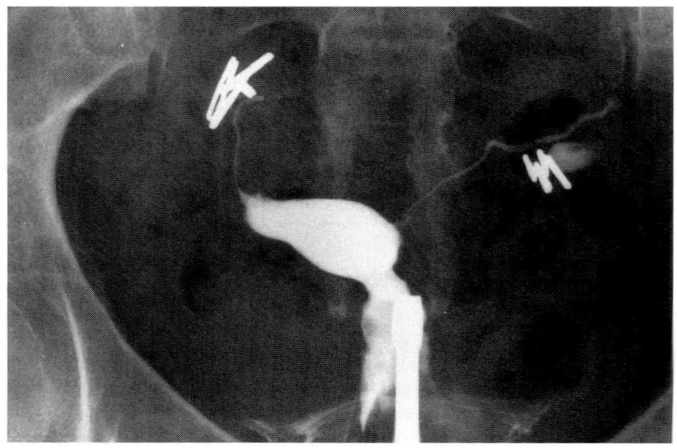

Fig. 9-12. HSG: Prior tubal sterilization. There are four clips at the sterilization site on each side.

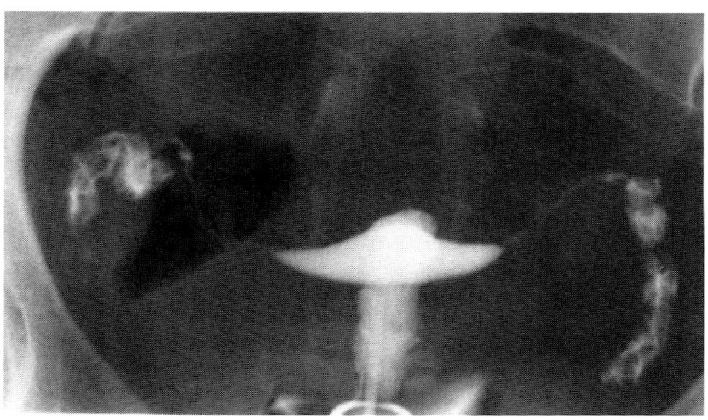

Fig. 9-13. HSG: Severe intratubal adhesions producing a honeycomb appearance.

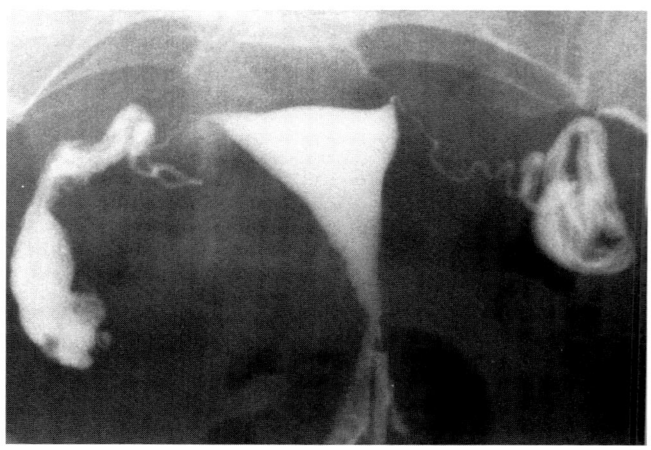

Fig. 9-14. HSG: Bilateral hydrosalpinx, demonstrating the presence of longitudinal folds in one of the tubes *(left)*.

topic pregnancy may result in isthmic obstruction, although such occlusions are more frequent in the proximal ampulla near the ampullary-isthmic junction.[36]

Abnormalities of the ampulla. Ampullary and isthmic occlusions tend to have the same etiology. Endosalpingeal infections may produce intraluminal adhesions. Patchy filling defects (leopard skin appearance) indicate the presence of intraluminal adhesions (Fig. 9-13). Tubal pregnancies may arrest and may even calcify and cause an obstruction, usually in the proximal ampulla. If not absorbed, they may be associated with a round "tumor-like" image.[37] The most frequent site for occlusion associated with tuberculosis salpingitis is the proximal ampulla.

Abnormalities of the infundibulum. The most common site of tubal occlusion is at the fimbriated end. Most forms of pelvic inflammatory disease, including those caused by chlamydia and gonorrhea, as well as pelvic sepsis resulting from extragenital infections, primarily obstruct the distal end of the oviduct. Such obstructions are usually bilateral (Fig. 9-14) but may be unilateral.

The film obtained during the early filling phase of the tubes is most valuable for assessing the endotubal architecture properly. The presence of longitudinal tubal folds in a hydrosalpinx (Fig. 9-14) is associated with a more favorable postoperative prognosis, whereas extensive intratubal adhesions or a "leopard skin" (Fig. 9-13) pattern represent a contraindication to corrective surgery. Such detail may be obscured once the tubes are distended with contrast material. When later in the performance of the HSG the tubes are distended to determine the ampullary diameter, the condition of their muscularis may be indirectly assessed.

Phimosis of the distal tubal ostium is accompanied by intraluminal retention of contrast medium and slow intraperitoneal spill from the stenosed tube. The greater the degree of phimosis, the slower will be the spill of contrast and the greater the retention of medium and intraluminal distension. In such cases, intratubal retention is frequently seen on the delayed film.

The hysterosalpingographic findings assist in deciding whether or not to recommend reconstructive surgery. A prognostic numeric grading system for distal tubal disease, which is highly correlated with subsequent pregnancy rates, has recently been produced by the American Fertility Society[38] (see Table 9-3).

Table 9-3. The American Fertility Society classification of distal tubal occlusion

Patient's Name ________________ Date ________ Chart ________

Age ______ G ______ P ______ Sp Ab ______ VTP ______ Ectopic ______ Infertile Yes ______ No ______

Other Significant History (i.e., surgery, infection, etc) ________________

HSG ________ Sonography ________ Photography ________ Laparoscopy ________ Laparotomy ________

Distal ampullary diameter	<3 cm	3-5 cm	>5 cm
L	1	4	6
R	1	4	6
Tubal wall thickness	Normal/Thin	Moderately Thickened or	Thick & Rigid
L	1	Edematous	6
R	1	4	6
		4	
Mucosal folds at neos-tomy site	Normal/ >75% Preserved	35% to 75% Preserved	<35% Preserved
		4	Adherent Mucosal Fold
L	1	4	6
R	1		6
Extent of adhesions	None/Minimal/Mild	Moderate	Extensive
L	1	3	6
R	1	3	6
Type of adhesions	None/Filmy	Moderately Dense (or	Dense
L	1	vascular)	4
R	1	2	4
		2	

Prognostic Classification for Terminal Salpingostomy (Salpingoneostomy)

	LEFT		RIGHT
A. Mild	_____	5-8	_____
B. Moderate	_____	9-10	_____
C. Severe	_____	>10	_____

Additional Findings: ________________

From Gomel V: *Fertil Steril* 49:946-948, 1988.

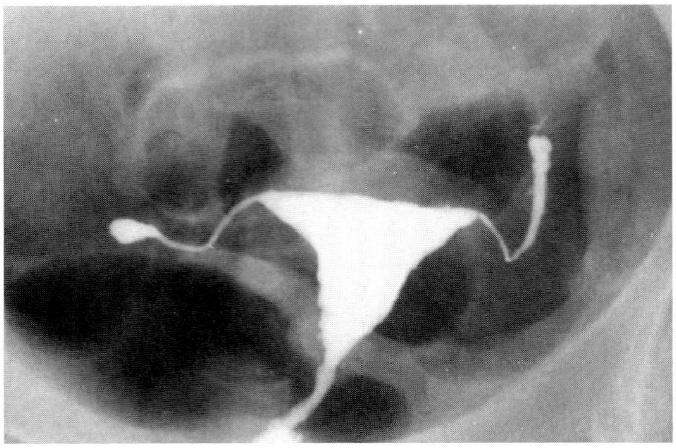

Fig. 9-15. HSG: The tubes appear rigid and are opacified only until the proximal ampulla where a sacculation can be noted.

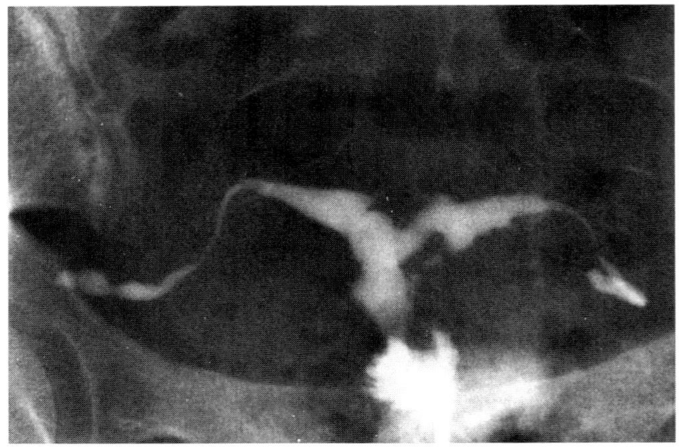

Fig. 9-16. HSG: The proximal segments of the tubes that opacify show alternating segments of dilatation and stenosis. The uterine cavity has filling defects that represent synechiae.

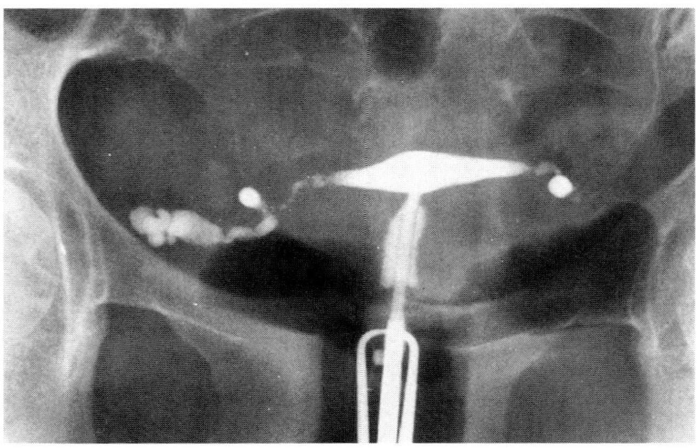

Fig. 9-17. HSG: One of the tubes, which opacifies almost completely, has dilated or constricted sections and terminates in the form of a Maltese cross.

Abnormalities of intraperitoneal spread. Passage of the contrast into the peritoneal cavity and its dispersal must be observed closely. Perifimbrial and peritubal adhesions may cause localized pooling and loculation of the contrast medium around the distal ends of the oviducts, with limited intraperitoneal spread or perhaps pooling in the pouch of Douglas. Manipulation of the uterus with the cannula may help in better assessment of such pooling.

Radiographic images of pelvic tuberculosis. Sequelae of genital tuberculosis are usually associated with typical radiographic images:

1. Golf-club appearance: the tube appears rigid (pipe-like) and shortened with a sacculation at the occlusion site, located usually in the proximal ampulla (Fig. 9-15).
2. Cotton wool image: the tube appears rigid and shortened (as in 1) with a distal image that resembles cotton wool.
3. Beaded appearance: the tube shows alternating segments of stenosis and dilatation (Fig. 9-16).
4. The Maltese cross appearance: the tube which is almost completely filled appears rigid, often dilated irregularly, and terminates in the form of a Maltese cross (Fig. 9-17) that is frequently surrounded by a halo.
5. Leopard skin appearance: the ampullary portion of the tube is irregularly opacified. This results from the penetration of the contrast material between adherent thick mucosal folds.

Frequently, uterine synechiae are also present (Fig. 9-16). Intravasation of the contrast material may also be noted. The presence of calcified pelvic lymph nodes and/or calcified inclusions in the tubal lumen associated with any of these changes serves further to strengthen the diagnosis.

Limitations

It must be emphasized that HSG has limitations. Its predictive value for diagnosing periadnexal adhesive disease or endometriosis is very low. It is associated with false-positive findings for cornual occlusion. It frequently does not divulge the exact nature of intrauterine lesions.

Selective salpingography and tubal cannulation

Selective salpingography refers to the injection of contrast medium directly into the uterine tubal ostium. This is achieved by the use of a special radiopaque cannula that is introduced through the cervix and directed toward the desired tubal ostium. The tube itself may be cannulated using a special flexible wire guide and narrow gauge cannula introduced through the larger initial cannula (Figs. 9-18 and 9-19).

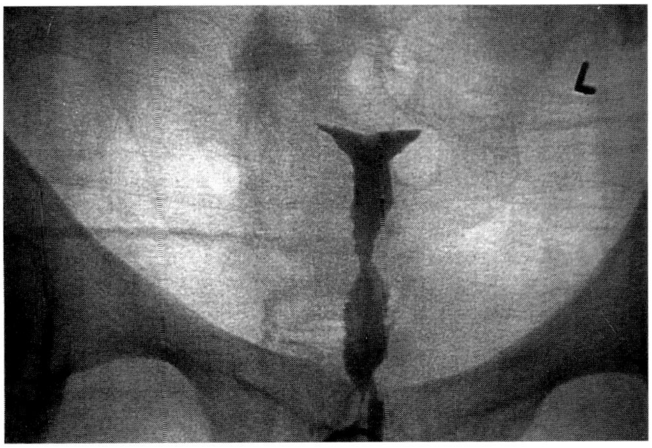

Fig. 9-18. HSG: Bilateral proximal tubal occlusion in the cornual region.

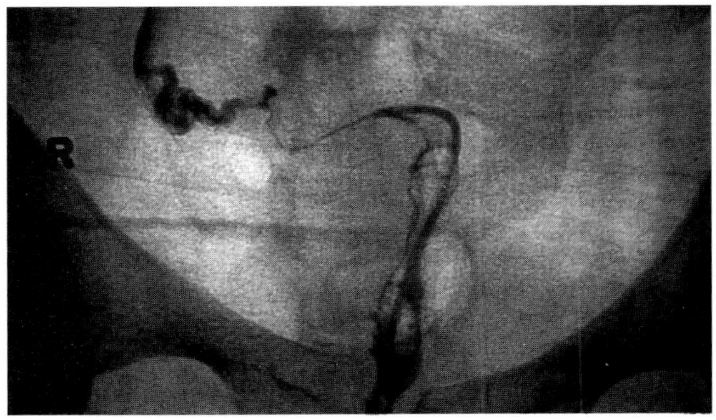

Fig. 9-19. HSG, tubal cannulation (same patient as Fig. 9-18): the cannulated right tube opacifies.

Selective salpingography and tubal cannulation may be useful in differentiating true from false cornual occlusion. Both selective salpingography and tubal cannulation may dislodge intraluminal amorphous material or separate intratubal synechia that may be responsible for the obstruction.[39] However, it is doubtful that these techniques provide a therapeutic effect in occlusions due to lesions such as salpingitis isthmica nodosa, endometriosis, obliterative fibrosis, and chronic follicular salpingitis. These techniques may provide a means of differentiating a functional obstruction from true occlusion requiring reconstructive microsurgery or in vitro fertilization.

Radionuclide hysterosalpingography

Radionuclide hysterosalpingography is a scintigraphic procedure evaluating the spontaneous pro-ovarian transport of microspheres in the genital tract. It is still experimental. A solution containing technetium^{99}m-labeled albumen microspheres is placed in the upper vagina and external cervical os. The subsequent transport of the microspheres through the cervix, uterus, and oviducts to the peritoneal cavity is monitored by a gamma-camera equipped with a pinhole collimator. The transport of microspheres depends not only on anatomic patency of the genital tract but also on the "functional integrity" of the uterus and oviducts.[40] This test is designed to assess the sperm transport function of the uterus and fallopian tubes. However, the procedure does not assess the capability of the oviduct to transport ova and embryos in the opposite direction.

LAPAROSCOPY

Laparoscopy and chromopertubation are used to visualize directly the internal reproductive organs and to test tubal patency. It is an invasive procedure for which general anesthesia is usually necessary. Laparoscopy is the most accurate way to identify periadnexal adhesive disease and endometriosis.

Periadnexal adhesions, if occurring in the presence of patent tubes, are not an absolute cause of sterility. Adhesions reduce the liklihood of pregnancy.[41] Whether they interfere with oocyte pick-up by encasing the ovary and/or the tube or restricting tubal movement or are simply a visible indicator of more subtle damage to the function of the tube is unclear. It is probable that both mechanisms are contributory.

The relationship between endometriosis and infertility will be discussed in detail in Chapter 11.

Laparoscopy is frequently used to confirm abnormal hysterosalpingographic findings. It has been argued that immediate recourse to laparoscopy should supersede hysterosalpingography.[42,43] An analysis of 18 published series has revealed that there is good congruence between laparoscopic and hysterosalpingographic findings. From these collected data the sensitivity of the HSG was found to be 76% and the specificity 83%.[44] These studies represent a selected population of patients in whom the aggregate prevalence of tubal occlusion was 38%. This prevalence figure falls to 10% in studies of large numbers of unselected patients,[45,46] which more accurately reflects the general population.

If these sensitivity and specificity figures are applied to a hypothetical group of 100 patients, in whom 10% have tubal obstruction, the calculations indicate that in the average patient a normal HSG will be followed by an abnormal laparoscopy in only 3% of cases and thus provides about 97% confidence that an immediate laparoscopy is not required. A normal test result would occur in the majority of patients.

On these grounds alone it would seem that hysterosalpingography should be the preliminary investigation. There is a caveat, however: A properly performed HSG can be of inestimable value. A poorly performed HSG is of little value to the patient or the physician.

Further advantages of initial HSG include the identification of uterine anomalies, intrauterine lesions, and cornual occlusion and/or lesions, even in the presence of cornual patency. HSG also allows immediate identification of distal tubal occlusion and assessment of intratubal architecture, which is of prognostic significance. Finally, there is increasing ability among surgeons to perform corrective laparoscopic surgery for tubal and adnexal disease. Such surgery is most likely to be successful if the uterine cavity, cornua, and intratubal architecture are normal. Prior hysterosalpingography confirming uterine and intratubal normalcy will encourage the surgeon who confirms the presence of such lesions at laparoscopy to proceed to immediate laparoscopic correction.

It is evident, therefore, that hysterosalpingography, laparoscopy, and hysteroscopy are complementary and not competitive investigative procedures.

Assessment of tubal and peritoneal factors

After the completion of the preliminary investigations described earlier in the chapter, the patients fall into one of three categories: (1) the apparently ovulatory woman whose partner is normal; (2) the apparently ovulatory woman whose partner is severely oligo- or azoospermic; and (3) the anovulatory woman.

The apparently ovulatory woman and normozoospermic man. In this instance, the next logical step is to investigate the uterine, tubal, and peritoneal factors.

If the preliminary hysterosalpinography is normal in all respects, any endoscopic evaluation should be delayed for 4 to 6 months, since pregnancy occurs spontaneously in many of these patients. If hysterosalpingography demonstrates evidence of tubal disease, the patient can be scheduled for laparoscopy. If the hysterosalpingogram demonstrates evidence of intrauterine lesions, hysteroscopy is indicated and should preferably be combined with laparoscopy.

While these comments apply to the younger infertile patient, it is advisable that endoscopic evaluation should rapidly follow even a normal hysterosalpingogram in women in their later reproductive years and those with a history that suggests the presence of uterine and/or peritoneal factors.

The apparently ovulatory woman and the man in whom cause for infertility has been determined. With oligozoospermic patients, in conjunction with ovarian stimulation, timed intrauterine insemination may be undertaken using appropriately prepared husband's sperm. In most of the more severe cases, treatment of the male is not very effective and many couples may decide to enter a therapeutic donor insemination (TDI) program. Considering the effort and cost associated with these treatment methods, if there are clinical grounds to suspect the presence of tubal and/or peritoneal disease or if the woman is of advanced reproductive age, it is appropriate to perform a preliminary hysterosalpingography before such treatments are initiated. If there are no indications for preliminary investigations, hysterosalpingography and laparoscopy should be delayed until 4 to 6 months of treatment cycles have failed to result in pregnancy. Endometriosis and adhesive disease are commonly detected in this latter group of women.

The anovulatory woman. Despite early enthusiasm for endoscopic evaluation of the ovaries in such patients, a better understanding of the endocrinology of anovulation and more sophisticated hormonal assays and ovulation induction techniques have relegated laparoscopy to a secondary role.

Premature menopause is diagnosed by the finding of consistently elevated follicle-stimulating hormone (FSH) levels in young women with secondary amenorrhea who are chromosomally normal. The differentiation between pure gonadal dysgenesis, premature ovarian failure, and the resistant ovary syndrome is made initially by laparoscopic visualization of the ovaries. The typical streak ovaries of pure gonadal dysgenesis are easily recognized. With normal appearing ovaries, adequately taken biopsies should be examined histologically. If follicles are present, a diagnosis of resistant ovary syndrome is substantiated. If no follicles are present the patient is suffering from premature ovarian failure. While estrogen-deficient women will probably require estrogen replacement therapy, those with premature ovarian failure may have a variety of associated autoimmune disorders and endocrine deficiencies that may require further investigation and follow-up.

In rare cases of intersex or primary amenorrhea, noninvasive imaging techniques and hormonal studies may fail to provide sufficient data. If such is the case, laparoscopy may be required to visualize the gonads and intrapelvic structures.

If it appears necessary to induce ovulation with gonadotrophins, a preliminary laparoscopy is recommended. In view of the risks and expense of exogenous gonadotropin therapy, a clear knowledge of the state of the patient's pelvis is indicated prior to institution of such treatment. When other methods of induction of ovulation are used (e.g., clomiphene or clomiphene and hCG or GnRH), it is appropriate to delay endoscopic evaluation until several ovulatory cycles have failed to result in a pregnancy unless there are clinical grounds to suspect tubal, peritoneal, or uterine lesions.

The role of laparoscopy in the investigation of the infertile women

Having discussed the indications of laparoscopy in the infertile patient, it is appropriate to examine its role in more detail.

In principal it is laparoscopy that permits the following questions to be answered:

1. Is the pelvic architecture normal?
2. Is there evidence of endometriosis? (see Chapter 11)
3. If the tubes are damaged should treatment be carried out?
   Laparoscopically
   Microsurgically
   By assisted reproductive techniques

These matters will be discussed in detail in Chapter 15.

Laparoscopy in the patient with a normal hysterosalpingogram. The role of laparoscopy in the patient with a normal hysterosalpingogram is either to confirm normality or to detect periadnexal adhesive disease or endometriosis, both of which frequently are missed by hysterosalpingography. Properly performed hysterosalpingography rarely misses intrauterine lesions; however, there is a wide discrepancy between hysteroscopic findings and those at hysterosalpingography if the latter has been inadequately carried out. If the surgeon has reason to believe that a so-called normal hysterosalpingogram has been inadequately performed, it is appropriate to combine hysteroscopy with the laparoscopic evaluation.

Laparoscopy in the patient with an abnormal hysterosalpingogram. The role of endoscopy in the patient with an abnormal hysterosalpingogram is dependent on the abnormality apparently detected.

Periadnexal adhesive disease. Well-performed hysterosalpingography may suggest that there is periadnexal adhesive disease. The exact nature and severity of such a condition can be assessed only laparoscopically. The laparoscopic evaluation will confirm or refute the presence of such adhesions. If adhesions are detected, their nature and severity can be noted and usually they will be amenable to laparoscopic surgical correction, as will be described in Chapter 15. In rare circumstances the type, extent, and severity of adhesions, even in the presence of patent tubes, may be sufficient to be a contraindication to reparative surgery.

Distal tubal disease. If hysterosalpingography suggests distal tubal phimosis or demonstrates the presence of a hydrosalpinx, laparoscopy is indicated. Laparoscopy will determine whether or not a fimbrial phimosis does indeed exist. It permits the assessment of any hydrosalpinx, the nature and extent of associated periadnexal adhesive disease, and/or other intrapelvic lesions.

Distal tubal occlusion may be partial or complete. Partial occlusion results from agglutination of the fimbria (fimbrial phimosis) or from stenosis at the level of the abdominal tubal ostium located at the apex of the infundibulum (prefimbrial phimosis). The fimbrial end may also be covered by fibrous tissue. When the distal tube is totally occluded this is termed hydrosalpinx, as it usually contains clear fluid. Particular attention must be paid to the extent of tubal distention, thickness, and rigidity of the tubal wall. The severity and nature of any associated pelvic and periadnexal adhesions must also be noted.

These factors have been used to develop a numeric scoring system by which the likely surgical outcome can be estimated[38] (see Table 9-3 on p. 107).

Proximal tubal disease. When hysterosalpingography suggests cornual occlusion or proximal tubal disease, laparoscopy serves to confirm or refute the presence of occlusion by chromopertubation and may identify abnormal morphologic changes in the proximal tube. Enlargement in the cornual region is usually due to salpingitis isthmica nodosa or rarely endometriosis. Laparoscopy will also enable the assessment of the remainder of the tube with particular reference to the status of the fimbriated end and determination of the presence or absence of any periadnexal adhesive disease or other pathologic processes.

The endoscopic survey in infertility

"No surgical procedure is entirely without risk and the endoscopic evaluation of the infertile patient should not be undertaken lightly, nor should it be performed unless it is done so in a fashion which will provide the maximum amount of information."[1] It is the purpose of this section to describe in detail the thorough endoscopic survey of the infertile patient.

As described in Chapter 5, after the laparoscope has been inserted, the entire peritoneal cavity including the upper abdomen is inspected. Particular attention is paid in the lower abdomen to the parietal peritoneum and any obvious omental adhesions. The patient is then placed in the Trendelenberg position to improve access to the pelvic cavity. The bowel is displaced by manipulating the uterus with the uterine cannula, as previously described. A thorough infertility survey cannot be performed unless a probe is inserted through a second puncture cannula. After the probe has been inserted, any residual bowel in the pelvic cavity is gently displaced with this probe. If this step is not undertaken, it is frequently impossible to visualize fully the pouch of Douglas.

A systematic survey is carried out as follows: A general panoramic inspection of the pelvic contents is first performed with the laparoscope at some distance from the pelvic organs. Such a general inspection will allow an immediate impression of the pelvis to be formed. The uterine manipulator should be used to elevate the uterus, particularly in cases of uterine retroversion, and to mobilize the adnexae.

Once a general impression has been formed, the laparoscope is advanced and systematic viewing of the pelvis undertaken, commencing with the uterus. The manipulator is used to position the uterus in retroversion, and its anterior surface and the uterovesical reflection are scrutinized. Unless this step is taken, areas of endometriosis may be missed. The uterus is moved into anteversion and its fundus and posterior surface assessed.

The amount of fluid in the pouch of Douglas and its nature is noted and any evidence of scarring or endometriosis ascertained. The appearance of endometriosis is very variable and will be discussed in greater detail in Chapter 11. Peritoneal fluid can be aspirated by replacing the probe with a suction cannula. Aspiration may be required if the fluid is of such nature or quantity as to obscure visualization of the cul-de-sac and uterosacral ligaments. Further, such aspirated fluid may be of value in biochemical or microbiologic studies. Each uterosacral ligament is viewed so that endometriosis and scarring can be detected.

Each adnexa in turn is thoroughly scrutinized. A proper evaluation of the adnexa requires the visualization of all of the surfaces and this is achieved by the use of the probe. The anterior surface of the ovary is inspected. The ovary is then elevated with the probe and flipped toward the tube. However, on some occasions this can be achieved by the systematic displacement of the pelvic organs with the uterus, by appropriately manipulating the uterine cannula. The inferior surface of the ovary and the posterior leaf of the broad ligament to the level of the uterosacral ligament are evaluated.

The tube is inspected systematically. The fimbria are visualized and manipulated gently with the probe and viewed *en face*. Attention is paid to the fimbria ovarica and its length. The tube is examined throughout its length from its distal to its proximal segment. Particular attention is paid to any evidence of distal tubal occlusion (hydrosalpinx), fimbrial phimosis, or fusiform swelling at the uterotubal junction. The latter is usually caused by salpingitis isthmica nodosa or endometriosis. Any evidence of endometriosis of the tube is sought. The other adnexa is similarly assessed.

At this point of the evaluation, chromopertubation is performed by injecting dilute methylene blue or indigo carmine solution through the uterine cannula. It is essential that the seal between the uterine cannula and the cervix is watertight. The passage of dye solution is followed through the uterotubal junction and along the isthmus and ampulla. The fimbria should once again be gently manipulated with the probe so that they can be viewed *en face* to determine whether or not there is free spill of the dye. The presence or absence of prefimbrial phimosis or fine fimbrial adhesions that may impede ovum pickup should be noted.

The description thus far has assumed easy access to the pelvis. In the presence of significant pelvic adhesive disease, visualization of the pelvic structures may be much more difficult.

Omental adhesions. Particularly in patients who have undergone previous lower abdominal surgery, the omentum may be adherent to the scars and hang like a curtain between the laparoscope and the pelvic structures. In order to achieve pelvic visualization, it may be necessary to seek a lateral route around this curtain or, in many cases, in order to visualize both adnexa, it may be necessary to adopt a bilateral lateral approach. In other circumstances, the omentum may be adherent to the entire circumference of the pelvic brim entirely occluding access. It is usually possible to identify a thin avascular area through which the tip of the telescope may be thrust; otherwise separation may be achieved by use of the blunt probe or preferably laparoscopic scissors (see Chapter 7).

Periadnexal adhesive disease. The presence of periadenxal adhesive disease may prevent visualization of the ovaries or of the oviducts, especially at their distal portions. It may be necessary to introduce other ancillary instruments to dissect these adhesions before visualization can be achieved. This technique of dissection will be described in Chapter 15.

Endometriosis. Following panoramic viewing of the pelvis, apparent normalcy may be detected. However, when the probe is introduced below the ovary it may be impossible to free it from the pelvic sidewall. In this event, even if no other evidence of endometriosis is detected, in the absence of a history of prior pelvic surgery or evidence of periadnexal adhesive disease, it is probable that such patients do indeed suffer from endometriosis. If the ovaries are adherent to the pelvic sidewall, an endeavor should be made to separate them with the blunt probe. If separation occurs, areas of endometriosis are usually noted on the posterior surface of the ovary and the lateral pelvic sidewall. If the ovary is enlarged or appears to contain an endometrioma and is intimately adherent, force should not be used in an attempt to separate it from the pelvic sidewall. If undue force is applied, the endometrioma may rupture or bleeding may be caused. Similarly, ovarian manipulation should be carried out gently in the presence of an early corpus luteum, as such structures are extremely fragile and can bleed profusely. These matters are considered in greater detail in Chapter 11.

Assessment of the woman requesting reversal of sterilization

Prior to endoscopic evaluation of a woman requesting reversal of a sterilization, the operative and pathology reports should be obtained to ensure that the previous procedure does not preclude a reversal as, for example, in cases of subtotal salpingectomy. The fertility status of the male partner and the other fertility parameters of the woman should be determined.

A preliminary hysterosalpingogram is performed to assess the uterine cavity, the cornual regions, and the length, internal patency, and architecture of the proximal tubal segments (see Fig. 9-12). A subsequent laparoscopy will permit the assessment of the pelvis to detect adhesions or any additional lesions. Laparoscopy also permits the assessment of the length and status of the distal tubal segments including the fimbria. This information is essential for advising the patient about the prognosis and in planning the reconstructive surgical procedure.

In certain circumstances, when the sterilization has been performed with occlusive devices such as clips and rings, which are associated with relatively little destruction of the oviducts, and in the operative report the pelvic structures have been described in detail as being normal, especially with women in the same union and/or if a great deal of time has not elapsed since the sterilization procedure, the surgeon may dispense with the preliminary laparoscopy.

Timing of laparoscopy during the menstrual cycle

Endoscopic evaluation of the infertile patient can be performed during the follicular or luteal phase. Patients with suspected intrauterine disease are best examined during the follicular phase, since concurrent hysteroscopy is more easily performed at this time. In addition, if cornual occlusion is suspected, the cornua can be better visualized by hysteroscopy and chromopertubation is less likely to give false positive results

Laparoscopy performed in the luteal phase offers the advantage of inspecting the ovaries for the presence of corpora lutea and ovulation stigmata. In addition, endometrial biopsy samples to determine presumptive evidence of ovulation can be obtained. Endoscopy performed in the luteal phase has certain disadvantages. Hysteroscopic interpretation is more difficult, and the procedure may be performed despite an unsuspected pregnancy. In addition, laparoscopic manipulations are made more difficult by the presence of the fragile hemorrhagic corpus luteum.

For most surgeons, the ability to time such procedures accurately is difficult due to operating room schedules. Nevertheless, every attempt should be made to assess those patients believed to have cornual occlusion or intrauterine lesions during the early follicular phase.

SUMMARY

1. Laparoscopy and hysterosalpingography play complementary roles in the investigation of the infertile female.
2. Hysterosalpingography is of value only if properly performed.
3. Laparoscopic investigation of the female genital tract should be performed *after* all other appropriate tests for both partners have been concluded.
4. Hysterosalpingography should be the primary method of investigation, offering as it does the advantages of:
   Identification of uterine anomalies and intrauterine lesions
   Identification of probable cornual occlusion and/or cornual lesions even in the presence of cornual patency
   Immediate identification of distal tubal occlusion and an assessment of the intratubal architecture
   Selection of certain patients for planned laparoscopic fertility-enhancing surgery
5. Hysterosalpingography is less effective than laparoscopy (or hysteroscopy where appropriate) in:
   Assessing uterine lesions
   Detecting periadnexal adhesions and endometriosis
6. The finding of an abnormal hysterosalpingogram should be followed by endoscopic evaluation.
7. Except in the reproductively older woman, endoscopy should be delayed 4 to 6 months in cases where the hysterosalpingogram is apparently normal.
8. Unless the endoscopic pelvic survey is performed meticulously, it is of limited value. Pelvic contents should be scrutinized thoroughly and systematically. This survey cannot be performed adequately without the aid of a uterine manipulator and a calibrated probe.
9. Hysterosalpingography and laparoscopy should be performed in the majority of women requesting reversal of sterilization before a laparotomy is undertaken for reconstructive surgery. Hysterosalpingography alone may be sufficient for many patients who have undergone clip or ring sterilization.

REFERENCES

1. Gomel V, Taylor PJ, Yuzpe AA, Roux JE: Laparoscopy and hysteroscopy in gynecologic practice. Chicago, 1986, Year Book Medical Publishers.
2. Leader A, Taylor PJ, Daudi FA: The value of routine rubella and syphilitic serology in the infertile couple. *Fertil Steril* 42:140, 1984.
3. Rosenfeld DL, Garcia CR: A comparison of endomentrial histology with simultaneous plasma progesterone determinations in infertile women. *Fertil Steril* 27:1256-1266, 1976.
4. Marik J, Hulka J: Luteinized unruptured follicle syndrome: a subtle cause of infertility. *Fertil Steril* 29:270-274, 1978.
5. Koninckx PR, Ide P, Vandenbroucke W, Brosens IA: New aspects of the pathophysiology of endometriosis and associated infertility. *J Reprod Med* 24:257-260, 1978.
6. Jones GES: Some newer aspects of the management of infertility. *JAMA* 141:1123-1129, 1949.
7. Lenton EA, Landgren B-M, Sexton L: Normal variation in the length of the luteal phase of the menstrual cycle: identification of the short luteal phase. *Br J Obstet Gynaecol* 91:685-689, 1984.
8. Marshall J: Thermal changes in the normal menstrual cycle. *Br Med J* 1:102-104, 1963.
9. Shoupe D, Mishell jun DR, Lacarra M, et al: Correlation of endometrial maturation with four methods of estimating day of ovulation. *Obstet Gynecol* 73:88-92, 1989.
10. Balasch J, Creus M, Marquez M, Burzaco I, Vanrell JA: The significance of luteal phase deficiency on fertility: a diagnostic and therapeutic approach. *Hum Reprod* 1:145-147, 1986.
11. Glazener CMA, Kelly NJ, Hull MGR: Luteal deficiency not a persistent cause of infertility. *Hum Reprod* 3:213-217, 1988.

12. Taylor PJ, Collins JA: Unexplained infertility. New York, 1992, Oxford Medical Publications.
13. Griffith CS, Grimes DA: The validity of the postcoital test. *Am J Obstet Gynecol* 162:616-620, 1990.
14. Deleted in proofs.
15. Templeton AA, Mortimer D: The development of a clinical test of sperm migration to the site of fertilization. *Fertil Steril* 37:410-415, 1982.
16. Taylor PJ, Graham G: Is diagnostic curettage harmful in women with unexplained infertility? *Br J Obstet Gynecol* 89:296-298, 1982.
17. Pauerstein CJ, Turner T, Eddy CA: A technique for evaluating functional patency of the oviduct. *Fertil Steril* 28:777-780, 1977.
18. Uher J, Rypacek F, Presl J: Transport of novel ovum surrogates in the human fallopian tube: a clinical study. *Fertil Steril* 54:278-82, 1990.
19. Brosens IA, Vasquez G: Fimbrial microbiopsy. *J Reprod Med* 16:171-178, 1976.
20. Gomel V: Microsurgery in female infertility. Boston, 1983, Little Brown.
21. Rosenfeld DL, Seidman SM, Bronson RA, Scholl GM: Unsuspected chronic pelvic inflammatory disease in the infertile female. *Fertil Steril* 39:44-8, 1983.
22. Collins JA, Wrixon W, Janes LB, Wilson EH: Treatment-independent pregnancy among infertile couples. *N Engl J Med* 309:1201-1206, 1983.
23. Hull MGR, Glazener CMA, Kelly NJ, et al: Population study of causes, treatment, and outcome of infertility. *Br Med J* 291:1693-1697, 1985.
24. Kliger BE: Evaluation, therapy and outcome in 493 infertile couples. *Fertil Steril* 41:40-46, 1984.
25. Stumpf PG, March CM: Febrile morbidity following hysterosalpingography: identification of risk factors and recommendations for prophylaxis. *Fertil Steril* 33:487-492, 1980.
26. Westrom L: Effect of acute pelvic inflammatory disease on fertility. *Am J Obstet Gynecol* 121:707-713, 1975.
27. Dan U, Oelsner G, Gruberg L, et al: Cerebral embolization and coma after hysterosalpingography with oil-soluble contrast medium. *Fertil Steril* 53:939-940, 1990.
28. DeCherney AH, Kort H, Barney JB, DeVore GR: Increased pregnancy rate with oil-soluble hysterosalpingography dye. *Fertil Steril* 33:407-410, 1980.
29. Schwabe MG, Shapiro SS, Haning jun RV: Hysterosalpingography with oil contrast medium enhances fertility in patients with infertility of unknown etiology. *Fertil Steril* 40:604-606, 1983.
30. Johnson JV, Montoya IA, Olive DL: Ethiodol oil contrast medium inhibits macrophage phagocytosis and adherence by altering membrane electronegativity and microviscosity. *Fertil Steril* 58:511-517, 1992.
31. Alper MM, Garner PR, Spence JEH, Quarrington AM: Pregnancy rates after hysterosalpingography with oil- and water-soluble contrast media. *Obstet Gynecol* 68:6-9, 1986.
32. Musset R: An atlas of hysterosalpingography. Quebec, 1979, Les Presses de l-Universite Laval.
33. Leeton J, Salwood T: The tortuous tube: pregnancy rate following laparoscopy and hydrotubation. *Aust NZ J Obstet Gynaecol* 18:259, 1978.
34. Glazener CMA, Loveden LM, Richardson SJ, et al: Tubo-cornual polyps: their relevance in subfertility. *Hum Reprod* 2:59-62, 1987d.
35. Gordts S, Boeckx W, Vasquez G, Brosens I: Microsurgical resection of intramural tubal polyps. *Fertil Steril* 40:258-259, 1983.
36. Urman B, Gomel V, McComb P, Lee N: Midtubal occlusion: etiology, management, and outcome. *Fertil Steril* 59:747-750, 1992.
37. Gomel V, Filmar S: Arrested tubal pregnancy. *Fertil Steril* 48:1043-1047, 1987.
38. Gomel V: Distal tubal occlusion. Fertil Steril 49:946-948, 1988.
39. Thurmond AS: Selective salpingography and fallopian tube recanalization. *AJR* 156:33-38, 1991.
40. Brundin A, Dahlborn M, Ahlberg-Ahre E, Lundberg HJ: Radionuclide hysterosalpingography for measurement of human oviduct function. *Int J Gynecol Obstet* 28:53, 1989.
41. Tulandi T, Collins JA, Burrows E, et al: Treatment-dependent and treatment-independent pregnancy among women with periadnexal adhesions. *Am J Obstet Gynecol* 162:354-357, 1990.
42. Taylor PJ, Cumming DC: Laparoscopy in the infertile female. *Curr Probl Obstet Gynecol* 2:3-59, 1979.
43. Templeton AA, Kerr MG: An assessment of laparoscopy as the primary investigation in the subfertile female. *Br J Obstet Gynaecol* 84:760-762, 1977.
44. Taylor PJ, Collins JA: Unexplained infertility. Oxford, 1992, Oxford University Press.
45. Collins JA, Wrixon W, Jans LB, Wilson EH: Treatment-independent pregnancy among infertile couples. *N Engl J Med* 309:1201-1206, 1983.
46. Hull MGR, Glazener CMA, Kelly NJ, et al: Population study of causes, treatment and outcome of infertility. *Br Med J* 291:1693-1697, 1985.

Chapter 10

PELVIC PAIN

The relief of pain is one of the most urgent and pressing requests that a patient can make of any physician. For the gynecologic patient, this pain tends to be located in the lower abdomen and pelvis. While frequently the cause is obvious and the treatment clear cut, in other clinical situations the diagnosis remains elusive.

Pain is a symptom that may or may not be associated with obvious organic findings. Furthermore, pain is subjective. In each case, the psychologic and organic aspects may be extremely difficult to separate. The main function of the laparoscopic evaluation is to detect the presence or absence of an obvious organic lesion. The often difficult role of the physician is to relate these endoscopic findings to the total picture of the patient and attempt to devise a successful course of treatment. In some situations this treatment may be effected by laparoscopic means.

The anatomic distribution of pain fibers to the pelvis is still not clearly understood and the initiation, transmission, and perception of painful stimuli continue to be a source of research endeavor for the neurophysiologist.

This chapter will briefly describe the anatomy of the nerve supply of the pelvis and physiology of pain transmission and perception. Acute and chronic pelvic pain states will be classified. The symptoms and signs will be described, not by disease state, but rather as how they will be encountered in the office or emergency room. Discussions of the diagnosis and management options for patients suffering from both acute and chronic pelvic pain will follow. The role of laparoscopy in the diagnostic process will be highlighted. Laparoscopic surgical approaches will be mentioned briefly, but the details of their performance will be found in the appropriate chapters in Section IV.

ANATOMY AND PHYSIOLOGY

Nerve supply

The anterolateral muscles of the lower abdominal wall (the internal and external oblique, rectus abdominus, transversus, and pyramidalis) are innervated from the anterior primary rami of the lower three thoracic and first lumbar nerves (T10-11-12 and L1) of the central nervous system.

The visceral structures are supplied by fibers derived from the autonomic nervous system. The uterus is supplied by motor nerves of sympathetic and parasympathetic origin arising from the spinal roots T5 to L2. Preganglionic fibers coalesce to form the greater, lesser, and the lowest splanchnic nerves. The preganglionic fibers synapse in the celiac, aorticornual, and inferior mesenteric branch of the hypogastric ganglia. The preganglionic fibers from L1 and L2 also synapse in the hypogastric ganglion. The postganglionic fibers travel in close proximity to the aorta. Those supplying the pelvic structures form the two hypogastric (presacral) nerves. These nerves eventually intermingle to form the hypogastric plexus. From the hypogastric plexus, the right and left pelvic (Frankenhauser's) plexus form. Preganglionic parasympathetic fibers from S2 and S3 join Frankenhauser's plexus. Those fibers which supply the uterus run along the course of the internal iliac arteries and uterine arteries. The fundus of the uterus and the fallopian tubes receive postganglionic sympathetic motor neurons from the renal plexus. The sensory nerve supply of the ovaries, fallopian tubes, and uterus is derived from the spinal roots T11 and T12.[1] Afferent fibers from the cervix run with the uterine artery in the base of the broad ligament through the pelvic plexuses and eventually to the spinal cord through S2, 3, and 4. Fibers from the fundus of the uterus, tubes, and ovaries reach the dorsal roots through the ovarian and renal plexus.

The pelvic colon, rectum, and anus receive a sympathetic nerve supply from the lumbar part of the sympathetic trunk and the hypogastric plexus. The parasympathetic supply, in the form of preganglionic fibers, is derived in part from the pelvic splanchnics.

The parietal peritoneum has a sensory nerve supply derived from the sympathetic nervous system. The distribution of this supply is roughly equivalent to the distribution of somatic sensory nerves in the abdominal surface. Pain caused by irritation of the parietal peritoneum is appreciated in a dermatome that is supplied by somatic nerves. This description of the neuroanatomy is heavily dependent on the work of Coote and Crawford.[2]

Pain transmission

Of all sensations, pain is the least well understood. It is recognized that it is induced by tissue-damaging stimuli. These stimuli cannot be measured with the same degree of accuracy as, for example, thermal or auditory stimuli. Classically, pain is described as occurring in two forms. "First pain" is related temporally to the stimulus, but as it is experienced only in the skin it is not relevant to the pain experienced due to lesions of the pelvic organs. "Second pain" is felt in the skin and deep tissues. It is poorly localized, conducted slowly, and often persists after the nocioreceptive stimulus has been removed. This is the type of pain experienced from the internal organs.

When a tissue-damaging stimulus occurs, it affects the pain receptors, which are bare nerve endings located within the viscera. These are nonspecific nociceptors and will respond to a variety of damaging stimuli. From the receptors, the stimulus is conducted to the spinal cord and ascends to higher centers. A large number of neurotransmitters have been implicated in the production of the painful stimulus and include glutamic acid, substance P, somatostatin, cholecystokinin-like peptide, vasoactive intestinal peptide, and angiotensin.[3] Numerous other neurotransmitters have been identified within the dorsal horn neurons and in the supraspinal regions.

Afferent fibers which supply the pelvic organs terminate in the posterior horn of the gray matter of the spinal cord. The posterior horn neurons which relay painful inputs are found predominantly in laminae 1 and 5. The ascending projection from these neurons goes through the lateral spinothalamic tract to the opposite side, although a small number of fibers ascend ipsilaterally. These pathways seem to project to the ventral posterior nuclei of the thalamus, where the capability to recognize and localize pain sensation is found. They probably handle more first pain than second pain. It is possible also that these ascending pathways project to nonspecific thalamic nuclei as well as the reticular formation of the lower brainstem, the hypothalamus, limbic system, frontal lobes, and aqueductal gray matter of the midbrain.

Despite the fact that pelvic pain is the second most common presenting gynecologic symptom, it is recognized that the uterus, tubes, ovaries, and gut are insensitive to many of the stimuli that result in pain in the skin and superficial tissues. Thermal, chemical, and tactile sensations are not appreciated from the pelvic structures. To explain this anomaly of neurophysiology, visceral pain is described as referred and splanchnic.

The same spinal cord segment that supplies the autonomic fibers to a pelvic organ also innervates a dermatome with somatic nerves. The concept of *referred pain* suggests that autonomic impulses arising in the diseased organ set up an irritable focus within the spinal cord thereby exciting the cells that receive impulses from the somatic area. These stimuli are then transmitted to the corresponding central nervous system sites and the pain is appreciated in the referred superficial area. True *splanchnic* or *visceral pain* is best illustrated by the discomfort of dysmenorrhea or the pain of a distended viscus, where the nociostimulus is indeed appreciated in the specific organ from which it arises. Stimuli that can produce pain from lesions within the pelvis include (1) inflammation of the nerves secondary to inflammation or neoplastic processes, (2) ischemia, (3) irritation of the parietal peritoneum, (4) stretching of the capsule of a solid organ, and (5) distention and contraction of the muscles of a hollow viscus.

Pain perception

The physical locations wherein pain is perceived centrally are not fully defined. The role of the central neurotransmitters and particularly the endogenous opiate peptides is under very active investigation. The interested reader is referred to the review by Jessel.[3] It must be remembered that there is a major affective component to pain perception[4] and that the patient's emotional state can greatly influence the manner in which a particular painful stimulus is appreciated.

CLASSIFICATION OF PELVIC PAIN

The following is simple classification of pelvic pain:

1. acute pelvic pain
2. chronic pelvic pain
   - cyclic
   - constant

Each category may be further subdivided into:

1. arising from the reproductive tract
2. arising from other organ systems

and each of these may be:

1. obviously organic in origin
2. possibly organic in origin
3. probably psychogenic in origin

CLINICAL PRESENTATION

The first steps toward establishing a working diagnosis are the history and physical examination. Attention should be paid to the nature of the presenting symptom, the relationship of the pain with the menstrual cycle, any associated symptoms, and the physical findings.[5]

The nature of the presenting symptom

The patient should be questioned about the onset of the pain, its character, intensity, and duration.

Onset. Pain of sudden onset may be indicative of an acute intraperitoneal event that has led to soiling of the peritoneum with either blood, pus, contents of bowel, or the contents of an ovarian cyst or to ischemic infarction of an intrapelvic structure. Pain of sudden onset may also be due to acute colic of the urinary or gastrointestinal tracts. It may occur in the absence of any obvious organic lesion. Differentiation between the pain of colic and that of an intraperitoneal event is made by examination of the second quality of the pain, its character.

Character. Pain may be constant or intermittent, sharp or dull. Constant acute pain usually presupposes peritoneal irritation or ischemia of an intra-abdominal or pelvic organ. Colicky pain suggests increased contractions of a distended hollow organ such as the ureter, bowel, fallopian tube, or uterus. Sharp pain tends to occur when there is obstruction of a hollow viscus or an acute intraperitoneal catastrophe. Dull pain is more likely to be associated with an inflammatory process.

Intensity. The intensity of the pain can be assessed by evaluation of the patient's subjective feelings, which can be extremely unreliable, or by the assessment of objective criteria. A patient who is smiling but complaining of unbearable pain is unlikely to be suffering from a major organic complaint. The pale, drawn, sweating patient must be considered to have an organic lesion. Further objective criteria relating organic lesions to the severity of the patient's complaint will be detected by physical examination and will be described later.

Duration. Whether the pain is acute or chronic in nature, it is important to establish the length of time that the patient has suffered. When the presentation is acute, it is unusual for the patient to have experienced the symptom for more than 48 hours. While some conditions such as acute appendicitis may begin with a slow onset of gradual aching pain that progresses to an acute episode, others may begin suddenly and acutely as when an ovarian cyst ruptures. The duration of the symptoms of chronic pelvic pain is extremely variable. Such a symptom may have been present for a few weeks or for several years before the patient draws it to the attention of her physician.

Relationship of pain to the menstrual cycle

The pain may bear a direct temporal relationship to menstrual function or may be completely unrelated. Pain occurring with menstruation is usually one or other form of dysmenorrhea (see later). Midcycle pain (mittelschmerz) may be coincident with ovulation. Pain occurring in a patient during the reproductive years following a short period of amenorrhea must be regarded as a complication of early pregnancy until proved otherwise. All other causes of pelvic pain bear no such temporal association, except coincidentally.

Associated symptoms

Associated symptoms will be dependent upon the cause of the pain and the involvement of adjacent structures. Pain of gastrointestinal origin may be associated with anorexia, vomiting, diarrhea, tenesmus, and painful defecation. However, these symptoms may also occur if blood or pus invest the lower gastrointestinal tract. Blood in the stool is indicative of a bowel lesion.

Frequency, dysuria and strangury are symptoms associated with lesions of the urogenital tract but may all be provoked if adjacent organs are involved in an inflammatory or hemorrhagic process. For example, blood lying on the dome of the bladder will cause acute pain each time the patient voids. It is unusual for hematuria to have a source other than from the urogenital tract.

Fainting attacks frequently accompany small amounts of intraperitoneal bleeding. The mechanism is not understood. Irritation of the undersurface of the diaphragm will be appreciated as shouldertip pain. The diaphragm may be irritated by large quantities of blood or fluid within the peritoneal cavity or by the inflammatory process of perihepatitis, a condition seen in association with acute salpingitis.

There will be many instances in which differentiation is still difficult. Attention should be paid to any helpful antecedent history. It is impossible to provide an exhaustive list of all those conditions in the antecedent history, which may provide valuable clinical clues. However, an example might be the patient who has had a documented attack of acute pelvic inflammatory disease (PID). She may well be suffering from a recurrence and is at greater risk of an ectopic pregnancy as is the woman who has had previous tubal reparative surgery, or assisted reproduction (ART). A history of prior appendectomy can be invaluable; clearly, such a patient does not suffer from the same condition at this presentation.

The physical findings

The physical signs of those conditions that may lead to a complaint of pelvic or lower abdominal pain are too numerous to mention individually. In general terms, however, once the general physical examination has been completed, attention should be paid to the examination of the abdomen and the pelvis. The abdomen should be examined by the classic method of inspection, auscultation, palpation, and percussion. Such an approach will permit localization of the site of maximum tenderness; the presence or absence of guarding, rebound, and reflex rigidity; the presence or absence of bowel sounds, which may be indicative of intestinal obstruction or ileus; the presence or absence or ascitic fluid; and the presence or absence of a palpable abdominal mass.

The subsequent pelvic examination will permit thorough

inspection of the lower genital tract. In almost all such patients, the bimanual examination will undoubtedly provoke the complaint of tenderness. Such patients may be differentiated into those with and those without an obvious palpable mass. Pain triggered by cervical movement (cervical excitation pain) points toward the affected adnexa. In cases of ectopic pregnancy, this excitation pain was eloquently described by Munro Kerr as "yelling tenderness."[6]

By the time the history has been taken and the physical examination performed, it may be possible to establish a firm diagnosis. Under these circumstances, no special investigations will be required and management may be implemented. In other cases, the physician should have arrived at a working differential diagnosis and on this basis implement appropriate investigations. In a final patient category, a clear working differential diagnosis cannot be established, despite the application of clinical acumen.

The application of these basic principles to the specific patient with either acute or chronic pelvic pain will be discussed in the subsequent sections.

ACUTE PELVIC PAIN

Acute pelvic pain, arising in the reproductive tract, usually presents with sudden onset, starts in the lower abdomen, and ultimately may involve the entire abdomen. The pain may be associated with anorexia, vomiting, diarrhea, or urinary symptoms, depending on the cause and involvement of adjacent structures. There also may be vaginal bleeding. Diaphragmatic irritation will be perceived as shoulder pain.

The clinical presentation of acute pelvic pain of nonreproductive tract origin is beyond the scope of this book and should be familiar to the reader. The more common causes of acute pelvic pain are listed in the box at right and must be considered in the differential diagnosis. In addition, acute pelvic pain may present in patients in whom no organic cause is found.

In cases of acute pelvic pain, it is essential to determine:

1. What, if any, immediate supportive steps are required?
2. Is the patient pregnant? And if so, is the pregnancy:
   Within the uterus and the primary source of the pain?
   Within the uterus, but associated with some other source of pain?
   Without the uterus (ectopic pregnancy)?
3. If the patient is not pregnant, what is the most likely cause of the pain?

This is also the time to decide whether the patient must be taken directly to the operating room or whether a conservative approach should be followed.

In the days before laparoscopy one of our teachers used to define such patients as "operating sick" and "watching sick." Those in the former category require immediate surgical intervention and include patients with an obvious hemoperitoneum and clinically apparent torsion of an ovarian cyst. It is in the second group, in which the diagnosis is less evident, that laparoscopy is of great assistance.

Acute pelvic pain

Reproductive tract causes	*Nonreproductive tract causes*
PREGNANCY RELATED	GASTROINTESTINAL TRACT
Abortion	Appendicitis
Ectopic pregnancy	Meckels diverticulitis
OVARY	Inflammatory bowel disease
Ovarian hyperstimulation	Mesenteric adenitis
Ruptured cyst	Performation
Torsion of a cyst	Obstruction
Bleeding corpus luteum	URINARY TRACT
Mittelschmerz	Acute infection
TUBES	Renal calculus
Torsion	VASCULAR
Torsion of a stump following sterilization	Mesenteric vascular disease
	Aortic aneurysm
UTERUS	INTEGUMENT
Degeneration of a fibroid	Rectus hematoma
Torsion of a fibroid	Herpes zoster
Pyometra	METABOLIC
Dysmenorrhea	Porphyria
Retrograde menstruation	Sickle cell crisis
ACUTE PELVIC INFLAMMATORY DISEASE	
NO EVIDENT ORGANIC ABNORMALITY	NO EVIDENT ORGANIC ABNORMALITY

Immediate supportive measures

The need for immediate supportive measures will be dictated by the patient's condition. Obvious hypotension, particularly associated with tachycardia, should raise suspicion of either overt or covert blood loss. Hypotension if associated with a high fever will direct attention toward the possibility of bacteremia shock. At this time appropriate laboratory blood samples should be drawn concurrent with the insertion of a wide-bore intravenous system. Initial fluid replacement may be given with any physiologic fluid while waiting for whole blood to be cross-matched. If necessary, the patient's feet can be elevated and oxygen administered. Such an acutely ill patient in whom the diagnosis is evident will require immediate surgical and/or medical treatment and is unlikely to require endoscopic evaluation.

For the less ill patient, the insertion of a wide-bore intravenous system is a wise precaution. The decision whether or not to cross-match blood will be based on the clinical presentation. It is always better to err on the side of caution.

Disorders of early pregnancy

Once satisfied that the patient's general condition is stable and immediate surgery is not required, the next step is to differentiate between patients who are pregnant and those who are not; a differentiation simply made by measuring the βhCG level.

If the pregnancy is within the uterus and appears to be the primary source of the patient's pain, she may be experiencing the abortion of either a pregnancy or a hydatidiform mole. A history of amenorrhea immediately preceding the onset of pain, with or without subjective symptoms of pregnancy, should arouse such a suspicion. The pain associated with a threatened or inevitable abortion is typically intermittent and occurs at regular intervals. The interval between pains decreases as the abortion progresses. There also is vaginal bleeding. Abdominal examination may elicit mild tenderness. If the uterus is larger than the patient's length of amenorrhea would suggest, a diagnosis of multiple or molar pregnancy should be entertained.

The vaginal examination serves to confirm the diagnosis in most cases of abortion. There is obvious bleeding, the cervix is soft and may be dilated, and products of conception may have been expelled. The uterus is soft and enlarged.

If the clinical diagnosis is either inevitable or incomplete abortion, the uterus should be evacuated. There is no need for extensive investigation. In those cases in which the clinical evaluation is suggestive of abortion but doubt exists, ultrasonography and measurement of the βhCG may be of value and will be discussed later. Laparoscopy has no place in the investigation of abortion.

Acute pain in the presence of an intact intrauterine pregnancy. If the pregnancy is within the uterus but does not appear to be the source of pain, nonreproductive tract causes, particularly urinary infection and acute appendicitis, should be excluded. Clinical evaluation may be complemented by ultrasonography, which would confirm the presence of an intact intrauterine gestation. In addition, it will identify ovarian and uterine masses.

Unless there are obvious reasons for operative intervention (e.g., acute appendicitis, clinical evidence of hemoperitoneum) such patients are best managed by observation and appropriate medical treatment. The pain usually subsides. If the pain does not subside and the diagnosis cannot be made by noninvasive means, laparoscopy or laparotomy may be required. The choice of procedure is dependent on the condition of the patient, the size of the uterus, and the experience of the surgeon. When the uterus is larger than 16 weeks in size, it is safer to perform an exploratory laparotomy. There is a real risk to the pregnant uterus, especially after the twelfth week of gestation, from the Veress needle and the laparoscopic trocars. In the hands of an experienced laparoscopist, this risk can be reduced if the insufflation is carried out by the introduction of the Veress needle subcostally on the left. In addition, the abdomen should be overdistended as described in Chapter 5 and the laparoscopic trocar and cannula inserted in the midline but above the umbilicus. If laparoscopy is undertaken, no intrauterine manipulators should be used.

Acute pain in the absence of an intrauterine pregnancy. In the patient with acute pain and no intrauterine pregnancy, the differential diagnosis must include:

Ectopic pregnancy
Pelvic inflammatory disease
Other reproductive tract causes (see box on p. 118)
Nonreproductive tract causes (see box on p. 118)
No obvious organic cause

The temptation to proceed to immediate laparoscopy should be resisted in many of these patients. A useful rule of thumb is to perform laparoscopy to confirm diagnoses formulated clinically, particularly if the condition will be amenable to laparoscopic treatment. When the clinical presentation is unclear, 24 to 36 hours of observation may lead to resolution of the symptoms.

The pitfalls to be avoided include missing a diagnosis of organic disease or, on the basis of inadequate information, appending an unjustified diagnostic label to a patient. Every gynecologist is familiar with the woman who has been admitted repeatedly and has undergone many courses of antibiotic therapy because at some stage an erroneous diagnosis of acute PID was made.

An article written in preultrasound days, which outlined the clinical presentation and diagnosis of unruptured ectopic pregnancy, appeared in *Munro Kerr's Operative Obstetrics*.[6] He described this patient as "the woman who suffers for some time from abdominal uneasiness, pain, occasional faintings, and hemorrhagic vaginal discharge." Early diagnosis of ectopic pregnancy in any patient presenting with acute pelvic pain, particularly in those women with a history of acute pelvic inflammatory disease and/or ectopic pregnancy, who are using an intrauterine contraceptive device or have undergone reconstructive tubal surgery or have been sterilized may be made before these classic symptoms appear. In addition, infertile patients, particularly those who have undergone ART or one of its variants, are at greater risk.

Pelvic inflammatory disease should be suspected if the patient presenting with acute lower abdominal pain has in addition two or more of the findings listed in the box on p. 120. Fever is an important diagnostic criterion.

Other reproductive tract causes of acute pelvic and lower abdominal pain may present with any combination of symptoms and a variety of pelvic findings, from an apparently normal pelvis to one with an obviously palpable mass. A working diagnosis of "other pelvic cause" should be enter-

Signs of pelvic inflammatory disease in the patient with acute lower abdominal pain

Purulent vaginal discharge
Fever
Menstrual irregularity
Urinary symptoms
Symptoms of proctitis
Marked tenderness of pelvic organs during bimanual examination
Palpable adnexal masses
Increased erythrocyte sedimentation rate

tained only after ectopic pregnancy and acute PID have been excluded.

On many occasions, despite the best application of clinical acumen and ancillary testing, such differentiation is impossible.

Ectopic pregnancy

There has been a significant increase in the occurrence of ectopic pregnancy. In the United States in 1985, 78,400 ectopic pregnancies occurred. This represents a greater than fourfold increase since 1970.[7] Of even greater significance, ectopic pregnancy is now among the leading causes of maternal death. The most common presenting symptom of this condition is acute pelvic and lower abdominal pain. The earlier part of this chapter has described in general terms how the condition may be differentiated from other causes of pain. This section will describe in detail the diagnosis of ectopic pregnancy.

A minority of patients with ectopic pregnancy will present with acute onset of abdominal pain, collapse, and obvious signs of hemoperitoneum. They do not pose a diagnostic dilemma and will not be discussed further. It is in the patient with the unruptured or leaking ectopic pregnancy that diagnositic difficulties may arise. In such patients, early diagnosis permits prompt treatment and thus markedly reduces the mortality and morbidity associated with this condition. In addition, the shortened hospital stay leads to considerable financial savings. Furthermore, early diagnosis prior to extensive tubal destruction permits medical or surgical interventions designed to conserve the oviduct in those patients who wish to retain their fertility potential.

While a high index of suspicion along with a thorough history and physical examination are the key to early diagnosis, a range of modern ancillary measures can greatly facilitate this task. These measures include β-subunit human chorionic gonadotropin (βhCG) and serum progesterone assays, ultrasonography, and laparoscopy. The former noninvasive investigations and increasing interest in nonsurgical treatment are reducing the need to perform laparoscopy in all cases of ectopic pregnancy.

βhCG assay. This highly specific assay is positive only in the presence of tissue that is actively secreting hCG. If the βhCG assay result is negative, pregnancy can be excluded.

If the qualitative βhCG assay is positive it is necessary to ascertain the absolute levels by using a quantitative assay (radioimmunoassay or enzyme-linked immunoabsorbant assay—ELISA). The ELISA method is accurate and the results can be obtained more rapidly. The initial baseline levels will be of value if it becomes necessary to observe the patient for some time prior to establishing the diagnosis. As will be discussed in Chapter 14, it may also be necessary to monitor the βhCG levels during treatment and follow-up.[8-9]

Serum progesterone assay. A single determination of the serum progesterone levels is a useful diagnostic adjunct. Normal intrauterine pregnancies will show values greater than 15 ng/ml. Lesser concentrations will be noted in cases of ectopic and failing intrauterine pregnancies.[10] Taken in conjunction with low rates of increase in βhCG levels, abnormal progesterone concentrations have been shown to have positive predictive value of 1.0 for the presence of pathologic pregnancy.[11]

Ultrasonography. The use of high-resolution ultrasonography, particularly transvaginal ultrasonography, has significantly improved our ability to diagnose ectopic pregnancy. If the pregnancy is sufficiently advanced that a mass can be identified in which there is an obvious heart beat in the adnexal region, the diagnosis is beyond doubt. Unfortunately, this occurs in only 10% of ectopic pregnancies.[12] If the ectopic pregnancy cannot be visualized directly the diagnosis becomes one of exclusion. If an intrauterine gestation is observed, the likelihood of a coexistent tubal pregnancy lies in the range from 1:3899 to 1:15000.[13] Heterotopic pregnancies are more common in women who have been treated with induction of ovulation, or have undergone one of the methods of assisted reproduction.

Making the diagnosis. If no intrauterine sac is identified and βhCG is positive, either the patient has an ectopic pregnancy or the scan has been performed at too early a gestational age to identify the gestation sac. An intrauterine sac can be identified using a transvaginal scan as early as 35 days after the last menstrual period. This is 7 to 10 days earlier than can be expected if a transabdominal method is used.[14] When ultrasonography is used in conjunction with the βhCG values, transabdominal scanning is unlikely to identify an intrauterine pregnancy if the βhCG levels are less than 6500 mIu. Transvaginal ultrasound is accurate with levels as low as 1500 mIu/ml.[14]

Intelligent use of endocrine assays and ultrasonography will allow division of patients into four categories: (1) those with a clearly identifiable intrauterine pregnancy, (2) those with a clearly identifiable extrauterine pregnancy, (3) those in whom a diagnosis of tubal pregnancy is probable and, (4) those in whom the diagnosis is still in doubt.

Role of laparoscopy in early pregnancy. The diagnostic role of laparoscopy is diminishing. It may have a limited place in those in whom an intrauterine pregnancy has been identified ultrasonographically, but their pelvic pain persists. In these patients, serial evaluation of βhCG levels cannot identify the presence of a concurrent tubal pregnancy, as production from the intact intrauterine gestation will mask any changes derived from the ectopic gestation. Laparoscopy may enable identification of the source of the patient's pain.

In patients in whom a firm diagnosis of ectopic pregnancy has been made by ultrasonographic means, laparoscopy for purely diagnostic purposes is superfluous. This statement is also relevant in cases of heterotopic gestations if both the intrauterine and extrauterine pregnancies have been identified.

When the diagnosis of ectopic pregnancy is probable, a choice must be made between laparoscopic confirmation, expectancy, or medical treatment. Details of management will be discussed in Chapter 14. The decision whether or not to perform laparoscopy should be based upon the progression of the clinical picture, especially the severity of the pain, the patient's wishes, and the degree of diagnostic probability.

The same principles are applied when the diagnosis is in doubt. Management of these patients can be achieved by monitoring the clinical progress, the use of serial βhCG assays, and ultrasonography. If the βhCG fails to achieve its normal rate of doubling, the patient may have either a threatened abortion or an ectopic pregnancy. The diagnosis may become evident from developments in the clinical presentation or when the fetus attains the gestational age at which ultrasonography in conjunction with βhCG levels may clarify the picture.

Acute pelvic inflammatory disease

Acute pelvic inflammatory disease (PID) is an infection caused by the ascent of micro-organisms that locate in the cervix and spread along the mucosal surfaces to the uterus and fallopian tubes. Intraperitoneal dissemination may lead to pelvic peritonitis, generalized peritonitis, and/or abscess formation.

Incidence. Acute PID has been estimated to occur at a rate of 10 cases per 1,000 women per year in the age group of 15 to 39 and in the high-risk age group (15 to 24) at a rate of 20 cases per 1,000 women per year.[15]

Etiology. The classic concept presupposed that the disease was caused by organisms that normally inhabited the cervix or the vagina, but ascended through the genital tract. It is now evident that most if not all attacks of acute PID are caused by sexually transmitted organisms. The most frequently isolated are *Chlamydia trachomatis, Neisseria gonorrhea,* and *Mycoplasma hominis.* Currently *Chlamydia trachomatis* is the most frequently identified.[16] While these organisms would appear to account for the majority of primary invasion, in as many as 15% to 60% of cases of acute PID, aerobic or anaerobic bacteria can also be identified.[17] The most common aerobic isolates include nonhemolytic *Streptococci, Escherichia coli,* and *Hemophilus influenzae.* The most common anaerobes are *Peptococci, Peptostreptococci,* and *Bacteroides.* Patients with the most severe clinical findings often have both aerobic and anaerobic infection. Anaerobic bacteria are almost always present in abscesses secondary to PID.

Certain women are at greater risk of contracting PID. Clearly, the number of sexual partners will increase the risk. The intrauterine contraceptive device (IUD) is believed by the public and physicians alike to be a potent cause of acute PID. Several critical reanalyses[18-21] have challenged this belief. It is clear that the early studies suffered from methodologic flaws. In these recent reanalyses many of the serious consequences of IUD use were minimized if the performance of the Dalkon Shield was excluded. With regard to the latter device a major overview analysis has demonstrated no evidence of an increased risk of PID when compared with other IUDs used in the same historic era.[22] All of these studies seem to show that if PID is to occur because of IUD use, it will do so immediately after insertion and that the apparent increase in PID among IUD users was more a reflection of the worldwide epidemic of sexually transmitted diseases.[16] This latter statement is given added credence when it is recognized that there is no significant increase in the risk of PID in parous IUD users living in a monogamous sexual relationship.[16]

A previous episode of PID predisposes to subsequent attacks. Medical procedures such as hysterosalpingography, chromopertubation, hydropertubation, and D&C facilitate the ascent of pathogens located in the vagina or cervix to the upper genital tract.[23-24]

Clinical manifestations. Clinically, acute pelvic inflammatory disease can vary from an almost asymptomatic condition to a life-threatening event. Serious illness occurs in about 3% of patients.[25] Acute PID is often preceded by lower genital tract infection (LGTI). The latter often passes unnoticed. The first symptom of ascending infection is usually bilateral lower abdominal or pelvic pain. The pain initially is subacute and of dull character. The onset of lower abdominal pain at the time of menstruation is twice as likely to be due to the gonococcus than to nongonococcal organisms. The pain associated with gonococcal salpingitis is more severe than that associated with *Chlamydia* or *Mycoplasma.* Dyspareunia is a frequent concomitant complaint. Intermenstrual spotting, urinary frequency, and dysuria are commonly reported in association. In mild and moderately severe cases of PID, nausea and vomiting, proctitis, and right upper quadrant pain occur in 10%, 7%, and 5%, respectively.[25] The right upper quadrant pain is caused by the development of perihepatitis.

The most important physical finding is fever. Fever is more common in patients who are infected with the gonococcus. Abdominal findings are very variable and are dependent on the degree of involvement of the peritoneum.

The greater the degree of peritoneal involvement, the greater the tenderness, guarding, and rebound tenderness. The most frequent pelvic findings are purulent cervical discharge and bilateral tenderness, particularly if the cervix is moved and the adnexa palpated. Regrettably, this classical picture of pelvic inflammatory disease occurs in less than 50% of affected patients. Indeed, many patients are completely asymptomatic. Gomel has observed that more than 50% of patients found to have a hydrosalpinx when investigated for infertility give no previous history of an acute attack of pelvic inflammatory disease.[26] This observation has been confirmed in a more recent study.[27]

Laboratory investigation. A simple office procedure is to perform a wet mount using material obtained from the cervix. A large number of inflammatory cells will invariably be demonstrated in mounts prepared from patients with LGTI. This is an important associated finding in the diagnosis of PID.[25] The erythrocyte sedimentation rate (ESR) will be elevated in the majority of patients both with acute PID and those with a simple LGTI. It is of limited value. The peripheral leukocyte count (WC) will be increased in two-thirds of patients with pelvic inflammatory disease but at least one-third of patients with a LGTI. Acute appendicitis and acute complications of ovarian cysts may similarly affect the ESR and the WC. Serum antichymotrypsin, orosomucoid, and/or C-reactive protein values are elevated in both patients with PID and LGTI and are of limited value. Culdocentesis, however, may be of inestimable value. The white cell content in the peritoneal fluid will generally exceed 30,000/mm^3 in cases of PID but will be less than 1,000 in women who are free from infection.[25]

Role of laparoscopy in pelvic inflammatory disease. The acronym PID, while properly standing for "pelvic inflammatory disease," has also been used to connote "pus in dere" or more recently "pretty inadequate diagnosis." The latter is an accurate remark! Using the strict clinical criteria described earlier in this chapter (see also the box on p. 120), Jacobson and Westrom submitted 814 patients to diagnostic laparoscopy. The minimal criteria for the laparoscopic diagnosis of acute salpingitis included the presence of three signs: pronounced hyperemia of the tubal serosa, edema of the tubal wall, and the presence of a sticky exudate. In 532 patients (65%), acute salpingitis was visually confirmed; in 184 (23%), no pathologic changes were detected; in a further 98 (12%), other pathologic conditions were noted including acute appendicitis, intrapelvic hemorrhage, and pelvic endometriosis. In another group of patients, 91 cases of acute salpingitis were found unexpectedly by laparoscopy although some other clinical diagnosis had been made. This work served to highlight the relative inaccuracy of the clinical diagnosis.[28] More recently, Westrom[25] has remarked "the classic concept of PID is woefully inadequate." This statement is regrettably accurate, particularly in view of its impact on subsequent fertility.

Whether or not all patients in whom the diagnosis of PID is suspected should undergo diagnostic laparoscopy is controversial. In women in whom the differential diagnosis is in question and includes surgical emergencies such as appendicitis, ectopic pregnancy or other reproductive tract disorders, laparoscopy is indispensable in providing a prompt and accurate diagnosis. Bacteriologic sampling can be performed directly from the oviducts, if necessary.

Treatment. Once a diagnosis of acute PID has been established, treatment will be dependent on the severity of the disease. If the woman has an IUD in place, the device should be removed once appropriate antibiotic coverage has been instituted.

Those patients who have suffered a catastrophic rupture of a pelvic abscess will require antibiotic therapy and pelvic drainage. A pelvic abscess that is unruptured should be surgically drained (see Chapter 16). Ultrasonographic evaluation helps in the diagnosis of abscess formation. Such abscesses have also been drained transabdominally by the insertion percutaneously of ultrasonographically directed catheters.[29] In view of the endocrine importance of the ovaries and the progress achieved in in vitro fertilization techniques, it would appear prudent to attempt to conserve ovaries unless their removal is unavoidable.

The remaining less severely ill patients should be treated conservatively. The use of antibiotic regimens effective against anaerobic bacteria and particularly *Bacteroides fragilis* has significantly reduced the need for surgical intervention for this condition.

The sequelae of acute PID with respect to the patient's subsequent fertility can be disastrous. Antibiotic therapy must be aggressive and take into account the polymicrobial nature of the infection. The antibiotic regimens and doses recommended by the Centers for Disease Control and Prevention[30] are listed in the box on p. 123.

It is noteworthy that the subsequent infertility rate was reported to be identical among women who received antibiotics of widely differing spectra.[31] The most predictive parameter of subsequent infertility, however, was the stage of tubal damage noted at laparoscopy when antibiotic therapy was instituted.[32] It is evident that the aim should be the prevention of salpingitis by public education and early recognition and treatment of lower genital tract infections.

Other causes of acute pain within the reproductive tract

If neither ectopic pregnancy nor acute PID can be implicated as the cause of the patient's pain, some other organic cause should be sought either within or without the reproductive tract.

If there is reasonable suspicion that the pain arises from the reproductive tract, differentiation must be made between *complications of ovarian cysts*, a *bleeding corpus luteum*, the *rare torsion of a tube or a fragment thereof*, *degeneration or torsion of a fibroid*, and *retrograde menstruation*.

Treatment of pelvic inflammatory disease

Centers for Disease Control and Prevention recommendations—1993[30]

INPATIENT TREATMENT

Experts have experience with both of the following regimens. Also, there are multiple randomized trials demonstrating the efficacy of each regimen.

REGIMEN A

Cefoxitin 2 g IV every 6 hours or cefotetan 2 g IV every 12 hours

PLUS

Doxycycline 100 mg IV or orally every 12 hours.

Note: This regimen should be continued for at least 48 hours after the patient demonstrates substantial clinical improvement, after which doxycycline 100 mg orally 2 times a day should be continued for a total of 14 days. Doxycycline administered orally has bioavailability similar to that of the IV formulation and may be administered if normal gastrointestinal function is present.

Clinical data are limited for other second- or third-generation cephalosporins (e.g., ceftizoxime, cefotaxime, and ceftriaxone), which might replace cefoxitin or cefotetan; although many authorities believe they also are effective therapy for PID. However, they are less active than cefoxitin or cefotetan against anaerobic bacteria.

REGIMEN B

Clindamycin 900 mg IV every 8 hours

PLUS

Gentamicin loading dose IV or IM (2 mg/kg of body weight) followed by a maintenance dose (1.5 mg/kg) every 8 hours

Note: This regimen should be continued for at least 48 hours after the patient demonstrates substantial clinical improvement, then followed with doxycycline 100 mg orally 2 times a day or clindamycin 450 mg orally 4 times a day to complete a total of 14 days of therapy. When tubo-ovarian abscess is present, many health care providers use clindamycin for continued therapy rather than doxycycline because it provides more effective anaerobic coverage. Clindamycin administered intravenously appears to be effective against *C. trachomatis* infection; however, the effectiveness of oral clindamycin against *C. trachomatis* has not been determined.

ALTERNATE INPATIENT REGIMENS

Limited data support the use of other inpatient regimens, but two regimens have undergone at least one clinical trial and have broad-spectrum coverage. Ampicillin/sulbactam plus doxycycline has good anaerobic coverage and appears to be effective for patients with a tubo-ovarian abscess. Intravenous ofloxacin has been studied as a single agent. A regimen of ofloxacin plus either clindamycin or metronidazole provides broad-spectrum coverage. Evidence is insufficient to support the use of any single agent regimen for inpatient treatment of PID.

OUTPATIENT TREATMENT

Clinical trials of outpatient regimens have provided little information regarding intermediate and long-term outcomes. The following regimens provide coverage against the common etiologic agents of PID, but evidence from clinical trials supporting their use is limited. The second regimen provides broader coverage against anaerobic organisms but costs substantially more than the other regimen. Patients who do not respond to outpatient therapy within 72 hours should be hospitalized to confirm the diagnosis and to receive parenteral therapy.

REGIMEN A

Cefoxitin 2 g IM plus probenecid, 1 g orally in a single dose concurrently, or ceftriaxone 250 mg IM or other parenteral third-generation cephalosporin (e.g., ceftizoxime or cefotaxime),

PLUS

Doxycycline 100 mg orally 2 times a day for 14 days

REGIMEN B

Ofloxacin 400 mg orally 2 times a day for 14 days,

PLUS

Either clindamycin 450 mg orally 4 times a day, or metronidazole 500 mg orally 2 times a day for 14 days

Clinical trials have demonstrated that the cefoxitin regimen is effective in obtaining short-term clinical response. Fewer data support the use of ceftriaxone or other third-generation cephalosporins, but, based on their similarities to cefoxitin, they also are considered effective. No data exist regarding the use of oral cephalosporins for the treatment of PID.

Ofoxacin is effective against both *N. gonorrhoeae* and *C. trachomatis*. One clinical trial demonstrated the effectiveness of oral ofloxacin in obtaining short-term clinical response with PID. Despite results of this trial, there is concern related to ofloxacin's lack of anaerobic coverage; the addition of clindamycin or metronidazole provides this coverage. Clindamycin, but not metronidazole, further enhances the gram-positive coverage of the regime.

ALTERNATIVE OUTPATIENT REGIMENS

Information regarding other outpatient regimens is limited. The combination of amoxicillin/clavulanic acid plus doxycycline was effective in obtaining short-term clinical response to one clinical trial, but many of the patients had to discontinue the regimen because of gastrointestinal symptoms.

FOLLOW-UP

Hospitalized patients receiving IV therapy should show substantial clinical improvement (e.g., defervescence, reduction in direct or rebound abdominal tenderness, and reduction in uterine, adnexal, and cervical motion tenderness) within 3 to 5 days of initiation of therapy. Patients who do not demonstrate improvement within this time period usually require further diagnostic workup or surgical intervention, or both.

If the provider elects to prescribe outpatient therapy, follow-up examination should be performed within 72 hours, using the criteria for clinical improvement previously described.

Because of the risk for persistent infection, particularly with *C. trachomatis*, patients should have a microbiologic reexamination 7 to 10 days after completing therapy. Some experts also recommend rescreening for *C. trachomatis* and *N. gonorrhoeae* 4 to 6 weeks after completing therapy.

On occasion, women, particularly young women, may present with a very severe episode of mittelschmerz (ovulation pain) or dysmenorrhea. Such a diagnosis should also be considered and usually can be confirmed by the menstrual history and a short period of observation. These latter two conditions will be discussed in the section on chronic pelvic pain.

English authors eloquently describe complications that occur as "accidents" to the pathologic ovary. These accidents include bleeding into or from the surface, rupture, infection, and torsion. While these accidents happen in pathologic ovaries, torsion can occur on rare occasions in a normal ovary.

The pain associated with *rupture of an ovarian cyst* is dependent on the character of the cyst's contents and whether or not there is bleeding. The onset of pain tends to be sudden and violent. If the contents of the cyst are irritant, a chemical peritonitis with signs of generalized peritonism and fever will develop.

If there is *bleeding into the interior of a cyst,* the onset of pain is less sudden. The pain is of a more boring or throbbing nature and is usually unilateral and constant. Pelvic examination will reveal the cystic mass, which is exquisitely tender to the touch.

Torsion of an ovarian cyst is a puzzling condition and may be intermittent. The onset of the pain frequently follows intercourse. The pain is colicky and may be associated with nausea and vomiting. There may be low-grade fever.

Primary infection of the ovary is a rare event but may accompany mumps when it is associated with an aching pain. With the increasing ability to needle ovarian follicles and cysts using ultrasound guidance, postoperative infection in a small number of cases is inevitable and ovarian abscesses may develop. The pain is similar to that experienced by the patient with an intracystic hemorrhage, but the systemic signs, particularly of fever and toxemia, are much more pronounced.

Although *ovarian tumors* including malignant neoplasms are usually asymptomatic, malignancy in an ovarian tumor may be associated with a chronic, gnawing lower abdominal ache.

Ovarian hyperstimulation is associated with acute abdominal pain and is seen in patients who have been treated with high doses of exogenous gonadotropins. The diagnosis is not difficult as the pain occurs within 3 to 4 days following hCG administration. The ovaries become extremely enlarged, tender, and fragile. There are marked fluid shifts with the development of ascites and, on occasion, pleural effusion. There is hyperviscosity of the circulatory system, which can lead to intravascular thrombosis.

A significant number of patients will be found to suffer from no obvious organic lesion even after complete evaluation, including laparoscopy. When such patients are examined clinically, the presence or absence of a pelvic mass should be sought. If a mass is detected, ultrasonography may help to define its nature and allows selection of those patients who may be managed laparoscopically. If no mass is palpated, ultrasonography can be used routinely. A more selective approach is to use ultrasonography only in those in whom obesity or tenderness have rendered the examination unsatisfactory or when there is reason to suspect presence of fluid in the pelvis.

The decision to proceed to laparoscopy is predicated upon the patient's general condition and whether or not a reasonable working diagnosis has been made. It is worth repeating the dictum that laparoscopy should be performed only to confirm an already formulated diagnosis. For the remaining patients, a period of observation may lead to resolution. If such a patient's symptoms do not resolve, the clinical picture worsens, or she requires a subsequent admission, it is appropriate to perform a laparoscopy. By this means the organically normal pelvis can be differentiated from one involved in a pathologic process.

Many of these conditions can be managed laparoscopically as will be described in later chapters. If a cyst has ruptured, a corpus luteum is bleeding, or there is retrograde menstruation, the pelvic cavity can be irrigated with warm, heparinized Ringer's lactate and the washings aspirated through a second-puncture cannula. If the affected organ is bleeding, electrocoagulation with a bipolar forceps is usually possible.

If laparoscopic evaluation reveals a normal pelvis, it may be that no organic disease exists. It is always imperative to inspect the appendix, the ileum, and the entire peritoneal cavity.

Non–reproductive tract causes of acute pain

Acute appendicitis. Acute appendicitis is a disease of many guises.[33] When laparoscopy is performed in patients with pelvic and abdominal pain, it is mandatory that the appendix be inspected. This is best achieved with the patient in the Trendelenburg position. The cecum is manipulated with the probe so that the whole appendix, even when retrocecal, can be inspected throughout its entire length. On occasion this maneuver will reveal an organ that, although apparently healthy at its tip, is distended and clearly inflamed in its proximal segment, a finding that would have been missed if the entire appendix had not been visualised. This thorough inspection is imperative considering the complications associated with ruptured appendicitis and the disastrous effects on the subsequent reproductive function of young women.

Other causes. Other non–reproductive tract causes of acute lower abdominal and pelvic pain have been listed in the box on p. 118. In all of these conditions the diagnosis should have been made by clinical and ancillary methods and appropriate consultation sought.

If laparoscopy has been performed, a thorough survey of the peritoneal cavity may elicit a non–reproductive tract cause for the patient's pain. Even if such is not the case, the detection of normality is an important finding. During this thorough survey, evidence of acute cholecystitis, acute perihepatitis, Meckels diverticulitis, and regional ileitis may be discovered. In rare instances malignant metastatic lesions may be noted on the serosal surfaces, omentum, or parietal peritoneum.

Acute pain in a normal pelvis

The patient complaining of acute abdominal pain in whom no obvious cause is found presents a dilemma. Her management is similar to that of the patient with chronic pelvic pain without organic findings and will be discussed later in this chapter.

CHRONIC PELVIC PAIN

Chronic pelvic pain is experienced over a long period. It may be cyclic and clearly related to menstrual function or bear no obvious temporal relationship to the menstrual cycle. The box at right lists the most common causes of chronic pelvic pain. Each will be discussed in turn.

Causes of chronic pelvic pain

Cyclic	*Acyclic*
Mittelschmerz	**Causes outside the reproductive tract**
Dysmenorrhea	**Causes within the reproductive tract**
Primary	
Secondary	Pelvic adhesive disease
	Endometriosis
Lesions of the lower genital tract or uterus	Ovarian tumors
	Pelvic varicosities
	No organic cause

Chronic cyclic pelvic pain

Chronic cyclic pelvic pain includes mittelschmerz, dysmenorrhea, and lesions of the lower genital tract and uterus.

Mittelschmerz. Classically occurring at midcycle, mittelschmerz is a sudden, occasionally severe, episode of lower abdominal pain believed to accompany follicular rupture at the time of ovulation. It is usually unilateral and despite the recognition that ovulation occurs randomly from each ovary, is frequently experienced in the same side in every cycle by some individual patients. The most usual presentation is that of a patient who will draw this symptom to the attention of a physician while her visit initially is for some other gynecologic complaint. The diagnosis under these circumstances is clinical and largely based on the clearly recognizable history, confirmation being achieved when pelvic examination fails to reveal any palpable abnormality. Treatment consists of reassurance and, when necessary, suppression of ovulation, usually with an oral contraceptive. Resolution of the symptoms in the latter instance confirms the diagnosis.

Occasionally a severe attack of mittelschmerz may bring a patient to the emergency department with a complaint of acute pelvic pain. As previously discussed, such an episode must be differentiated from all other causes of acute pelvic pain, including ectopic pregnancy.

Dysmenorrhea. Dysmenorrhea describes the pain that accompanies menstruation. It may be primary or secondary. The term "primary" describes painful menstruation in the absence of any obvious organic pelvic lesions. "Secondary" dysmenorrhea is usually the result of organic pelvic disease.

A varying degree of menstrual discomfort is experienced by 52% of postpubescent females.[34] Ten percent are incapacitated for 1 to 3 days each month. In 1978 it was calculated that 140 million working hours are lost annually in the United States[35] due to dysmenorrhea. Since the publication of that study, many more women have joined the work force and this figure currently greatly underestimates the socioeconomic impact of this common condition.

Primary dysmenorrhea. Primary dysmenorrhea almost invariably accompanies ovulatory cycles and usually begins to appear with the establishment of regular ovulation following menarche. As ovulatory cycles are usually established within 2 years of this event, the young woman who has been pain free in excess of this time may well be suffering from some organic pelvic lesion, the most frequent of which is endometriosis.

The pain is spasmodic and usually located in the lower abdomen. It may radiate to the lower back or the front of the thighs. Its onset is usually concurrent with the onset of menstrual loss and its duration is rarely longer than 24 hours. On occasion, the pain may persist for two to three days but generally lessens as time passes. Fifty percent of patients experience additional symptoms which include low backache, nausea and vomiting, diarrhea, headache, and fatigue. In the most severe cases, syncope may occur and as with severe mittelschmerz these patients may present as acute emergencies. The diagnosis of primary dysmenorrhea is made clinically by careful evaluation of the presenting symptoms and the finding of an apparently normal pelvis by bimanual and rectovaginal examination.

Pathophysiology. The causation of the pain is complex and as with all aspects of human pain there is to a greater or lesser degree a psychological component. The psychological component is no more unique to dysmenorrhea than to any other kind of pain. While cervical stenosis may cause secondary dysmenorrhea, it is no longer believed to contribute to the primary variety. The hormonal milieu is important as primary dysmenorrhea accompanies only ovulatory cycles and hence will only occur in a uterus that has been influenced by sequential estrogen and progesterone. Circulating vasopressin levels are increased during the menstrual phase in women with dysmenorrhea. This hormone gives rise to dysrhythmic uterine contractions.[36]

Current interest has centered on the effects of the prostaglandins. The prostaglandins are C-20–hydrocarbon lipids derived initially from arachadonic and prostanoic acids. When the serum progesterone falls following the cessation of corpus luteum function, the lysosomes within the endometrial cells break down and release an enzyme, phospholipase A_2. The action of this enzyme upon the lipid cell membrane generates free arachadonic acid. A family of enzymes known collectively as prostaglandin synthetase convert arachadonic acid to prostaglandin E_2 and prostaglandin F_2. Prostaglandins can be shown to influence uterine muscular contractility and it is probable that increased uterine contractions, which may also be dysrhythmic, produce decreased uterine blood flow and ischemia. The ischemia itself is painful and it would also appear that the threshold of the nerve terminals within the myometrium to the action of both chemical and physical stimuli is lowered by the presence of prostaglandins.

Support for these arguments may be found in the literature. Women with primary dysmenorrhea demonstrate abnormalities in uterine activity that include elevated uterine basal tone, elevated intrauterine active pressure, increased frequency of uterine contractions, and incoordinate uterine activity.[37] Furthermore, there is a close relationship between the degree of pain and the quantity of prostaglandins in the menstrual fluid.[38] This increased level of prostaglandins can also be correlated with the reduction in uterine blood flow. The greatest amount of prostaglandins are released during the first 48 hours of menstrual flow, which is usually the maximum duration of symptoms of primary dysmenorrhea.[38,39] Levels of the metabolite of prostaglandin F_2 (15 keto-13, 14-dihydroPGH_2) in the peripheral plasma are higher in women with primary dysmenorrhea compared with those in normal women.[40] Lastly, prostaglandin synthetase inhibitors have been shown to be effective in the treatment of primary dysmenorrhea.[41-43]

Treatment. With a better understanding of the causative mechanism, a more logical treatment has been developed for this debilitating symptom. No longer must the patients be subjected to the following:

> "blisters of the iliac regions, bromide of potassium, glycerine plugs, and hot vaginal douches. Order a hot hip bath or the feet to be put in mustard and water. On no account whatsoever allow alcohol in any form to be given. If the mother has been giving whisky and water or gin and water, at once point out the risk the patient is running. A change of air where requisite is ordered."[44]

Treatment rests upon the foundations of (1) dialogue and discussion, (2) suppression of ovulation with oral contraceptives, (3) prostaglandin synthetase inhibitors, (4) laparoscopic search for organic causative factors, and (5) other measures.

DIALOGUE AND DISCUSSION. That the nature of dysmenorrhea and the patient's feelings about this symptom should be discussed is more than a simple motherhood statement. Dawood has demonstrated that objective reduction in symptoms can be obtained by this simple measure.[45]

SUPPRESSION OF OVULATION. If simple reassurance fails, further management will be dependent upon the suitability of prescribing oral contraceptives and the patient's needs in this regard. As primary dysmenorrhea tends to be a disease of younger women, the requests to deal with the dysmenorrhea and provide effective contraception are frequently concurrent. As primary dysmenorrhea occurs only in ovulatory cycles, the abolition of ovulation is the major mechanism whereby such medications are effective. It can be noted that the prostaglandin level in menstrual fluid in women taking oral contraceptives is also reduced.[46] Clearly, oral contraceptives should not be prescribed for those women in whom exists a contraindication. These contraindications have been extensively reviewed elsewhere.[47] Relief of symptoms within 3 to 4 months can be expected in 90% of patients.

PROSTAGLANDIN SYNTHETASE INHIBITORS. Prostaglandin synthetase inhibitors may be employed in addition to oral contraceptives or in their place, if the use of the latter is inappropriate. On occasion a trial of up to 6 months may be required before relief is obtained. Five families of prostaglandin synthetase inhibitor are available and have been extensively reviewed by Chan.[48] Table 10-1 demonstrates these families and the medications that belong to each family.

Clinical research has demonstrated that the most effective medications which have the least incidence of side effects are the fenamates or arylpropionic acid derivatives. Both families of drugs are contraindicated in patients known to have gastrointestinal ulcers or hypersensitivity. Side effects may include those related to the gastrointestinal tract and the central nervous system. Other nonspecific side effects such as allergic reactions, skin rash, edema, or bronchospasm and some hematologic abnormalities may occur. The side effects are reviewed extensively by Dawood.[45] Whichever medication is used, it should be started just prior to or immediately concurrent with the onset of menstrual

Table 10-1. Prostaglandin synthetase inhibitor familites and corresponding drugs

Family	Specific drug
Benzoic acid derivatives	Aspirin
Indoleacetic acid derivatives	Indomethacin
Buterophenones	Phenylbutazone
Fenamates	Mefenamic acid
Arylpropionic acid derivatives	Ibuprofen
	Naproxen
	Ketoprofen

flow and continued for 3 days. The two most widely used preparations are naproxen sodium (Anaprox or Naprosyn 275 mg 4 times daily) and mefenamic acid (Ponstan 250 to 500 mg 3 to 4 times daily).

LAPAROSCOPY. If simple reassurance, suppression of ovulation, and/or the use of prostaglandin synthetase inhibitors fails to relieve the complaint of primary dysmenorrhea, an organic cause must be excluded. Laparoscopy should be undertaken, particularly in those patients with a family history of endometriosis. In most cases an organic cause, most commonly endometriosis, will be found and treatment should be directed to this entity.

OTHER MEASURES. In rare cases an apparently normal pelvis is noted by laparoscopy. While the use of calcium antagonists such an Nifedipine appear promising,[49] little further rational organic treatment can be offered. The empiric performance of dilatation and curettage is without scientific foundation. Such patients should receive the benefit of counselling, as will be described later during the discussion of the management of the patient with chronic pelvic pain with no apparent organic pelvic lesion.

There is an upsurge of interest in laparoscopic segmental ablation of the uterosacral ligaments and presacral neurectomy. This subject will be addressed in detail in Chapter 20.

Secondary dysmenorrhea. Secondary dysmenorrhea tends to occur later in life and is usually the result of an acquired disease. Painful periods that have their onset more than 2 years after the menarche, can be traced to some antecedent medical event such as pelvic infection or pelvic surgery, accompany anovulatory cycles, or occur in young women with a family history of endometriosis should be suspected of having an organic basis. It is also worth noting that the use of an intrauterine contraceptive device can produce quite marked secondary dysmenorrhea. One exception to the rule of thumb that secondary dysmenorrhea does not accompany menarche is in the patient with a congenital anomaly of the lower genital tract. This may present as a complete blockage to outflow, as in the case of imperforate hymen or congenital absence of the cervix. It may also rarely be seen in the patient with a noncommunicating functioning uterine horn. In later life acquired stenosis of the cervix can occur following cone biopsy or extensive cautery. The common causes of secondary dysmenorrhea are shown in the box at right.

Common causes of secondary dysmenorrhea

Lower genital tract

Imperforate hymen
Transverse vaginal septum
Congenital cervical absence
Acquired cervical stenosis

Uterus

Noncommunicating horn
Adenomyosis
Pedunculated submucous myoma
Endometrial polyp
Intrauterine adhesions
IUD usage
Membranous dysmenorrhea

Pelvis

Endometriosis
Chronic pelvic inflammatory disease
Postsurgical adhesive disease

Prostaglandins. The role of prostaglandins in secondary dysmenorrhea is unclear. The levels in the endometrium are certainly higher in the patient with an IUD.[50,51] Moon et al. have demonstrated prostaglandin levels to be higher in peritoneal fluid in women suffering from endometriosis.[52]

Whether these elevated prostaglandin levels can be invoked as the major source of the pain in such patients is difficult to ascertain. The use of Ibuprofen and Naproxen have both been shown to relieve the associated dysmenorrhea and menorrhagia in IUD wearers.[53,54] In studies of the use of prostaglandin synthetase inhibitors in endometriosis, however, Kaupil and co-workers were unable to demonstrate any relief from pain in patients suffering from endometriosis who were treated with tolfenamic acid, indomethacin, and acetyl salicylic acid.[55]

Treatment. The management of secondary dysmenorrhea will be dependent upon establishing the nature of the pain and treating the organic cause. The previous history, current history, and physical findings may all be of assistance. Any suggestion of the occurrence of one of the conditions listed in the box above should lead immediately to the suspicion of secondary dysmenorrhea, particularly when the current history is one of late onset of pain in a previously pain-free patient. Typically, the pain of secondary dysmenorrhea may precede the onset of bleeding and generally lasts longer than that of primary dysmenorrhea. The pain will gradually wane as the period progresses. In some cases of endometriosis the pain actually worsens as menstruation progresses.[56]

The rare condition of membranous dysmenorrhea has a familial incidence. The endometrium, instead of being shed normally, may be passed as an entire cast of the uterine cavity or in very large fragments. The passage of this material is preceded by intense uterine contractions and severe cramps. This condition does not interfere with conception and pregnancy and is not cured by childbearing. It is refractory to all treatment including curettage, although occasionally suppression of ovulation may be effective.

On physical examination, in contradistinction to primary dysmenorrhea, palpable pelvic findings are frequent. The rectovaginal examination must not be ignored as endometriosis is frequently palpable in the cul-de-sac and rectovaginal septum. Final diagnosis of the nature of the underlying lesion will be dependent upon vaginal examination, hysteroscopy, and, most importantly, laparoscopy.

Lesions of the lower genital tract and uterus

Congenital lesions. The young patient in whom there is a failure of connection between the uterine corpus and the vagina may present with cyclic lower abdominal pain in the absence of menstrual loss. If the condition has been prolonged, the patient may also complain of abdominal swelling. Vaginal examination will reveal either the presence of an imperforate hymen, in which case there will be a hematocolpos proximal to the hymen, or congenital absence of the cervix. Cruciate incision and drainage of the imperforate hymen is generally curative, but such patients are particularly prone to develop endometriosis and subsequent infertility.

Congenital absence of the cervix presents a more thorny problem. While surgical reconstruction may be attempted, the outcome is usually poor. Rock et al. have described eight such women.[57] In two patients a fibrous cord with islands of endocervical glands was noted. This was treated successfully by creation of a cervicovaginal fistula. In the other six patients, complete absence of the cervical stroma required a uterovaginal anastomosis. Only one patient continued to menstruate. Ultimately, four of the six women with complete congenital absence of the cervix required hysterectomy. Although it proved possible to maintain menstrual function in these patients after repeated surgery, no pregnancies occurred and significant dysmenorrhea led to the removal of the uterine corpus for symptomatic relief.

Acquired lesions. Acquired lesions are usually encountered in mature women.

Uterine lesions. Acquired cervical stenosis may require dilatation. The pain associated with adenomyosis can be described as "gnawing" and there is a sensation of weight and fullness in the pelvis. The uterus is tender, enlarged, and bulky to bimanual palpation. The final diagnosis of this condition is rarely achieved until uterine tissue has been extirpated. While estrogen suppression can be attempted with either GnRH agonists or Danazol, the definitive approach in the older patient will be hysterectomy.

Lesions lying within the uterine cavity such as pedunculated submucous myomata, endometrial polyps, and intrauterine adhesions can specifically be identified only by hysteroscopy, although a hysterosalpingography will demonstrate their presence. The discrepancies between hysterosalpingography and hysteroscopy have been described in detail.[58] Similarly, although ultrasonography may suggest the presence of an intrauterine filling defect, the nature of this defect can be determined accurately only if the lesion is directly visualized. Such lesions can be treated successfully through the hysteroscope.

Intrapelvic lesions. While the clinical finding of fixity, tenderness, and nodularity within the pelvis may be suggestive of endometriosis, chronic pelvic inflammatory disease, or postsurgical adhesive disease, the final diagnosis can be made only by laparoscopy. Indeed, in one study the error in clinical assessment depending on the diagnosis ranged from 22% to 71%.[59] Once a firm diagnosis has been established, appropriate medical or surgical treatment should be undertaken.

Chronic acyclic pelvic pain

Undoubtedly one of the most puzzling clinical problems for patient and gynecologist alike is the symptom of prolonged intractable pelvic pain that is unrelated to menstrual function. It is particularly in this group of patients that the disentanglement of the psychogenic from the somatic often presents almost insurmountable difficulties. The classification described earlier of obviously organic in origin, possibly organic in origin, and probably psychogenic in origin must consistently be borne in mind.

Organic sources of chronic lower abdominal and pelvic pain may lie within or without the reproductive tract. Those lying without the reproductive tract include disorders of the nervous, musculoskseltal, and gastrointestinal and urinary tracts.

When the gynecologist is approached by a patient with such a complaint, it must first be determined whether further investigation and management should be carried out or the patient referred to a specialist in the appropriate discipline. An excellent method of triage is suggested by Basu[60]:

> "The following clinical features may point to the existence of nongynecologic disorders: (1) Coexisting symptoms such as nausea, vomiting, and alteration of bowel habits suggest the possibility of gastrointestinal disorders. (2) Pain located in the lower abdomen or lower back is usually of gynecologic origin. Pain located entirely in the lumbar or lumbosacral region is probably of orthopedic origin. Pain located in the upper abdomen may be due to a general surgical cause but may also be associated with pelvic pathology such as diverticulitis, ulcerative colitis, or malignancy associated with intestinal obstruction. (3) Spasm or rigidity of muscles especially those of the vertebral column suggest nongynecologic diseases such as orthopedic, neurologic, or rheumatic lesions. (4) In cases of hyperalgesia of the abdominal wall or back, pain is usually of somatic origin in either the muscles or joints. (5) Relationship to activity, backache of gynecologic origin is made worse as the day progresses, whereas backache of rheumatic origin is worst in the morning."

If, however, the gynecologist believes the pain to be of gynecologic origin, the varying roles of the psyche and the soma must be investigated.

The patient should be examined thoroughly with particular attention being paid to the pelvic and rectovaginal examinations. If an obvious pelvic mass is detected, ultrasound may identify its nature. Unless there is evidence of malignancy or the mass is very large, laparoscopy may be required to reach a final diagnosis. Fibromyomata and ovarian tumors, unless they have undergone an accident or degenerative change, are usually pain free. As in the case of the patient with secondary dysmenorrhea, fixity and nodularity of the pelvis should give rise to a suspicion of endometriosis or chronic pelvic inflammatory change. If fixity and nodularity are detected, laparoscopy should be performed to determine the nature of the palpable lesion. Such organic causes as pelvic adhesions and endometriosis may be amenable to lysis or ablation during the laparoscopy. The treatment of endometriosis will be dependent on the severity of the lesion and the patient's desire for future fertility; it may be medical with either Danazol, Depo-Provera, or GnRH analogs, surgical (either conservative or extirpative), or a combination of both.

In those patients without evidence of a palpable lesion, when the chronic pain has been sufficiently severe, persistent, or has required several consultations, laparoscopy is indicated to establish the status of the patient's pelvis and peritoneal cavity. It must be recognized, however, that the finding of an organic lesion does not necessarily presuppose cause and effect with respect to the patient's complaint of pain. For example, endometriosis and pelvic adhesive disease are classically stated to be the cause of this chronic pain. However, the number of patients attending for infertility investigations who are quite devoid of painful symptoms in whom are discovered extensive adhesive disease or endometriosis is impressive.

Further, when laparoscopy is performed in patients without clinical pelvic findings, the rate of discovery of unsuspected organic lesions is relatively low. Table 10-2 summarizes the findings from large published series in which laparoscopy was performed in patients with chronic pelvic pain.[61-65] It will be noted that in the majority of these series, normal pelves were found in close to or in excess of 50% of women. In only one, that of Frangenheim and Kleindienst, was a remarkably high pickup rate of 93% for organic lesions reported.[61] In this latter series of 302 cases, endometriosis accounted for 83 and adhesions for 80. There were 80 cases of myomata that, while being definite lesions, are not believed to cause pain. Fourteen patients were thought to suffer from the Allen and Masters syndrome, a peculiar condition where a rent appears in the base of the broad ligament.[66] The suggestion that this particular condition is a cause of pain subsequently has been refuted and it would appear to be an incidental finding that may be related to endometriosis.

In the largest published series, the laparoscopic findings in 1,194 patients are described.[59] Three hundred fifty-five (29%) had evidence of a laparoscopically normal pelvis. Regrettably, that article does not clarify whether or not the patients examined with a complaint of pain were suffering from pain of the acute or chronic variety. It does serve to underline, however, that a complaint of pain may frequently occur in the absence of any obvious organic lesion. Of further interest, a total 749 of these patients had a normal pelvic examination prior to the diagnostic laparoscopy. Of these, 479 (63%) had abnormal findings. Of 445 patients with abnormal pelvic examinations, 401 (82.5%) had abnormal findings at the time of laparoscopy.

Table 10-2. Laparoscopic findings in patients complaining of pelvic pain

	No. of patients	No. with organic cause (%)	No. with no cause (%)
Frangenheim and Kleindienst[61]	302	281 (93)	21 (7)
Sememchyshyn and Strickler[62]	198	67 (34)	131 (66)
Pent[63]	38	20 (53)	18 (47)
Lundberg[69]	95	55 (54)	40 (46)
Liston et al.[65]	134	32 (24)	102 (76)

It must be apparent that many women with a complaint of chronic pelvic pain have such a complaint in the absence of any obvious macroscopic intrapelvic lesion. Some other mechanism must be sought. To suggest that the cause may be psychogenic is "an affront to self respect."[67] Further, in today's arena of sexual politics, for a male gynecologist to make such a suggestion is fraught with risk of the accusation that this is yet another example of the uncaring male chauvinist determined to prove that women are neurotic creatures.

If these distracting side issues can be ignored, there are elegant data to suggest that indeed psychogenic causes do play a large part in the etiology of pelvic pain in women.[68] These studies have disposed of the concept of Allen and Masters syndrome. Nor is the psychogenic basis of pain restricted to women. Dodge concluded that in 95% of children referred to a hospital clinic for abdominal pain the symptoms were emotionally determined.[69] Gomez and Dally examined both men and women who attended outpatient clinics for recurrent or persistent abdominal pain for which no organic cause was apparent.[70] They concluded that psychiatric factors were primarily responsible for the pain in at least 84% of these patients; the women to men ratio was 2:1. Organic changes can be detected in response to emotional stress. Duncan and Taylor have demonstrated fluctuations in pelvic blood flow induced by acute mood changes such as anxiety, depression, and resentment.[71]

Beard and co-workers compared 18 women with pelvic pain but no demonstrable pathology with 17 women with a similar complaint but some form of pelvic pathology, and a control group of nine women with no gynecologic problems.[72] The findings of this study confirmed the view that women who complain of pelvic pain but have no demonstrable organic cause are as a group psychologically different from women without pelvic pain. They tended to be more neurotic, to have abnormal attitudes toward their own and their partner's sexuality, and to form less rewarding relationships. Fifteen of the 18 women without organic lesions had a sexual component to their emotional disturbance.

Renaer and co-workers evaluated 108 patients with chronic pelvic pain; 28 of these were diagnosed as chronic pain without obvious pathology.[73] Psychometric tests were administered to three groups of patients, which included: (1) 15 of the above 28 with chronic pain without clear organic cause, (2) 22 patients with chronic pelvic pain and endometriosis, and (3) 23 pain-free control patients. All three groups were compared with a normative population for the psychometric instruments used. Interestingly, both groups of patients with pain, that is those with and without organic lesions, had inflated scores for hypochondriasis, depression, and hysteria when assessed by the Minnesota Multiphasic Personality Inventory (MMPI). The Amsterdam biographic questionnaire[74] showed that after univariate analysis, patients with pelvic pain without clear organic cause displayed a stronger neurotic tendency. The interpersonal relations questionnaire[75] showed that the patients with no organic lesion had a much worse relationship with their husbands than patients in the other groups. After very detailed multivariate analysis of the data, the authors concluded that there was not a significant difference between the variables concerning psychic function in patients with chronic pelvic pain but no clear organic cause and those with chronic pain with an organic cause. They concluded that chronic pelvic pain with organic cause could lead to neurotic reactions. A similar finding has been reported in patients with back pain.[76] Nevertheless, when patients with chronic pelvic pain but no organic lesion were compared with the normative population, they exhibited neurotic symptomatology with heightened scores for hypochondriasis, depression, hysteria, and repression and lower scores on ego strength with heightened scores of neurotic instability.

Stenchever evaluated 50 patients with chronic pelvic pain and no organic findings and compared them with 30 control subjects.[77] He noted the following occurred more frequently in the study group at the $p < 0.01$ level:

1. In childhood: sexual assault/rape, need for mental health evaluation, arrests/detention, did not complete high school
2. In adulthood: moved frequently, rape, not working, on welfare.

Those events associated with statistically significant difference of $p < 0.05$ were:

1. In childhood: use of drugs, was physically abused, witnessed physical abuse
2. In adulthood: had several marriages/live-in partners.

When the MMPI was administered, somatomisation disorders occurred in the studied patients in 26% and only 6.7% of controls. Depression was seen in 22% of patients and none in the controls. Borderline personality was seen in 28% of patients and 3.3% of controls.

The above data would support the contention that psychological components play a large part in the makeup of the woman complaining of chronic pelvic pain, particularly in those with no obvious organic lesion. Nor must it be forgotten that continuous chronic pain of organic cause can lead to significant emotional upset.

Management of chronic acyclic pelvic pain. Management of the patient with chronic acyclic pelvic pain should be aimed at assessing the severity of the pain and the degree to which this pain interferes with the patient's daily activities and attempting to determine the cause of the pain. Subsequent treatment will be directed at the cause. As described previously, the history and physical examination are the first steps to differentiating between pain on an organic basis within and without the reproductive tract. If it is believed that the pain arises in an organ system without the reproductive tract, appropriate referral and consultation should be sought.

If a non–reproductive tract cause can reasonably be excluded, a simultaneous approach aimed at differentiating the psychic from the somatic should be undertaken. In an ideal setup, the gynecologist should work in conjunction with a specially trained behavioral counsellor who would concurrently, with the gynecologic investigations, begin probing for any underlying psychological difficulties.

In those patients with no palpable pelvic abnormalities, the gynecologist should await the outcome of psychological screening. It is probable that many of these patients ultimately will undergo laparoscopy. The gynecologist will receive little thanks from the patient who may indeed have underlying psychological difficulty and yet harbors an organic lesion if this lesion is not detected early in the course of management. The combined approach will mean, however, that appropriate psychotherapeutic measures will have already begun and if, as is quite possible, the laparoscopic findings are negative, steps will already have been taken to begin to help the patient resolve her difficulties.

It has been demonstrated that optimal results for such patients are achieved when physicians and counsellors work in close consort in the same geographic location.[72-76]

CONCLUSION

While many causes of pelvic pain are obvious and the management clear cut, such a happy outcome is not invariably achieved. The physician dealing with patients complaining of pelvic pain must be technically competent and empathetic and in addition must be possessed of the ability to deal with failure. A cure will not and indeed cannot be achieved in all patients. It is with these patients that some of the greatest challenges in gynecologic practice exist.[78]

REFERENCES

1. Cleland JEP: Paravertebral anesthesia in obstetrics. *Surg Gynecol Obstet* 57:51, 1933.
2. Coote JH, Crawford JS: Neuroanatomy and neurophysiology of the female genitalia. In Phillip EE, Barnes J, Newton M, editors: Scientific Foundations of Obstetrics and Gynaecology, Chicago, 1986, Year Book Medical Publishers.
3. Jessel TM: Neurotransmitters and CNS disease. Pain. *Lancet* 2:1084, 1982.
4. Keele CA, Neil E: Samson Wright's Applied Physiology, London, 1971, Oxford University Press.
5. Gomel V, Taylor PJ, Yuzpe AA, Rioux JE: Laparoscopy and Hysteroscopy in Gynecologic Practice. Chicago, 1986, Year Book Medical Publishers.
6. Kerr M: In Chassar-Noir J, ed: Munro Kerr's Operative Obstetrics. London, 1964, Balliere Tindall and Cox.
7. Centers for Disease Control: Ectopic pregnancy. United States 1984-1985, *MMWR*. 37:637-639, 1988.
8. Sauer MV, Vermesh M, Anderson RE, et al: Rapid measurement of urinary pregnandiol glucuronide to diagnose ectopic pregnancy. *Am J Obstet Gynecol* 159:1531-1535, 1988.
9. Batzer FR, Schlaff S, Goldfarb AB, et al: Serial β subunit human chorionic gonadotropin doubling time as a prognosticator of pregnancy outcome in an infertile population. *Fertil Steril* 35:307, 1981.
10. Yeko TR, Gorrill MJ, Hughes LH, et al: Timely Dopnosis of early ectopic prenancy using a single blood progesterone measurement. *Fertil Steril* 48:1048-1050, 1987.
11. Hahlin M, Sjoblom P, Lindblom B: Combined use of progesterone and human chronic gonadotrpin determiuations for differential diagnosis of very early ectopic pregnancy. *Fertil Steril* 56:492-496, 1991.
12. Coleman BG, Arger PH: Ultrasound in early pregnancy complications. *Clin Obstet Gynecol* 31:3-18, 1988.
13. Bello G, Schonhal D, Mosipur J, et al: Combined pregnancy, The Mount Sinai Expereince. *Obstet Gynecol Furv* 41:613, 1986.
14. Fossum GT, Davajan V, Kletzky OA: Early detection of pregannсy with trausvaginal ultrasound. 49:788-791, 1988.
15. Westrom L: Incidence, prevalence and trends of acute pelvic inflammatory disease and its consequences in industrialized countries. *Am J Obstet Gynecol* 138:880, 1980.
16. Westrom L: Pelvic Inflammatory disease and other sexually transmitted diseases. *Cur Op Obstet Gynecol* 1:5-10, 1989.
17. Cunningham FG, Hauth JC, Gilstrap LC: The bacterial pathogenesis of acute pelvic inflammatory disease. *Obstet Gynecol* 52:161, 1978.
18. Edelmann DA: The use of intrauterine contraceptive devices, pelvic inflammatory diseaes, and *Chlamydia trachomatis* infection. *Am J Obstet Gynecol* 158:956-959, 1988.
19. Lee NC, Rubin GL, Borucki R: The intrauterine device and pelvic inflammatory disease revisited: new results from the women's health study. *Obstet Gynecol* 72:1-6, 1988.
20. Kessel E: Pelvic inflammatory disease with intra-uterine device use: a reassessment. *Fertil Steril* 51:1-11, 1989.
21. Kirshorn B, Poindexter AN III, Spitz MR: Pelvic adhesions in intrauterine device users. *Obstet Gynecol* 71:251-254, 1988.
22. Mumford SD, Kessel E: Was the Dalkon Shield a safe and effective introuterine device? The conflict between case control and clinical trial study findings. *Fertil Steril* 57:1115-1176, 1992.
23. Measday B: An analysis of the complications of hysterosalpingography. *J Obstet Gynaecol Br Commw* 67:663, 1960.
24. Taylor PJ, Graham: Is diagnostic curettage harmful to women with unexplained infertility? *Br J Obstet Gynaecol* 89-296, 1982.
25. Westrom L: Clinical manifestations and diagnosis of pelvic inflammatory disease. *J Reprod Med* 28(Suppl) 703, 1983.
26. Gomel V: Microsurgery in Female Infertility. Boston, 1983, Little, Brown & Company.
27. Sellors J W, Mahony JB, Chernesky MA, Rath DJ: Tubal factor infertility: an association with prior chlamydial infection and asymptomatic salpingitis. *Fertil Steril* 49:451-457, 1988.
28. Jacobson J, Westrom L: Subjectivized diagnosis of acute pelvic inflammatory disease. *Am J Obstet Gynecol* 105:1088, 1969.
29. Derzof ST, Robins AG, Johnson WC, et al: Percutaneous catheter drainage of abdominal abscess—a five year experience. *N Engl J Med* 305:653, 1981.
30. Centers for Disease Control, *MMWR* 52:75-81, 1993.
31. Westrom L, Iosif S, Svensson L, et al: Infertility after acute salpingitis: results of treatment with different antibiotics. *Curr Ther Res* 26:752, 1979.
32. Westrom L: Effect of acute pelvic inflammatory disease on fertility. *Am J Obstet Gynecol* 121:707, 1975.
33. Bongard F, Landers DV, Lewis F: Differential diagnosis of appendicitis and pelvic inflammatory disease—a prospective analysis. *Am J Surg* 150:90, 1985.
34. Dawood MY: Dysmenorrhea. *Clin Obstet Gynecol* 26:719, 1983.
35. Ylikorkala O, Dawood MY: New Concepts in Dysmenorrhea. *Am J Obstet Gynecol* 130:833, 1978.
36. Akerlund M, Stromberg P, Gorsling MD: Primary dysmenorrhea and vasopressin. *Br J Obstet Gynaecol* 86:484, 1979.
37. Csapo AI, Pulkkinen MO, Henzl MR: The effects of naproxin sodium on the intrauterine pressure and menstrual pain of dysmenorrheic subjects. *Prostaglandins* 13:193, 1977.
38. Dawood MY: Prostaglandins, hormones in dysmenorrhea. In Dawood MY editor: Dysmenorrhea. Baltimore, 1981, Williams & Wilkins.
39. Chan WY, Dawood MY, Fuch SF: Prostaglandin in primary dysmenorrhea: comparison of prophylactic and nonprophylactic treatment with Ibuprofen and use of oral contraceptives. *Am J Med* 75:35, 1981.
40. Lundstrom V, Green K: Endogenous levels of prostaglandin F_2 and its main metabolites in plasma and endometrium of normal and dysmenorrheic women. *Am J Obstet Gynecol* 130:640, 1978.
41. Pulkkinen MO, Csapo AI: The effect of Ibuprofen on the intra-uterine pressure and menstrual pain in dysmenorrheic patients. *Prostaglandin* 15:1055, 1978.
42. Lundstrom V, Green K, Viqvist M: Prostaglandins indomethacin and dysmenorrhea. *Prostaglandins* 11:893, 1976.
43. Henzl MR, Buttram V, Segre EJ, Bessler S: The treatment of dysmenorrhea with naproxen sodium: a report of two double-blind trials. *Am J Obstet Gynecol* 127:818, 1977.
44. Berry Hart D, Barbour AHF: Manual of Gynecology. Toronto, 1902, J.A. Carveth & Co.
45. Dawood MY: Overall approach to the management of dysmenorrhea. In Dawood MY, editor: Prostaglandins, Hormones in Dysmenorrhea. Baltimore, 1981, Williams & Wilkins.
46. Chan WY, Dawood MY: Prostaglandin levels in menstrual fluid of nondysmenorrheic and dysmenorrheic subjects with and without oral contraceptive or Ibuprofen therapy. *Adv Prostaglandin Thromboxane Res* 81:443, 1980.
47. Greydanus DE, McAnamey ER: Menstruation and its disorders in adolescents. *Curr Prob Ped* 12:22, 1982.
48. Chan WY: Prostaglandin inhibitors and antagonists in dysmenorrhea therapy. In Dawood MY, (editor): Dysmenorrhea. Baltimore, 1981, Williams & Wilkins.
49. Sandahl B, Ulmsten U, Andersson KE: Trial of calcium antagonists and Nifedipine in the treatment of primary dysmenorrhea. *Arch Gynecol* 227:147, 1979.
50. Hillier K, Kason JM: Prostaglandin E and F concentrations in human endometrium after insertion of intra-uterine contraceptive device. *Lancet* 1:15, 1976.
51. Chandhuri D: Release of prostaglandins by the IUCD. *Prostaglandins* 3:773, 1973.
52. Moon YS, Leung PCS, Ho Yuen B, Gomel V: Prostaglandin F in human endometriotic tissue. *Am J Obstet Gynecol* 141:344, 1981.
53. Anderson ABM, Guillebaud DJ, Haynes PJ, Turnbull AC: Reduction in menstrual blood loss by prostaglandin synthetase inhibitors. *Lancet* 1:774, 1976.

54. Davies AJ, Anderson AB, Turnbull AC: Reduction by naproxen of excessive menstrual bleeding in women using intra-uterine devices. *Obstet Gynecol* 57:74, 1981.
55. Kaupil A, Puolakka J, Ylikorka AO: Prostaglandin biosynthesis inhibitors in endometriosis. *Prostaglandins* 18:665, 1979.
56. Jeffcoate TNA: Dysmenorrhea, in Principles of Gynecology, London, 1967, Butterworths.
57. Rock JA, Schlaff WD, Zacur HA, Jones HW Jr: The clinical management of congenital absence of the uterine cervix. *J Gynecol Obstet* 22:231, 1984.
58. Cumming DC, Taylor PJ: Combined laparoscopy and hysteroscopy as the initial investigation of the ovulatory infertile female. *Fertil Steril* 33:475, 1980.
59. Cunanan RG, Courey NG, Lippes J: Laparoscopic findings in patients with pelvic pain. *Am J Obstet Gynecol* 146:587, 1983.
60. Basu HK: Major common problems, pelvic pain. *Br J Hosp Med* 150, 1981.
61. Frangenheim H, Kleindienst W: Chronic pelvic disease of unknown origin. *J Reprod Med* 13:23, 1974.
62. Semchyshyn S, Strickler RC: Laparoscopy: is it replacing clinical acumen? *Obstet Gynecol* 48:615, 1976.
63. Pent D: Laparoscopy: its role in private practice. *Am J Obstet Gynecol* 113-459, 1972.
64. Lundberg WI, Wall JE, Mathers JE: Laparoscopy in evaluation of pelvic pain. *Obstet Gynecol* 42:872, 1973.
65. Liston WA, Bradford WP, Downie J, Kerr MG: Laparoscopy in a general gynecologic unit. *Am J Obstet Gynecol* 113:672, 1972.
66. Allen WM, Masters WH: Traumatic lacerations of uterine support. *Am J Obstet Gynecol* 70:500, 1975.
67. Editorial: *Lancet* 19:617, 1981.
68. Renaer M: Chronic pelvic pain without obvious pathology in women: personal observations and a review of the problem. *Eur J Obstet Gynecol Reprod Biol* 10:415, 1980.
69. Dodge JA: Recurrent abdominal pain in children. *Br Med J* 1:385, 1976.
70. Gomez J, Dally P: Psychological mediated abdominal pain in surgical and medical outpatient clinics. *Br Med* J 1:1451, 1977.
71. Duncan CH, Taylor HC: A psychosomatic study of pelvic congestion. *Am J Obstet Gynecol* 64:1, 1952.
72. Beard RW, Belsey EM, Lieberman BA, Wilkinson JCM: Pelvic pain in women. *Am J Obstet Gynecol* 128:566, 1977.
73. Renaer M, Vertommen H, Nij SP, et al: Psychologic aspects of chronic pelvic pain in women. *Am J Obstet Gynecol* 134:75, 1979.
74. Wilda GJS: Neurotische Labiliteit Gemeten Volgens de Vragenlijstmethode Amsterdam Vanrossem, 1963.
75. Vertomme H, Rochet EF: Vragenlijst Internpersonnlijke Relaties: Vir. Amsterdam, 1978, Swetz and Zeitlinger.
76. Sternbach RA, Wolf SR, Murphy RW, Akeson WH: Aspects of chronic lower back pain. *Psychosomatics* 14:52, 1973.
77. Stenchever MA: ACOG postgraduate course gynecology update. Lake Louise, June 1985.
78. Taylor PJ, Gomel V: Pelvic Pain. *Curr Prob Obstet Gynecol Fertil* 9:393-437, 1987.

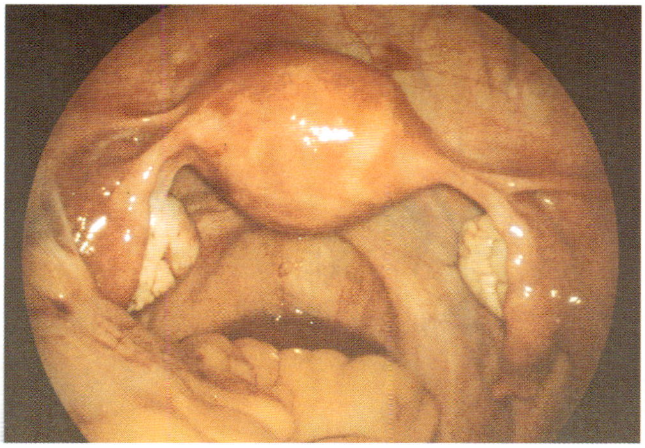

Initial inspection of the pelvis.

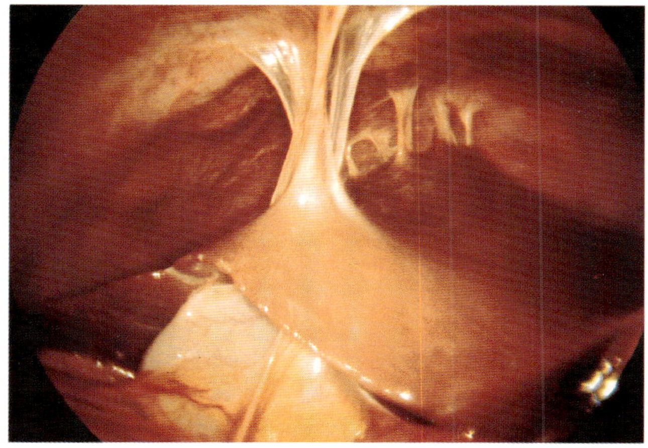

The gall bladder and right lobe of the liver with adhesions extending from the liver to the parietal peritoneum.

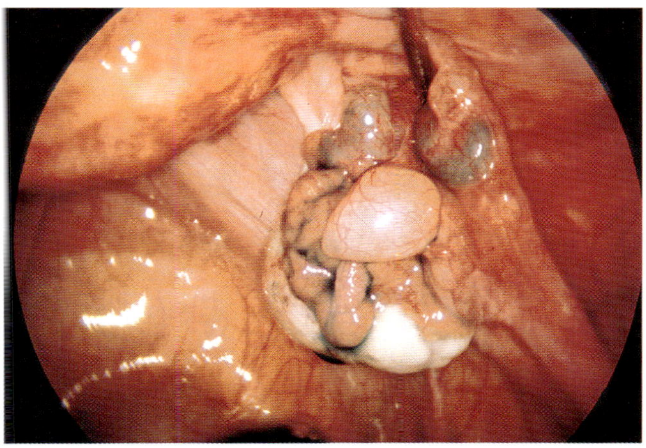

The fimbriated extremity of the tube viewed *en face*. Healthy fimbria, escape of dilute dye solution, and a small hydatid of Morgagni are noted.

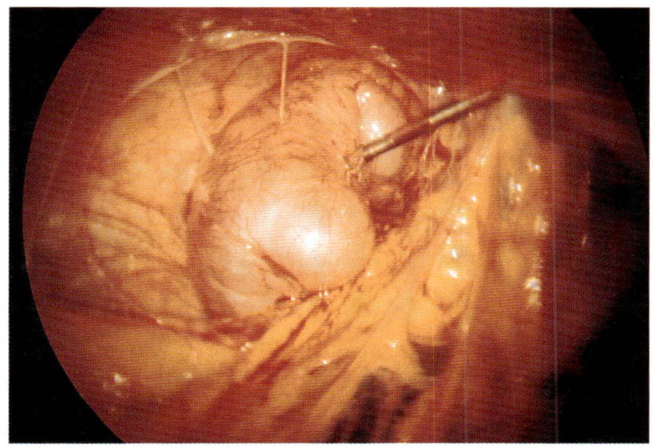

Large thin walled hydrosalpinx with extensive omental adhesions.

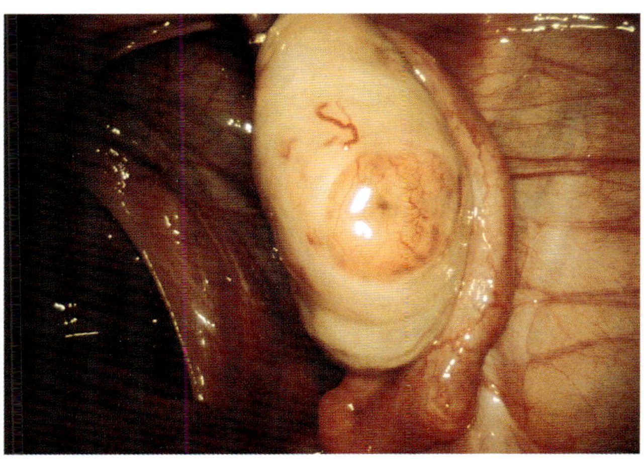

Ovary with an early corpus luteum and ovulation stigma.

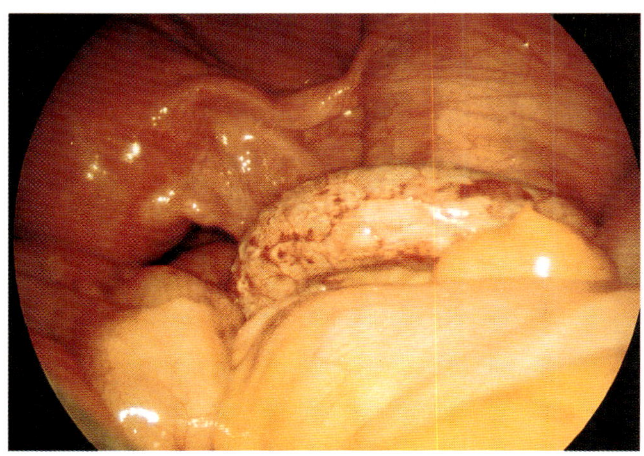

Acute appendicitis.

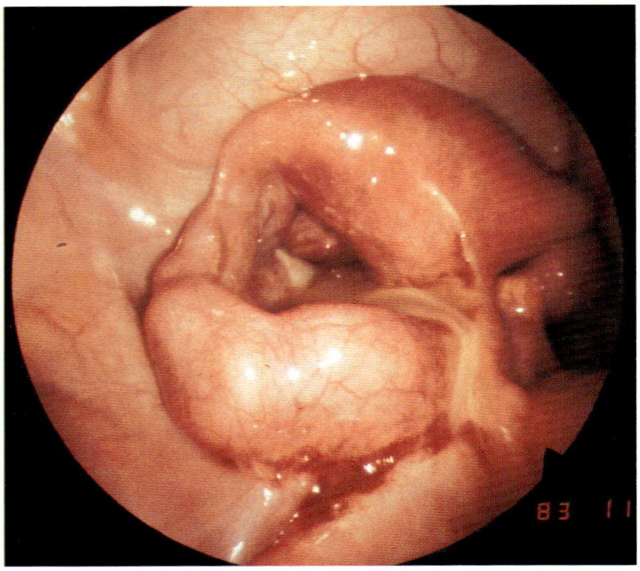

Pelvic inflammatory disease: pus draining from abscess.

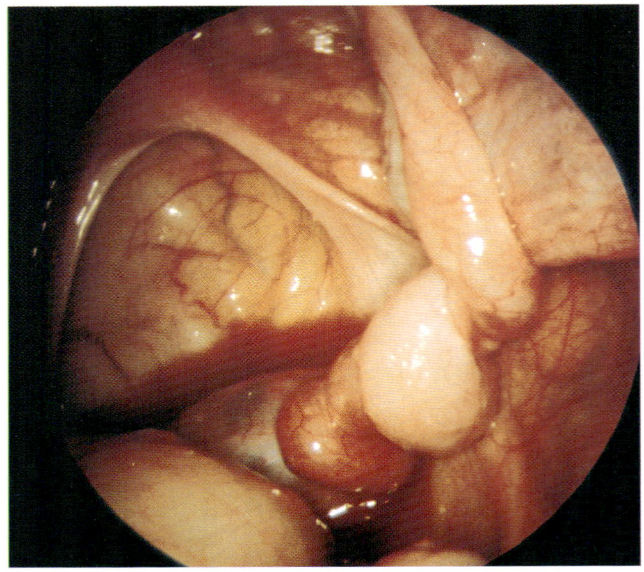

Torsion of the fallopian tube.

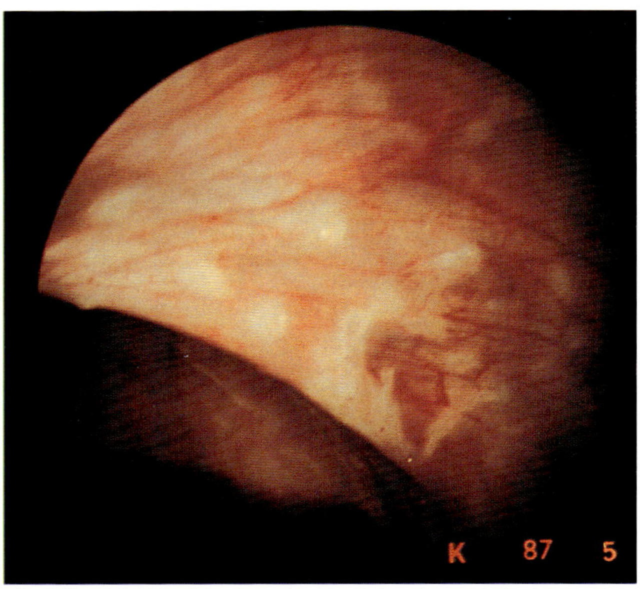

Endometriosis: clear lesions (courtesy Dan Martin).

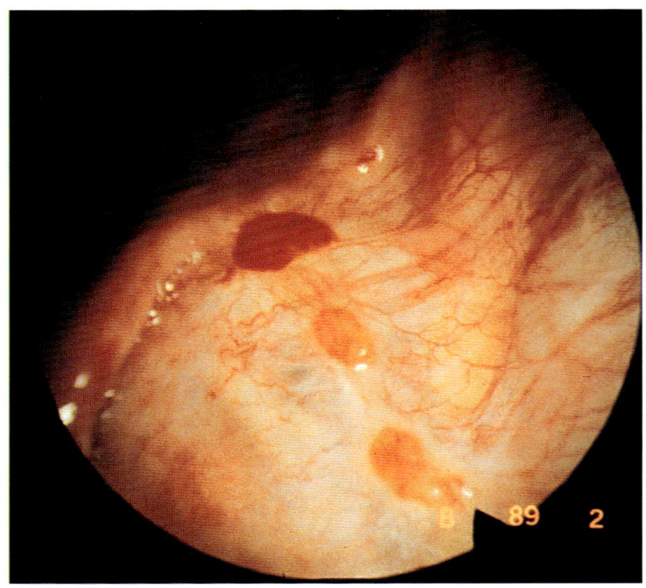

Endometriosis: red lesions (courtesy Dan Martin).

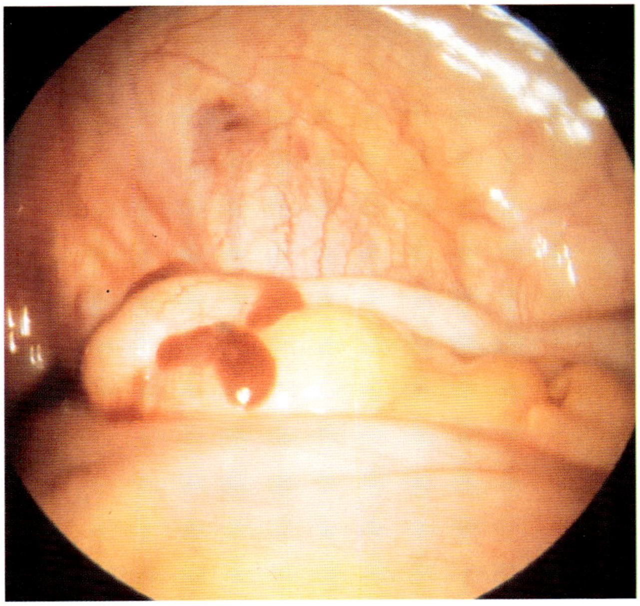

Endometriosis affecting the appendix.

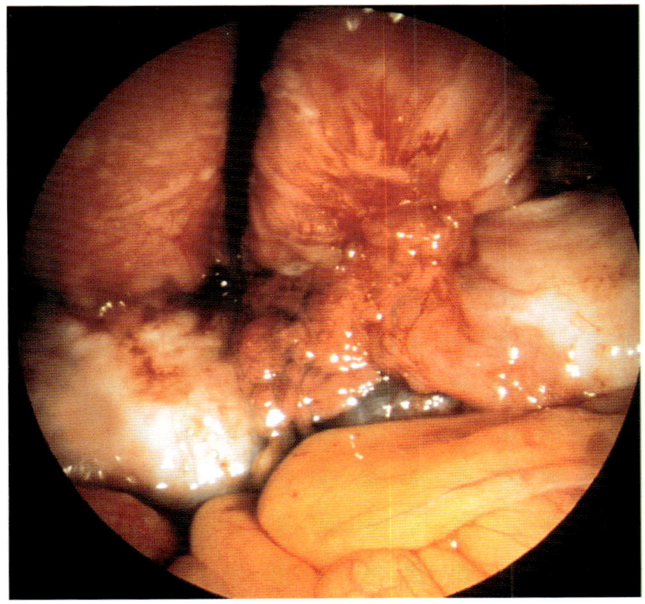

Severe endometriosis with enlarged ovaries adherent to one another (kissing ovaries) and the posterior surface of the uterus.

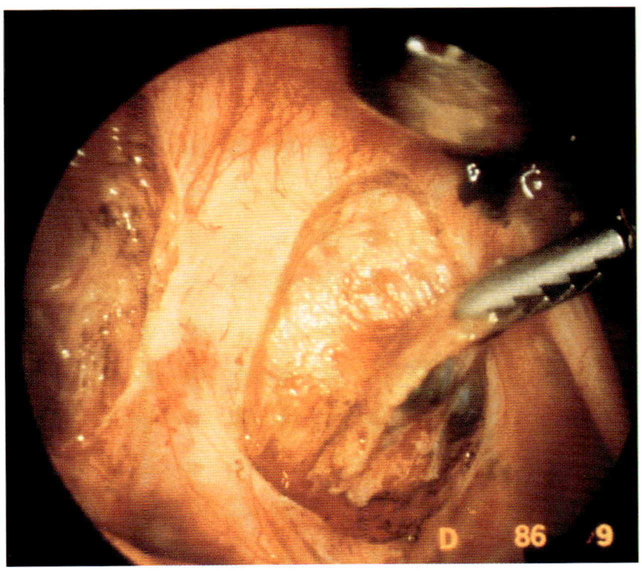

Excisional biopsy of typical purple-black endometriotic lesions (courtesy Dan Martin).

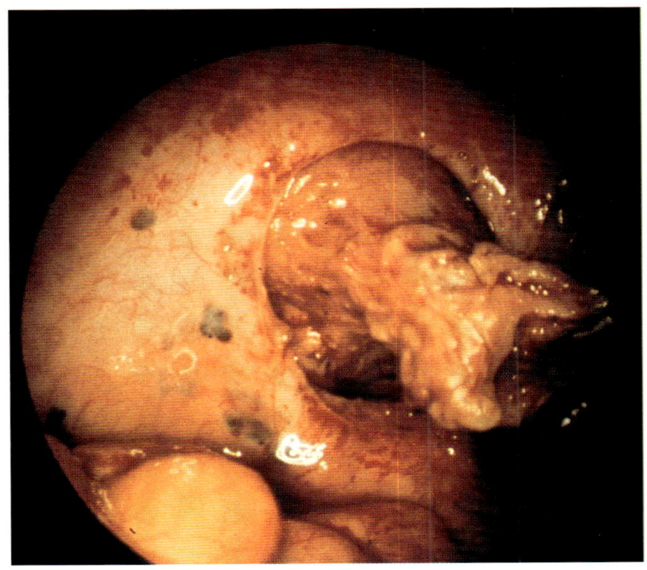

Excision of deeply infiltrating cul de sac endometriosis (courtesy Dan Martin).

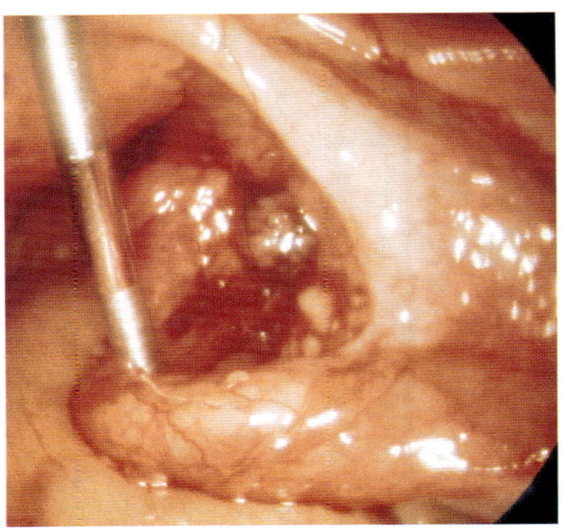

Carcinoma of the fallopian tube.

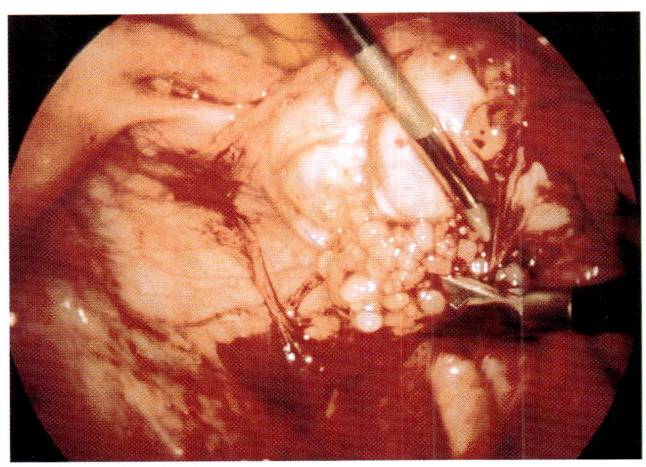

Ovarian carcinoma of low malignant potential discovered during salpingo-ovariolysis for infertility.

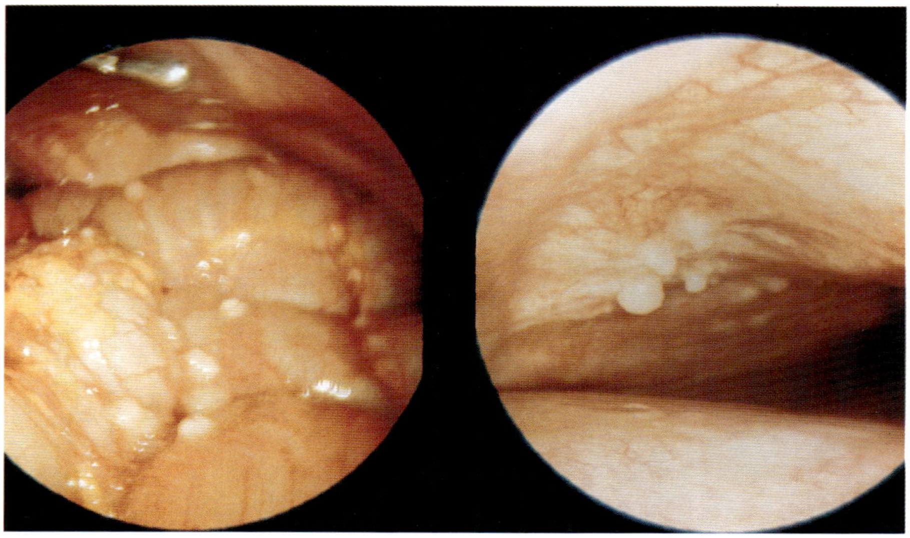

Disseminated intra-peritoneal carcinomatosis.

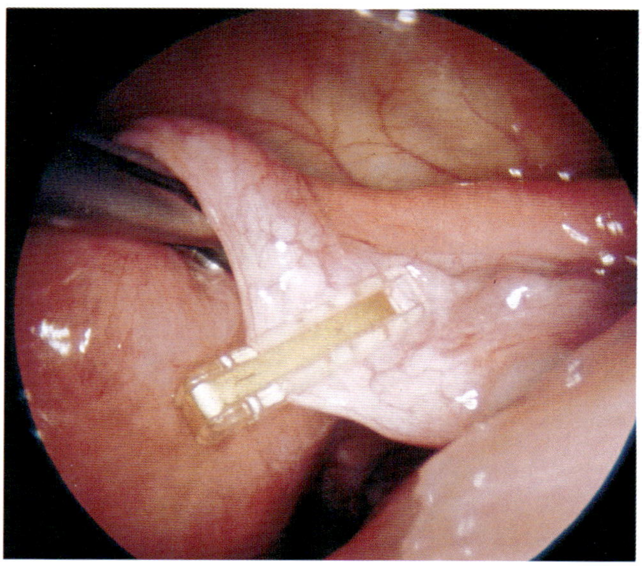

Tubal sterilization with the Hulka clip.

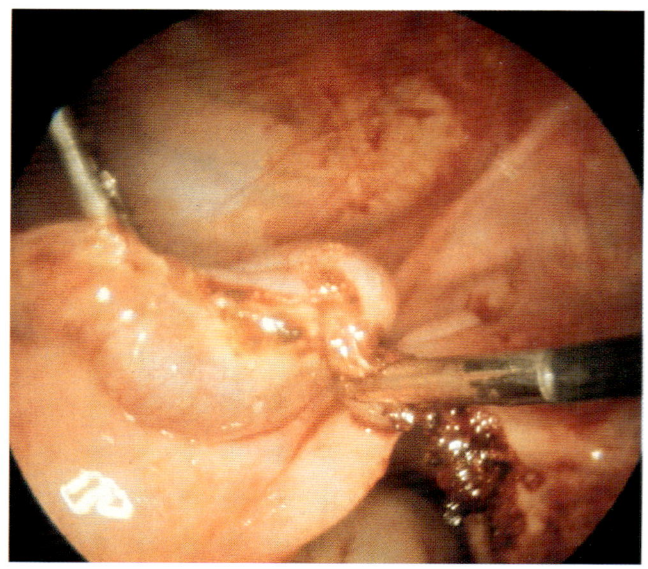

Segmental excision of tubal pregnancy: electrodesiccation and division of the mesosalpinx of the affected segment.

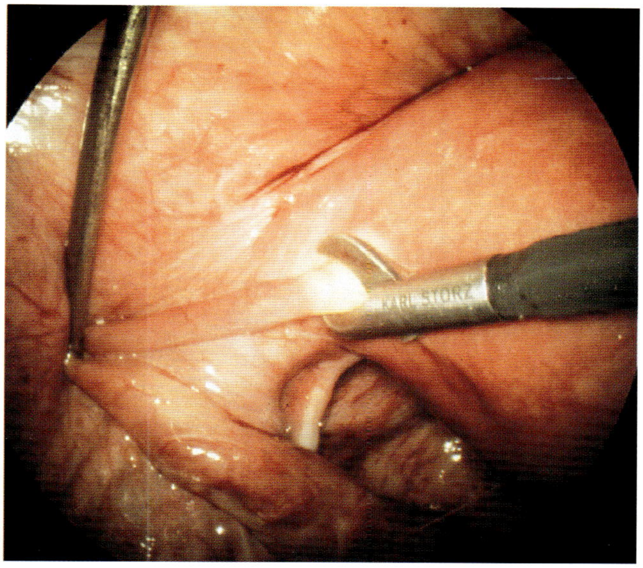

Salpingectomy for tubal pregnancy: electrodesiccation and division of the tube at the uterotubal junction.

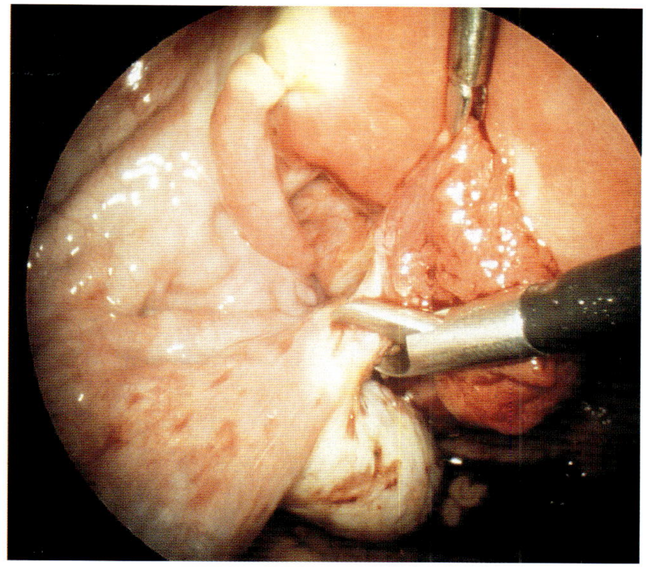

Salpingectomy: electrodesiccation and division of the tubo-ovarian ligament.

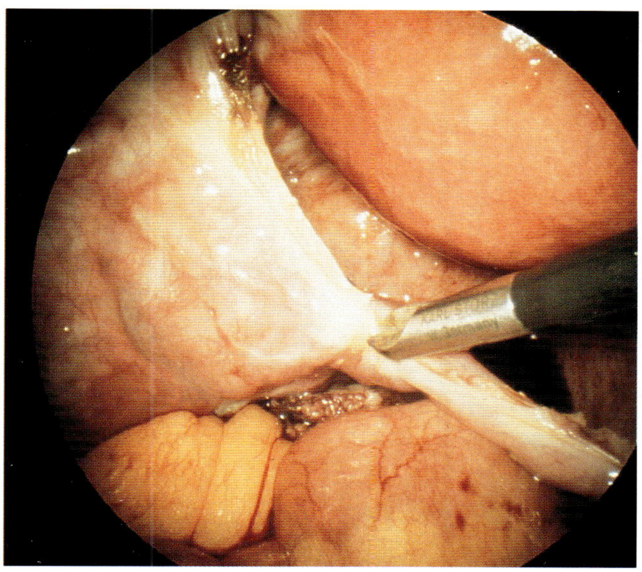

Salpingectomy: the tube is excised by the division of the intervening mesosalpinx.

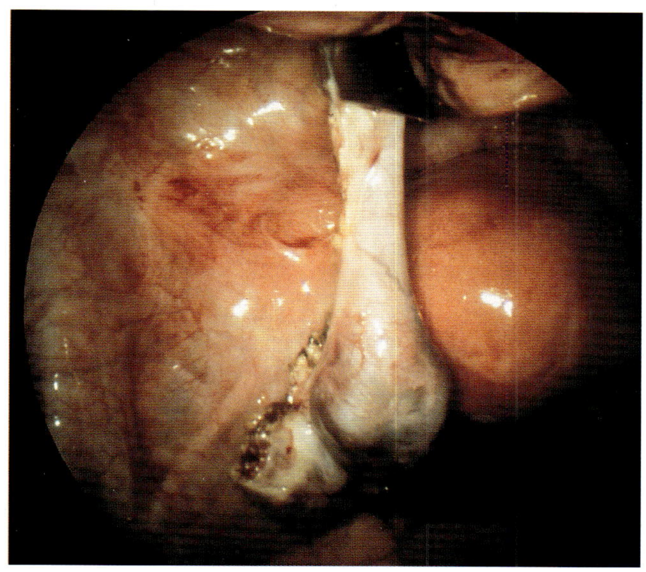

Salpingectomy: the tube is removed through an 11 mm cannula.

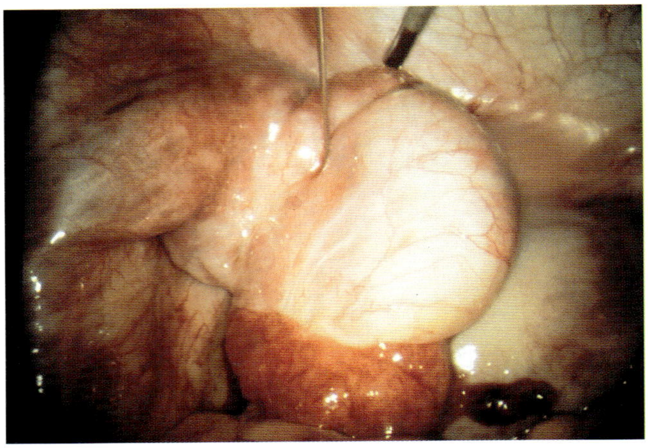

Linear salpingotomy: injection of dilute vasopressin solution under the serosa of the mesosalpinx adjacent to the gestational site.

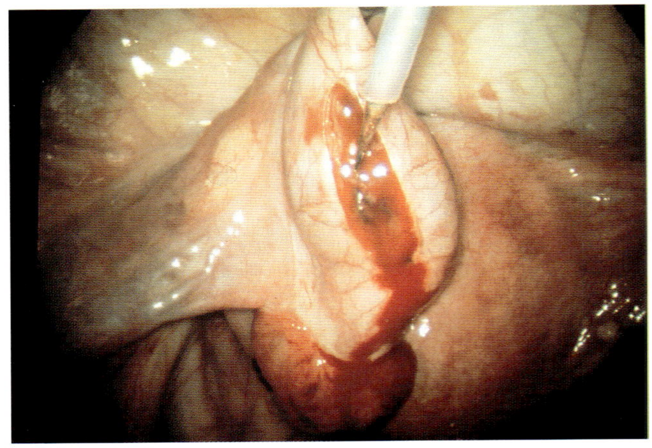

Linear salpingotomy: an incision has been placed over the implantation site.

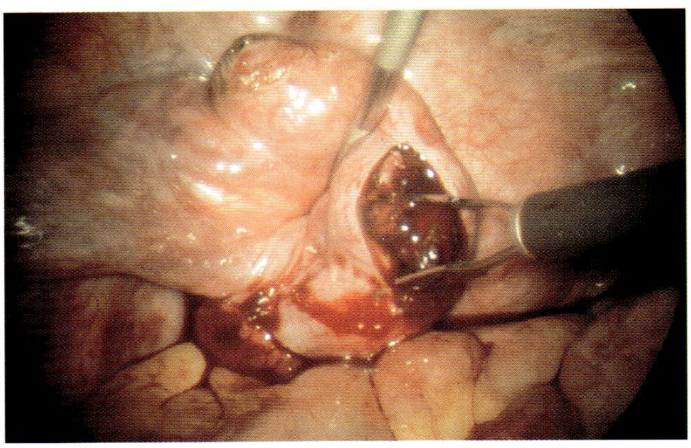

Linear salpingotomy: gestational products are teased out.

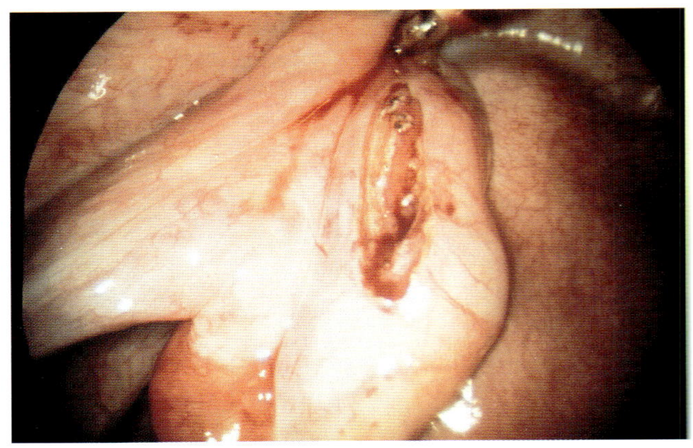

Linear salpingotomy: final inspection.

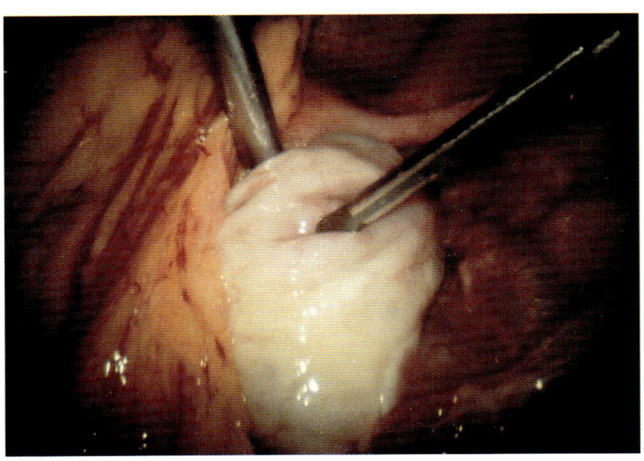

GIFT procedure: oocyte recovery.

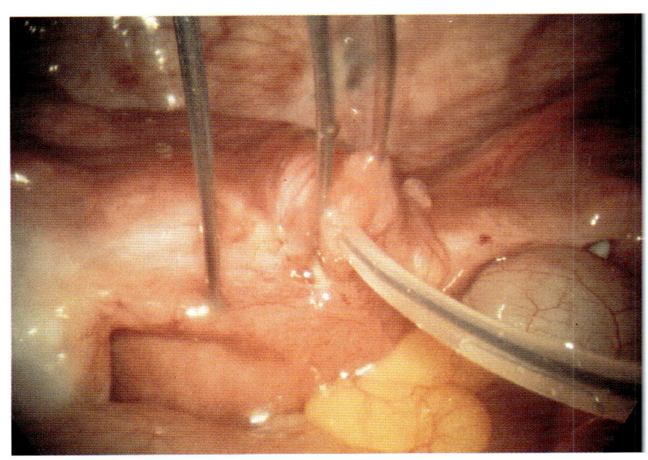

GIFT procedure: transfer of gametes into the ampullary portion of the tube.

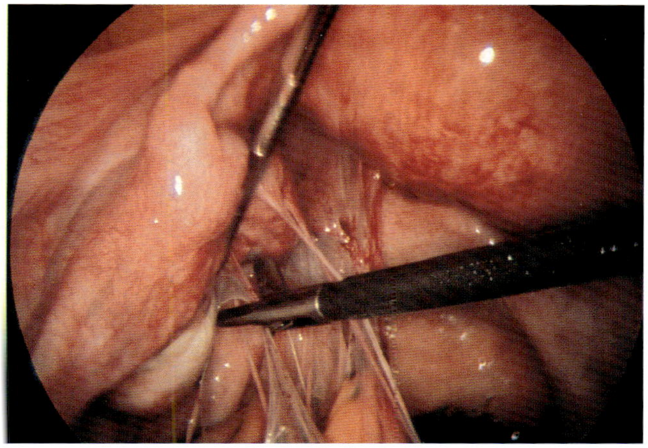

Salpingo-ovariolysis: adhesions are divided one layer at a time along the organ of interest.

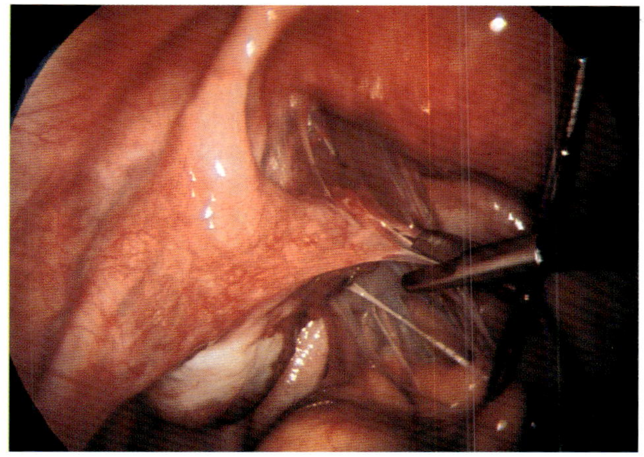

Salpingo-ovariolysis: adhesions between the tube and the bowel are progressively divided.

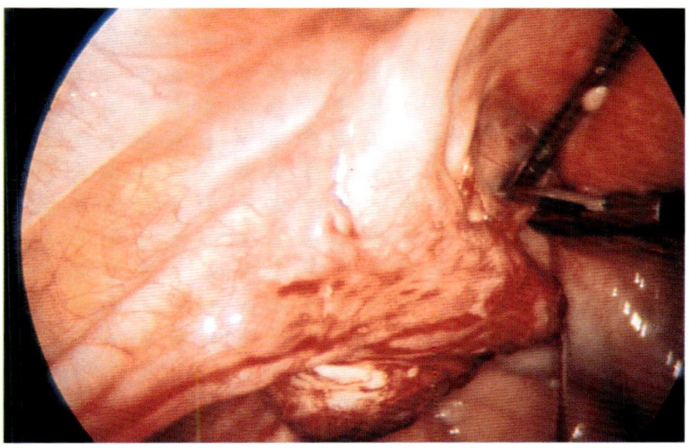

Salpingo-ovariolysis: The inferior aspect of the tube has been cleared. Adhesions between the fimbriated end of the tube, the ovary, and the uterus are being removed.

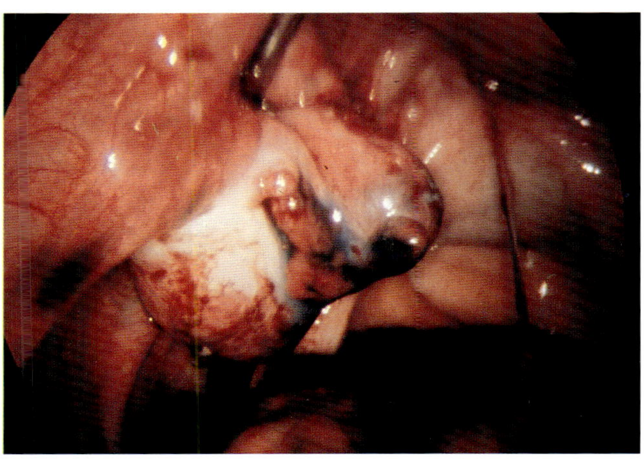

Salpingo-ovariolysis: the tube and ovary are now free. Passage of dilute methylene blue solution is noted.

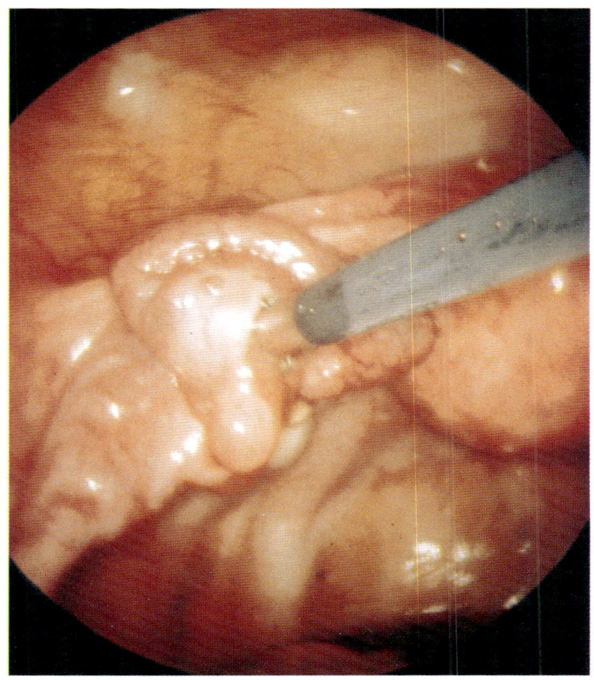

Tubal phimosis: disagglutination of fimbria.

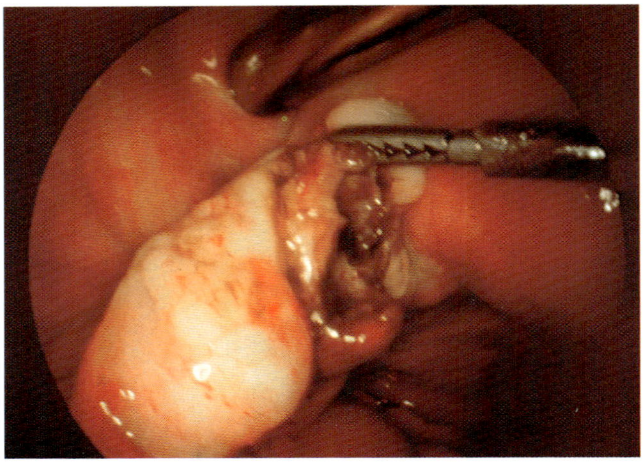

Excision of endometrioma: the endometrioma has been fenestrated and is being dissected from the ovary (courtesy Dan Martin).

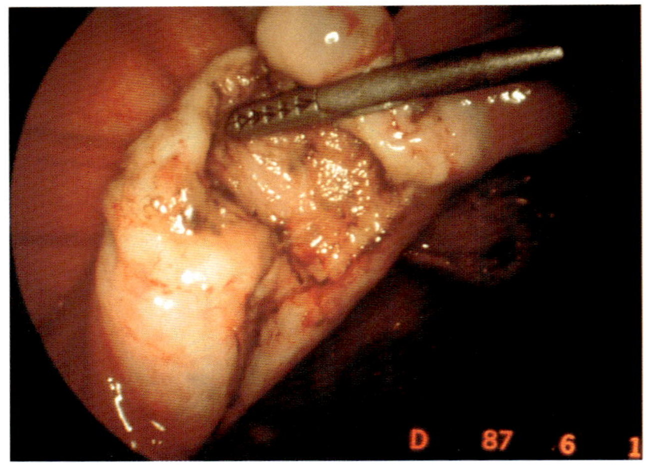

Excision of endometrioma: the excision site is inspected and hemostasis obtained (courtesy Dan Martin).

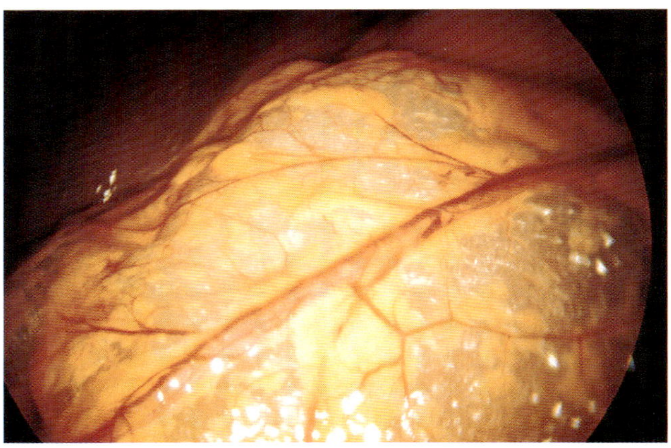

Pneumo-omentum.

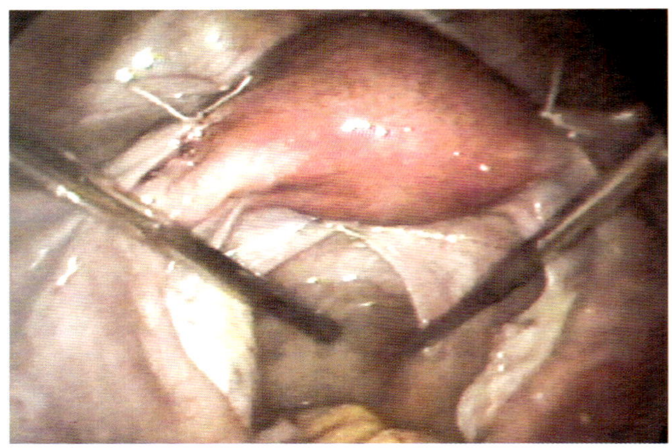

Uterine suspension: Gargiulo's three stitch technique (courtesy Tige Gargiulo).

Chapter 11

ENDOMETRIOSIS

Endometriosis, the presence of endometrial glands and stroma at sites other than the endometrial cavity, was first described by Sampson in 1921.[1] Despite more than 70 years of intense interest in the condition, it is probably true to say that we are no closer today to comprehending its pathogenesis, relationship to either pelvic pain or infertility, or the optimum form of management.

For a reasoned, concise, and contemporary consideration of all these matters the reader is referred to the proceedings of the Canadian Consensus Conference on Endometriosis.[2] This chapter will be confined to a discussion of the diagnosis of the disorder, with particular reference to the role of diagnostic laparoscopy.

In order to make any diagnosis, the physician must understand the prevalence of the condition, the symptoms and signs with which it is usually associated, and the investigations that can be used to confirm its presence.

PREVALENCE

Prevalence studies are impossible to perform. A final diagnosis can be made only by examination of biopsy specimens, which must be obtained by invasive methods. Thus large populations of asymptomatic women cannot be screened. All currently available information is based on data derived from specific populations. Much of these data are from retrospective studies, which introduces another level of bias. To compound the issue, until recently the significance of the pleomorphism of the endometriotic lesions has largely been overlooked. Nonclassically appearing lesions may, nevertheless, contain the histologic markers of the disease. Thus the following details of apparent prevalence must be read in light of the preceding caveats.

It would be of supreme importance if the true prevalence among asymptomatic women of proved fertility were known. Attempts to derive these figures from observations of women undergoing sterilization have produced percentages ranging from two to 20.[3-6] Two common symptoms leading to the finding of endometriosis are pain and infertility. In the former patients the lesions have been identified in from 5% to 21%.[7-11] In adolescent patients undergoing laparoscopy for a complaint of pain this figure may rise to an amazing 53%.[12] The reported range in infertile women is from 20% to 50%.[3-6] All of these percentages may err conservatively. Histologic appearances of stroma and glands have been detected in biopsy specimens obtained from normal-looking peritoneum in from 6% to 13%.[13,14]

SYMPTOMS AND SIGNS

Pain is a very common presenting symptom[15,16] (See box on p. 134). It is usually expressed as dysmenorrhea, particularly resistant to nonsteroidal anti-inflammatory agents and/or deep dyspareunia. Less frequently the patient may complain of chronic pelvic pain, rectal pain, or low back pain. Frustratingly there is no clear-cut relationship between the severity of the pain and the extent of the visible lesions.[17,18]

Infertility must always raise the suspicion that endometriosis is present, although the cause and effect relationship is extremely unclear.[19] Menstrual disturbances can occur and include menorrhagia, premenstrual spotting, and hypermenorrhea. Bleeding from either the urinary or gastrointestinal tracts may be reported and should be taken as presumptive evidence that endometriosis is present if it is related temporally to menstruation. Other bladder or bowel dysfunction may also occur at this time. Finally there is a greater likelihood of finding the disorder if there is a history of endometriosis in a first-degree relative.[2]

It is important to remember that the physical examination may be absolutely normal. Suspicious findings include fixed retroversion of the uterus, tender nodularity of the uterosacral ligaments, cul-de-sac, and back of the uterus, and/or the presence of a tender adnexal mass. Colored le-

Symptoms and signs of endometriosis

Pain
Infertility
Menorrhagia
Premenstrual spotting
Hypermenorrhea
Bleeding from urinary or gastrointestinal tracts
Bladder or bowel dysfunction
History of endometriosis in a first-degree relative
Fixed retroversion of uterus
Tender nodularity of the uterosacral ligaments, cul de sac, and back of uterus
Tender adnexal mass
Colored lesions of umbilicus, vulva, vagina, and cervix
Tender masses in episiotomy scars
Tender masses in abdominal scars of previous uterine surgery

sions of the umbilicus, vulva, vagina, and cervix or tender masses in episiotomy scars or abdominal scars of previous uterine surgery may, on occasion, be noted.

INVESTIGATIONS

The search continues for noninvasive methods to detect endometriosis. Regrettably none of the measurements of chemical markers are of sufficient sensitivity or specificity nor are the powers of resolution of the various imaging techniques adequate.

The cell surface antigen, CA-125, is present in many normal tissues including the pleura, pericardium, peritoneum, fallopian tube, endometrium, and cervix. It can be assayed from the peripheral plasma, and levels may be elevated in association with ovarian cancer, pregnancy, acute pelvic inflammatory disease, and endometriosis[20] (see Chapter 17). It is also present in the menstrual effluent in concentrations that are considerably higher than those found in the plasma. These menstrual blood levels were found to be elevated in women with endometriosis when compared with controls.[21]

Other avenues of investigation have concerned evaluation of the levels of circulating antibodies to endometrium[22] and the endometrial secretory protein PP14.[23]

Ultrasound is valuable for delineating more clearly the nature of any ovarian cysts. Regrettably, this technique, just as computer-assisted tomography (CAT) and magnetic resonance imaging (MRI), is unable to detect adhesions or peritoneal implants. The gold standard of diagnosis remains direct visualization, usually achieved laparoscopically, and examination of biopsy specimens.

THE ROLE OF LAPAROSCOPY IN ENDOMETRIOSIS

In view of the inaccuracy of clinical methods, peripheral markers, or imaging techniques, no woman should be told that she does or does not have endometriosis, nor should she be treated for this condition until at least a visual and, preferably, a histologic diagnosis has been made.

Indications

As described in Chapter 9 laparoscopy should be carried out in the infertile woman once the simpler investigations have been completed and have been shown to be normal or following failure of a short course of treatment if an easily correctable cause of the infertility had been detected. This advice is valid only if there is no other clinical reason to suspect the presence of endometriosis. This reason may be an association of any of the other symptoms of the disorder or abnormal physical findings. In these cases treatment should be deferred until a laparoscopy has been performed.

If the complaint is one of pain, the symptom must be analyzed to determine whether laparoscopy is indicated immediately or could reasonably be deferred. Immediate visualization of the pelvis should be performed if the pain is of recent onset, associated with other symptoms that are suggestive, or exists in concert with abnormal pelvic findings. In the younger woman, particularly if it seems that she is suffering from primary dysmenorrhoea, an empiric trial of prostaglandin synthasese inhibitory medication or oral contraceptives should be considered. If after three months of such a therapeutic trial there has been no symptomatic improvement, the internal pelvic organs must be inspected.

Timing of laparoscopy

Diagnostic laparoscopy may be performed at any time during the menstrual cycle. If endometriosis is suspected clinically, it may be preferable to perform the procedure during, or a day or so before, the onset of menstruation. At that time, the endometriotic lesions are more pronounced and may even be seen to be bleeding actively. In addition, evidence of retrograde menstruation with blood dripping from the fimbria may be observed. Not only do these findings facilitate the diagnosis but they may also explain why some women experience such severe symptoms despite the presence of relatively few small implants.

The laparoscopic survey

The need for and technique of the thorough pelvic survey, aided by a blunt, calibrated probe and a uterine manipulator, have been discussed in Chapter 5. Every aspect of the pelvic peritoneum must be scrutinized if small lesions are not to be overlooked. The initial survey should be performed by observation through the laparoscope with the naked eye because direct visualization permits discrimination between subtle shades of color. If a significant amount of fluid is present in the pelvis, this must be aspirated to properly visualize the peritoneal surfaces of the cul-de-sac and uterosacral ligaments. Apparently healthy but adherent ovaries must be regarded with suspicion and gentle separation attempted. The appendix must be inspected in every case.

The magnifying power of the laparoscope, particularly when combined with a high-resolution video system, can be used to advantage. With the distal lens held practically in contact with the peritoneal surface,[24] identification of lesions as small as 180 μ can be achieved; indeed carbon particles as small as 40 μ, the result of previous laser and electrosurgery, were identified.[25]

Biopsy

Biopsy of suspected areas of endometriosis should provide a definitive histologic diagnosis. To be conclusive the pathologist must identify the presence of both endometrial glands and stroma. Such biopsies should be taken only from safe areas where vital structures are not exposed to damage and when the risk of bleeding is deemed to be minimal. The floor of the cul-de-sac or the uterosacral ligaments and the ovarian surface are ideal sites from which to obtain such biopsies. Electrocoagulation of the biopsy sites is rarely necessary.

The importance of these biopsy specimens cannot be overemphasized. The detection rate was increased from 42% in 1982 to 72% in 1988 by the simple expedient of taking multiple biopsies.[26-28] In 1982 samples were taken only from 13% of patients, a figure that had risen to 100% by 1988. Of even greater interest, whereas 62% of the specimens were positive in 1982, an accuracy of 98% had been achieved by the later date.[28,29]

In some instances, it will not be possible to obtain an adequate biopsy specimen or the specimen will not show the pathognomic histologic features. Under these circumstances a presumptive diagnosis must be made from the morphologic appearance of the lesions—a presumptive diagnosis that can be inaccurate.

Morphologic appearance of the lesions

The appearance of endometriosis varies enormously and can be confused with other lesions (see the box at right). Three types of morphologic change may be noted: superficial implants, ovarian endometriomata, and adhesions.

Implants. Implants are the most common and are most frequently found in the dependent parts of the pelvis. The uterosacral ligaments, peritoneal surfaces of the pouch of Douglas, the vesicouterine pouch, the ovarian fossae, and the lateral pelvic side walls are the usual sites. It has been postulated that these areas are most frequently affected because of the effect of the force of gravity on endometrial tissue entering the pelvis at the time of retrograde menstruation. Implants may also be noted on the surfaces of the ovaries and oviducts. The appendix must be visualized since the disease process may involve this organ in a small percentage of cases.

It would appear that implants have a temporal natural history. The earliest lesions are clear or pinkish blebs or vesicles. As the disease progresses they become flame colored. The final stage is represented by the "gunpowder burn" or "mulberry" lesions. It is probable that the younger lesions are more biologically active.[17] Implants may be solitary or occur in clumps, with the diameter of the individual lesions varying from 2 to 5 mm. They may actually be seen to be bleeding when laparoscopic examination is performed in the immediately premenstrual or menstrual phase of the cycle.

> **Lesions with which endometriosis may be confused[28-32]**
>
> Epithelial inclusions
> Reactions to oil-based contrast material
> Remnants of trophoblast
> Malignant metastases
> Carbon deposits from electrosurgery or laser surgery
> Residue of suture material
> Psammoma bodies
> Ovarian cancer
> Hemangioma

Although these lesions may appear to be superficial, the depth to which they extend is extremely variable. This feature has caused some authors to refer to the superficial lesions as merely "the tip of the iceberg." Sometimes, either in association with these lesions or independently, scarring, puckering, and hemosiderin staining of the peritoneum may be observed, especially over the uterosacral ligaments.

Peritoneal defects (small areas of reduplication without any other associated findings) have also been suggested to represent old, burned-out lesions. This finding does not exclude the possibility of active areas of endometriosis located at the base of the defect; these are not always readily accessible to laparoscopic visualization. Larger peritoneal defects have, in the past, been referred to as the Allan and Masters syndrome and were believed to be due to spontaneous rupture or splitting of the posterior leaf of the broad ligament following childbirth trauma. When the inner margins and the base of these defects are exposed, areas of endometriosis may be encountered. The frequent observation of such peritoneal defects in nulliparous women has weakened significantly the theory of childbirth trauma as their cause.

When the disease process is more extensive, there is greater involvement of the ovaries, fallopian tubes, round, broad, and uterosacral ligaments, and even the serosal surfaces of the sigmoid colon, rectum, and bladder. Superficial lesions undergo recurrent cyclic bleeding into the peritoneal cavity. The resultant inflammatory response causes adhesion formation and adherence of the pelvic structures. The ovaries tend to become fixed to the ovarian fossa, uterus, posterior leaves of the broad ligaments, and the pelvic floor. If an adherent ovary is freed using a blunt probe, there is almost always evidence of endometriosis along with a marked peritoneal inflammatory reaction and bleeding at the site of dislodgement.

Ovarian endometriomata. Ovarian endometriosis may become cystic and lead to the formation of endometriomas that vary in size and may exceed 10 cm in diameter. The affected ovary, which is usually adherent on at least one of its surfaces, has a smooth glistening appearance. Endometriomas may rupture, causing an episode of acute abdominal pain.

Ovarian endometriomas are frequently bilateral. They may become adherent in the cul-de-sac, to the pelvic sidewalls, to the posterior aspect of the uterus, or bowel. Enlarged but visually normal ovaries may adhere to one another behind the uterus ("kissing ovaries"). Although there may be no other overt evidence of endometriosis, this finding in the absence of prior pelvic surgery is pathognomic.

Endometriosis may directly affect the oviducts. Extensive involvement of the other pelvic structures may incorporate parts or the whole of the tubes within the severe adhesive process. The tubes themselves usually remain patent.

Adhesions. In more advanced cases, the rectum becomes densely adherent to the posterior surface of the uterus, partially or completely obliterating the cul-de-sac. The adhesive process between the uterus and bowel may enclose the entire adnexa. These observations confirm the progression and extent of inflammation associated with this disease. The severity of the disease must be recorded, both in the dictated operative report and by using a scoring system.

Scoring systems

That most frequently used is the revised American Fertility Society (rAFS) system. This is a multipoint scoring system which allows for a very detailed description and the subdivision of cases into four degrees of severity; stages 1, 2, 3, and 4. A proposed stage 5 may be added for very severe disease. Further revision is needed to take into consideration the morphologic differences of the individual lesions and prospective correlations with infertility and pain.

CONCLUSIONS

Diagnostic laparoscopy with visualization of the lesions combined with directed biopsy is the gold standard of the diagnosis of endometriosis. The physician who wishes to manage such cases must be completely familiar with the clinical manifestations of endometriosis, the varied appearances of the lesions, and the techniques by which tissue samples are obtained. The treatment of endometriosis will be discussed in Chapter 18.

REFERENCES

1. Sampson JA: Perforating haemorrhagic (chocherate) cysts of the ovary, *Arch Surg* 3:245, 1921.
2. Canadian Consensus on Endometriosis, *J.S.O.G.C.* 15:(Suppl)1-37, 1993.
3. Mahmood TA, Templeton AA: Prevalence and genesis of endometriosis, *Hum Reprod* 6:544, 1991.
4. Schweppe K-W: Etiology, pathogenesis and natural history of endometriosis. In Genazzani AR, Petralglia F, Volpe A et al, editors: *Advances in gynecological endocrinology.* Carnforth, 1988, Parthenon Publishing.
5. Strahy JH, Molgaard Ca, Coulam CB: Endometriosis and infertility: a laparoscopic study of endometriosis among fertile and infertile women, *Fertil Steril* 38:667-, 1982.
6. Rawson JM: Prevalence of endometriosis in asymptomatic women, *J Reprod Med* 36:513, 1991.
7. Liston WA, Bradford WP, Downie J et al: Laparoscopy in a general gynecologic unit, *Am J Obstet Gynecol* 113:672, 1972.
8. Talbot HM, Leeton J. The role of laparoscopy in 1400 patients, *Med J Aust* 1:36, 1974.
9. Duignan NM, Jordan JA, Coughlan BM et al: One thousand consecutive cases of diagnostic laparoscopy, *J Obstet Gynaecol Br Commonw* 79:1016, 1972.
10. Kleppinger RK: One thousand laparoscopies in a community hospital, *J Reprod Med* 13:13, 1974.
11. Hasson HM: Incidence of endometriosis in diagnostic laparoscopy, *J Reprod Med* 16:135, 1976.
12. Goldstein DP, de Cholnoky C, Evans SJ et al: Laparoscopy in the diagnosis and management of pelvic pain in adolescents, *J Reprod Med* 24:251, 1980.
13. Jansen RPS, Russell P: Nonpigmented endometriosis: clinical, laparoscopic and pathologic definition, *Am J Obstet Gynecol* 155:1154-1159, 1986.
14. Nisolle M, Paindaveine B, Bourdon A, et al: Histologic study of peritoneal endometriosis in infertile women, *Fertil Steril* 53:984, 1990.
15. Rock JA, Markham SM: Pathogenesis of endometriosis, *Lancet* 340:1264-1267, 1992.
16. Mahmood TA, Templeton AA, Thomson L et al: Menstrual symptoms in women with pelvic endometriosis, *Br. J Obstet Gynecol* 98:558-563, 1991.
17. Stout AL, Steege JG, Dodson WC et al: Relationship of laparoscopic findings to self-report of pelvic pain, *Am J Obstet Gynecol* 164:73-79, 1991.
18. Fedele L, Parazzini F, Bianchi S, et al: Stage and localization of pelvic endometriosis and pain, *Fertil Steril* 53:155-158, 1990.
19. Taylor PJ, Collins JA: Unexplained Infertility. Oxford, 1992, Oxford University Press.
20. Pittaway DE: CA-125 in women with endometriosis, *Obstet Gynecol Clin N Am* 16:237, 1989.
21. Takahashi K, Nagata H, Susa A, et al: Clinical usefulness of CA-125 levels in the menstrual discharge in patients with endometriosis, *Fertil Steril* 54:360-362, 1990.
22. Wild RA, Shivers CA: Antiendometrial antibodies in patients with endometriosis, *Am J Reprod Immunol* 8:84, 1985.
23. Telimaa S, Kauppila A, Ronnberg L et al: Elevated serum levels of endometrial secretory protein PP14 in patients with advances endometriosis, *Am J Obstet Gynecol* 161:866, 1989.
24. Redwine DB: The distribution of endometriosis in the pelvis by age groups and fertility, *Fertil Steril* 47:173, 1987.
25. Martin DC, Redwine DB, Reich H et al: Laparoscopic appearance of endometriosis, ed 2: Memphis, 1992, Resolle Press.
26. Stripling MC, Martin DC, Chatman DL, et al: Subtle appearance of endometriosis, *Fertil Steril* 49:427, 1988.
27. Stripling MC, Martin DC, Poston WM: Does endometriosis have a typical appearance? *J Reprod Med* 33:879-884, 1988.
28. Martin DC, Hubert GD, Vader Zwagg R et al: Laparoscopic appearances of peritoneal endometriosis, *Fertil Steril* 51:63-67, 1989.
29. Martin DC, Vander Zwaag R: Excisional techniques with the Co_2 laser laparoscopie, *J Reprod Med* 32:753, 1987.
30. Jansen RPS, Russell P: Nonpigmented endometriosis: clinical laparoscopic, and pathologic definition, *Am J Obstet Gynecol* 155:1154, 1986.
31. Martin DC, Diamond MP: Operative laparoscopy: comparison of lasers with other techniques, *Curr Prob Obstet Gynecol Fertil* 9:564, 1986.
32. Stovall TG, Ling FW: Splenosis: report of a case and review of the literature, *Obstet Gynecol Surv* 43:69, 1988.

Chapter 12

NEOPLASIA

with
Denis Querleu
Eric Leblanc

Diagnostic laparoscopy has four major applications in gynecologic oncology: (1) assessment of ovarian tumors, (2) diagnosis and staging of ovarian cancer, (3) monitoring therapy of ovarian cancer, and (4) lymph node staging. Laparoscopy for these four indications should be undertaken only by gynecologic oncologists working with skilled laparoscopic surgeons or surgeons with combined training in both fields.

Laparoscopy provides visual access to and a magnified view of the pelvis and peritoneal cavity. It is particularly valuable for looking into difficult regions, including the pouch of Douglas and the subdiaphragmatic areas. Biopsies and material for cytologic evaluation may be obtained with minimal surgical trauma. Successive laparoscopies over time enable the oncologist to monitor the evolution of the disease. Pelvic lymph node sampling by a retroperitoneal endoscopic approach has been described.[1] Progress in laparoscopic surgery has since provided the opportunity to perform a surgically satisfactory pelvic and paraaortic lymphadenectomy.[2,3] This chapter will include descriptions of initial assessment of adnexal tumors, indications for laparoscopy, staging of ovarian carcinoma, including indications for lymph node biopsy and the place of elective lymphadenectomy for staging various gynecologic cancers. The techniques of specific surgical procedures will be covered in Chapter 25. The reader must be aware that exploratory laparoscopy is in many instances inadequate if not complemented by operative procedures.

GENERAL PRINCIPLES

Abdominal exploration in gynecologic oncology requires observation of every aspect of the abdominal cavity, the entire surface of the parietal peritoneum, and the surfaces of the intraperitoneal organs. Material for peritoneal cytologic examination must be obtained. Lymph node assessment is also mandatory in most cases.

Positioning of the patient

The patient must give informed consent to the laparoscopic procedure and be ready for a laparotomy if technical difficulties or complications arise. She is given a general anesthetic with endotracheal intubation. The patient is placed in the supine position without any flexion of the hips, as the flexed legs may limit the movements of the instruments. The legs are placed at 30 degrees, so the surgeon may stand between them when exploring the upper quadrants of the abdomen. The senior surgeon usually stands at the left side of the patient, but it may be useful when exploring the left lateral part of the abdomen and pelvis to stand on the right side. Alternatively, two surgeons may work together. It is advisable to use two monitor screens, one caudad and one cephalad.

Placement of cannulas

A cannula is placed in the uterus unless there is a cervical or endometrial tumor, although the cannula is not necessary for the completion of lymphadenectomy, even in the pelvic area, or for exploration of the abdominal cavity. A cannula is obviously not used in case of previous hysterectomy.

A pneumoperitoneum is created and a 10 mm laparoscope is introduced through an umbilical incision. The video camera is attached. After preliminary observation of the liver surface, the appendix, and the internal genitalia, at least two ancillary 5 mm incisions are made through which ancillary cannulas are introduced. A sample of peritoneal fluid is taken as soon as possible so the cytologist can receive a sample which has not been contaminated with blood (see below).

The placement of the ancillary portals is important and must not be influenced by esthetic considerations. The goal is to achieve optimal use of the instruments in different areas of the pelvis and abdomen. When the diagnostic procedure is limited to the pelvis, the incisions are made in the right and left lower quadrants, approximately 4 cm above the inguinal ligament. When peritoneal samples are to be taken from the diaphragmatic surface, the incisions are made in the upper quadrants. In fact, four portals may be necessary for the pelvic and abdominal exploration of ovarian carcinomas. Sometimes, the anatomy of the patient allows access to both the pelvis and the diaphragm through a single incision: two 5 mm incisions are in these cases made approximately 10 cm lateral to the umbilicus. This placement of the portals is advised for paraaortic node sampling and usually allows access to the pelvic area.

The number of portals is also a function of the operative requirements. The exploratory and operative procedure requires the use of 4.5 mm scissors, grasping forceps, an irrigation-aspiration device, and coagulation forceps. Microbipolar forceps are used to obtain fine hemostasis close to the ureter, the bowel, or large vessels. An additional portal is sited, usually in the midline above the symphysis pubis, and a 12 mm cannula is placed to accommodate an endoscopic clip applicator or sometimes GIA staplers. This portal will later serve to remove lymph nodes from the abdomen with a three-arm retractable Dargent forceps (Lépine, Lyon, France) or with an endoscopic bag. It is essential to avoid even minimal contamination of the abdominal wall with potentially malignant tissue. If it is necessary to retract bowel, a 5 mm cannula will accommodate a probe or forceps. An endoretractor (Endoretract USSC, Norwalk, Conn.) must be introduced through the larger cannula.

Endoscopic examination

A magnified view is obtained when the tip of the endoscope is placed close to the peritoneum. The normal peritoneum shows a fine microvascular network and a transparent smooth surface. Papillary growth, thickening of the peritoneum, whitish areas, or enlarged capillaries suggest the presence of malignancy. The pattern of the involved peritoneum is quite similar to the colposcopic view of a malignant tumor of the cervix. In fact, the magnified laparoscopic view of the peritoneum is superior to standard inspection at the time of conventional surgery. Biopsies are taken with the help of two instruments: the suspect area is grasped with a forceps and removed with scissors. We do not advise the use of standard biopsy forceps. They are traumatic and remove only small specimens.

The pelvis is first thoroughly inspected. The patient is placed in a slight (10 degrees) Trendelenburg position. The entire surface of the ovaries is observed. Ovarian masses are carefully manipulated to avoid rupture and subsequent spillage, but their external surface must be thoroughly inspected (see following part of this chapter). The peritoneal surfaces of the uterus, broad ligaments, and anterior and posterior cul-de-sac are inspected. The cervix and cardinal ligaments may be palpated with the help of the instruments. The ureters are identified and their caliber is assessed. The pelvic lymph nodes under the peritoneum are palpated. The peritoneum may be opened for the purpose of node sampling or node dissection.

The exploration of the upper abdomen follows, mainly in cases of ovarian malignancy (see corresponding part of this chapter for details). The operating table is tilted to the left. The video monitor is placed at the head of the operating table, and the surgeon either stands on the side of the patient or between her legs. Although some surgeons advise a suprapubic approach, we use the transumbilical approach for the placement of the endoscope. The abdominal cavity is thoroughly explored, including the surface of the diaphragm, the liver, the omentum, the mesentery, the colon, the appendix, and the small bowel. Every loop of the small bowel must be carefully moved and sequentially inspected, from the ileocecal junction up to the duodenojejunal junction. The bowel is then placed in the left upper quadrant, and the posterior peritoneum covering the aorta and vena cava is inspected. Enlarged para-aortic nodes may then be identified and managed, as will be described. Elective para-aortic lymphadenectomy may be carried out at this time.

Exploration of the pelvic and abdominal nodes is an essential part of staging. Elective pelvic or para-aortic lymphadenectomy may be included in the staging procedure (see Chapter 25). If elective node dissection is not required, other diagnostic procedures may be undertaken. Enlarged nodes may be identified by inspection or palpation of the nodal areas. However, enlargement is not specific for malignancy and specimens for microscopic evaluation must be taken. The peritoneum overlying the suspect node is opened with scissors. Fine needle aspiration under direct vision may be useful, as it may be immediately processed and read by the pathologist. Otherwise, biopsy of the node is required. We advise against partial biopsy, unless the node is fixed to the vessel. Partial biopsy will leave the remaining tumor in permanent contact with the peritoneal cavity or the retroperitoneal tissues. Sampling of the entire node is preferable and is carried out as follows. The node is gently grasped, bluntly separated from the surrounding structures, and removed through a large port or with a bag. Clips may be applied to unresectable nodes for later radiologic localization. After simple observation, selective lymph node sampling, or lymph node dissection, the peritoneum is left open.

The operation ends by ensuring that hemostasis is complete and by copious lavage of the peritoneal cavity. The ancillary incisions are also washed to avoid tumor grafting, especially in case of peritoneal disease.

OVARIAN TUMORS

Preliminary investigation and laparoscopic diagnosis of ovarian masses

Preoperative workup. Adnexal masses are one of the most controversial indications for laparoscopic surgery. The problem lies between the overtreatment by laparotomy of benign masses and the undertreatment by laparoscopy of ovarian cancers. To avoid the occurrence of unsuspected ovarian cancer found during a laparoscopy done by surgeons not qualified in gynecologic oncology, all adnexal masses must be investigated preoperatively. Measurement of plasma Ca-125 levels and ultrasound examination, including color Doppler imaging, are mandatory. Only cases with Ca-125 levels below 35 mUI/ml and benign ultrasound patterns should undergo laparoscopy in nonspecialized settings. Solid masses should not be managed laparoscopically, except by experienced gynecologic oncologists.

Laparoscopic examination of ovarian masses. The sensitivity and specificity of ultrasound, Doppler, and Ca-125 levels are not ideal. Laparoscopic surgery is in this context a satisfactory diagnostic tool for early ovarian malignancy, with a false negative rate of less than 1% in experienced hands.[4,5]

On the other hand, false positive cancer diagnosis is not uncommon in the preoperative work-up of adnexal masses. Screening for ovarian cancers may lead to a number of unnecessary laparotomies, impairing the cost efficiency of the screening program; laparoscopy should thus be included in the management of selected adnexal masses. Patients may benefit from laparoscopy when it is used as a tool to define the need for laparotomy and plan the line of incision. An obviously malignant tumor must be operated on by a midline incision, while an obviously benign tumor can be correctly managed through a suprapubic incision or by laparoscopy.

The visual findings suggesting malignancy are papillary or solid growth on the external surface of the ovary and suspicion of metastatic peritoneal implants. When the ovarian and peritoneal surface are normal, the diagnosis of cancer is not yet totally excluded. We advise aspiration and lavage of the cyst with a minimum of spillage. The internal surface of the cyst is then inspected in search of papillary growth. If papillary growth is found on either surface of the cyst, the simple cystectomy procedure must be aborted.

When an unsuspected ovarian cancer is found, biopsies of the ovarian surface may be of help, but the diagnostic value of frozen sections is questionable. Four choices are possible, depending upon the availability of a trained gynecologic oncologist, the level of training of the surgeon in advanced operative laparoscopy, and the degree of informed consent given by the patient.

The first option is to consult a gynecologic oncologist. A laparotomy with comprehensive staging and radical surgery of the ovarian carcinoma is performed. The second option is to take biopsies, without rupturing the cystic portion of the tumor, and to await the results of permanent sections before definitive therapy or referral of the patient. The third option is to perform, laparoscopically or by laparotomy, a salpingo-oophorectomy (see Chapters 17 and 25) for definitive pathologic examination of the entire ovary. The fourth option is limited to the rare surgeon trained in gynecologic oncology and skilled in laparoscopic surgery. After frozen section examination, definitive laparoscopic surgery can be performed for ovarian carcinoma, which includes total hysterectomy and bilateral salpingo-oophorectomy (or unilateral salpingo-oophorectomy in selected cases), pelvic and para-aortic node sampling, and abdominal staging.

If the laparoscopic approach is chosen, great care must be taken to avoid or limit spillage of cystic fluid and to remove the specimen without any contact with the abdominal wall to avoid implantation of tumor grafts. The use of an endoscopic bag is mandatory, as well as copious lavage of the abdominal cavity and of the trocar ports.

Hazards of laparoscopic surgery of ovarian masses. Laparoscopic surgery may lead to spillage of tumour cells, aggravating the prognosis if there is a delay between diagnosis and definitive therapy.[6,7] If some part of the tumor is removed without special precautions being taken, tumoral grafts to the abdominal wall are to be anticipated.[8] Radical surgery must be carried out as soon as possible after laparoscopic diagnosis and, ideally, at the time of primary surgery. As a consequence, the laparoscopic surgeon must be aware of the macroscopic features of ovarian cancer.

Staging of ovarian cancer

General principles. The rules of staging of ovarian cancer are well established. The 1988 FIGO classification (see the box on p. 140), still in use, takes into account several pathologic prognostic factors that must be observed during staging procedures. Material for peritoneal cytologic examination must be obtained either by aspiration of existing peritoneal fluid or peritoneal washings in the pelvis and paracolic gutters. The entire surface of the parietal peritoneum, the external surface of the intraperitoneal organs, the appendix and the omentum must be searched for tumor implants. Samples must be taken from all suspicious areas and blind biopsies obtained from every part of the abdomen. When indicated, appendectomy and omentectomy are performed; these represent large peritoneal biopsy specimens. A pelvic and para-aortic node dissection or sampling of enlarged nodes is also performed. Since our first publication of infrarenal paraaortic lymphadenectomy,[9] all of these goals may be achieved by laparoscopy. Thorough examination of the diaphragmatic peritoneum is easier to perform laparoscopically than it is by laparotomy. Laparoscopic restaging or laparoscopic second-look procedures may in this regard spare the patient a laparotomy and reduce the discomfort of surgical monitoring of therapy of ovarian carcinomas, while strictly adhering to the rules of oncologic surgery.

FIGO staging in primary carcinoma of the ovary (1985, revised 1988)

Stage I	Growth limited to the ovaries.
Ia	Growth limited to one ovary; no ascites. No tumor on the external surface; capsule intact.
Ib	Growth limited to both ovaries; no ascites containing malignant cells. No tumor on the external surfaces; capsules intact.
Ic	Tumor either Stage Ia or Ib, but with tumor on surface of one or both ovaries; or with capsule ruptured; or with ascites present containing malignant cells, or with positive peritoneal washings.
Stage II	Growth involving one or both ovaries with pelvic extension.
IIa	Extension and/or metastases to the uterus and/or tubes.
IIb	Extension to other pelvic tissues.
IIc	Tumor either Stage IIa or IIb, but with tumor on the surface of one or both ovaries; or with capsule(s) ruptured; or with ascites present containing malignant cells, or with positive peritoneal washings.
Stage III	Tumor involving one or both ovaries with peritoneal implants outside the pelvis and/or positive retroperitoneal or inguinal nodes. Superficial liver metastasis equals Stage III. Tumor is limited to the true pelvis, but with histologically proved malignant extension to the small bowel or omentum.
IIIa	Tumor grossly limited to the true pelvis with negative nodes but with histologically confirmed microscopic seeding of abdominal peritoneal surfaces.
IIIb	Tumor involving one or both ovaries with histologically confirmed implants of abdominal peritoneal surfaces none exceeding 2 cm in diameter. Nodes are negative.
IIIc	Abdominal implants greater than 2 cm in diameter and/or positive retroperitoneal or inguinal nodes.
Stage IV	Growth involving one or both ovaries with distant metastases. If pleural effusion is present, there must be positive cytology to allot a case to Stage IV. Parenchymal liver metastasis equals Stage IV.

Technique for staging or monitoring laparoscopy of intraperitoneal disease in ovarian cancers. The general principles of laparoscopic exploration in gynecologic malignancy have already been addressed, as well as the requirements for the staging of ovarian cancers. It remains to define the steps of the laparoscopic staging procedure.

Peritoneal fluid samples for cytologic examination are obtained first. Sampling of peritoneal fluid is easy and must be done at the beginning of the procedure with an aspiration needle, ideally on blood-free pelvic fluid. In the absence of significant peritoneal fluid, the peritoneum must be lavaged in the pouch of Douglas and the parietocolic gutters by injection of isotonic saline using a syringe attached to an aspiration needle; the fluid is then aspirated into the same syringe.

The peritoneal cavity is then inspected and a search made for obvious tumor deposits. If tumor growth is immediately noted in the abdominal cavity, the diagnosis of stage III tumor (requiring primary laparotomy or chemotherapy) or chemotherapy-resistant tumor is established. If no tumor is identified at first glance, a throrough examination of the entire peritoneal cavity is needed. Samples are taken from suspicious areas. When the peritoneum looks normal, blind biopsies are obtained from every part of the abdomen.

After previous surgery, adhesions between the loops of bowel frequently obscure the view. Virtually any of these abdominal adhesions can be divided. With the help of two atraumatic forceps unrolling one loop at a time, the bowel can be examined from the ileocecal junction to the duodenum. The two surfaces of the mesentery can be examined in the same way and samples taken.

Biopsy specimens are obtained as follows: The suspicious peritoneal area or the area chosen for a blind biopsy is superficially grasped with a forceps (we use the Manhes grip-pince, Microfrance, Bourbon-l'Archambault, France), forming a fold. The fold is incised for about 2 mm. The edge of the incision is grasped and the sample is elevated. Once the retroperitoneal space is visible the undersurface of the peritoneal patch is freed by blunt dissection. The peritoneal sample is then excised by sharp incision of the dissected area, avoiding injury to retroperitoneal structures, namely the ureter, vital vessels, or diaphragmatic or mesenteric vessels. Moderate bleeding of the peritoneal edge may occur but usually stops spontaneously. If it does not it can be electrodesiccated with the help of a fine bipolar forceps (1 mm broad tip). The pelvic and laterocolic peritoneum may be sampled through the suprapubic ports. To obtain biopsy specimens from the diaphragmatic peritoneal surfaces, additional ancillary portals must be placed in the upper quadrants. For this part of the procedure, the videomonitor is moved to the head of the patient and the surgeon changes sides. Bleeding of the diaphragm may occur and usually stops in a few minutes. Otherwise hemostasis is obtained with bipolar electrodesiccation.

In case of primary surgery, or during second-look laparoscopies, the contralateral ovary may be present. Its surface can be thoroughly inspected through the endoscope. The magnified view allows identification of even minimal disease, which can be biopsied. Biopsy of a normal ovarian surface is not necessary.

Diagnostic laparoscopic infracolic omentectomy is feasible by using dessication and section (see Chapter 25). Appendectomy is also performed routinely.

Rationale for lymphadenectomy in ovarian cancers. The technique of pelvic and of para-aortic lymphadenectomy will be addressed in Chapter 25.

Lymph node assessment is an essential part of the surgical staging of early ovarian carcinoma. The incidence of positive lymph nodes may be as high as 24% in stage I patients.[10] Although its therapeutic value is highly arguable, it is not acceptable to neglect node dissection up to the level of the renal veins in the staging of ovarian carcinoma. Cases of invasive ovarian adenocarcinoma referred with unsatisfactory staging information or early ovarian carcinomas treated by laparoscopy (whether conservatively or by radical operation) must be offered node sampling. This indication is more controversial with borderline tumors. We presently restage serous borderline tumors but not mucinous tumors.

Laparoscopy may, in the future, offer an opportunity to obtain the necessary information about the para-aortic nodal status without the need for a midline incision and its inherent cost, pain, and complications. In the same way, para-aortic node sampling may be included as part of a second-look laparoscopy after therapy for stage III ovarian carcinoma, when no residual intraperitoneal disease is visible, in order to identify disease-free patients. However, the potential risk of complications, including unintended laparotomy, and the general acceptance of the lack of therapeutic value of second-look operations leaves this indication open to debate.

Indications for laparoscopic staging of ovarian cancers. Staging is mandatory during primary surgery, but may also need to be completed during early (restaging) second-look procedures. A recent trend in favor of laparoscopic staging of advanced ovarian cancer before neoadjuvant chemotherapy will also be addressed.

Primary laparoscopic surgery of ovarian cancers will be adressed in Chapter 25. Primary surgery must obviously include a staging procedure, including peritoneal and nodal sampling. (See box at right.) Staging procedures are most important for early ovarian cancer, especially when the disease is apparently limited to one ovary. In such cases, inadequate surgical exploration may ignore peritoneal or nodal involvement and consequently lead to undertreatment, as it is generally accepted that only stage Ia and Ib patients do not need adjuvant chemotherapy.

Laparoscopy is also useful in the follow-up and restaging of ovarian carcinomas. Restaging procedures are most important for early ovarian cancer, especially when the disease is apparently limited to one ovary. In such cases, inadequate surgical exploration may ignore peritoneal or nodal involvement and consequently lead to undertreatment. The case of the referred patient with unsatisfactory staging, whether treated by laparoscopy or by laparotomy, is not uncommon and may be managed laparoscopically, combining staging and additional surgery such as hysterectomy and contralateral oophorectomy.[11]

Some investigators advise neoadjuvant chemotherapy in obviously inoperable ovarian tumors. In this regard, laparoscopy may help to identify those patients with massive involvement of the diaphragmatic surface, the gastrocolic ligament and the lesser sac, and the entire surface of the small bowel in whom optimal surgery is impossible. The planned laparotomy is cancelled and a monitoring laparoscopy is planned after three courses of chemotherapy. Only patients who respond will benefit from optimal or suboptimal surgery.

Indications for laparoscopic staging in ovarian cancer

Primary surgery	Peritoneal and nodal sampling to plan treatment
Follow-up	To monitor results of surgery and to restage
After chemotherapy	To identify inoperable patients who have responded to chemotherapy and who might now benefit from surgery

Specific precautions for monitoring second-look procedures. Monitoring the extent of residual disease is the primary goal of second-look procedures after therapy for ovarian carcinoma when no residual intraperitoneal disease is demonstrated by a preoperative work-up, including CT scan and measurement of Ca-125 blood levels.

Laparoscopy carries a higher risk in the patient who has had prior abdominal and pelvic surgery. There may be intraperitoneal adhesions and bowel loops may be adherent to the anterior abdominal wall. When laparoscopy is undertaken in such patients, specific precautions must be observed. The absence of adhesions below the umbilical area must be tested by a syringe test before the introduction of the umbilical trocar (see Chapter 5). The additional ports for ancillary instruments are ideally placed, in the absence of adhesions to this area, lateral to the umbilicus. This placement allows the surgeon, in a majority of cases, to reach every point of the abdominal cavity. However, the presence of adhesions of bowel to the abdominal wall must lead the surgeon to modify the placement of these portals. If adhesions are present, they must be first divided to examine the entire peritoneal surface. Care must be exercised to avoid surgical trauma to the bowel or other vital structures. A bowel injury may require laparoscopic repair (see Chapter 26) if a laparotomy is not indicated. At every step the laparoscopic approach must be abandoned if large tumor grafts are visible or if the staging procedure cannot be completed in accordance with proper oncologic standards. In such cases, the surgeon must shift to a conventional laparotomy or forgo the second-look procedure.

The value of a negative second-look laparoscopy has been questioned. In earlier reports only a limited view of the abdominal cavity was possible. The negative predictive

Table 12-1. FIGO staging of cervical carcinoma

Stage	Description
I	Cervical carcinoma confined to uterus (extension to corpus should be disregarded)
Ia	Preclinical invasive carcinoma, diagnosed by microscopy only
Ia1	Minimal microscopic stromal invasion
Ia2	Tumor with invasive component 5mm or less in depth, taken from the base of the epithelium, and 7 mm or less in horizontal spread
Ib	Tumor larger than Ia1 and Ia2
II	Tumor invades beyond uterus but not to pelvic wall or to lower third of the vagina
IIa	Without parametrial invasion
IIb	With parametrial invasion
III	Cervical carcinoma extends to pelvic wall and/or involves the lower third of the vagina and/or causes hydronephrosis or nonfunctioning kidney
IIIa	Tumor involves lower third of the vagina, no extension to pelvic wall
IIIb	Tumor extends to pelvic wall and/or causes hydronephrosis or nonfunctioning kidney
IVa	Tumor invades mucosa of bladder or rectum and/or extends beyond true pelvis. Note: The presence of bullous edema is not sufficient evidence to classify a tumor stage IV
IVb	Distant metastasis

value of second-look laparoscopy was obviously low, as a significant amount of persisting tumor may be hidden under adhesions or located in the retroperitoneal space. In experienced hands, after thorough examination of the entire abdominal cavity using the techniques of laparoscopic surgery as needed, the accuracy of a negative second-look is similar for laparoscopy and laparotomy.[12] However, the therapeutic role of second-look procedures has been questioned and this indication remains open to discussion. It should be used only in selected cases or to monitor new drugs in investigational programs. In this regard, the use of office laparoscopy may prove less expensive and more convenient to the patient in the future.[13]

CERVICAL CARCINOMA

Clinical staging of cervical carcinomas is still the mainstay of classification (Table 12-1). Intravenous pyelography and cystoscopy are also routinely performed. None of these investigations evaluates the lymph node status. Node involvement is, however, a major prognostic factor of cervical cancer. The sensitivity and specificity of imaging techniques (CT scan, ultrasound, MRI) in the detection of nodal involvement is low. Histologic examination is the only reliable method for appraising the status of lymph nodes. However, samples are usually taken either during a presurgical staging laparotomy, adding significant morbidity, or during the surgical step of treatment, at a time when primary decisions about treatment have already been taken. The rationale for laparoscopic pelvic lymphadenectomy stems from this.

General principles

Pelvic node involvement is the most significant single factor in the prognosis of early cervical carcinomas. The risk of "skip" metastases to the para-aortic area is negligible in patients with tumors smaller than 3 cm and negative pelvic nodes.[14] As a consequence, stage Ib to IIb cases with negative pathologic staging may be cured by local therapy (brachytherapy* alone or radical hysterectomy). On the other hand, radical hysterectomy does not seem justified when metastatic nodes are present,[15] and our node-positive patients are offered radiation therapy only. In addition, some stage Ia2 cervical carcinomas without pelvic node metastasis can be treated by cervical conization alone.

The risk of para-aortic node involvement is significant in patients with locally advanced cervical carcinomas[16,17] and in patients with pelvic nodal metastases.[18] Para-aortic nodal metastases may also occasionally be observed even in the absence of positive pelvic nodes in patients with stage I and II large cervical tumors. Sampling of the para-aortic lymph nodes has been suggested as a means of identifying those patients with extrapelvic spread and in whom standard therapy involving pelvic surgery or radiation fields would fail.

The risk-benefit assessment of surgical staging has been debated. The potential perioperative and late complications and the difficulties of treating patients with para-aortic nodal metastases do not favor routine surgical staging. It is necessary, however, to assess the para-aortic nodal status of high risk patients in therapeutic trials involving para-aortic irradiation and/or systemic chemotherapy. A proportion of patients without metastatic para-aortic nodes in the presence of advanced pelvic tumors undergo unnecessary extended-field irradiation, with subsequent complications and questionable therapeutic value. The probability that extended-field radiation without documentation of the para-aortic node status will improve therapy is expected to be no more than 4%,[19] which justifies some sort of surgical staging.

In recurrent or central stage IVa cervical carcinomas, pelvic exenteration is considered. Such a risky and incapacitating operation is not indicated in the presence of peritoneal disease, involved para-aortic nodes, or fixed pelvic nodes. A thorough abdominal exploration and nodal survey is usually done during laparotomy for exenteration. The finding of a contraindication led to cancellation of the procedure in 111 of 394 cases (28%) in the Miller series.[20] The majority of aborted procedures could have been identified by a diagnostic laparoscopy, as peritoneal disease was found

*Radium or cesium therapy.

in 46 patients, nodal disease in 45 patients, and bowel or hepatic involvement in 5 patients, even though significant intraperitoneal adhesions could have impeded an adequate laparoscopic diagnosis in 28 patients.

In conclusion, an elective pelvic lymphadenectomy provides satisfactory staging in the majority of early cervical carcinomas. In addition, low para-aortic lymphadenectomy may benefit patients with advanced cervical carcinomas (see Figs. 12-1 and 12-2).

Technical considerations

From the technical point of view, pelvic node dissection for the staging of early cervical carcinomas may be limited to the lymphatics of the "interiliac" area, including the obturator nodes and the nodes located between the external and internal iliac arteries.[1]

Extended dissection for staging advanced cervical carcinomas must include removal of the common iliac and para-aortic nodes. The surgical landmark of nodal dissection for cervical carcinomas is usually the origin of the inferior mesenteric artery. The aortic dissection must not be extended to the level of the renal vein, as removal of the nodes related to the origin of the ovarian vessels is not necessary. Section of ovarian arteries and of the right ovarian vein is not necessary, and the identification of the left renal vein is not required. The dissection is extended from the first 2 cm of the common iliac arteries up to the level of the inferior mesenteric artery between the right and left ureter.

History of laparoscopic lymphadenectomy in cervical carcinomas

Minimal access surgery is better adapted to the concept of a staging procedure than laparotomy. Laparoscopy may offer the opportunity to assess the nodal status before considering the extent of therapy of cervical cancer and allow time for psychological and medical preparation prior to exenteration.

Dargent and Salvat[1] in 1987 described a panoramic retroperitoneal approach for removal of the interiliac nodes. In 1989 we described the technique of interiliac pelvic lymphadenectomy by laparoscopy.[2] Following earlier descriptions of para-aortic node samplings or of dissection of the lower two centimeters of the aorta,[21,22] Childers et al. described the first low elective para-aortic lymphadenectomies.[3]

This operation is not difficult for an experienced oncologic surgeon and may be routinely carried out by laparoscopy. The proportion of patients in whom the operation can be satisfactorily completed by this new approach is well over 90% in the experience of three of the leading teams in this field [Childers, Querleu, Dargent, personal communications]. This procedure may spare the node-negative patient unnecessary pelvic or para-aortic irradiation and the node-positive patient unnecessary pelvic primary surgery or exenteration for pelvic recurrence.

Results of laparoscopic pelvic lymphadenectomy in early cervical carcinomas

Laparoscopic pelvic lymphadenectomy appears to yield a satisfactory assessment of pelvic nodes with a minimum of surgical trauma. The number of nodes removed in the obturator area and the medial chain of the external iliac nodes (average 5 to 7[2,3,23]) is comparable to the number removed by laparotomy (average 4.7 to 5.2 nodes in the obturator area[24]).

Dargent[23] reported 51 cases of cervical cancer managed with retroperitoneal lymphadenectomy and radical vaginal hysterectomy. The 3-year survival rate was 95.5% in node-negative stage Ib and IIa patients and 80% in node-negative early IIb patients.

In our series, up to 5-year follow-up is available for 106 patients with early cervical carcinomas managed with laparoscopic pelvic lymphadenectomy. The quality of the pelvic dissection has been checked by laparotomy in 68 patients. No residual positive node has been found. At the time of writing, the 4-year lifetable survival rate is 83% for the whole group and is similar to the survival rate of a historic group matched for age, stage, and therapy [personal unpublished results]. All recurrences were observed in high-risk patients (young women with bulky tumors or adenocarcinoma). We have observed three recurrences in the lateral pelvic area alone in 84 surgically treated node-negative patients. This 4%, purely lateropelvic recurrence rate, suggesting a growth of missed lymph nodes, is similar to the rate observed after laparotomy (5% of 467 patients[25], 2% of 733 patients[26]). The procedure is thus safe and accurate and may be included in the staging and therapeutic strategy for early cervical cancers (Fig. 12-1). Its use in bulky or advanced cervical carcinomas (Fig. 12-2) is still investigational.

ENDOMETRIAL CARCINOMA

Laparoscopic pretherapeutic staging of stage I endometrial carcinomas is not very useful insofar as surgery is indicated whatever the nodal status. However, staging is an essential part of surgical therapy, as peritoneal or node disease may modify the prognosis and define adjuvant therapy, although the therapeutic value of lymphadenectomy has been questioned.

The indication and extent of lymph node dissection should be tailored to the spread pattern (Table 12-2).

The prevalence of lymph node metastases depends on the histologic grade and depth of invasion.[28] The rate of pelvic node involvement is as low as 1% when no myometrial invasion is found (stage Ia) and 3% in grade 1 tumors. As a consequence, the prevalence of node disease is almost zero in stage Ia grade 1 cases, and we do not advocate lymphadenectomy in such cases.

The prevalence of para-aortic node disease is only 2% when the pelvic nodes are negative and 38% when the pelvic nodes are positive.[27] We recommend performing an in-

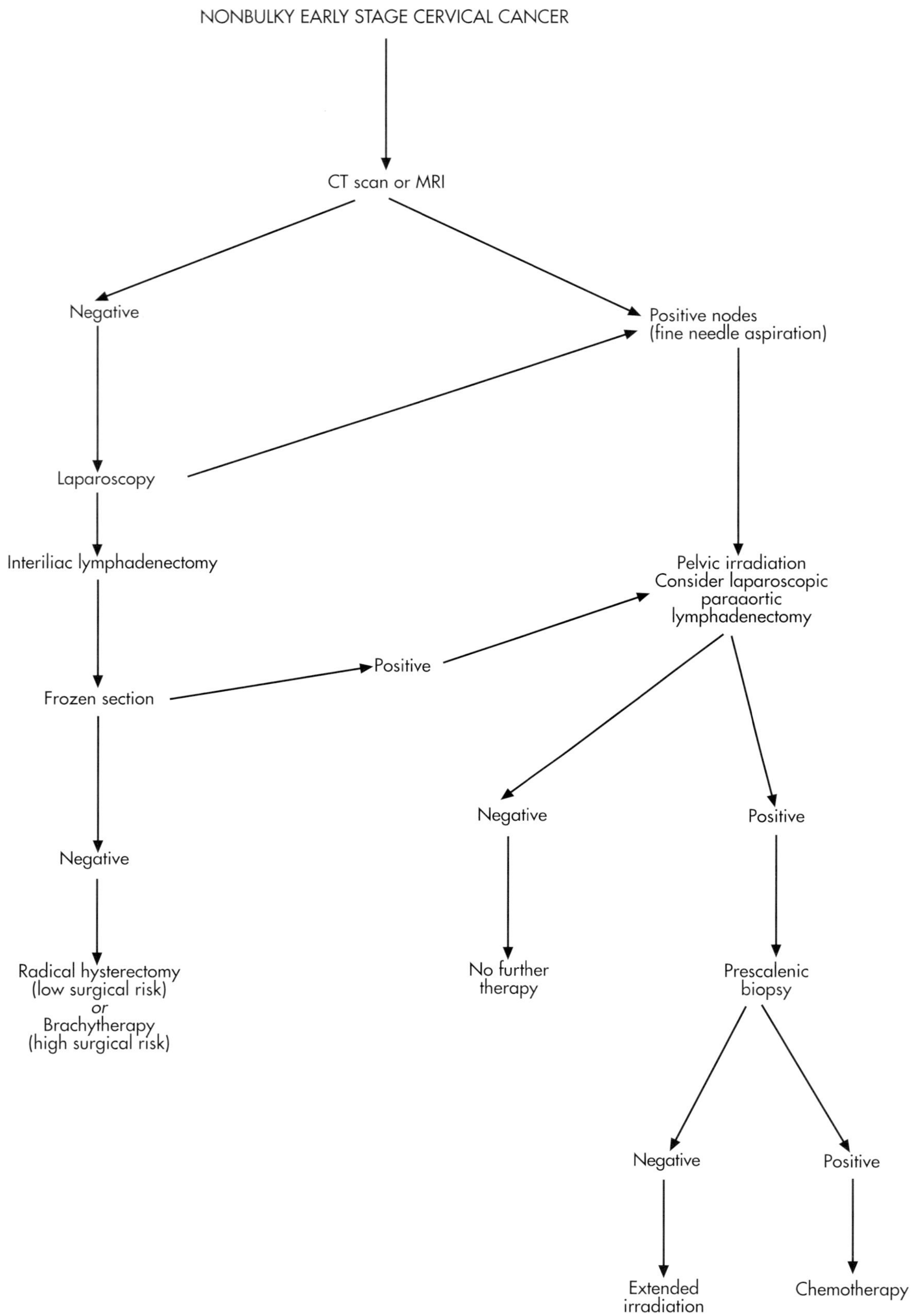

Fig. 12-1. Management of nonbulky early stage cervical carcinoma.

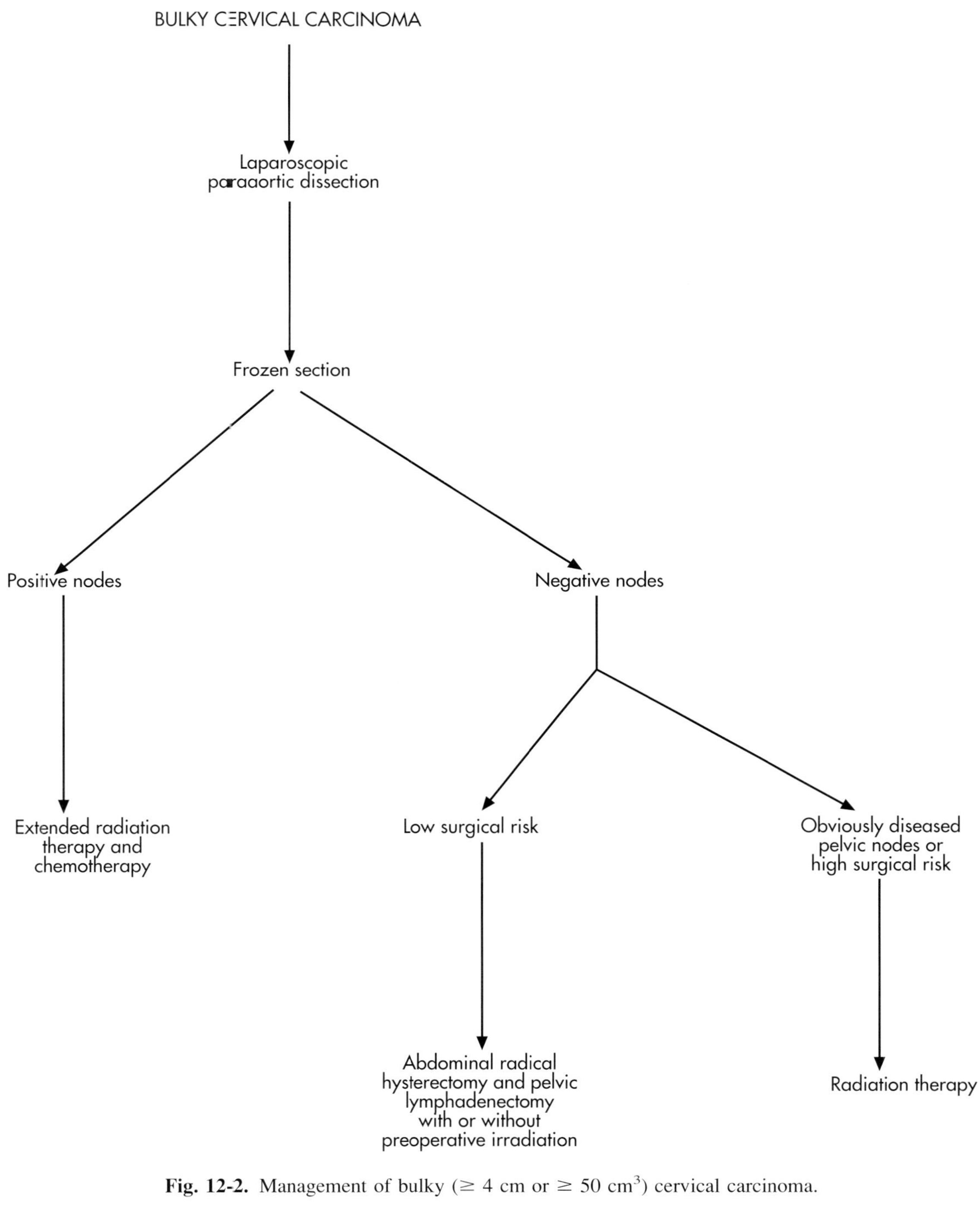

Fig. 12-2. Management of bulky ($\geq$ 4 cm or $\geq$ 50 cm^3) cervical carcinoma.

Table 12-2. Classification of endometrial carcinoma (FIGO Revision, 1988)

Stage	Description
0	Carcinoma in situ
I	Carcinoma limited to the corpus, including the isthmus
	Ia Limited to the endometrium
	Ib Invasion of up to half the myometrium
	Ic Invasion of more than half the myometrium
II	Spread to the corpus and cervix, but not beyond the uterus
	IIa Involvement of the endometrial glands only
	IIb Spread to the cervical stroma
III	Spread beyond the uterus, but not beyond the cervix
	IIIa Spread to the serosa of the uterus and/or into the adnexae and/or positive peritoneal cytology
	IIIb Vaginal metastases
	IIIc Positive pelvic and/or paraaortic nodes
IV	Spread beyond the true pelvis or into the mucosa of the bladder and rectum

teriliac pelvic lymphadenectomy first and using frozen section examination to identify the node-positive patients who will need para-aortic node dissection.

Laparoscopic lymphadenectomy may be included as part of the surgical treatment in association with vaginal surgery when obesity or a large tumoral volume or a narrow vagina do not preclude laparoscopy or vaginal surgery. Childers et al. have used laparoscopically assisted surgical staging in 59 patients with stage I endometrial cancers.[28] They found intraperitoneal disease in six patients. Lymphadenectomy was not indicated in 22 grade 1 patients. Obesity precluded the use of laparoscopic lymphadenectomy in only two patients. Extrauterine metastases was found in seven of 29 grade 2 and 3 patients.

Childers et al.[28] and Dargent[23] proposed a surgical strategy based on the preoperative assesment of the tumor grade. Patients with grade 1 lesions first undergo LAVH; if frozen section of the uterus shows deep myometrial invasion (over 50%), laparoscopic lymphadenectomy is performed. Patients with grade 2 and 3 lesions have laparoscopic lymphadenectomy first; LAVH is done only in node-negative patients, while node-positive patients are offered irradiation. The drawbacks of this strategy are:

1. Node involvement may be found in grade 1 patients with less than 50% myometrial invasion,
2. There are discrepancies between the preoperative and postoperative assesment of tumor grade,
3. Hysterectomy may benefit even the patient with node involvement,
4. Paraaortic lymphadenectomy is needed only in pelvic node-positive patients

As a consequence, we propose a modification of this strategy, taking into account both a preoperative workup including ultrasonography and MRI and examination of a frozen section to assess the degree of myometrial invasion and both a preoperative and frozen section evaluation of tumor grade (Fig. 12-3). Vaginal hysterectomy is performed first only in the patient with a grade 1 tumor with no myometrial invasion suspected at the preoperative workup. In such cases, laparoscopy is performed only if the frozen section examination shows a grade 2 or 3 tumor or some degree of myometrial invasion or if the ovaries cannot be removed from below.

Laparoscopy is performed first in patients with grade 2 to 3 tumor or with suspected myometrial invasion. Peritoneal examination and pelvic lymphadenectomy are carried out. In patients with peritoneal disease, we suggest surgical therapy by laparotomy followed by chemotherapy. In patients without pelvic node involvement as assessed by frozen section, the infundibulo-pelvic pedicles are divided laparoscopically and LAVH is performed. In patients with pelvic node involvement, we suggest adding a paraaortic lymphadenectomy; postoperative external irradiation is limited to the pelvic area if the para-aortic nodes are intact and extended to the para-aortic area if the para-aortic nodes are involved.

This strategy may be modified in case of surgical difficulty: laparoscopy and/or vaginal surgery may be impossible in some obese or nulliparous patients. Laparotomy is used if both laparoscopy and vaginal surgery are not feasible. Total laparoscopic hysterectomy is used if laparoscopy is feasible, but vaginal steps of LAVH, other than specimen removal, are impossible. In some cases, pelvic lymphadenectomy is feasible, but para-aortic lymphadenectomy is felt to be risky; as the therapeutic value of para-aortic dissection is not fully established, the operation is aborted and para-aortic irradiation is offered to pelvic node-positive patients.

In the same way, laparoscopic lymphadenectomy along with oophorectomy may be an adequate management of unsuspected endometrial adenocarcinomas found in hysterectomy specimens, unless there are only grade 1 stage Ia tumors.

DIAGNOSTIC LAPAROSCOPY IN OTHER AREAS OF ONCOLOGY

Although no clinical experience has been published, laparoscopic lymphadenectomy could in theory be used for staging vulvar carcinomas, vaginal carcinomas, and in some gynecologic malignancies of childhood or adolescence (clear-cell adenocarcinoma, endodermal sinus tumor, rhabdomyosarcoma of the vagina and/or cervix).

Diagnosis of intraperitoneal neoplasia was proposed as early as 1910 and was even the first application of laparoscopy in the human.[29] In a series of 112 patients presenting

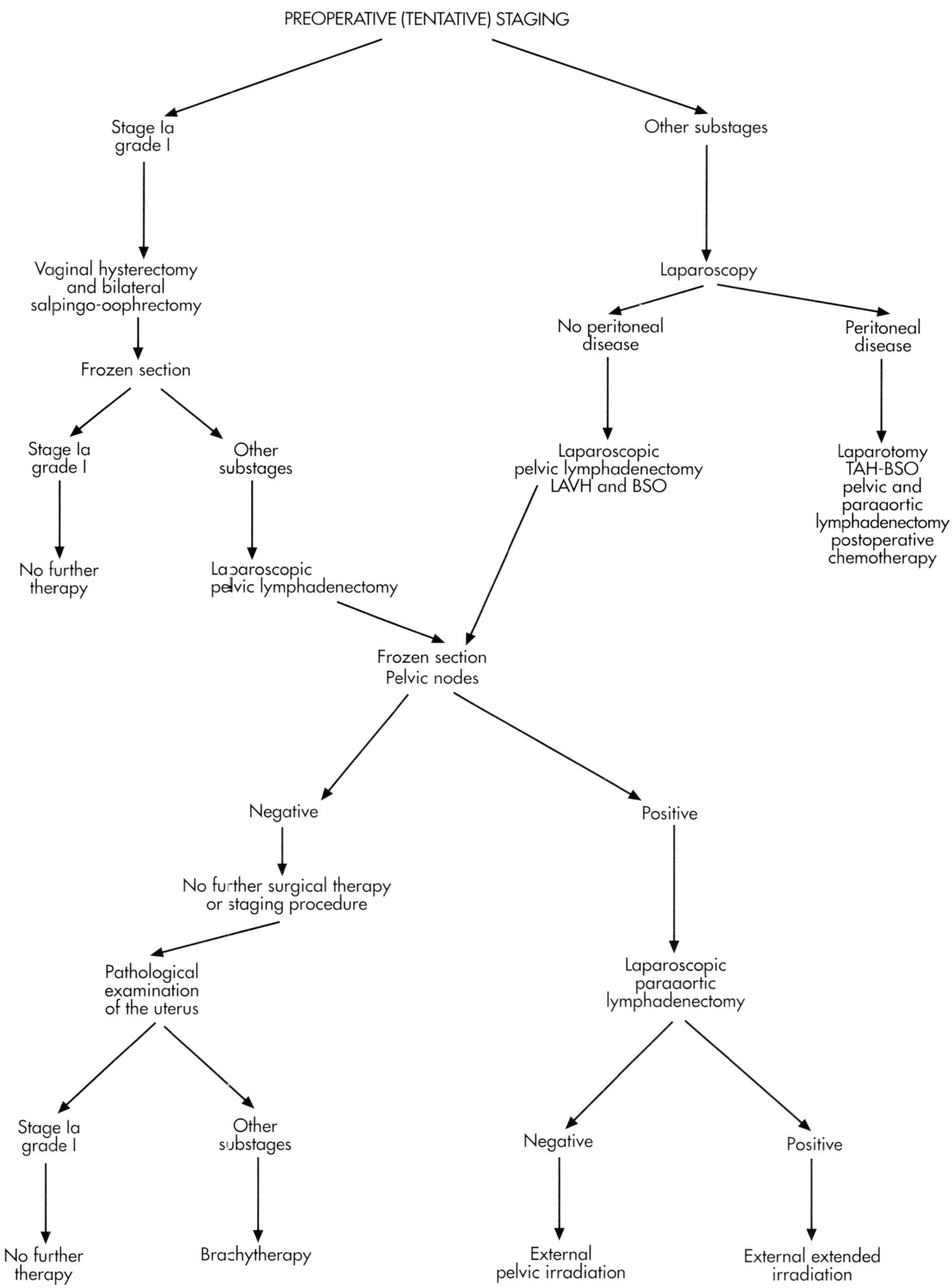

Fig. 12-3. Management of stage I endometrial cancer.

with carcinoma of the stomach, bowel, and pancreas, Canossi et al., in 1975, reported that 40% of patients were spared a laparotomy. [29] Laparoscopy is a useful tool for the diagnosis of the cause of malignant ascites from unknown primary carcinoma. It has also been used in the staging of bladder, prostate, or testicular cancer. Laparoscopic diagnosis or staging of lymphomas has also been suggested to replace laparotomy.[22]

CONCLUSION

Laparoscopic staging of malignancies, particularly gynecologic tumors, is not only feasible[1-3,9] but safe and accurate,[23,30] but only in the hands of surgeons experienced both in advanced laparoscopic surgery and gynecologic oncology. The data found in the current literature and in our own series show that if the standards of oncology are followed, the outcome of patients is not compromised by the use of minimal access surgery for staging. It remains to be seen if the introduction of laparoscopy in the management of gynecologic tumors will be followed by a lowering of the costs of treatment.

REFERENCES

1. Dargent D, Salvat J: L'envahissement ganglionnaire pelvien. Paris, 1989, MEDSI.
2. Querleu D, Leblanc E, Castelain B: Laparoscopic pelvic lymphadenectomy, *Am J Obstet Gynecol* 164:579-581, 1991.
3. Childers JM, Hatch K, Surwit EA: The role of laparoscopic lymphadenectomy in cervical carcinoma, *Gynecol Oncol* 47:38-43, 1992.
4. Nezhat F, Nezhat C, Welander CE et al: Four ovarian cancers diagnosed during laparoscopic management of 1011 women with adnexal masses, *Am J Obstet Gynecol* 167:790-796, 1992.
5. Mage G, Canis M, Manhes H et al: Laparoscopic management of adnexal cystic masses, *J Gynecol Surg* 6:71-79, 1990.
6. Maiman M, Seltzer V, Boyce J: Laparoscopic excision of ovarian neoplasms subsequently found to be malignant, *Obstet Gynecol* 77:563-566, 1991.
7. Benifla JL, Hauuy JP, Guglielmina JN et al: Kystectomie percoelioscopique: découverte histologique fortuite d'un carcinome ovarien, *J Gynecol Obstet Biol Repr* 21: 45-49, 1992.
8. Hsiu JG, Giveen FT, Kemp GM: Tumor implantation after diagnostic laparoscopic biopsy of serious ovarian tumors of low malignant potential, *Obstet Gynecol* 68(Suppl):90S-93s, 1988.
9. Querleu D: Laparoscopic paraaortic lymphadenectomy. A preliminary experience, *Gynecol Oncol* 49:24-29, 1993.
10. Burghardt E, Girardi F, Lahousen M et al: Patterns of pelvic and paraaortic lymph node involvement in ovarian cancer, *Gynecol Oncol* 40:103-106, 1991.
11. Querleu D, Leblanc E: Laparoscopic infrarenal lymphadenectomy in the staging of carcinomas of the ovary and fallopian tubes, *Cancer* 1994 (In press.)
12. Canis M, Chapron C, Mage G et al: Technique et résultats préliminaires du second look per-coelioscopique dans les tumeurs épithéliales malignes de l'ovaire, *J Gynecol Obstet Biol Repr* 21:655-663, 1992.
13. Childers JM, Hatch KD, Surwit EA: Office laparoscopy and biopsy for evaluation of patients with intraperitonal carcinomatosis using a new optical catheter, *Gynecol Oncol* 47:337-342, 1992.
14. Patsner B, Sedlacek TV, Lovecchio JL: Para-aortic node sampling in small (3 cm or less) stage IB invasive cervical cancer, *Gynecol Oncol* 44:53-54, 1992.
15. Potter ME, Alvarez RD, Shingleton HM et al: Early invasive cervical cancer with pelvic lymph node involvement: to complete or not to complete radical hysterrectomy, *Gynecol Oncol* 37:78-81, 1990.
16. Berman M , Keys H, Creasman W et al: Survival and patterns of recurrence in cervical cancer metastatic to periaortic lymph nodes. A Gynecologic Oncologic Group study, *Gynecol Oncol* 19:8-16, 1984.
17. Buschbaum HJ: Extrapelvic lymph node metastases in cervical carcinoma, *Am J Obstet Gynecol* 133:814-824, 1979.
18. Downey G, Potish R., Adcock L et al: Pretreatment surgical staging in cervical carcinoma: therapeutic efficacy of pelvic lymph node resection, *Am J Obstet Gynecol* 160:1055-1061, 1989.
19. Heaps JM. Berek JS: Surgical staging of cervical cancer, *Clin Obstet Gynecol* 33:852-862, 1990.
20. Miller B, Morris M, Rutledge F et al: Aborted exenterative procedures in recurrent cervical cancer, *Gynecol Oncol* 50:94-99, 1993.
21. Nezhat CR, Burrell MO, Nezhat FR et al: Laparoscopic radical hysterectomy with paraaortic and pelvic node dissection, *Am J Obstet Gynecol* 166:864-865, 1992.
22. Childers JM, Surwit EA: Laparoscopic para-aortic lymph node biopsy for diagnosis of a non-Hodgkin's lymphoma, *Surg Laparoscopy Endoscop* 2:139-142, 1992.
23. Dargent D: Laparoscopic surgery and gynecologic cancer, *Curr Opin Obstet Gynecol* 5:294-300, 1993.
24. Girardi F, Pickel H, Winter R: Pelvic and parametrial lymph nodes in the quality control of the surgical treatment of cervical cancer, *Gynecol Oncol* 50:330-333, 1993.
25. NG HT, Kan YY, Chao KC et al: The outcome of the patients with recurrent cervical carcinoma in terms of lymph node metastasis and treatment, *Gynecol Oncol* 26:355-363, 1987.
26. Webb MJ, Symmonds RE: Site of recurrence of cervical cancer after radical hysterectomy, *Amer J Obstet Gynecol* 138:813-817, 1980.
27. Creasman WT, Morrow CP, Bundy BN et al: Surgical pathologic spread patterns of endometrial cancer. A Gynecologic Oncology Group study, *Cancer* 60:2035-2041, 1987.
28. Childers JM, Brzechffa PR, Hatch KD et al: Laparoscopically assisted surgical staging (LASS) of endometrial cancer, *Gynecol Oncol* 51:33-38, 1993.
29. Marlow JL: Laparoscopy. In Coppleson M, editor: Gynaecologic Oncology, vol 1. New York, 1981, Churchill Livingstone.
30. Childers JM, Hatch KD, Tran AN et al: Laparoscopic paraaortic lymphadenectomy in gynecologic malignancies, *Obstet Gynecol* 82:741-747, 1993.

Chapter 13

TUBAL STERILIZATION

For the woman who has decided that she no longer wishes to bear children, laparoscopy offers a safe, dependable form of sterilization. For most gynecologists, sterilization is the first operative laparoscopic procedure that they will learn. It can be performed inexpensively as an interval procedure on an outpatient basis.

Clearly the decision to be sterilized must rest with the woman. Nonetheless, it is incumbent upon any surgeon who may be asked to carry out the sterilization to ensure that the patient has been fully informed about alternative forms of contraception, male sterilization, and the risks and benefits of tubal interruption. Despite advances in microsurgical techniques that can be used in the hopes of reversing a previously performed operation, sterilization should not be offered as potentially reversible. Those who wish to be sterilized should be as sure as is humanly possible that they will not change their minds. This chapter will review the various techniques of laparoscopic tubal sterilization and elaborate on their specific advantages and disadvantages.

Anderson, in 1937, first suggested that a laparoscopic technique could be used for female sterilization.[1] Four years later, two other Americans, Powers and Barnes, were first to perform perlaparoscopic electrocoagulation of the fallopian tubes.[2] Palmer's experience with tubal electrocoagulation and the technique that he published in 1962 attracted little initial attention. Using a biopsy drill forceps of his own design (see Fig. 13-1) and unipolar electrodesiccation, he destroyed a portion of the isthmic segment of the oviduct.[3] This technique became widely accepted, particularly in the English-speaking world, after the publication of the monograph on laparoscopy by Steptoe, in 1967.[4]

Since the early 1970s, the quest for even safer and more effective methods of laparoscopic sterilization has led to the development of the various techniques listed at right.

- Electrical Methods
  - Electrosurgery
    - Unipolar
    - Bipolar
  - Thermocoagulation
- Mechanical Methods
  - Clips
    - Hulka
    - Filshie
  - Falope ring

Laparoscopic tubal sterilization is currently the most common method of interval tubal occlusion in North America. Approximately 200,000 such procedures are performed in the United States annually. In the last decade there has been much greater use of mechanical methods of sterilization. These confer a measured destruction on the fallopian tube.

The laparoscopic approach has proved safe and effective overall. In a multicenter study of 5,342 women who underwent interval tubal sterilization by laparoscopy, 51 required an unintended laparotomy. Twelve of these were performed to manage complications (perforated viscus, 4; hemorrhage, 4; and other complications, 4) and 39 because of technical problems (due to adhesions or other anatomic distortion, 32; difficulty of entering the peritoneal cavity, 7). Women with prior abdominal or pelvic surgery were at increased risk.[5]

Irrespective of the sterilization technique used, the incidence of subsequent intrauterine and ectopic pregnancy rate is between two and eight cases per thousand, within a follow-up period of 2 to 3 years. Large studies report a contraceptive failure rate of approximately 5.4 per thousand.[6,7]

GENERAL PRINCIPLES

Laparoscopic sterilization, while a fundamentally sound procedure, has led to more medicolegal difficulties than any other gynecologic operation. Risk to the patient and to the physician can be kept to an irreducible minimum only by meticulous attention to detail.

Although the principles of all laparoscopic surgery have been described in Chapter 7, it is worth reviewing those principles common to all types of laparoscopic sterilization procedures before dealing with the specific aspects of each technique. The bladder must be empty. We prefer to use the lithotomy position and to have a rigid uterine cannula in place, both to displace the bowel and to facilitate access to the tubes. Proper pneumoperitoneum and an adequate degree of Trendelenburg position are essential. Clear identification of the oviducts and their anatomic components is mandatory before the sterilization is attempted. The surgeon must be completely familiar with the instruments to be used.

It is technically possible to perform most laparoscopic sterilizations through a single puncture by introducing the operative instrument through the operative channel of the laparoscope. We prefer the use of the double-puncture technique for sterilization. The separation of the operative axis from the visual axis increases the accuracy and the safety of the procedure. All of the sterilization procedures described in this chapter are performed by us using a multiple-puncture approach. The techniques are essentially the same when a single puncture is used, the only difference being the site of introduction of the operative instrument.

SURGICAL TECHNIQUES

Electrical Methods

Tubal sterilization may be achieved electrosurgically by using unipolar or bipolar current.

Unipolar current. This method employs a unipolar technique to (1) occlude and transect a segment of oviduct, (2) occlude and excise a portion, or (3) simply occlude a segment of tube. These techniques have lost favor and are now employed in very few centers.

Desiccation and transection. Unipolar desiccation and transection of an oviductal segment was the first widely employed laparoscopic tubal sterilization technique.[3] The isthmus is grasped, desiccated, and transected; the cut edges are grasped individually and recoagulated.

The instruments most commonly employed for this purpose are the Palmer biopsy drill forceps and the Frangenheim hook punch forceps. The Palmer instrument is equipped with flexible prongs that open when advanced from, and close when retracted into, an external circular sheath. This sheath has at its distal extremity a circular cutting blade which can be advanced by rotating the sheath (Fig. 13-1). The Frangenheim instrument is a punch biopsy forceps. The mobile upper jaw fits within the cavity of the fixed lower jaw, which possesses sharp parallel cutting edges.

The ancillary instrument, the Palmer biopsy forceps, or Frangenheim forceps is introduced through a second puncture located usually in the midline and 3 cm above the symphysis pubis to avoid the bladder.

The grasping jaws of the Palmer forceps are extended, and the tube is grasped in the midisthmic section, then the jaws are retracted and the snugly held tube is pulled away from the surrounding structures. Current is applied. This method concentrates electrical energy at the site at which the jaws of the forceps grasp the fallopian tube. The damaged tissues become blanched. A popping sound may be heard. The degree of tissue damage extends beyond the blanched area. After adequate desiccation of an appropriate tubal length (2.5 to 3 cm) and adjacent mesosalpinx, division of the oviduct is undertaken by twisting downward the circular knife of the Palmer forceps. A section of tube remains within the forceps.

If the Frangenheim hook-punch forceps is employed, the tube is loosely held within the forceps and desiccated. Once adequate desiccation is achieved, the tube is squeezed within the jaws of the forceps. This divides the tube between the parallel jaws of the forceps and a 3 mm desiccated section remains within the jaws.

Irrespective of the forceps used, the cut edges are examined. If they appear to have been inadequately coagulated or if there is bleeding, they are coagulated further.

Desiccation alone. Desiccation without tubal transection is equally effective provided complete destruction of the tubal segment is achieved. The tube is similarly grasped in the midisthmus with unipolar forceps. It is tented up away from the surrounding organs. Current is applied until blanching of a 2.5 cm segment of tube and adjacent mesosalpinx is obtained.

Bipolar current. Rioux, in 1973, developed a bipolar technique for tubal sterilization.[8] This system differs from the unipolar method in that the operating forceps carries both the active and the return electrode. The jaws are completely isolated from one another, so that high-frequency current passes through one jaw and is retrieved and returned to the generator through the other jaw. The current therefore passes selectively through the grasped tissue and travels only the short distance between the jaws of the forceps (Fig. 13-2).

The tube is identified and grasped at the midisthmus, 2 cm from the uterotubal junction (Fig. 13-3, *A*). The tube is tented up and, after ensuring that the forceps are not in contact with any other structure, the current is applied. The tube blanches and bubbles may form as desiccation proceeds. The end-point is more difficult to determine because the burn is localized to a small segment of tube. Tissue destruction must be adequate to achieve permanent obstruction (Fig. 13-3, *B*). While unipolar current spreads through the mesosalpinx and compromises the vascular supply of the affected segment ensuring its total destruction, bipolar current may spare the mucosa. If the burn is inadequate, pregnancy may subsequently occur.

It is our practice initially to use coagulating current to secure hemostasis. The procedure is completed using blended current. The addition of the cutting current, which

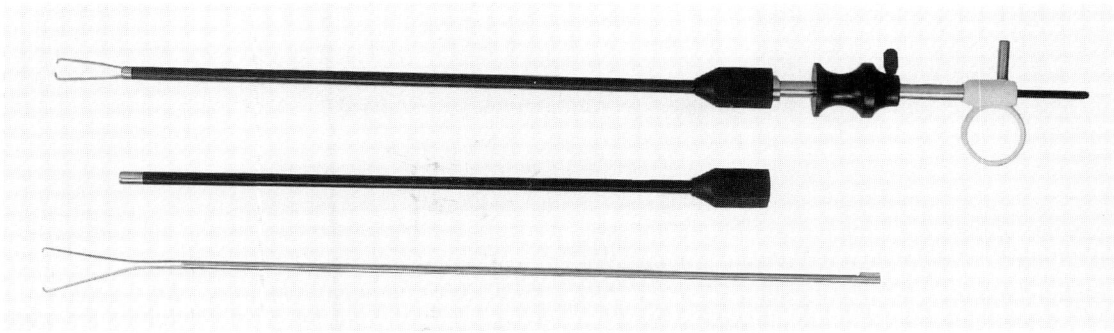

Fig. 13-1. The Palmer biopsy drill forceps.

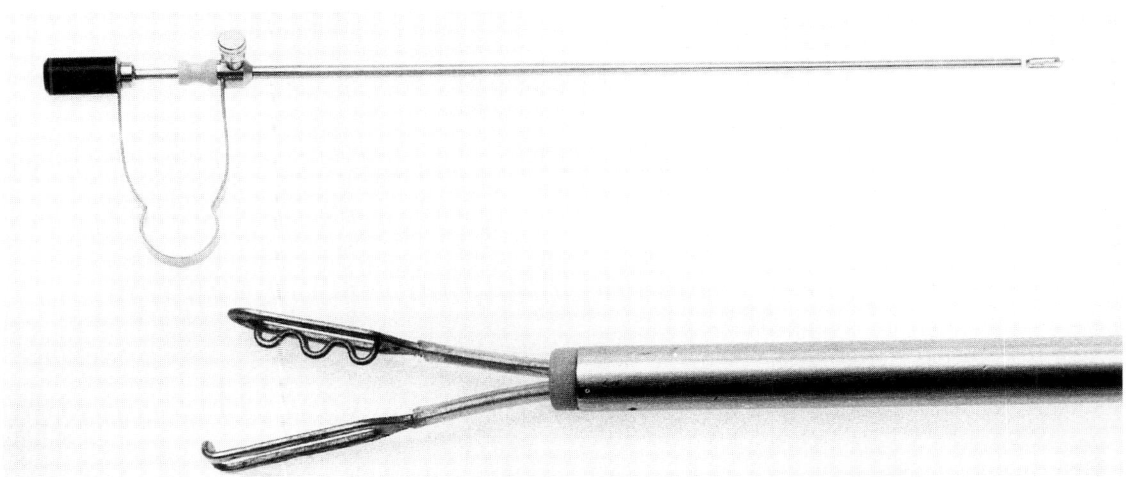

Fig. 13-2. Bipolar forceps.

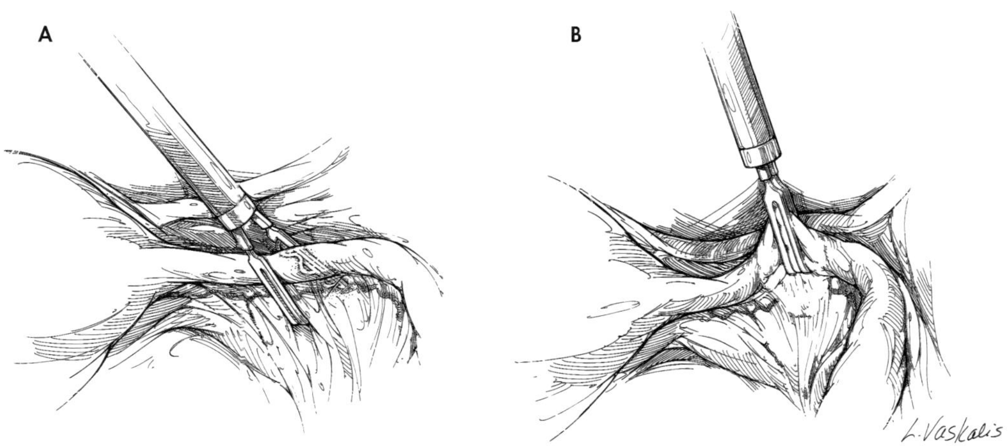

Fig. 13-3. Sterilization using bipolar electrodesiccation. **A,** The tube is grasped at the midisthmus. **B,** Tissue destruction has been achieved.

is more deeply penetrating, ensures destruction of the mucosa. The tube is regrasped and desiccated at an immediately adjacent site. When properly performed, the failure rate with this technique is similar to that associated with the unipolar method (approximately two per 1000 cases).

The introduction of low-voltage, high-frequency generators, the better training of physicians and operating room personnel, and the increased understanding of electrosurgery have contributed to the decrease in electrosurgical accidents.

Thermocoagulation. To avoid any introduction of electric current, the procedure of thermocoagulation was developed. Crocodile jaw forceps which operate on the copper soldering bolt principle are used. The current heats the forceps jaws but is not transmitted through the patient's tissues. Only tissue touched by the forceps will be heated. The isthmus is grasped and tented away from the surrounding structures. It is heated to 100°C for 20 seconds. A second contiguous burn is effected. The forceps are replaced with scissors and the center of the destroyed area is transected. In view of the fact that heat transmission is limited to a depth of 2 mm, it is essential to recoagulate the cut edges. The commercially available endocoagulators are equipped with an audible signal. A hum of increasingly higher frequency indicates that the preselected temperature has been reached in the tubal tissues. An automatic timer switches off the coagulator. This is coupled to a decreasing high-frequency hum.

We have limited experience with this technique, which is being used in many European centers.

Mechanical Methods

The mechanical devices currently used are the result of long developmental processes. Both the Hulka and the Filshie clips, for example, went through several versions; the applicators were continuously improved and simplified. The mechanical techniques are designed to occlude oviducts by either clips or rings. Although they aim to avoid the use of electricity for the purpose of sterilization, it is essential to have an electrosurgical unit in the theater when such a mechanical procedure is undertaken. Inadvertent trauma to the oviduct or its mesentery during the procedure may result in bleeding, which may require electrocoagulation for its control.

The Hulka clip. The Hulka clip was designed to be applied at a right angle to the isthmic portion of the tube.[(9)] The clip itself consists of two toothed jaws of lexan plastic joined by a metal hinge pin. The lower jaw possesses a distal hook. A gold-plated spring maintains the clip in an open position. When completely advanced the spring closes and locks the jaws.

The applicator is 7 mm in diameter with a three-ring configuration at the proximal end. The central ring, designed to accommodate the thumb, steadies the instrument. The paired lower two rings, designed to accommodate the index and middle fingers, control the clip application mechanism. The distal end of the applicator has a fixed lower jaw to accommodate the clip. A mobile upper jaw, when retracted, permits placement of the open clip and, when advanced, closes the clip. A center piston when totally advanced locks the spring (Fig. 13-4).

Once the tubes have been identified laparoscopically and the surgeon is satisfied that clip sterilization is technically feasible, the second puncture cannula is inserted. A clip is placed in the open jaws of the applicator. By moving the paired lateral rings down to their first position, the upper jaw is advanced. This action closes the clip to permit passage through the cannula. Retraction of the rings will open the clip within the peritoneal cavity. Manipulation of the uterus with the rigid uterine cannula is used to enhance tubal exposure.

The open clip is advanced at right angles to the isthmus approximately 2 to 2.5 cm from the uterotubal junction, and the hook of the lower jaw is placed against the posterior mesosalpinx (Fig. 13-5, *A*). The tube is slightly tented and the clip is closed by advancing the rings once again to their first position. The shaft of the applicator is gently rotated to permit confirmation of proper clip application. If the surgeon is dissatisfied, the clip is opened and reapplied. Once a satisfactory application is seen, the rings are further advanced to their second position driving the piston, which forces the gold-plated clip forward, thus locking the clip. The rings are fully retracted, opening the jaws of the applicator, which is freed from the clip. The clip is once again inspected to ensure its accurate placement (Fig. 13-5, *B*). The applicator is withdrawn from the abdomen and reloaded. The contralateral tube is treated in the same fashion.

The criteria of correct application are complete inclusion of the isthmus within the jaws, perpendicular application to the tube, a clip that is securely locked, and no evidence of bleeding or tears of the tube or mesosalpinx.

If the clip has not been satisfactorily applied, a second clip is placed immediately alongside the first. The tube is crushed by the clip and some hours elapse before complete occlusion occurs.

Failures of the Hulka clip should not exceed two to three per 1000, which is an acceptable rate for all female sterilization methods. To achieve this, the applicator must be in perfect working condition, the clips must have passed all quality control tests, and, most importantly, the surgeon must place the clips at "the right place, on the right structure and at a right angle."[8]

The Filshie clip. The Filshie clip is made of titanium lined with silastic rubber. Titanium is a nonreactive and sturdy metal. The silastic rubber lining permits complete compression of the tube without its being lacerated. The clip consists of two jaws joined by a hinge pin. The jaws are kept open by a spring mechanism. The lower jaw is straight and possesses a hooked tip. The upper jaw is curved. When the jaws are closed gently, a space remains between the

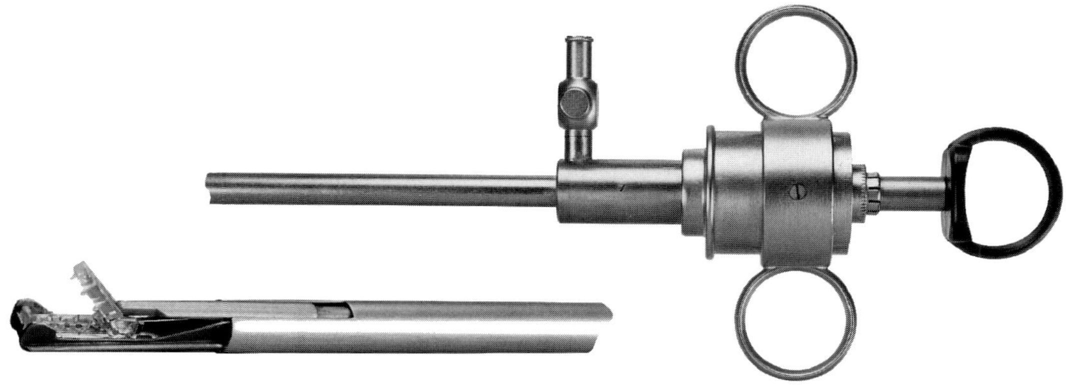

Fig. 13-4. Hulka clip and applicator.

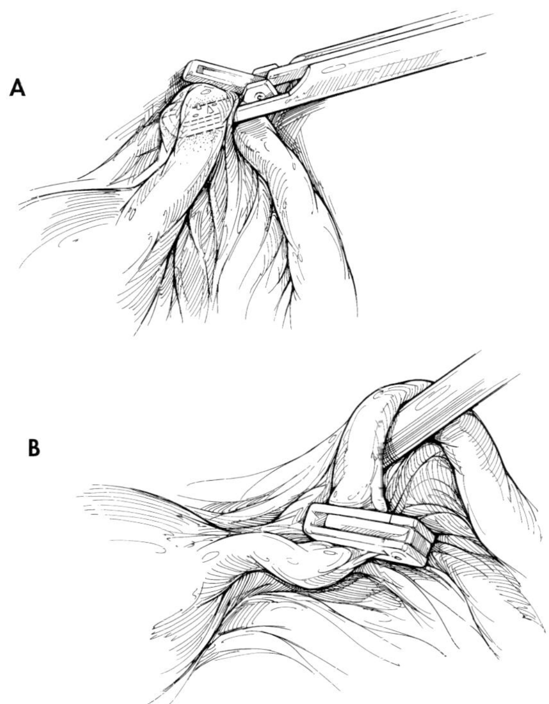

Fig. 13-5. Sterilization using the Hulka clip. **A,** The lower jaw is placed against the posterior mesosalpinx. **B**, Inspection of the clip to ensure proper placement.

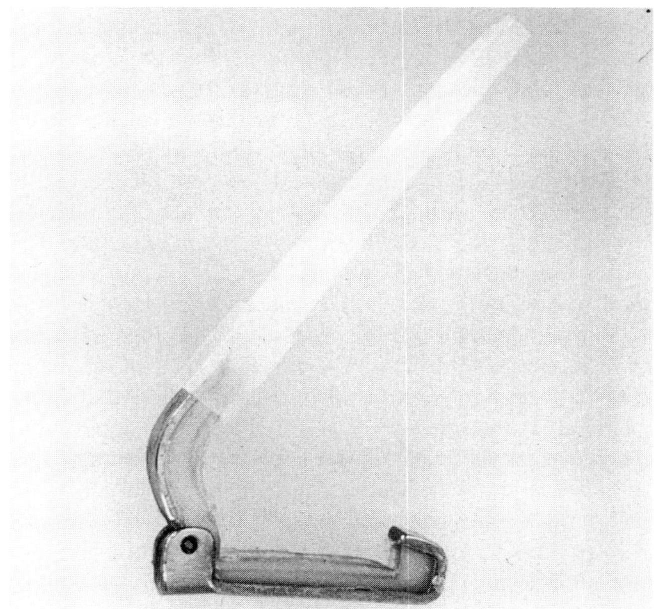

Fig. 13-6. The Filshie clip. Note the plastic loading handle.

straight lower and the concave upper jaw. A plastic loading handle has been preattached to the tip of the upper jaw of the clip (Fig. 13-6).

The applicator is 7 mm in diameter and has a squeeze mechanism at its proximal end with a finger bar which is perpendicular to the shaft. The distal end of the applicator has a fixed lower jaw that accommodates the clip (Fig. 13-7). A mobile shorter upper jaw when open permits the placement of the clip. When the upper jaw is closed gently, the clip closes but may be reopened by allowing the upper jaw of the applicator to open. When the upper jaw of the applicator is closed firmly, the curved upper jaw of the clip is flattened, the clip locks, and the opening that existed between the silastic lining of the jaws is eliminated.

Once the oviducts have been identified laparoscopically and the surgeon is satisfied that clip sterilization is feasible, the second-puncture cannula is inserted. The clip is grasped by the plastic loading handle and placed in the lower jaw of the open applicator until it snaps into position. The lower jaw of the clip must be flat within the appropriate space on

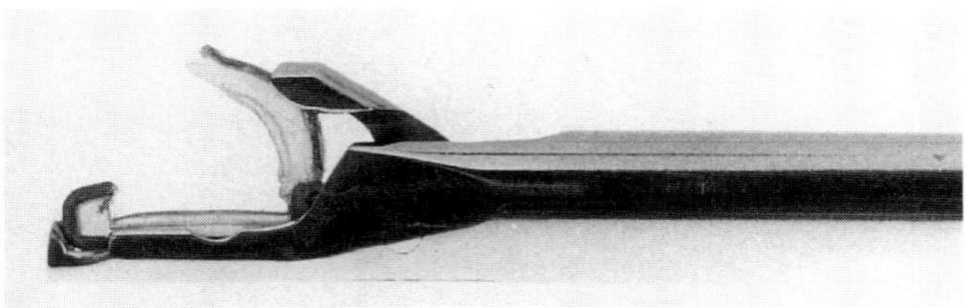

Fig. 13-7. The Filshie clip loaded in the applicator.

the lower jaw of the applicator. The loading handle is removed by pulling it upward.

The proximal end of the applicator is held within the hand, placing the upper short bar in the palm and the four fingers around the finger bar with the index and ring finger on one side and the fourth and fifth fingers on the other side of the shaft of the applicator. Gentle squeezing of the finger bar closes the upper jaw and, in turn, the clip. This action permits passage through the cannula. It is possible to manipulate the tube with the clip in this closed position for the purpose of identification. Relaxation of the finger bar will open the clip within the peritoneal cavity.

With the tube properly exposed—as described before—the open clip is advanced at right angles to the isthmus approximately 2 to 2.5 cm from the uterotubal junction. The adjacent area in the mesosalpinx should be seen to be relatively avascular. The clip is advanced until the tube is at the back end of the clip, close to the hinge. The finger bar is squeezed gently to close the clip. The shaft of the applicator is rotated to permit confirmation of proper clip application. If the surgeon is dissatisfied with the application, the finger bar is relaxed and the open clip is reapplied. If the application is satisfactory (as for the Hulka clip), the finger bar is squeezed slowly and firmly. This action depresses further the upper jaw of the applicator, which in turn flattens the upper jaw of the clip, locking it in place.

The finger bar is relaxed opening the jaws of the applicator, which is freed from the clip. Using the closed empty applicator as a probe, the clip is once again inspected to ensure its accurate placement (as for the Hulka clip). The finger bar is once again gently squeezed closing the jaws of the forceps. The applicator is withdrawn from the abdomen and reloaded. The contralateral oviduct is treated in the same fashion.

If the clip has not been satisfactorily applied, a second clip is placed alongside the first. If the tube is transected inadvertently, a second clip is applied on the proximal (uterine) side of the laceration.

The Falope ring. The falope ring is made of nonreactive silicone rubber.[10] To permit radiologic identification, 5% barium sulfate is incorporated. The ring is 2.2 mm thick with an outer diameter of 3.6 mm and an inner diameter of 1 mm. If not stretched for more than 6 mm, it possesses a specific elastic power with a recovery of 90% to 100%. The applicator consists of two concentric cylinders, the inner one of which contains grasping prongs at its distal end (Fig. 13-8). The movement of these cylinders may be controlled by proximal rings or by a pistol grip. Two rings can be fitted to the outer surface of the inner cylinder. They are first placed on a conical tip that stretches them sufficiently to permit transfer to the applicator (Fig. 13-9).

Once the tubes are identified and the surgeon is satisfied that ring application is technically feasible, the second-puncture cannula is inserted. The preloaded ring applicator is passed into the peritoneal cavity. The tube is grasped approximately 2.5 cm distal to the uterotubal junction by extending the grasping prongs. The prongs are retracted within the inner cylinder to a depth of 1 cm. The outer cylinder is advanced using the proximal control mechanism so that the first ring is transferred from the applicator to the loop of tube (Fig. 13-10, *A*). By reversing the proximal control mechanism the jaws of the forceps are extended and opened, permitting the ringed knuckle of tube to fall free. These manipulations can tear the mesosalpinx or transect the tube. It is essential to inspect the freshly banded tube to ensure correct application over a sufficient length of tube and note the absence of any complications (Fig. 13-10, *B*). The procedure is repeated on the contralateral tube.

Currently, the failure rate of the tubal ring is 3.3 per 1000 procedures. This is quite acceptable considering the simplicity of the procedure and its low complication rate.

REVERSAL OF STERILIZATION

Although sterilization should be offered only as a permanent form of contraception, some women will request reversal at a later date. While it is impossible to predict this for a specific individual, there are, however, certain traits that are common to women who request reversal. Women who have had their sterilization at a young age, when they were in an unstable relationship (poor marriage, separation, divorce), during the puerperium (either because they were influenced in their decision by difficulties with the current pregnancy or because of the loss of the child in the succeeding few months), or together with a voluntary termination of pregnancy appear particularly vulnerable. Whereas remarriage is a frequent reason for requesting reversal, at the time of sterilization a significant proportion of these women were in an unstable relationship. Psychologic reasons and tragedies such as the death of a partner or of a child represent other but rare causes that lead to this request.[11,12]

While the decision as to which technique should be used must be individualized, it is preferable to use a procedure that is effective yet associated with limited tissue destruction. The sterilization techniques that lend themselves best to reversal are those which destroy a small segment of the tubal isthmus.[13] These include the clip methods and simple bipolar electrocoagulation as described in this chapter. The falope ring, while destroying only about 3 cm of tube, often

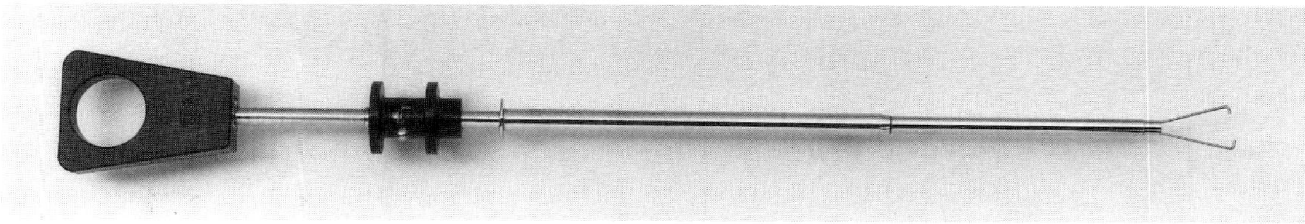

Fig. 13-8. The Falope ring applicator.

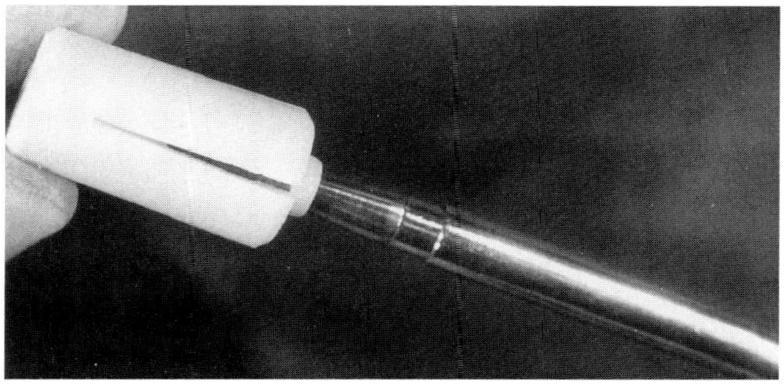

Fig. 13-9. Loading the falope ring onto the applicator.

involves a portion of the proximal ampulla, but is still associated with a good reversal prognosis.

SUMMARY

1. Despite advances in microsurgical reversal techniques, female tubal sterilization must be offered only to the patient as a permanent form of contraception.
2. Before sterilization it is appropriate for the physician to discuss all of the possible contraceptive choices with the woman or couple.
3. Once the patients have decided to undergo female sterilization, the physician's primary concern should be for safety and efficacy. The potential for reversal should be a secondary consideration.
4. If laparoscopic sterilization is to be the method of choice, the surgeon must be completely familiar with the instrumentation and the specifics of the techniques to be utilized.
5. Currently the most commonly-performed laparoscopic sterilization techniques are: bipolar electrocoagulation, clip application, and ring application.
6. Bipolar electrocoagulation is an effective method of sterilization when performed properly and complete destruction of the segment achieved.
7. Clip methods are effective. The clip must be applied at right angles to the isthmus and must include the entire circumference of the tube. When applied correctly, clips are effective, safe, and potentially reversible. The Filshie and Hulka clips are the devices of choice.

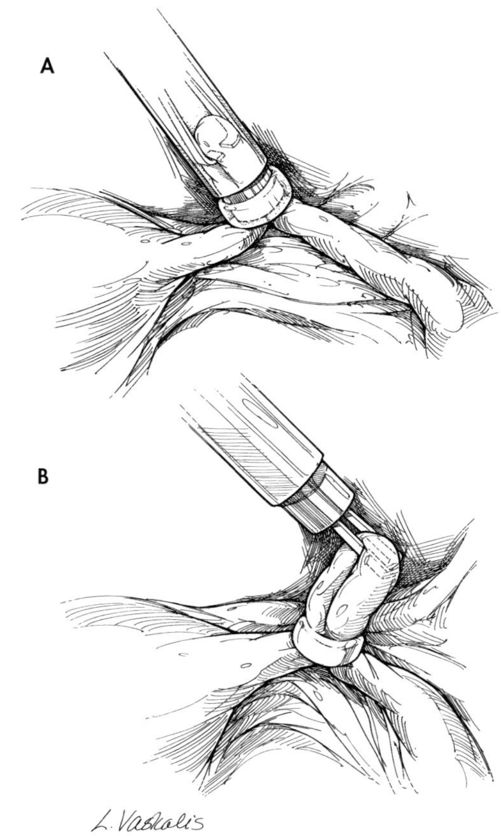

Fig. 13-10. Application of the falope ring. **A,** The ring is transferred to the tube. **B,** The banded tube is inspected.

8. The falope ring is easy to use, safe, and as effective as the clips and bipolar electrocoagulation methods.
9. Any laparoscopic sterilization method can be performed under general or local anesthesia, by a single or double puncture approach. Our preference is for the double puncture approach.

REFERENCES:

1. Anderson ET: Peritoneoscopy, *Am J Surg* 35:136, 1937.
2. Power FH, Barnes AC: Sterilization by means of peritoneoscopic tubal fulguration: a preliminary report, *Am J Obstet Gynecol* 41:1038, 1941.
3. Palmer MR: Essais de sterilisation tubaire coelioscopique par electrocoagulation isthmique, *Bull Fed Soc Gyn Obst* 14:298, 1962.
4. Steptoe PC: Laparoscopy in gynaecology. Edinburgh, 1967, E & S Livingston Ltd.

5. Franks AL, Kendrick JS, Peterson HB: Unintended laparotomy associated with laparoscopic tubal sterilization, *Am J Obstet Gynecol* 157:1102-5, 1987.
6. Bhiwandiwala PP, Mumbord SD, Feldblum PJ: A comparison of different laparoscopic sterilization occlusion techniques in 24,939 procedures, *Am J Obstet Gynecol* 144:319, 1982.
7. Cittadini E, LaSala G, Perino A: Endoscopy for contraception, *Acta Europ Fertil* 19:309-314, 1988.
8. Rioux JE, Yuzpe AA: Evaluation of female sterilization procedures. In Current Problems in Obstetrics and Gynecology, vol 11. Chicago, 1979, Year Book Medical Publishers.
9. Hulka JF: Studies in simpler tubocclusion methods, *Am J Obstet Gynecol* 122:137-347, 1975.
10. Yoon IB, King TM: A preliminary and intermediate report on a new laparoscopic tubal ring procedure, *J Reprod Med* 15:54-6, 1975.
11. Gomel V: Profile of women requesting reversal of sterilization, *Fertil Steril* 30:39-41, 1978.
12. Gomel V: Microsurgery in female infertility. Boston, 1983, Little, Brown & Co.
13. Gomel V: Microsurgical reversal of female sterilization: a reappraisal, *Fertil Steril* 33:587-597, 1980.

Chapter 14

TUBAL PREGNANCY

The rise in the rate of detection and the methods of diagnosis of tubal pregnancy have been described in Chapter 10. Ectopic pregnancy was regarded as inevitably fatal until Lawson Tait[1] in 1884 introduced timely surgical intervention and excision of the affected tube. Thirty-three of 40 women upon whom he operated survived both the ectopic pregnancy and the surgery. Salpingectomy remained the method of treatment for tubal pregnancy for nearly one century. Stromm[2] (1953) was the first to describe conservative surgical treatment of tubal gestation. By performing a salpingotomy he was able to remove the ectopic gestation without sacrificing the fallopian tube. Treatment of tubal pregnancy today may be expectant, medical, or surgical. This chapter will discuss the management of tubal pregnancy with particular reference to the use of operative laparoscopy.

EXPECTANT MANAGEMENT

In 1955 Lund[3] reported 215 cases of ectopic pregnancy treated between 1930 and 1946. Ninety-six of these patients displayed signs of extensive intraperitoneal hemorrhage and were treated by immediate operation. The remaining 119 were not acutely distressed, were termed "subacute cases," and were observed. They all had positive pregnancy tests (Aschheim-Zondek and, later, Friedmans test). Their treatment consisted of confinement to bed with close observation and inhibition of bowel activity by the administration of opium. The pregnancy test was repeated every 7 to 10 days and the patients examined regularly. They were kept in bed until the pregnancy test became negative and the pain ceased. The condition resolved in 68 of the 119 patients. The others (51 cases) required surgery, either because of evidence of intraabdominal hemorrhage or a persistent tender adnexal mass. Garcia et al.[4] reported 13 patients with unruptured tubal pregnancy who were managed expectantly. Inclusion criteria for expectant management were clinical stability, falling β-hCG titers, ultrasonographic evidence of an empty uterus, and no gross evidence of products of conception in the uterine curettings. If these prerequisites were satisfied, diagnostic laparoscopy was undertaken. Patients with a tubal mass under 4 cm in diameter and without active intraperitoneal bleeding were managed expectantly.

These selected patients were hospitalized and followed with daily measurements of serum β-hCG, hematocrit values, and ultrasonography. If they remained asymptomatic and the β-hCG levels declined for 5 consecutive days they were discharged from the hospital. Thereafter β-hCG levels were monitored three times per week until they fell below assay detectability on two successive occasions. One of the 13 patients required surgery. Her β-hCG level had remained constant for 11 days and she experienced increasing abdominal pain commencing on the ninth postlaparoscopy day. Ten of the 13 patients underwent hysterosalpingography (HSG) 3 months later. Seven had normal-appearing patent fallopian tubes and three had tubal occlusion at the site of the previous gestation.

Fernandez et al.[5] reported 14 patients with ampullary tubal pregnancy confirmed by laparoscopy and managed expectantly. The pregnancy resolved spontaneously in nine patients but surgical intervention was necessary in four; in two because of rising β-hCG titers and in two because of pain. The remaining patient, included in the series because of laparoscopic observation of an apparent tubal pregnancy, was ultimately found to have an ongoing intrauterine pregnancy. Spontaneous resolution occurred more frequently when the initial β-hCG concentration was less than 1000 mIU/ml. Hysterosalpingography was performed for six of the nine patients who had had spontaneous resolution. The tubes were patent in all, but one had an ampullary defect, 2 cm in diameter, at the previous gestational site.

Both of these small series of deliberately expectant management were associated with a high rate of residual tubal damage. This finding is not surprising in light of a previous report from our center[6] of five cases of tubal occlusion that had occurred at the site of undiagnosed ectopic pregnancies. Maymon et al.[7] have summarized 81 cases from eight publications, including those of Garcia[4] and Fernandez.[5] Sixty-two (76.5%) resolved spontaneously, but 19 (23.5%) required laparotomy. Twenty-nine patients underwent a follow-up HSG; 6 (20.7%) had tubal occlusion.

Once the diagnosis has been made by noninvasive means, expectant management may have a place in the treatment of tubal pregnancy in a patient who is asymptomatic, with low and dropping βhCG levels. Such management is protracted, worrying to the patient, and expensive if patients are observed in the hospital. Such an approach must also consider the initial high failure rate and the potential for tubal occlusion. In general clinical practice it would be difficult to justify expectant management once laparoscopy has been undertaken.

MEDICAL TREATMENT

It is obviously preferable to be able to treat any condition medically rather than surgically. A number of systemically and locally administrable compounds are under very active investigation.

Systemic agents

Chemotherapeutic agents that are known to destroy trophoblastic tissue and the antiprogestin RU486 have been used to treat tubal pregnancy. The results using RU486 have been disappointing. Methotrexate use seems to be more promising.

Medical therapy may be administered systemically or locally. Methotrexate has been used systemically, frequently in conjunction with citrovorum factor. Most protocols use intramuscular administration of methotrexate and citrovorum factor on alternate days, the former at a dosage of 1 mg/kg per day and the latter at a dosage of 0.1 mg/kg per day for 8 days. Failure is more likely to occur when the initial serum β-hCG level is above 6500 mIU/ml and when there is ultrasonographic evidence of cardiac activity or formed fetal elements.[8,9] Maymon et al.[7] have provided an extensive table summarizing the published experience with methotrexate. From this it was possible to identify 11 publications that described a variety of multiple-dose systemic treatments. Because of the heterogeneity of these data overview analysis was not possible. The following figures derived from these publications are the results of simple addition. Of eighty-six patients, 81 (92%) were treated successfully, five (8%) required laparotomy, and 22 (25.6%) experienced systemic side effects. Sixty of these patients underwent a follow-up HSG, in 19 (30.6%) tubal occlusion was noted.

The largest single series,[10] not included above, reports 100 patients. Of these four were treated because of persistent trophoblast following conservative surgery. The remaining 96 had primary administration of methotrexate. Ninety-two (95.8%) of these 96 were treated successfully and four (4.2%) required surgery. Five of the total group experienced minor systemic side effects. Fifty-eight patients underwent a follow-up HSG, and nine (15.5%) of these had tubal occlusion.

Methotrexate is a potent drug with many side effects, some which may be serious. It has several proved indications. However, considering other available proven, effective, and safe therapeutic options for tubal pregnancy and the failure rate, side effects, and rate of tubal occlusion, we view with scepticism the systemic use of methotrexate for the primary treatment of this condition. On the other hand, methotrexate has a distinct place in the treatment of retained trophoblast (after conservative surgical management); this requires the use of a much lower dosage, usually 50 mg given in a single injection. Systemic administration of methotrexate may also be useful in the treatment of pregnancies of rare ectopic location such as the cervix and the cornu.

Local medical therapy

Local medical therapy, injecting (under laparoscopic visualization) methotrexate,[11-13] prostaglandins F_{2a},[14] or hypertonic glucose solution[15,16] into the tubal gestation site (and the ovary containing the corpus luteum in the case of prostaglandins F_{2a}), appears to be effective in selected patients and is associated with few side effects. However the postoperative period is usually protracted. As long as it is necessary to resort to laparoscopy to administer the medication, we believe that it is preferable to remove the gestational products instead. Local medical treatment is promising, especially if the drug can be administered transvaginally under ultrasonographic control and local anesthesia.[17-19]

Fernandez et al. recently reported 100 patients with ectopic pregnancy treated by local administration of methotrexate transvaginally under sonographic control.[20] Patients who did not have a satisfactory response to the initial local injection were treated with intramuscular administration of the same agent. All of the 100 patients had clear evidence of an unruptured ectopic pregnancy on the basis of an adnexal mass visualized by transvaginal sonography. Methotrexate (1 mg/kg) was injected transvaginally using an 18 gauge needle. The procedure was performed either without anesthesia or local administration of 1% lydocaine to the posterior vaginal fornix. The ectopic sac was aspirated and the medication injected into the sac. An equal dose of methotrexate was administered intramuscularly, 1 week after the initial treatment, to those patients whose β-hCG levels remained the same or increased. After the initial local injection of methotrexate the patients were followed and the serum β-hCG levels assayed on days 2, 5, and 10 and then weekly until they returned to normal. Ninety-one of these

100 patients had a tubal pregnancy and nine a cornual pregnancy. The mean β-hCG levels of these patients was 4,930 mIU/ml with a range between 65 and 46,740. The diameter of the hematosalpinx averaged 21 mm with a range between 4 mm and 40 mm. Of the 100 patients, 83 were treated successfully. Fifty-five of these responded to the initial local injection of methotrexate, 23 required an additional intramuscular dose of methotrexate, and five patients required further intramuscular administration of the same agent. Among the 17 patients who failed to respond, four required emergency surgery for acute hemoperitoneum and the remaining 13 patients underwent surgery by laparoscopy because of inadequate regression of the β-hCG levels. Seventy-two of the 100 patients had an initial β-hCG level under 5000 mIU/ml, seven of these (9.7%) failed to respond to the treatment. Among the 28 patients whose initial β-hCG level was above 5000 mIU/ml, ten (35.7%) failed to respond. The length of time to resolution was 26.5 days and varied from 10 to 75 days. The ectopic gestations in 11 of the patients demonstrated cardiac activity, seven of these responded to the treatment and four failed.[20]

We began this section describing medical treatment of ectopic pregnancy by remarking that it is preferable to treat any condition medically rather than surgically. The failure rate of systemic medical treatment is high[7] and the post-treatment course may be protracted.[8,9,21] A compromise between systemic and surgical management is local injection into the gestational sac. An attempt has been made to compare such an approach with laparoscopic surgical treatment.[22] This study was prospective and randomized. However, it was discontinued because of poor results in the injection group after only 12 patients had completed the treatment protocol. While it is possible that more effective agents will become available for systemic and/or local administration, at the time of writing surgical management of tubal pregnancy continues to play the major role.

SURGICAL MANAGEMENT

Surgical access to a tubal pregnancy can be gained by laparotomy, minilaparotomy, or laparoscopy. Surgical management may be radical, that is by tubal excision, or conservative. Just as laparoscopy is rapidly becoming the method of access of choice, conservative procedures are being performed with increasing frequency.

Because most cases of tubal pregnancy are diagnosed before tubal rupture (see Chapter 10), the number of patients who present with acute abdominal pain in a state of surgical shock is rapidly diminishing. It is in these patients that active resuscitation and immediate life-saving surgery will be required. Only in a very few will conservation of the affected tube be feasible.

Unless it has been decided on the basis of the clinical and laboratory assessment alone to treat the patient medically, laparoscopy is used to confirm the diagnosis and select the best surgical approach. The decision whether to use radical or conservative surgery will depend upon the patient's desire for future fertility and the status of the oviducts at the time of the intervention. The conservative approach aims to remove all gestational tissue and obtain hemostasis while conserving as much healthy oviduct as possible with the use of an atraumatic technique.[23] The patient's wishes will have been determined preoperatively. If there is any doubt it is better to err on the side of preserving reproductive function, if possible. The oviducts and pelvis are assessed laparoscopically paying particular attention to:

- the site and size of gestation and the status of the affected tube,
- the ipsilateral ovary,
- the contralateral tube and ovary, and other pelvic structures.

Provided the affected tube can be shown to be free by gentle manipulation, access can be gained by minilaparotomy. The patient is left in the Trendelenberg position. A rigid uterine cannula is placed in the cervix and used to maneuver the uterine fundus forward and upward until it can be palpated through the abdominal wall. The minilaparotomy incision is made at this point. Further manipulation of the cannula will bring the affected tube under the incision. The definitive surgery is performed and the incision closed. This technique may be performed by experienced laparoscopists, on occasion, when necessary laparoscopic instruments are not available.

LAPAROSCOPIC SURGERY

Most tubal pregnancies are treated laparoscopically, by either salpingectomy, ablation of the gestational site, segmental excision, or salpingotomy.

Although tubal abortion (milking of the products of conception through the fimbriated end) enjoyed a brief vogue, it is no longer recommended. A gestation of infundibular location can be shelled out with relative ease and certainty of having removed all of the gestational products. With ampullary pregnancies, even of distal location, it is impossible to be assured of complete removal of gestational products since trophoblast frequently penetrates the lamina propria and muscularis of the tube and becomes extraluminal.[24] The incidence of postoperative bleeding from the tube after this approach is higher than that associated with other conservative procedures.

General principles

The laparoscope is usually introduced intraumbilically. The second puncture is normally placed suprapubically in the midline, with a 5 mm trocar and cannula that will accommodate instruments used both during the preliminary assessment and subsequent surgery. The third portal will be placed in one or other flank to provide the best angle of approach to the affected tube.

Cutting may be achieved using mechanical, electrosurgical, or laser energy. Hemostasis may be secured with electrosurgery, thermocoagulation, ligatures, sutures, or stapling devices. Injection of dilute vasoactive agents may be used as a hemostatic adjunct.

Removal of the specimen from the abdomen will depend on its size. Small pieces of tissue will fit through an ancillary cannula. Larger specimens may be removed intact by extending the suprapubic abdominal incision or through a colpotomy. Morcellation enables removal of some specimens piecemeal through the larger bore cannula. The lapsac can be used to reduce the risk of leaving islands of trophoblastic tissue (see Chapter 7). Thorough pelvic lavage and aspiration is carried out at the end of the procedure to remove all blood and fibrin and especially the trophoblastic tissue that may have entered the peritoneal cavity. Trophoblastic tissue retained in the peritoneal cavity may implant upon serosal surfaces and cause a postoperative rise in β-hCG levels.

Whereas some authors[25,26] routinely leave an intraperitoneal drain placed in the pouch of Douglas for 24 hours or longer, such has not been our practice.[27]

Salpingectomy

Salpingectomy is indicated in certain circumstances (see the box at right). If the patient has no interest in preserving fertility, salpingectomy is an option; indeed she may request that the contralateral tube be occluded to effect permanent sterilization. This procedure is also indicated if the tube is irreparably damaged or has been the site of previous gestation(s), or if the tubal gestation followed a salpingostomy for distal tubal occlusion.

We prefer to use a simple bipolar electrosurgical technique. The uterine cannula is used to position the uterus so that the affected tube is exposed. Immobilization of this tube and exposure of the immediate operative site is achieved with a probe, irrigation/aspiration cannula, or grasping forceps introduced through one of the ancillary portals. The tube, along with the adjacent mesosalpinx, is grasped, electrodesiccated (Fig. 14-1, *A* and *B*), and divided with scissors at the level of the uterotubal junction (Fig. 14-1, *C* and *D*). This obliterates one of the two major sources of blood supply to the tube from the ascending branch of the uterine artery. The tubo-ovarian ligament is then grasped, electrodessicated, and divided (Fig. 14-1, *E* and *F*). This obliterates the second major source of blood supply through the ovarian artery. The mesosalpinx is then electrodessicated and divided in a series of burns and cuts until complete excision of the tube has been achieved (Fig. 14-1, *G*, *H*, and *I*). The mesosalpinx may be electrodessicated in a selective manner, taking into account the vessels that reach the tube at the level of the ampullary isthmic junction. The specimen will be removed as described earlier.

Indications for salpingectomy

- Patient does not wish to preserve fertility
- Tube is irreparably damaged
- Tube has been site of previous gestation
- Tubal gestation followed salpingostomy for distal tube occlusion

This technique using bipolar electrosurgery may be safer than one using the monopolar mode, although the latter may be slightly faster. Endocoagulation may be used instead of electrosurgery. The Roeder loop can be used to ligate the mesosalpinx and tube proximal to the gestational site. Three ligatures are used. The first is loaded into the adaptor, which allows it to be passed through a 5 mm cannula without loss of the pneumoperitoneum. Grasping forceps are inserted through the other ancillary portal. The grasping forceps are passed through the loop. The tube is grasped with these forceps to help position the loop so that the distal end encircles the tubo-ovarian ligament and the knotted end lies proximal to the gestational site. Care must be taken not to include the ovary. The loop is tied and cut. These steps are repeated twice more so that the tube and mesosalpinx are triply ligated.[28] The forceps grasping the tube are used to expose the line of incision so that the mesosalpinx and tube can be divided with scissors without risk of cutting the ligatures. While this procedure is effective it is time consuming and leaves a large area of necrotic tissue. The ligatures are large and may provoke a foreign body reaction.

Ablation of gestational site

Ectopic pregnancies up to 1.5 cm in size located in the isthmus or proximal ampulla can be dealt with by electrodesiccation. The tube is grasped across the site of the ectopic pregnancy as far as the mesosalpinx with a bipolar electrosurgical forceps, and this segment is electrodesiccated.[27] To ensure destruction of the full thickness of the tube, including the inner part, blended or pure cutting current is used. Two or three contiguous burns will effectively destroy the ectopic pregnancy along with the segment of oviduct containing it. The end result is similar to that of a tubal sterilization by electrosurgery. Thus conservation of the remaining tube lends itself to subsequent microsurgical anastomosis should the need arise. The principal disadvantages of this technique are the absence of a specimen for histologic examination and the interruption of the functional integrity of the tube. In addition, although rare, it is possible for another ectopic pregnancy to occur in the blind distal portion of the tube.

Segmental excision

Segmental excision is the procedure of choice for gestations sited in the isthmus. This technique may also be used if after salpingotomy there is persistent bleeding, despite the

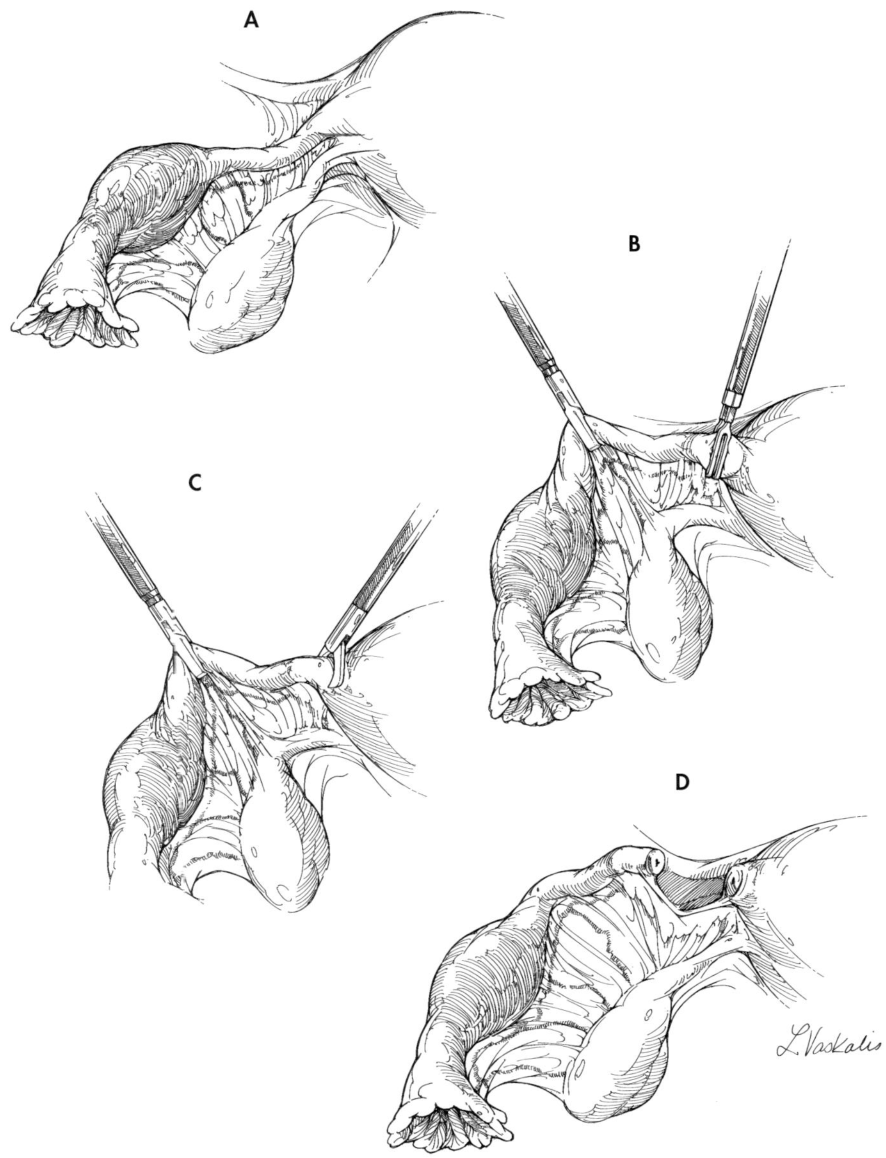

Fig. 14-1. Salpingectomy using electrodesiccation. **A,** Ampullary tubal pregnancy. **B,** Electrodesiccation of the tubocornual junction. **C** and **D,** Division of desiccated area in the tubocornual junction. *Continued.*

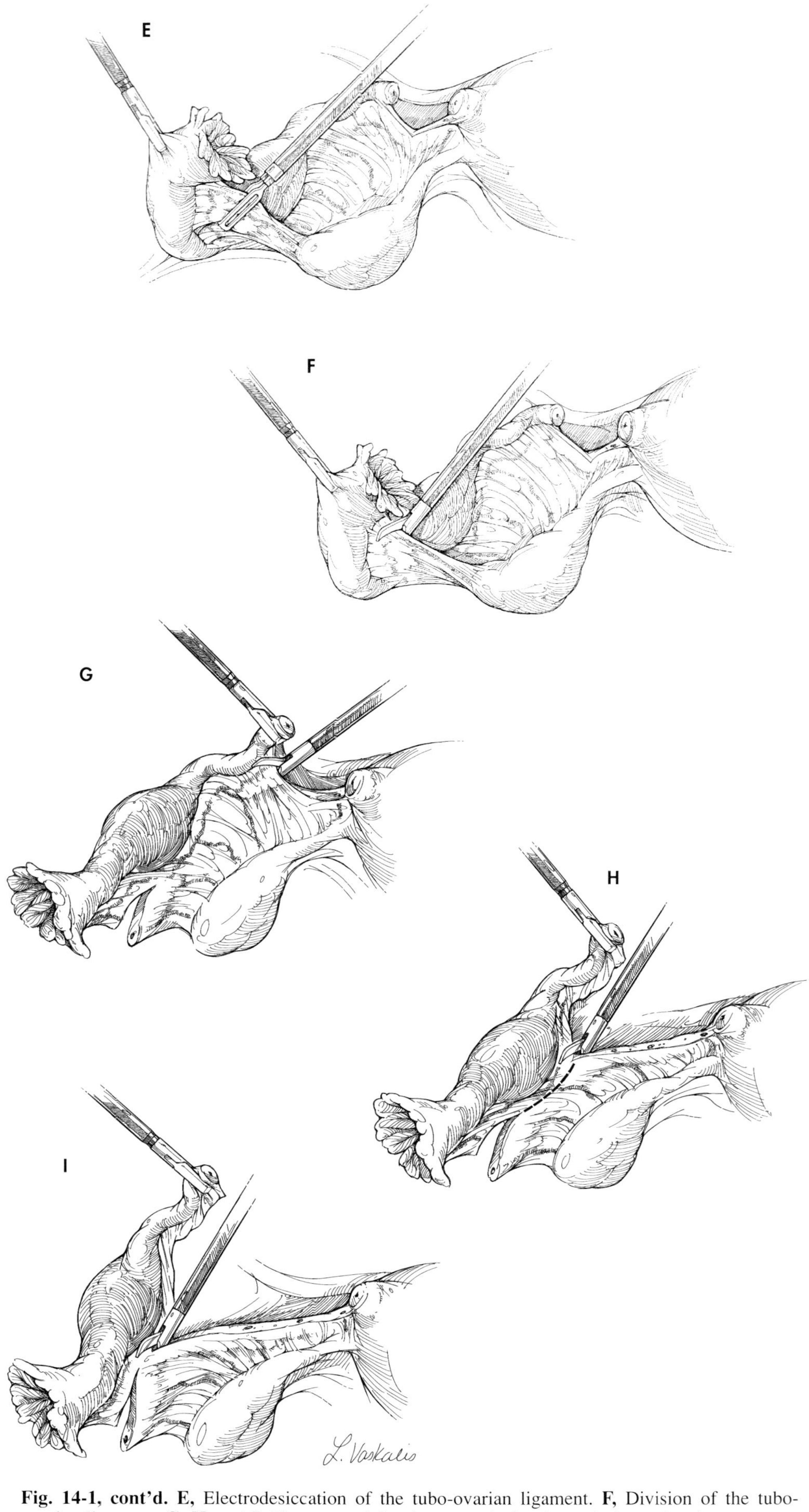

Fig. 14-1, cont'd. E, Electrodesiccation of the tubo-ovarian ligament. **F,** Division of the tubo-ovarian ligament. **G, H,** and **I,** The mesosalpinx is successively electrodesiccated and cut.

administration of vasopresin solution, and if tubal conservation is desired.

Segmental excision involves obliteration of the tube and its vasculature proximal and distal to the gestational site and the immediately underlying mesosalpinx and the excision of the involved tubal segment. Although the procedure may be effected using sutures, electrosurgery is faster and equally effective.[29,30]

When electrosurgery is used, the tube is grasped with bipolar electrosurgical forceps proximal to the pregnancy. The tube is elevated and blended or cutting current is passed until the tube and underlying vessels are completely desiccated (Fig. 14-2, *A*). This procedure is repeated immediately distal to the pregnancy (Fig. 14-2, *B*). The same forceps are used to elevate the affected segment and the previously dessicated regions are transected with scissors introduced through the second ancillary puncture site (Fig. 14-2, *C*). The scissors are removed and replaced with grasping forceps, which are used to hold one of the ends of the involved segment. Gentle traction with these forceps will expose the underlying mesosalpinx which is now grasped and desiccated (Fig. 14-2, *D*). The electrosurgical forceps are removed. The scissors are reintroduced and the mesosalpinx divided adjacent to the tube (Fig. 14-2, *E*).

If sutures are used, the tube is grasped to immobilize it. Sutures are placed through the mesosalpinx just beneath the vascular arcade and are tied to encompass the vessels and the tube at the proximal and distal limits of the implantation site. The needle holder is withdrawn and 5 mm scissors introduced. The tube is transected on the gestational side of the sutures. The mesosalpinx immediately beneath the transected tubal segment is now secured by a suture. The transected segment of the tube is elevated and the underlying mesosalpinx divided, adjacent to the tube, with scissors.

Irrespective of the technique used to excise the tubal segment, it is now important to inspect the site of excision and ensure that there is no bleeding. If a bleeding vessel is noted, hemostasis can be secured either with a suture or by electrodessication. The tubal segment is removed from the peritoneal cavity and pelvis lavage performed.

While this technique provides a specimen for histologic evaluation, it has all the other disadvantages of simple ablation.

Linear salpingotomy

The conservative surgical procedure of choice is linear salpingotomy when the pregnancy is in the ampulla.

The tube is stabilized with an atraumatic grasping forceps proximal to the implantation site and inspected. If the pregnancy is 3 cm or larger, a rapid rise in the β-hCG levels has been noted preoperatively, or ultrasound has detected cardiac activity, a vasoconstructive agent should be used. The mesosalpinx beneath the affected region of the tube is infiltrated with 2 ml of a dilute solution of vasopressin (10 IU diluted in 100 ml of saline). A 20 gauge spinal needle with the stilet in place is introduced through the abdominal wall. The stilet is removed and a 3 mm syringe containing the dilute vasopressin solution is attached to the needle. The tip of the needle is introduced just under the serosa of the mesosalpinx with the bevel of the needle facing the operator. The needle is advanced for a short distance immediately under the serosa, taking care to avoid penetration of any blood vessel (Fig. 14-3, *A*). Before injection of the solution, the plunger of the syringe is withdrawn further to confirm accurate placement. Use of a vasoconstrictive agent can be omitted if the lesion is small or inactive.

The next step is to incise the antimesosalpingeal border of the tube over the gestational site. The distended portion of the tube usually contains the ectopic gestation at its proximal end and clots distally. Therefore, the incision should be placed in the proximal portion of the distended area (Fig. 14-3, *B*). The incision can be made with scissors but there may be bleeding from the cut surfaces, particularly at the proximal angle of the incision. Laser energy is favored by some surgeons. The simplest approach is to use a monopolar fine needle electrode with the current set in the blended mode, which will provide both cutting and simultaneous hemostasis.

Once the tube over the site of implantation has been opened, extrusion of gestation products commences. Gentle compression of the tube with a probe or forceps enhances extrusion. The products are grasped with forceps and are slowly and gently teased out of the tube (Fig. 14-3, *C*). It is important to grasp gestational tissue only and not the endothelial fronds of the tube. Laceration of these fronds may cause bleeding that is difficult to control without significant damage to the endothelium. Furthermore, undue trauma to the endothelium may result in subsequent tubal occlusion at this site.[31] Hydrodissection can be used instead of grasping forceps to free the pregnancy from the tube.

Once removed, the products of conception can either be taken out of the peritoneal cavity immediately or placed in the vesicouterine pouch for subsequent removal. The lumen of the tube is irrigated to ensure that the tube is empty. The irrigation pressure will often dislodge any residual trophoblastic tissue, but if it does not the remaining fragments must be teased out with grasping forceps. Irrigation will also serve to identify any bleeding vessels which may require spot dessication. The tubal incision may safely be left to heal by secondary intention (Fig. 14-3, *D*).

Thorough pelvic lavage is especially important following linear salpingotomy because there is a greater risk of spill of trophoblastic tissue.

Tubal abortion

A distally sited tubal pregnancy may be expelled spontaneously from the tube, a condition referred to as tubal abortion. This occurs most frequently with infundibular implantations. Such tubal pregnancies can be

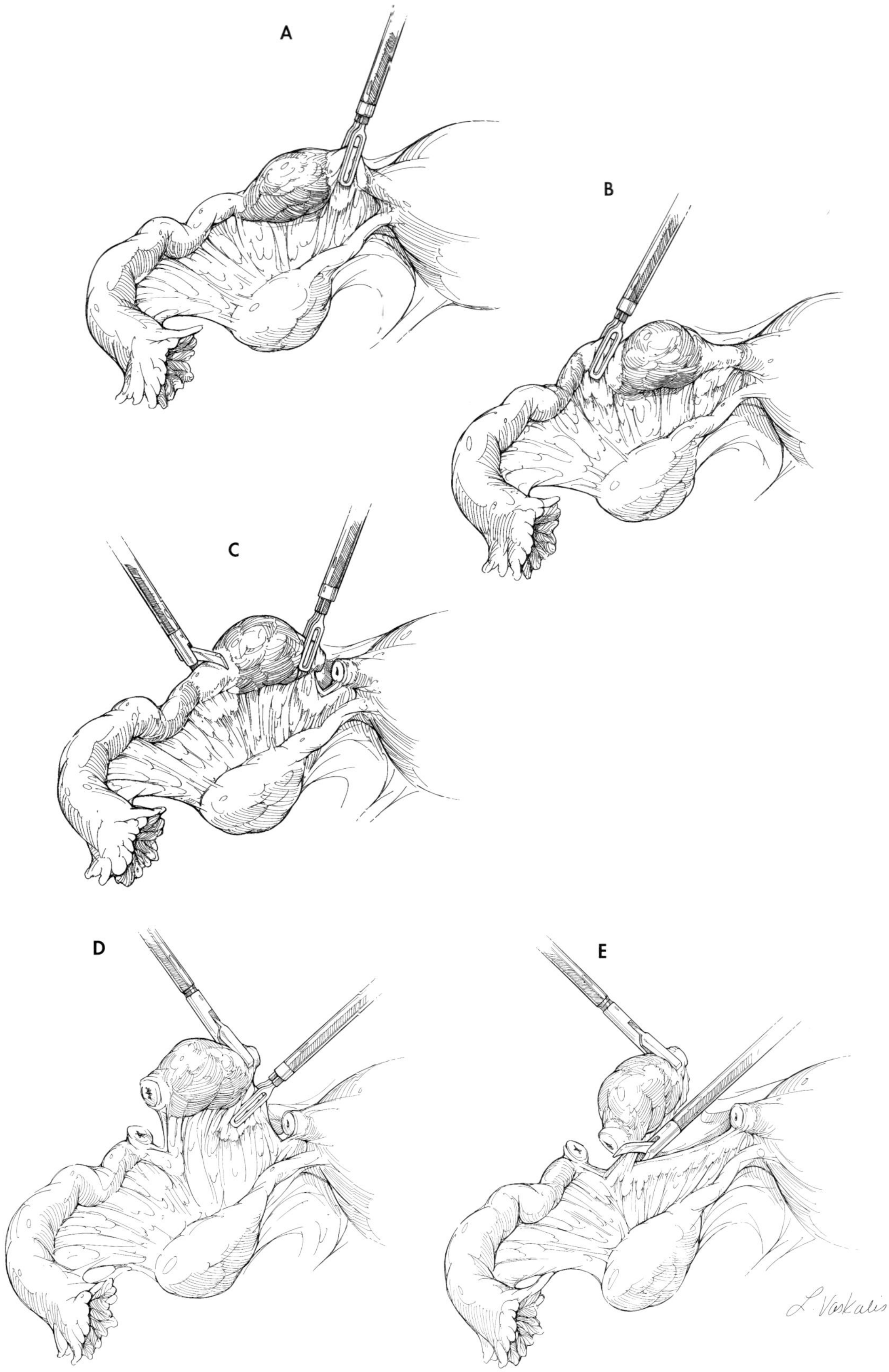

Fig. 14-2. Segmental excision with electrosurgery. **A,** The tube is grasped proximal to the pregnancy and electrodesiccated. **B,** The procedure is repeated immediately distal to the pregnancy. **C,** The desiccated regions are transected with scissors. **D,** The mesosalpinx of the affected tube is exposed and electrodesiccated. **E,** The mesosalpinx is divided.

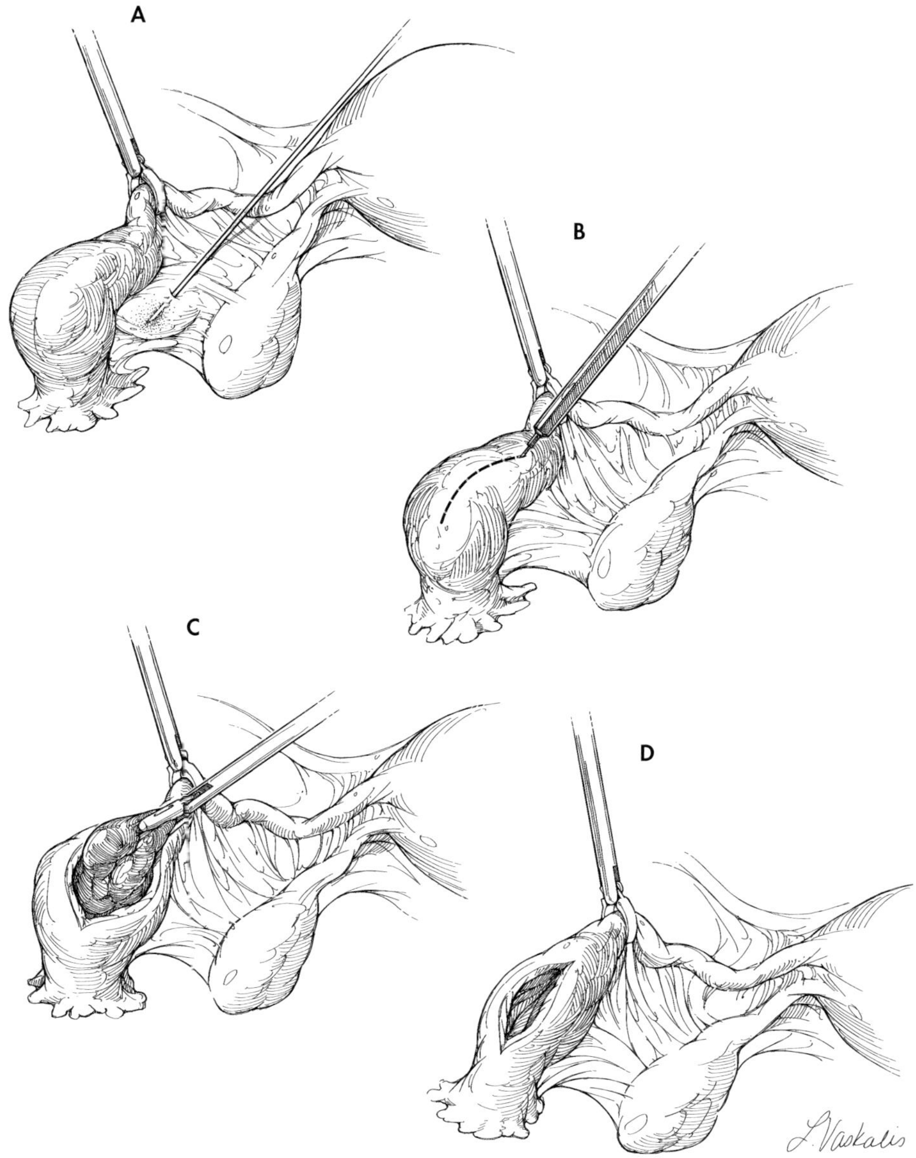

Fig. 14-3. Linear salpingotomy. **A,** The mesosalpinx, beneath the affected region of the tube, is infiltrated with approximately 2 ml of dilute vasopressin solution, using a spinal needle. **B,** The tube is stabilized and an incision made over the antimesosalpingeal border of the affected site. **C,** The products of conception protruding through the incision are grasped and teased out of the tube. **D,** The tubal incision is left open to heal by secondary intention.

shelled out with relative ease and certainty of having removed all the gestational products. Hydrodissection may facilitate removal. This approach has been shown to be effective for the management of infundibular pregnancies.[32]

Attempts to abort distal ampullary pregnancies by milking them from the tube have been less successful. There has been an unexpectedly high incidence of postoperative bleeding and persistent growth of retained trophoblastic tissue requiring subsequent intervention.[33] In these cases a linear salpingotomy is preferable. The incision extends from the gestational sac to the fimbriated end of the tube.

Cornual pregnancy

A technique similar to linear salpingotomy can be used for those rare cases of interstitial pregnancy. In these circumstances the first step is to infiltrate the surrounding myometrium with dilute vasopressin solution and to wait until blanching is noted. The affected cornual region is incised coronally using a monopolar needle electrode. The incision is carried down, through the uterine musculature, to the lumen of the interstitital segment of the tube. From this stage the operation is identical with linear salpingotomy described earlier. Once hemostasis is secured, the incision can be safely left to heal by secondary intention.

Any patient in whom laparoscopic surgery is planned should always be asked to give consent for laparotomy should it be necessary. This is particularly important in cases of cornual pregnancy in which profuse bleeding can occur. Because of the potential for myometrial infiltration by trophoblastic tissue, it is prudent to give these patients a single dose of 1 mg/kg methotrexate by intramuscular route.

Postoperative care

Patients are usually kept in the hospital for a few hours following laparoscopy and discharged home. We noted that the mean postoperative hospital stay of patients treated by laparoscopy was 0.87 days compared with 4.03 days in a control group (matched for gestational age, prior tubal pregnancy, tubal surgery or in vitro fertilization, clinical presentation, site of implantation, tubal rupture, and specific surgical procedure performed to treat the tubal pregnancy) treated via laparotomy.[34]

The patients must be followed postoperatively by serial biweekly quantitative β-hCG determinations until the levels reach nonpregnant values. This approach permits early detection of patients who have retained trophoblast. Such patients usually respond to a single dose of 50 mg methotrexate administered intramuscularly.[35]

JUSTIFICATION FOR CONSERVATIVE SURGICAL MANAGEMENT (REPRODUCTIVE OUTCOME)

Conservative surgical management for tubal pregnancy is undertaken principally to maintain the patient's reproductive potential. It is recognized that there will be some impairment of fertility in these patients. The degree of impairment will be influenced by a number of factors, which are listed in the box below. Furthermore, the woman who has had one ectopic pregnancy has an eightfold likelihood of a recurrence.

Factors influencing subsequent fertility in patients with ectopic pregnancy

Age
History of infertility
Parity
Previous abdominal surgery
Previous pelvic inflammatory disease
Status of tubes at time of intervention
Type of operative procedure
Number of prior ectopic pregnancies

We evaluated the risk factors by univariate and multivariate analysis. The number of prior tubal pregnancies and the status of the contralateral tube at the time of surgical intervention for tubal pregnancy proved to be the only two significant predictors of subsequent fertility outcome. The intrauterine and ectopic pregnancy rates subsequent to one tubal pregnancy were 61% and 7%, respectively; after two tubal pregnancies both intrauterine and tubal pregnancy rates became 28%; after three or more tubal pregnancies the intrauterine pregnancy rate was only 14%, whereas the rate of ectopic pregnancy rose to 72%.[36]

Irrespective of whether radical or conservative surgery is employed for the treatment of the initial tubal pregnancy, subsequent fertility is influenced by the status of the contralateral tube.[37,38] Earlier studies demonstrated no difference either in intrauterine or ectopic pregnancy rates subsequent to a tubal pregnancy whether treated radically or conservatively.[39,40] The value of conservative over radical surgery became evident in patients with single fallopian tubes. In one study 13 women with single fallopian tubes underwent conservative surgery for tubal pregnancy. One was lost to follow-up, another had intentionally avoided pregnancy. The remaining 11 patients all achieved term deliveries.[41] Other studies failed to report such optimistic outcomes. In one series, ten of 26 patients with single tubes who had a tubal pregnancy treated conservatively achieved a subsequent intrauterine pregnancy and five another tubal pregnancy.[42] Obviously, had these 26 patients been treated in a radical fashion, none of them would have conceived. In 15 patients with a tubal pregnancy each with only one "functional" fallopian tube who were treated by salpingotomy, a subsequent viable pregnancy rate of 53% with a recurrent ectopic pregnancy rate of 20% was reported.[43] In a similar study Oelsner et al. reported subsequent intrauterine and ectopic pregnancy rates of 48% and 43%, respectively.[44]

Microsurgical tubotubal anastomosis subsequent to an ectopic pregnancy, treated by segmental excision, was carried out in nine patients with single tubes. Five achieved a viable pregnancy and one a recurrent tubal pregnancy.[45] In a more recent survey of 17 such patients the same author noted that ten of them had achieved viable pregnancies and two had tubal pregnancies. It is noteworthy that none of these patients had prior reconstructive tubal surgery. The reproductive performance in patients with prior tubal surgery, in terms of intrauterine pregnancy subsequent to conservative treatment of tubal pregnancy in single remaining tubes, is disappointingly low and the tubal pregnancy rate very high.[36]

It would seem reasonable to conclude that conservative surgical management of tubal pregnancy offers greater hope of success to the woman who wishes to preserve reproductive potential, although she must accept the risk of recurrent ectopic pregnancy. The advantages are enhanced if the surgery can be performed laparoscopically.

In a study of 216 consecutive tubal pregnancies we found the operating time and the amount of postoperative analgesia to be significantly less with patients treated by laparoscopy compared with those treated by laparotomy. There was no difference in the rates of postoperative morbidity and retained trophoblast between the two groups. The subsequent fertility outcome was similar for both groups.[46] Other studies are confirmatory of these findings.[38,47] The laparoscopic approach is cosmetically preferable. The postoperative hospital stay is significantly shorter and has been estimated to result in average savings of $1,500 per patient.[47,48] In addition the patients usually return to full activity within 1 week of the surgery.

CONCLUSIONS

It is unclear whether or not some of the operative laparoscopic procedures to be described in the subsequent chapters offer any real advantage. The same cannot be said about the laparoscopic management of tubal pregnancy.

Despite advances in noninvasive diagnostic methods, recourse to laparoscopy may still be required in many instances where doubt exists. The laparoscopic surgery is relatively simple to perform, the results gratifying, and cost and recovery times are demonstrably reduced. Until more effective medical approaches have been developed, laparoscopic management will remain the approach of choice.

REFERENCES

1. Tait RL: Pathology and treatment of extrauterine pregnancy, *Br Med J* 2:317, 1884.
2. Stromme WB: Salpingotomy for tubal pregnancy, *Obstet Gynecol* 1:472, 1953.
3. Lund JJ: Early ectopic pregnancy, *J Obstet Gynecol Br Emp* 62:70, 1955.
4. Garcia AJ, Aubert JM, Sama J et al: Expectant management of presumed ectopic pregnancies, *Fertil Steril* 48:395-400, 1987.
5. Fernandez H, Rainhorn JD, Papiernik E et al: Spontaneous resolution of ectopic pregnancy, *Obstet Gynecol* 71:171-174, 1988.
6. Gomel V, Filmar S: Arrested tubal pregnancy, *Fertil Steril* 48:1043-1047, 1987.
7. Maymon R, Shulman A, Bar-Shira Maymon B et al: Ectopic pregnancy, the new gynecological epidemic disease: review of the modern work-up and the nonsurgical treatment option, *Int J Fertil* 37(3):146-164, 1992.
8. Sauer MV, Gorrill MJ, Rodi IA et al: Nonsurgical management of unruptured ectopic pregnancy: an extended clinical trial, *Fertil Steril* 48:752-755, 1987.
9. Stovall TG, Ling FW, Buster JE: Outpatient chemotherapy of unruptured ectopic pregnancy, *Fertil Steril* 51:435-438, 1989.
10. Stovall TG, Ling FW, Gray LA et al: Methotrexate treatment of unruptured ectopic pregnancy: a report of 100 cases, *Obstet Gynecol* 77:749-753, 1991.
11. Pansky M, Bukovsky I, Golan A et al: Local methotrexate injection: a nonsurgical treatment of ectopic pregnancy, *Am J Obstet Gynecol* 161:393-396, 1989.
12. Kooi S, Kock HCLV: Treatment of tubal pregnancy by local injection of methotrexate after adrenaline injection into the mesosalpinx: a report of 25 patients, *Fertil Steril* 54:580-584, 1990.
13. Wolf GC, Witt BR: Outpatient laparoscopic management of ectopic pregnancy with a local methotrexate injection, *J Reprod Med* 36:489-492, 1991.
14. Lindblom B, Hahlin M, Lundorff P: Treatment of tubal pregnancy by laparoscope-guided injection of prostaglandin F_{2a}, *Fertil Steril* 54:404-408, 1990.
15. Lang PF, Weiss PAM, Mayer HO et al: Conservative treatment of ectopic pregnancy with local injection of hyperosmolar glucose solution or prostaglandin F_{2a}: a prospective randomised study, *Lancet* 336:78-81, 1990.
16. Lang PF, Tamussino K, Honigl W et al: Treatment of unruptured tubal pregnancy by laparoscopic instillation of hyperosmolar glucose solution, *Am J Obstet Gynecol* 166:1378-1381, 1992.
17. Feichtinger W, Kemeter P: Conservative treatment of ectopic pregnancy by transvaginal aspiration under sonographic control and methotrexate injection, *Lancet* 1:381, 1987.
18. Timor-Tritsch I, Baxi L, Peisner DB: Transvaginal salpingocentesis: a new technique for treating ectopic pregnancy, *Am J Obstet Gynecol* 160:459-461, 1989.
19. Tulandi T, Atri M, Bret P, et al: Transvaginal intratubal methotrexate treatment of ectopic pregnancy, *Fertil Steril* 58:98-100, 1992.
20. Fernandez H, Benifla J-L, Lelaidier C et al: Methotrexate treatment of ectopic pregnancy: 100 cases treated by primary transvaginal injection under sonographic control, *Fertil Steril* 59:773-777, 1993.
21. Stovall TG, Ling FW, Gray LA: Single-dose methotrexate for treatment of ectopic pregnancy, *Obstet Gynecol* 77:754-757, 1991.
22. Mottla GL, Rulin MC, Guzick DS: Lack of resolution of ectopic pregnancy by intratubal injection of methotrexate, *Fertil Steril* 57:685-687, 1992.
23. Gomel V: Microsurgery in female infertility. Boston, 1983, Little Brown & Co.
24. Budowick M, Johnson TRB, Genadry R et al: The histopathology of the developing tubal ectopic pregnancy, *Fertil Steril* 34:169-171, 1980.
25. Mettler L, Semm K: Management of ectopic pregnancy: a shift from laparotomy to pelviscopy, *Int J Fertil* 33:389-392, 1988.
26. Donnez J, Nisolle M: Laparoscopic treatment of ampullary tubal pregnancy, *J Gynecol Surg* 5:157-162, 1989.
27. Gomel V, Taylor PJ, Yuzpe AA: Laparoscopy and hysteroscopy in gynecologic practice. Chicago, 1986, Year Book Medical Publishers, Inc.
28. Semm K: Operative manual for endoscopic abdominal surgery. Chicago, 1987, Year Book Medical Publishers, Inc.
29. Gomel V: La laparoscopia en el diagnostico y tratamiento de la gestacion ectopica, *Gine Dips* 2:85-87, 1978.
30. Stangel JJ, Gomel V: Techniques in conservative surgery for tubal gestation, *Clin Obstet Gynecol* 23:1221-1228, 1980.
31. Gomel V: Management of tubal pregnancy: transabdominal -In press.
32. Reich H, DeCaprio J, McGlynn F et al: Aquaexpresion for laparoscopic removal of distal tubal pregnancies, *Gyn Endo* 1:69-71, 1992.
33. Pouly JL, Mahnes H, Mage G, et al: Conservative laparoscopic treatment of 321 ectopic pregnancies, *Fertil Steril* 46:1093-1097, 1986.
34. Zouves C, Gomel V: Tubal pregnancy: management by operative laparoscopy versus laparotomy, *Infertil* 12:23-29, 1989.
35. Gomel V, Urman CB: Laparoscopic surgery, *Curr Op Obst Gynecol* 2:303-311, 1990.
36. Urman B, Zouves C, Gomel V: Fertility outcome following tubal pregnancy, *Acta Eur Fertil* 22:205-208, 1991.
37. Tuomivaara L, Kauppila A: Radical or conservative surgery for ectopic pregnancy? A follow-up study of fertility of 323 patients, *Fertil Steril* 50:580-583, 1988.
38. Silva PD, Schaper AM, Rooney B: Reproductive outcome after 143 laparoscopic procedures for ectopic pregnancy, *Obstet Gynecol* 81:710-715, 1993.
39. Timonen S, Nieminen U: Tubal pregnancy, choice of operative method of treatment, *Acta Obst Gynecol Scand* 46:327-339, 1967.
40. DeCherney A, Kase N: The conservative surgical management of unruptured ectopic pregnancy, *Obstet Gynecol* 54:451-455, 1979.
41. Valle JA, Lifchez AS: Reproductive outcome following conservative surgery for tubal pregnancy in women with a single fallopian tube, *Fertil Steril* 39:316-320, 1983.

42. Hallatt JG: Tubal conservation in ectopic pregnancy: a study of 200 cases, *Am J Obstet Gynecol* 154:1216-1221, 1986.
43. DeCherney A, Maheaux R, Naftolin F: Salpingostomy for ectopic pregnancy in the sole patient oviduct: reproductive outcome, *Fertil Steril* 37:619-622, 1982.
44. Oelsner G, Rabinovitch O, Morad J et al: Reproductive outcome after microsurgical treatment of tubal pregnancy in women with a single fallopian tube, *J Reprod Med* 31:483-486, 1986.
45. Gomel V: Microsurgery in female infertility. Boston, 1983, Little Brown & Co.
46. Zouves C, Urman B, Gomel V: Laparoscopic surgical treatment of tubal pregnancy. A safe, effective alternative to laparotomy, *J Reprod Med* 37:205-209, 1992.
47. Murphy AA, Nager CW, Wujek JJ, et al: Operative laparoscopy versus laparotomy for the management of ectopic pregnancy: a prospective trial, *Fertil Steril* 47:1180-1185, 1992.

Chapter 15

FERTILITY-PROMOTING PROCEDURES AND ASSISTED REPRODUCTIVE TECHNOLOGY

The investigation of the infertile couple has been described in Chapter 9. A preliminary hysterosalpingography and observation at laparoscopy, including chromopertubation, are complementary procedures in assessing the status of the fallopian tubes. With distal tubal disease this assessment can be refined further by performing a retrograde salpingoscopy. This chapter will describe in detail the performance of laparoscopic fertility-promoting procedures and will include a discussion of salpingo-ovariolysis, treatment of fimbrial phimosis, neosalpingostomy, and tubotubal anastomosis. The role of laparoscopy in assisted reproductive technology (ART) will be considered.

Fertility-promoting procedures were among the first operations for which operative laparoscopy was employed. Our center was very active in the development and application of both microsurgical and laparoscopic techniques to restore fertility.[1-4]

GENERAL PRINCIPLES

The goal of fertility-promoting surgery is to restore the functional integrity of the reproductive organs and to ensure that de novo postoperative adhesions and re-formation of adhesions are kept to an absolute minimum. Microsurgery represents the gold standard of reproductive surgery. It is essential to apply microsurgical principles to laparoscopic surgery. These principles include:

1. Tissue trauma is kept to a minimum by using as atraumatic a technique as possible, keeping serosal surfaces moistened to avoid drying, and preventing introduction of foreign substances into the peritoneal cavity.
2. Meticulous hemostasis with minimal adjacent tissue damage.
3. Complete excision of abnormal tissue.
4. Precise alignment and approximation of tissue planes.
5. Magnification permits appreciation of normal and pathologic morphologic details and facilitates the application of the preceding principles. Furthermore it enables the use of microsurgical instruments and sutures of fine gauge.[5]

Operative laparoscopy is performed within a closed peritoneal cavity, which largely prevents drying of the peritoneal surfaces. This protective effect will be eliminated if large volumes of gas are insufflated, as happens during the removal of smoke (plume) generated by the use of laser energy. Working within a closed environment eliminates the necessity to use packs and prevents the introduction of foreign materials such as lint and talcum powder. The laparoscope confers a degree of magnification that can be enhanced by the use of a magnification device attached to the proximal lens. In addition it is possible to bring the distal end of the laparoscope close to the area of interest and achieve excellent visibility and illumination. Intraoperative irrigation of tissues to keep them moistened and expose any bleeders is also a fundamental of laparoscopic surgery. Furthermore, the pressure effect of the pneumoperitoneum diminishes venous oozing and permits spontaneous coagulation of minor bleeders. The use of fine electrodes to achieve precise electrosurgical hemostasis is also possible.

Like microsurgery, laparoscopic procedures are performed with few instruments. But these laparoscopic instruments require still further refinement. Furthermore the length of these instruments and the cannula in the abdominal wall acting as a fulcrum increase the force applied to tissue by the working end of the instruments. This may generate undue trauma.

Laparoscopic suturing is awkward and more time consuming. The use of fine microsurgical sutures is difficult, which frequently leads to the use of larger sutures and the application of fewer sutures. The latter may compromise proper alignment and approximation of tissue planes, especially in tubo-tubal anastomosis. Many of these limitations are simply technical problems which will be overcome in time.

There are other limitations. Hand-eye coordination is somewhat hampered by the lack of stereoscopic vision. This and the less precise instruments in use hamper the surgeon's ability to handle tissues with the same degree of delicacy and accuracy that can be achieved by microsurgery.

It is difficult to assess the cumulative effect of these conflicting factors, although it is possible that some of the advantages of the laparoscopic approach are indeed compromised by the drawbacks. This is already evident with present laparoscopic techniques for tubotubal anastomosis.

SURGICAL TECHNIQUE

Immediate preoperative preparation

The hysterosalpingogram films are placed on the viewing box. Selective antibiotic prophylaxis (usually 1 gm cephazol) is administered preoperatively by intravenous route.

The anesthetized patient is placed in the lithotomy position, which permits access to the genital tract from below. The patient is prepared and draped. A rigid uterine cannula is attached to the cervix by means of a tenaculum (Fig. 15-1). The cannula permits both the performance of interoperative chromopertubation and the manipulation of the uterus during the procedure. Exposure may be enhanced by uterine manipulation, and the uterus can be made to support the adnexal structures upon which the surgeon is working.

The laparoscope is usually introduced intraumbilically and the abdomen and pelvis surveyed through the telescope. Two additional portals of entry are usually employed, one suprapubically in the midline and the other on the right at the McBurneys point. When necessary an additional third portal is placed in the left lower quadrant. After initial inspection the camera is attached to the laparoscope. The procedure is performed viewing the field on the television monitor.

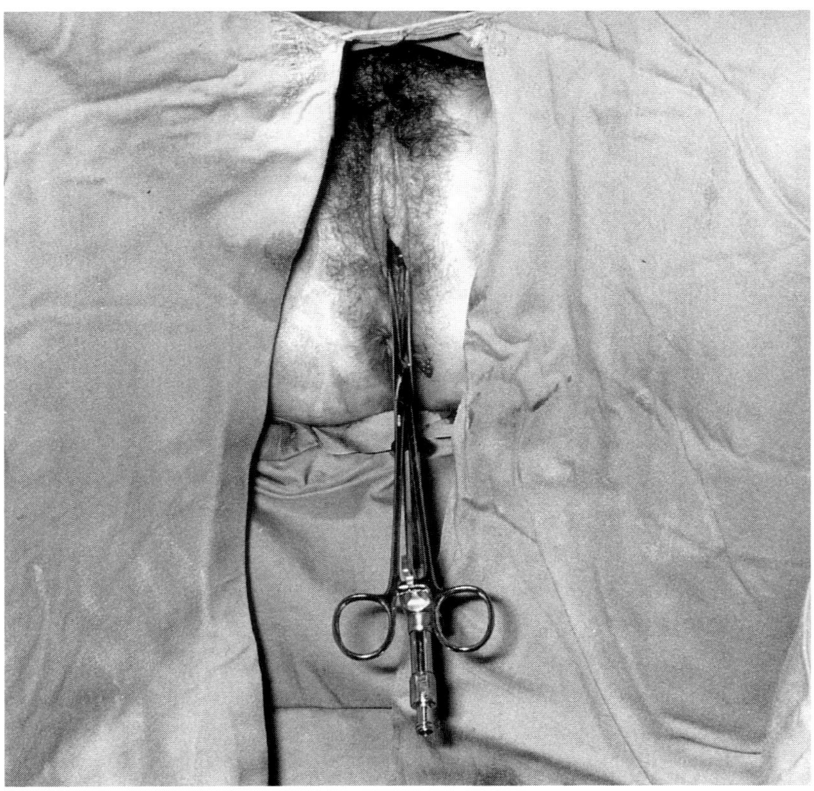

Fig. 15-1. A rigid uterine cannula is attached to the cervix by means of a tenaculum.

Adhesions may be present between the omentum and anterior abdominal wall. These may limit visualization of the pelvic organs. It will be necessary to lyse these adhesions first as has been described in Chapter 7.

Salpingo-ovariolysis

Periadnexal adhesions may be the sole abnormality and cause infertility by encapsulating the tubes, which themselves are normally patent, and/or the ovaries preventing the capture of the oocyte by the fallopian tube. Once the pelvic organs have been completely exposed they are thoroughly inspected. The location, extent, and nature of the periadnexal adhesions are assessed. Chromopertubation is performed to confirm tubal patency. Periadnexal adhesions frequently coexist with other tubal lesions, especially distal tubal occlusion. In such cases salpingo-ovariolysis becomes the first step of the reconstructive procedure.

The performance of effective and safe salpingo-ovariolysis requires clear identification and exposure of each adhesive layer that is grasped and retracted. Dissection should always begin in well exposed areas (Fig. 15-2, *A*). It is critical that the attachments of the adhesions are clearly identified and what lies behind recognized before dissection begins.

The layers of adhesions are exposed and divided along the organ of interest. One adhesive layer must be divided at a time. Adhesions that initially appear to be one single layer are frequently composed of two layers. Each layer may be affixed to the organ of interest at different sites. Identification of each of the separate layers permits transec-

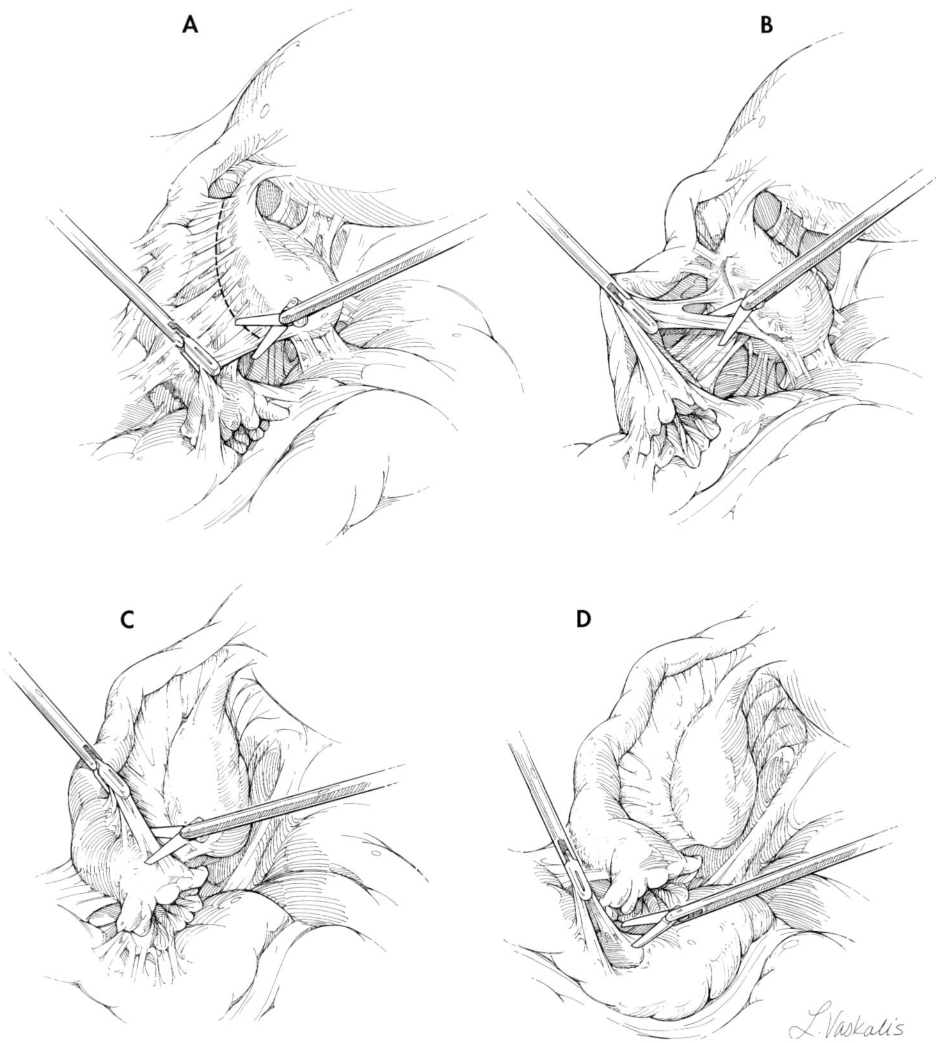

Fig. 15-2. Salpingo-ovariolysis. **A,** Division of adhesions commences in a well-exposed area. **B,** Adhesions are stretched and are divided one layer at a time parallel to the organ of interest. **C,** Broad adhesions are freed at all points and removed from the peritoneal cavity. **D,** Salpingo-ovariolysis being completed.

tion without damaging the serosal surface of the organ. Damage may well occur if two layers are divided at once.

There is a fixed sequence of steps. The adhesion is grasped with forceps at about its midpoint and gentle traction exerted, thus exposing one of its attachments. A small incision is made over a clear area to elucidate what lies behind the adhesion and determine whether it is composed of a single layer or double layers. The adhesion is divided parallel to the target organ, pausing to secure any obvious blood vessels prior to division (Fig. 15-2, *B*). The line of division should be as close to the serosa of the structure to which it is attached as is compatible with safety. Broad adhesions are dissected free at all points of attachment and removed through one of the ancillary portals (Fig. 15-2, *C*). Shallow adhesions are simply divided. The adhesiolysis continues until the normal pelvic anatomy has been restored (Fig. 15-2, *D*).

Transection can be achieved mechanically using sharp scissors, electrosurgically using a microelectrode, or with laser energy. We prefer the use of scissors and obtain hemostasis by desiccating any bleeders along the transection line, either with a monopolar electrode or with a microbipolar forceps. Larger vessels along the transection line are desiccated prior to division. With cohesive adhesions it will be necessary to identify the dissection plane by making a small incision and developing a tissue plane either by spreading the jaws of the scissors, by blunt dissection, or by hydrodissection. No thermal energy should be used in such cases.

Pelvic lavage is then carried out with irrigation solution (heparinized lactated Ringers) until the fluid is clear. The pelvis is then flooded with the irrigation solution, the pneumoperitoneum pressure reduced, and the region inspected with the distal lens of the telescope under the surface of the fluid. Any small bleeding vessels will be very obvious and can be dealt with. In addition, if the fimbria are inspected in this fashion, any fine interfimbrial adhesions can be seen and gently removed.

With fertility-promoting procedures many authors leave a physiologic solution or hyskon in the pelvis to reduce postoperative adhesions. At the close of the procedure we leave 150 to 200 ml of lactated Ringers containing 500 mg of hydrocortisone succinate in the pelvis.

Fimbrioplasty

This term is used to describe reconstruction of the existing fimbria of a partially or totally occluded fallopian tube. Tubal phimosis may be caused by the agglutination of the fimbria only. In this case a degree of patency will be noted. Chromopertubation will distend the ampulla before escape of the dye solution into the peritoneal cavity occurs. The agglutinated fimbrial end of the tube may also be covered by a fibrous layer, which may lead to complete occlusion. Less frequently, the tube is stenosed at the level of the abdominal tubal ostium located at the apex of the infundibulum (prefimbrial phimosis). In such cases the fimbriated end of the tube may have a normal appearance.

Frequently, periadnexal adhesions will be present. It will be necessary first to perform a salpingo-ovariolysis. Once the tube and ovary are totally freed of the adhesions, it will be possible to assess the condition of the tube. The tube is stabilized with an atraumatic grasping forceps or blunt probe and held either against the uterine fundus, which can be made to support it, or the pelvic side wall.

When the distal end of the tube is covered by a fibrous layer, the fibrous tissue must be either incised or removed to expose the agglutinated fimbria. Disagglutination of the fimbria can be accomplished using a 3 mm alligator jawed forceps. The forceps is introduced through the stenosed opening while the tube is distended by chromopertubation (Fig. 15-3, *A*). Once inserted, the jaws of the forceps are opened within the tube (Fig. 15-3, *B*) and gently withdrawn, while keeping the jaws open thus breaking down some of the adhesive process (Fig. 15-3, *C*). It will be necessary to repeat this step several times, altering the axis of insertion of the jaws, until the surgeon is satisfied that the fimbria have been completely disagglutinated. There is usually very little bleeding and if there are any small bleeding vessels they can be spot desiccated.

Correction of prefimbrial phimosis requires placement of an incision on the antimesosalpingeal border of the distal tube to relieve the stenosis. The tube is grasped in the midampullary region with an atraumatic forceps and immobilized by holding it against the uterine fundus. A second set of forceps is used to insert a narrow Teflon probe or stent through the ostium. An incision is placed along the antimesosalpingeal border of the tube electrosurgically using a needle electrode. The incision is started at the fimbriated end and continued into the distal ampulla past the divided stenotic ring (Fig. 15-4, *A* and *B*). Any bleeding vessels are spot desiccated with the needle. In an attempt to maintain tubal patency, it may be necessary to place 6-0 interrupted sutures (see Chapter 7) at the apices of each of the flaps that have been created (Fig. 15-4, *C*). Alternatively, the serosal aspect can be lightly dessicated as will be described immediately below.

Pelvic lavage and thorough inspection of the operative site is carried out as described earlier.

Salpingostomy (Salpingoneostomy)

If the distal end of the tube is completely occluded, resulting in the formation of a hydrosalpinx, its reconstruction will necessitate the creation of a new stoma (salpingoneostomy). The prognosis for such patients is very dependent on the structural, hence functional, integrity of the tubal epithelium. It is possible to evaluate the tubal epithelium, at least that of the ampulla, by performing an intraoperative, retrograde salpingoscopy, as will be described later.

A preliminary salpingo-ovariolysis will frequently be

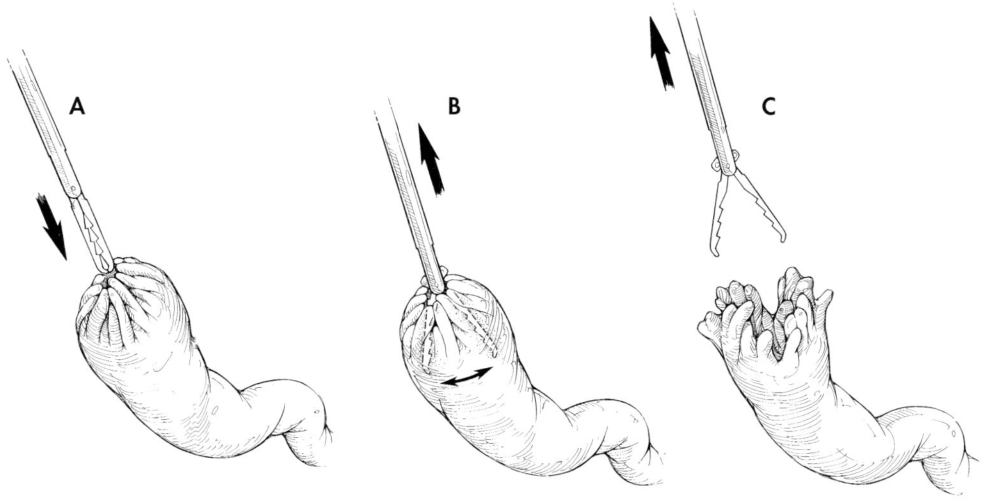

Fig. 15-3. Fimbrioplasty: Disagglutination of fimbria. **A,** The 3 mm alligator jawed forceps is introduced through the sterosed opening. **B,** The jaws of the forceps are opened within the tube. **C,** The forceps are gently withdrawn while keeping the jaws open.

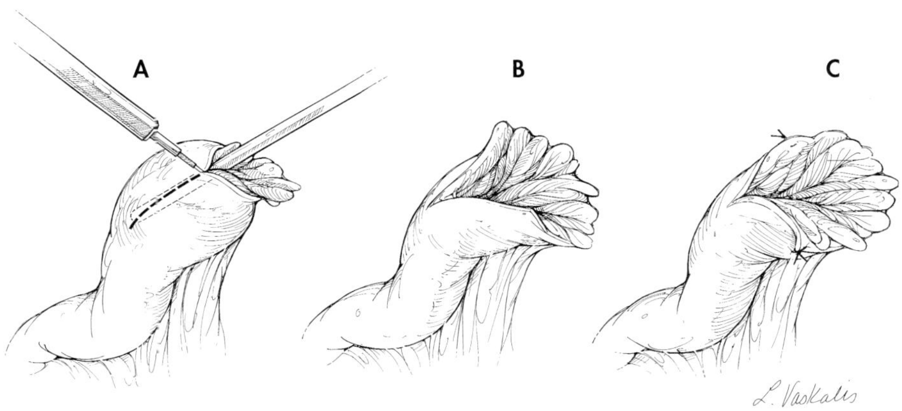

Fig. 15-4. Fimbrioplasty: correction of prefimbrial phimosis. **A** and **B,** An incision is placed at the antimesosalpingeal border of the tube. **C**, Completed procedure with flaps everted.

necessary, since periadnexal adhesions often coexist with distal tubal occlusion. Once this portion of the procedure is complete, the tube is inspected thoroughly. The surgeon must ensure that the distal tube is free. If it is adherent to the ovary, it will be necessary to free this portion of the tube from the ovary (Fig. 15-5). This is accomplished with sharp and blunt dissection. The dissection is continued until the tubo-ovarian ligament is visualized. Further dissection puts the vessels within this ligament at risk.

The tube is grasped near the occluded distal end with atraumatic forceps. Inspection of the free distal tube will often reveal a centrally placed avascular area (dimple) from which avascular scarred lines extend in a cartwheel manner (Fig. 15-6, *A*). Chromopertubation at this stage will confirm patency of the proximal tube, distend the ampulla, and facilitate observation of the described changes.

The technique employed to fashion a salpingostomy is adopted from that used in microsurgery. The tube is stabilized and a small incision is made into the lumen of the tube over the central dimple using scissors, electrosurgery, or laser energy. Once the lumen is entered the dilute dye solution will escape. It is now that salpingoscopy is carried out. If it is decided to continue with the salpingostomy, the atraumatic grasping forceps are moved to the edge of the small opening made over the central dimple. It will now be necessary to incise along the avascular areas radiating from

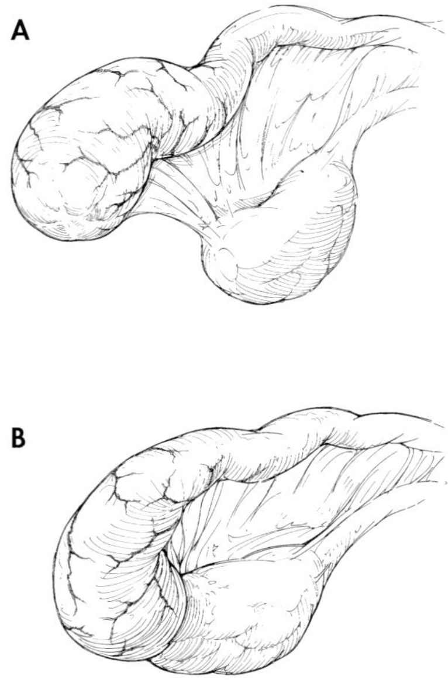

Fig. 15-5. Hydrosalpinx. **A,** The occluded distal tube is free. **B,** The occluded distal tube is adherent to the ovary.

this initial opening. The first incision is made along an avascular line toward the ovary to fashion a new fimbria ovarica (Fig. 15-6, *B*). The tube is now everted by regrasping the edge of the incision and exerting pressure on the serosal aspect of the tube about 1 cm proximal to the cut surface using the tip of a blunt instrument or the side of the scissors. By everting the tube the surgeon is able to visualize the distal tube from within and identify avascular areas between mucosal folds along the circumference of the tube. These avascular areas are incised from within the tube, thus avoiding cutting through the vascular mucosal folds, which will be fashioned as new fimbria (Fig. 15-6, *C*). This procedure is continued until a satisfactory new stoma has been created (Fig. 15-6, *D*).

There is no clear evidence that fixing the edges of this new stoma to the serosa of the tube improves the outcome. However, if eversion is desired, it can be accomplished either by desiccating the serosal aspect of the flaps created by the formation of the new stoma with low power electrical energy or with a defocussed laser. Alternatively two or three interrupted sutures may be applied using a 6-0 absorbably synthetic material (Vicryl, Dexon, or polysorb) (Fig. 15-6, *E*). At the end of the procedure the pelvic lavage is

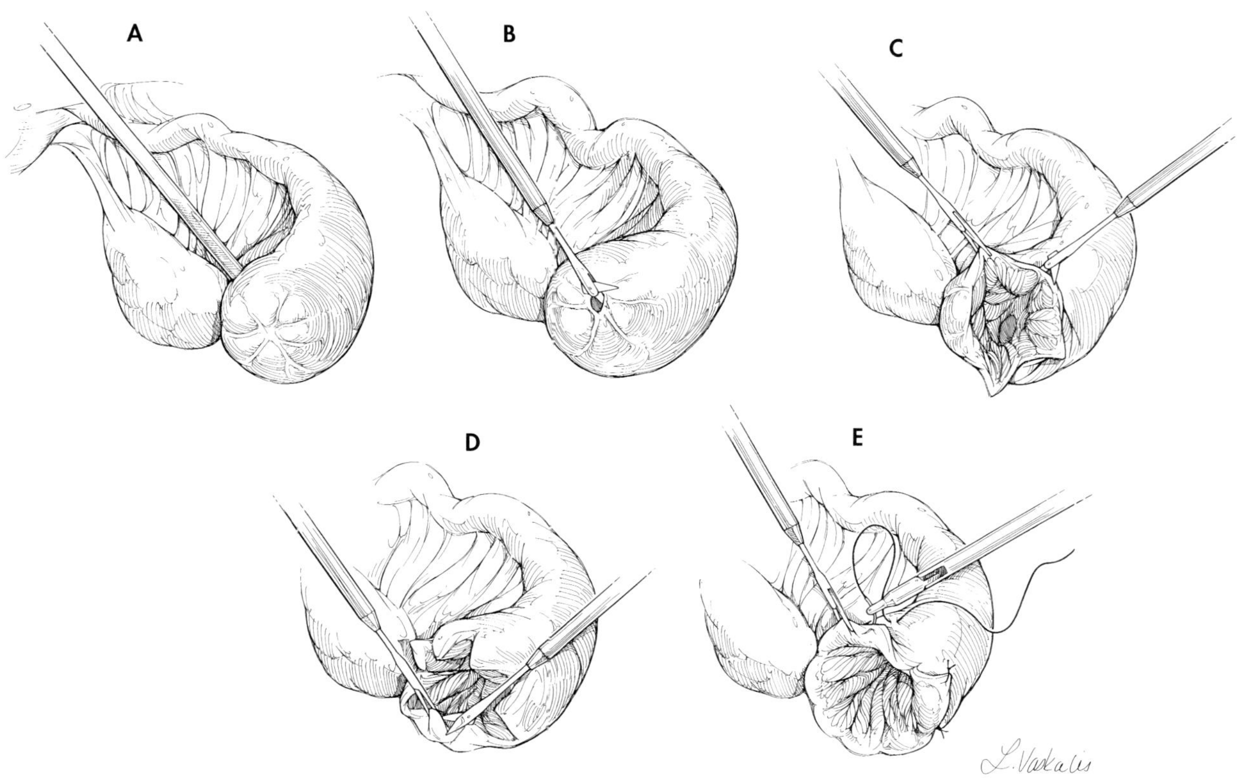

Fig. 15-6. Salpingostomy. **A**, The occluded distal end of the tube usually has a centrally placed avascular area from which avascular scarred lines extend in a cartwheel manner. **B**, The first incision is made along an avascular line toward the ovary. **C,** Avascular lines are incised viewing from within the tube along the circumference of the initial opening. **D**, Cutting along the avascular lines is continued until a satisfactory stoma is fashioned. **E**, The flaps may be everted by placement of two or three 6-0 absorbable synthetic sutures.

performed, the operative site inspected to ensure hemostasis has been achieved, and 150 to 200 mls of lactated Ringers containing 500 mg of hydrocortisone succinate is left in the pelvis.

Retrograde salpingoscopy

Retrograde salpingoscopy can be performed using a hysteroscope within its own sheath. This instrument is introduced into the peritoneal cavity through one of the ancillary portals. A small opening is made at the occluded outer end of the tube as described earlier. The tube is held with an atraumatic forceps in a way to enable the introduction of the hysteroscope into the fallopian tube. The tip of the hysteroscope is introduced through the small incision and the tube distended with a physiologic solution which is injected through the sheath of the hysteroscope. The ampullary epithelium is assessed by gradually advancing the hysteroscope through the tube. In this fashion it is possible to assess all of the ampulla by introducing the scope to the vicinity of the ampullary-isthmic junction. Extensive epithelial destruction or the presence of extensive intra-ampullary adhesions may be sufficient grounds to abandon any further attempt at tubal reconstruction. Based upon the findings, there may even be grounds to consider a salpingectomy. The information yielded by salpingoscopy will influence the decision to proceed with IVF sooner rather than later even if a salpingostomy had been performed.

RESULTS OF RECONSTRUCTIVE PROCEDURES FOR DISTAL TUBAL OCCLUSION

It is difficult to compare the results of many published series. In part this is due to enormous variations in classification of the lesions and in study design. For example, inclusion of fimbrioplasty cases in a salpingostomy series will produce an artificial improvement in the outcome. In addition, the only outcome of real value is the delivery of viable infant. Those reports which have simply recorded the crude pregnancy rates do not allow for the loss due to spontaneous abortion or, more importantly, ectopic pregnancies that occur following such procedures with discouraging frequency. Finally, if the tubes were patent prior to surgery, as is the case with periadnexal adhesive disease and tubal phimosis, the patient's infertility is not absolute. The Canadian Infertility Evaluation Study Group reported the results of the multicenter, controlled, randomized study on patients with periadnexal adhesions.[6] The aim of this study was to assess the treatment-dependent and treatment independent pregnancy rates. After a 2-year follow-up period the pregnancy rates were 45% among the 69 patients in the treated group and only 16% in the 78 patients in the untreated control group. This study demonstrates clearly the value of salpingo-ovariolysis for periadnexal adhesions.

Salpingo-ovariolysis

Laparoscopic salpingo-ovariolysis was first reported by Gomel in 1975.[3] In this study of 33 patients, 24 were followed for more than 1 year. The intrauterine pregnancy rate among these 24 patients was 59%. The same author later reported 37 patients followed for more than 18 months. Intrauterine pregnancies occured in 20 (57%) and tubal pregnancies in two patients.[7] In 1979, Mettler et al.,[8] reported crude pregnancy rates of 36% in 20 patients who had laparoscopic salpingolysis and 21% among 19 patients who had ovariolysis. Unfortunately the anatomic location and outcomes of these pregnancies were not specified.

Gomel, in 1983,[9] reported a series of 92 salpingo-ovariolysis patients. Seventy-nine of these patients had severe and 13 had moderate periadnexal adhesions, and ovum pick up by the fimbriae was deemed impossible or greatly hampered in all. All of the patients had at least 20 months of infertility. After a postoperative follow-up period of at least nine months, 57 of the 92 patients (62%) had intrauterine pregnancies; 54 patients (59%) had live births, and five had ectopic pregnancies. After the publication of this study, among those patients who could not be contacted and thus were reported as failures, we became aware of four additional patients who had live births. These results are similar to those yielded by microsurgical techniques.

A study from the United States[10] of 50 such patients reported an intrauterine pregnancy rate of 56% and another study from Europe[11] reported an intrauterine pregnancy rate of 52% among 93 patients. The outcome of these pregnancies was not specified. Similar results have been obtained in more recent reports.[12] The rate of ectopic pregnancies in these series (ranging from 4% to 7.5% of patients who had undergone surgery) clearly demonstrates that periadnexal disease is not an entity confined to periadnexal structures alone and that there must be concomitant damage of the tubal endothelium.

Fimbrioplasty

Very few investigators have classified fimbrioplasty as an independent procedure. In a study from our center of 40 such patients, viable pregnancies occurred in 19 (48%) patients. There were two ectopic gestations.[13] In the previously mentioned study by Mettler et al.,[8] the crude pregnancy rate was 31% among 51 women. Once again, the anatomic location or outcome of these pregnancies was not recorded. Dubuisson et al.[14] followed 31 women who were submitted to fimbrioplasty. After 18 months' follow-up eight patients (25.8%) achieved intrauterine pregnancies and ectopic pregnancies occurred in four (12.9%). The rate of intrauterine pregnancy in their fimbrioplasty group was inferior to that yielded in the salpingostomy group, which is surprising. Canis et al.[15] reported 32 such patients; 16 (50%) achieved intrauterine pregnancies but the outcome of these was not given. What is surprising in this group of patients is that no tubal pregnancies ensued. While all of these studies suffer from having been uncontrolled, the reported results approximate those yielded by microsurgical series.

Salpingostomy

The requirement is less stringent that studies of surgery for distal tubal occlusion be controlled, since the occurrence of pregnancy in such women, if untreated, would be highly unlikely.[16] It is reasonable to compare the results of laparoscopic surgery to those yielded by microsurgery for the same condition, even though such comparisons of one study with another do not satisfy the rigorous demands of properly conducted randomized prospective studies.

Laparoscopic salpingostomy was first described in 1977 in a small series of nine patients, eight of whom had previously undergone attempted tubal repair by laparotomy.[17] Four women conceived and later were delivered of live infants. The one patient in whom the laparoscopic approach was the primary surgery was included among the successes. In the previously cited study by Mettler et al.,[8] ten of 38 women achieved pregnancies after salpingostomy. Once again, the site and outcome of these pregnancies was not stated. Daniell and Herbert[18] reported the results in a group of 22 women who had salpingostomy performed using the CO_2 laser. Four of the patients achieved intrauterine pregnancies, one of which aborted spontaneously. Three patients (14%) had live births and one a tubal pregnancy. Dubuisson et al.,[14] in the previously cited publication, also reported 34 salpingostomy patients. There were ten (29.4%) intrauterine pregnancies (outcome not reported) and one tubal pregnancy. In a recent French study of 87 patients,[15] 29 achieved intrauterine pregnancies, the outcomes of which were not revealed, and six had tubal pregnancies. These 87 patients were subdivided into four groups according to the severity of the tubal damage. Closer scrutiny of this report demonstrates that stage 1, the most favorable group (32 patients) in their classification, refers to tubes demonstrating "partial occlusion (phimotic tube)." These were patients requiring a fimbrioplasty and not a salpingostomy and should have been reported as such. Sixteen of these 32 patients achieved intrauterine pregnancies; we have cited this group of patients earlier. Among the remaining 55 patients with completely occluded tubes in this series, 13 (22.8%) achieved intrauterine pregnancies and six (10.9%) tubal pregnancies. In a recent study of 22 salpingostomy patients from our center, 5 had viable births and one a tubal pregnancy.[19]

The American Fertility Society has approved a classification based upon those factors that clearly influence the prognosis for salpingostomy.[20] (See Fig. 9-15 for the AFS classification.) These factors include:

1. Distal ampullary diameter
2. Thickness of the tubal wall
3. Status of the tubal endothelium
4. Extent of any adhesions
5. Nature of the adhesions

Ninety patients underwent microsurgical salpingotomy of whom, based upon the AFS classification, 73 patients were severe (poor prognosis) and 17 mild (good prognosis). The intrauterine pregnancy rates were 18% and 71%, respectively ($p < 0.05$).[21]

The results yielded by laparoscopic salpingostomy appear to be somewhat inferior to those obtained by microsurgery. Therefore in very carefully selected cases it might be better to offer the patient microsurgery. We have been performing such microsurgical procedures through minilaparotomy incisions since 1986. Before and after the operation the site of the incision is infiltrated with a long-acting local anesthetic agent. Once the incision has been closed a regional nerve block is established. These patients are admitted on the same day for their surgery. Because of the smaller incision, the local anesthetic, and minimal bowel manipulation, only small amounts of postoperative systemic analgesics are required. These patients are discharged and return to normal activity almost as rapidly as those who have had procedures performed laparoscopically.[22] It will be obvious to the reader that we are enthusiastic proponents of laparoscopic surgery. Nevertheless we do not let this enthusiasm blind us to the possibility that some procedures may still be performed better by improvements in the traditional methods.

For the majority of patients, the laparoscopic procedure, which can be effected at the same time as the diagnostic laparoscopy, while offering a marginally reduced likelihood of successful pregnancy has distinct advantages because of the decreased cost and avoidance of a second procedure.

For those patients in whom the severity of the disease precludes any attempt at laparoscopic repair or who have undergone one attempted tubal repair unsuccessfully, irrespective of method, IVF is the best option for achieving a pregnancy and delivery.[23]

TUBOTUBAL ANASTOMOSIS

Tubotubal anastomosis is usually performed to reverse a previous sterilization and on rare occasions to correct a mid-tubal occlusion. The results which have been achieved using microsurgical techniques[22-24] are unlikely to be bettered laparoscopically. Furthermore, microsurgical repair is relatively easy to effect using the minilaparotomy local anesthesia technique described earlier in this chapter. We remain to be persuaded that the laparoscopic approach to tubotubal anastomosis offers any great advantages and describe it for the sake of completeness.

The principles of tubotubal anastomosis are well known.[25] The occluded segment must be excised until healthy tubal tissue is identified. Care must be taken to avoid compromizing the tubal vasculature. Hemostasis must be secured. The cut edges must be aligned accurately and rejoined with fine material, which will provoke the least inflammatory response. While each of these steps is now routine in microsurgical practice, they all present challenges to the laparoscopist.

Technique

Tubotubal anastomosis is performed using two or three ancillary portals. The tubes are examined in their entirety (Fig. 15-7, *A*). Any necessary salpingo-ovariolysis is performed. The proximal segment is distended by transcervical chromopertubation. The occluded end is grasped with fine forceps and held so that the fine scissors can approach the antimesosalpingeal border of the tube at right angles. The tube is transected taking care to avoid the vascular arcade (Fig. 15-7, *B*). The lumen will be identified as the dye solution escapes. The proximal cut surface is inspected with the laparoscope in close proximity to confirm that the tissues are healthy (Fig. 15-7, *C*). If such is not the case further incisions are made proximal to the first until normal tissues are encountered. In the case of an isthmic-isthmic anastomosis, the occluded distal stump is similarly treated. A fine polythene cannula introduced through one of the ancillary portals is guided into the fimbriated end and dye solution injected to confirm continuity of the distal tubal lumen.

At this point the occluded portion will be tethered by a short segment of mesosalpinx. This is now divided with a

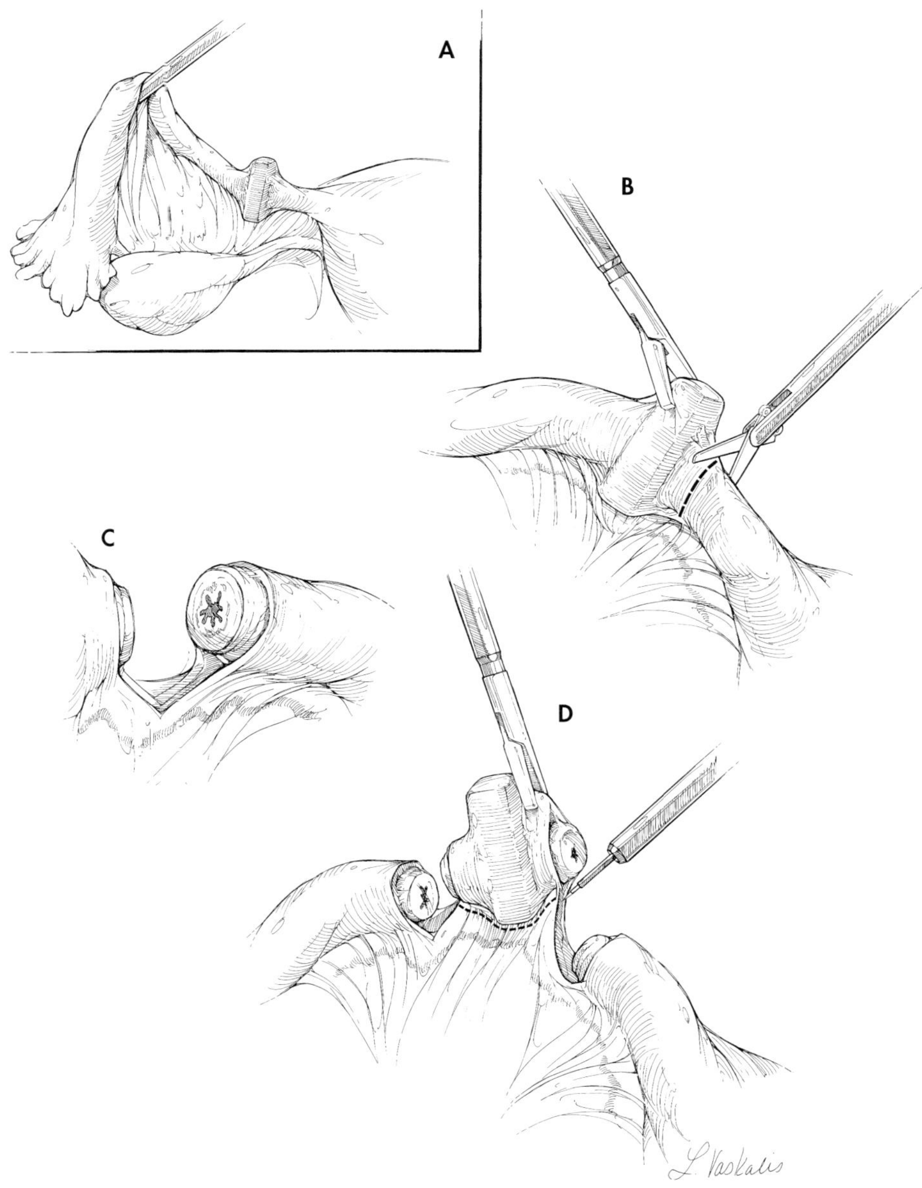

Fig. 15-7. Tubotubal anastomosis—isthmic-isthmic. **A**, Prior clip sterilization. **B**, The tube is elevated and transected at right angles with scissors. **C**, The cut surface is examined under magnification to ensure that it is normal. **D**, The occluded tube (including clip) is excised, remaining close to the tube, with a microelectrode. *Continued.*

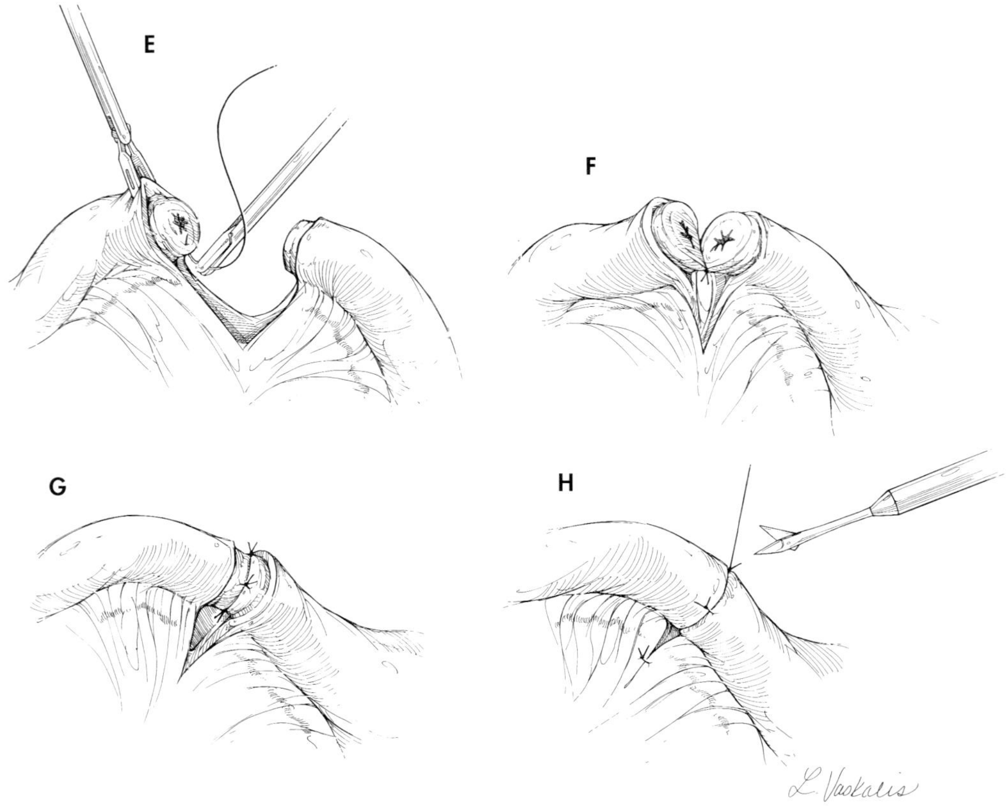

Fig. 15-7, cont'd. E and **F**, The first suture is placed at 6 o'clock position and tied. Knots remain external. **G**, Apposition of the muscularis and epithelium is completed by placement of additional sutures. **H**, The anastomosis is completed by apposing the serosa and mesosalpinx.

fine unipolar microelectrode. The incision is placed close to the tube to avoid the mesosalpingeal vessels (Fig. 15-7, *D*). The excised tissue is easily removed through the ancillary portal. Bleeding from the cut end of the tubes is exposed by irrigation and any vessels in the muscularis are dealt with using the microelectrode. Oozing from the epithelium is self-limiting and should not be desiccated.

Isthmic-ampullary anastomosis is technically more difficult because of the disparity in luminal caliber. It is necessary to introduce the polythene cannula and distend the distal tube. When the site of occlusion is so identified it is grasped with fine grasping forceps and elevated. Fine sharp scissors are used to incise the serosa, which is dissected to expose the underlying muscularis. The muscularis is regrasped at the tip of the occlusion and the scissors are used to fashion an opening which will correspond in size to the diameter of the lumen of the proximal tubal segment.

Irrespective of the site of anastomosis (isthmic-isthmic or isthmic-ampullary), apposition of the tubal segments is carried out as follows. A 7-0 Vicryl suture swaged to ⅜ curve needle is introduced into the peritoneal cavity and loaded in a needle driver. The first suture is placed at 6 o'clock, to include the muscularis and epithelium in such a way that when tied the knot remains peripheral (Fig. 15-7, *E* and *F*). The first suture is critical to the proper alignment of the two segments and must be placed accurately. All knot tieing is intracorporeal. This first suture apposes the two segments and facilitates placement of subsequent sutures. The number of additional sutures required will depend upon the circumference of the tubal lumina. Once the primary layer of sutures is completed, transcervical chromopertubation should reveal tubal patency (Fig. 15-7, *G*). The serosa and the defect in the mesosalpinx are now repaired with interrupted or continuous sutures using the same suture material (Fig. 15-7, *H*). The same technique is used to repair the other tube. Pelvic lavage is performed. Koh and Janik have presented a video of this technique.[26]

The technique just described differs little from microsurgery, although 7-0 rather than 8-0 sutures are used. While the description has not taken long there are significant technical difficulties with laparoscopic dissection and suturing.

Results

Most surgeons who have attempted tubotubal anastomosis using this technique have found that operating times are prolonged. In order to simplify the procedure, Sedbon et al. replaced suturing by inserting tubal stents and effecting tissue apposition with a biologic glue (Tissucol Immuno

Laboratoire France).[27] Pregnancy was not reported. Auld et al.[28] used a modification of Sedbon's technique and placed tubal stents by hysteroscopic guidance. The operating times ranged from 92 to 149 minutes. Of six patients so treated, two have achieved viable intrauterine pregnancies and one an ectopic pregnancy. All of these patients had been sterilized with Filshie clips and only one tube was treated. Clips of course are the simplest method of sterilization to reverse.[25] Reich et al. reported the results of laparoscopic tubotubal anastomosis on 22 patients.[29] Apposition of the tubal segments was achieved by placing two sutures, one at 6 o'clock and one at 12 o'clock. These sutures incorporated the serosa, muscularis, and often the endosalpinx. They used either 4-0 or 6-0 caliber sutures. Operating times ranged from 65 to 240 minutes despite the fact that only one tube per patient was repaired. Six women had at least one intrauterine pregnancy and three had at least one ectopic pregnancy. The authors concluded that "at this point, laparoscopic tubal anastomosis cannot approximate the results of laparotomy."

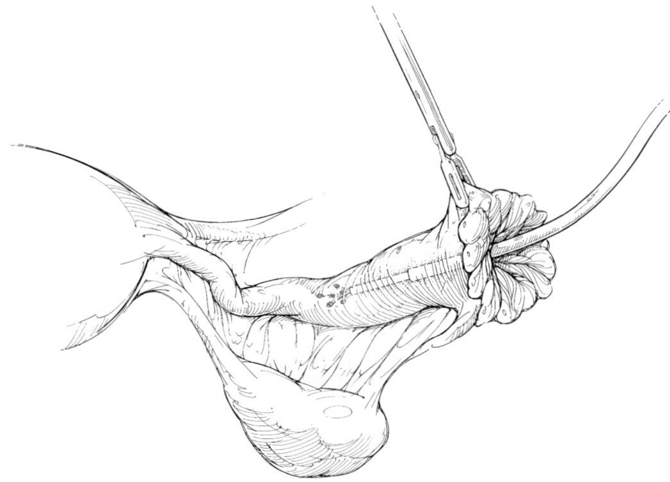

Fig. 15-8. Technique of gamete and pre-embryo replacement.

THE ROLES OF LAPAROSCOPY IN THE ASSISTED REPRODUCTIVE TECHNOLOGIES

Assessment and selection of treatment

The woman with tubal infertility has only two realistic options if she wishes to conceive: reconstructive tubal surgery or recourse to assisted reproductive technology (ART). A woman is entitled to be given the most accurate information so that she can decide which of these options is best suited to her needs. Usually these decisions will be made by the infertile couple after discussion with their medical advisor. The information which must be considered will be a combination of technical and nontechnical factors.[23] In many instances the laparoscopic assessment of the tubes and pelvic architecture will be critical to these discussions.

Nontechnical factors to be considered include the age of the woman (the success rates with in vitro fertilization (IVF) decline dramatically once she has reached her fortieth birthday), cost, and the wishes of the couple. The couple's decision will be greatly influenced by their perception of the relative risks and rates of success of their therapeutic options. The physician must provide this information based upon accurate data which are derived from the following technical factors.

The take home baby rate for IVF should be presented clearly and compared with the potential for success of any proposed tubal reconstructive procedures. This in turn will depend on accurate evaluation of the tubes and pelvis.

Under certain circumstances tubal surgery is not even an option and this may be apparent prior to any invasive investigation. These circumstances include:

1. Absence of the fallopian tubes
2. Destruction of the greater part of the distal ampulla
3. A history of prior reconstructive surgery for distal tubal disease
4. Prior pelvic tuberculosis, an absolute contraindication to tubal surgery. This diagnosis may not be made prior to the performance of an HSG (see Chapter 9).

In couples in whom there is a combination of severe male factor infertility and HSG evidence of tubal occlusion, laparoscopy may be superfluous, since IVF may be a better option. In most other couples the decision will hinge upon whether or not tubal surgery or IVF holds the best promise for success. For these women laparoscopy is critical, as it will complement the HSG findings to establish the prognosis.

Technical applications

The early years of IVF were made possible by the use of laparoscopic oocyte retrieval. This technique has been superseded by the ultrasonographic approach. The predominant technical role for laparoscopy in ART is the deposition into the fallopian tube(s) of gametes (gamete intrafallopian transfer, GIFT) pronuclear stage embryos (PROST), or zygotes (zygote intrafallopian transfer, ZIFT) in attempts to overcome long-standing infertility in couples in whom the female partner can be shown to have patent tubes.

The technique of gamete or early embryo replacement in the fallopian tube is simple. A laparoscopy is performed. Atraumatic grasping forceps are introduced through a 5 mm auxillary portal and the tube elevated so that access can be gained to the tubal ostium. A 3 mm second ancillary portal is placed through which is passed the transfer device composed of an external placement cannula and an internal sialastic catheter in which the gametes or early embryos have been preloaded. The external cannula is maneuvered through the tubal ostium and into the ampulla to a depth of 1.5 to 2 cm. The inner cannula is advanced for a further 1 to 2 cm and the contents deposited in the ampulla (Fig. 15-8).

The question must be answered: Are these procedures demonstrably better than conventional IVF, which is less invasive to the patient and less consumptive of the time of the medical staff? Despite the fact that uncontrolled studies of GIFT report success rates which range from 20% to 25%, these studies do not demonstrate its superiority.[(30)] Data from two small studies, one of which alternatively allocated patients to GIFT or IVF[31] and the other of which did randomize case allocation,[32] do not demonstrate any difference in outcome. Regrettably, neither study had sufficient statistical power to avoid the possibility that a type 2 error might have occurred.

A randomized prospective study from our center comparing the efficacy of ZIFT and IVF has failed to demonstrate any advantage of the former procedure.[33]

REFERENCES:

1. Gomel V: Tubal anastomosis by microsurgery, *Fertil Steril* 28:59, 1977.
2. Gomel V: Reconstructive surgery of the oviduct, *J Reprod Med* 18:181-190, 1977.
3. Gomel V: Laparoscopic tubal surgery in infertility, *Obstet Gynecol* 46:47, 1975.
4. Gomel V: Salpingostomy by laparoscopy, *J Repro Med* 18:265-267, 1977.
5. Gomel V: Microsurgery in female infertility. Boston, 1983, Little Brown & Co.
6. Tulandi T, Collins JA, Burrows E et al: Treatment-dependent and treatment-independent pregnancy among women with periadnexal adhesions, *Am J Obstet Gynecol* 162:354, 1990.
7. Gomel V: In Fertility surgery in laparoscopy. Phillips, JM, editor: Baltimore, 1977, Williams & Wilkins.
8. Mettler L, Giesel H, Semm K: Treatment of female infertility due to tubal obstruction by operative laparoscopy, *Fertil Steril* 32:384-388, 1979.
9. Gomel V: Salpingo-ovariolysis by laparoscopy in infertility, *Fertil Steril* 340:607-611, 1983.
10. Fayez JA: An Assessment of the role of operative laparoscopy in tuboplasty, *Fertil Steril* 39:476-479, 1983.
11. Bruhat MA, Mage G, Manhes H et al: Laparoscopy procedures to promote fertility: ovariolysis and salpingolysis results of 93 selected cases, *Acta Europ Fertil* 14:476-479, 1983.
12. Donnez J, Nisolle M, Casanas-Roux F: CO_2 laser laparoscopy in infertile women with adnexal adhesions and women with tubal occlusion, *J Gynecol Surg* 5:47, 1989.
13. Gomel V: Microsurgery in Female Infertility. Boston, 1983, Little Brown and Co.
14. Dubuisson JB, Borquet de Jolinière J, et al: Terminal tuboplasties by laparoscopy: 65 consecutive cases, *Fertil Steril* 54:410, 1990.
15. Canis M, Mage G, Pouly JL, et al: Laparoscopic distal tuboplasty: report of 87 cases and a 4-year experience, *Fertil Steril* 56:616-621, 1991.
16. Gomel V, McComb P: Unexpected pregnancies in women afflicted by occlusive tubal disease, *Fertil Steril* 36:529-530, 1981.
17. Gomel V: Salpingostomy by laparoscopy, *J Repro Med* 18:265-267, 1977.
18. Daniell JF, Herbert CM: Laparoscopic salpingostomy using the CO_2 laser, *Fertil Steril* 41:558-563, 1984.
19. McComb P, Paleologou A: The intussusception salpingostomy technique for the therapy of distal oviductal occlusion at laparoscopy. *Obstet Gynecol* 78:443-447, 1991.
20. Gomel V: Distal tubal occlusion, *Fertil Steril* 49:946-948, 1988.
21. Gomel V, Erenus M: The American Fertility Society, 46th Annual meeting. Program Supplement (Abstracts) P-097,S-106, 1990.
22. Gomel V, Taylor PJ: In Insler V, Lunenfeld B, editors: Reconstructive tubal surgery in the female in infertility, male and female. Edinburgh, 1993, Churchill Livingstone.
23. Gomel V, Taylor PJ: In vitro fertilization versus reconstructive tubal surgery, *JARGE* 9:306-309, 1992.
24. Gomel V: Microsurgical reversal of female sterilization: A reappraisal, *Fertil Steril* 33:587-597, 1980.
25. Gomel V: Microsurgery in female infertility. Boston, 1983, Little Brown & Co.
26. Koh CH, Janik GM. Presented at the American Fertility Society Annual Meeting, Montreal, October 1993.
27. Sedbon E, Bouquet Delajolinieres J, Boudouris O et al: Tubal desterilization through exclusive laparoscopy, *Hum Reprod* 4:158-159, 1989.
28. Auld BJ, Ahmed E, Wright JT et al: Laparoscopic reversal of sterilization facilitated by hysteroscopic tubal cannulation. Presented at the third biennial meeting of The International Society of Gynecologic Endoscopy, Washington, DC, June 1993.
29. Reich H, McGlynn F, Parents C, et al: Laparoscopic tubal anastomosis, *J Am Assoc Gynecol Laparoscop* 1:16-19, 1993.
30. In vitro fertilization/embryo transfer in the United States: 1990 results from the National IVF-ET registry, *Fertil Steril* 57:15-24, 1992.
31. Leeton J, Rogers P, Caro C et al: A controlled study between the use of gamete intrafallopian transfer (GIFT) and in vitro fertilizaton and embryo transfer in the management of idiopathic and male infertility, *Fertil Steril* 48:605-607, 1987.
32. Crosignani G, Walters DE, Soliani A: The ESHRE multicentre trial on the treatment of unexplained infertility: a preliminary report, *Hum Reprod* 6:953-558, 1991.
33. Fluker MR, Zouves CG, Bebbington MW: A prospective randomized comparison of zygote intrafallopian transfer and in vitro fertilization-embryo transfer for nontubal factor infertility, *Fertil Steril* 60:515-519, 1993.

Chapter 16

PELVIC INFLAMMATORY DISEASE AND TUBO-OVARIAN ABSCESS

with
Harry Reich

Pelvic inflammatory disease (PID) afflicts one million American women annually. Intravenous antibiotics have been the mainstay of treatment of the unruptured tubo-ovarian abscess, with surgical intervention reserved for those cases in whom antibiotic therapy was not effective. This may result in the formation of dense adhesions with consequent impairment of fertility. Immediate laparoscopy, which is the most accurate method of diagnosis, also allows the surgeon to drain the abscess and to perform an adhesiolysis before the adhesions have become organized and fibrous.[1,2]

Simpson, in 1909, suggested that early surgical intervention before the infection had resolved would lead to exaggerated tissue damage, and this belief has not been challenged until recently.[3] The observation of the ease of adhesiolysis during early second look laparoscopy led logically to the application of these techniques early in the genesis of acute pelvic inflammatory changes. Such laparoscopic surgery does not require a high degree of technical expertise and can readily be performed by any trained gynecologist, nor does it require the use of sophisticated equipment. The key to success is the use of gentle blunt dissection using either a blunt probe or an aquadissector.

This chapter will briefly review the use of laparoscopy for the diagnosis of acute pelvic inflammatory disease (see also Chapter 10) and pelvic abscesses. The management of tubo-ovarian abscesses and pelvic abscesses—where the former implies involvement of the adnexa alone and the latter that the inflammatory process has extended further into the pelvis—will be described.

Particular attention will be paid to the surgical techniques whereby laparoscopy can be used to deal with the entire spectrum of acute PID from acute tubal inflammation to the ruptured abscess. The rationale for this approach and the financial implications will be considered.

LAPAROSCOPIC DIAGNOSIS AND MANAGEMENT OF ACUTE PELVIC INFLAMMATORY DISEASE

The inaccuracy of the clinical diagnosis of acute PID has been described in Chapter 10. Recall Jacobson's and Westrom's report in which they noted that of 814 women in whom the diagnosis of acute PID was made by clinical criteria, laparoscopy was able to confirm this in only 65%. In 12% different lesions were identified. Twenty three percent were free from any evidence of organic disease.[4] Binstock collected ten reports in which a total of 1901 patients was described.[5] Acute PID was confirmed laparoscopically in 62% (range, 46% to 73%). No organic lesions were noted in 20%.

The findings from these studies, which were performed in large metropolitan centers, have also been observed in smaller centers in which initial diagnosis and treatment is often carried out by nongynecologists. In Reich's institution the diagnosis of active PID was confirmed laparoscopically in 20% of patients only, most of whom had pain, pyrexia, cervical tenderness, and a pelvic mass confirmed both by physical examination and by ultrasonography.

Until an accurate noninvasive method of diagnosis of acute PID is introduced, laparoscopy should be the diagnostic method of choice. Laparoscopy will also provide the means to obtain specimens for microbiologic evaluation. Furthermore, any exudates can be removed and adhesions lysed when they are soft and easily broken down. Aquadissection is used to separate the tube from the pelvic side wall and other tissues and the ovary can be similarly mobilized. The pelvis should be irrigated with copious amounts of Ringer's lactate.

PELVIC ABSCESS

Laparoscopy can also be used to establish the diagnosis of tubo-ovarian or pelvic abscesses. Clinically, apparently obvious abscesses may in fact be hemorrhagic corpora lutea, endometriomas, or the results of a ruptured appendix. The interpretation of ultrasound findings can be wrong. Gallium-67 and indium-111 labeled white blood cells can be used to enhance the image detected by computer-assisted tomographic scans. This is a complex approach. Laparoscopy can establish the final diagnosis with great accuracy and provide access for drainage if the presence of an abscess is confirmed.

Medical therapy

If it is to be argued that immediate laparoscopic intervention is preferable to the use of intravenous antibiotics, the results of such medical therapy must be considered. In general terms intravenous antibiotics, capable of penetrating the abscess and effective against the responsible organism or organisms, are used as a first-line treatment. If they are clearly ineffective, surgical drainage, unilateral salpingo-oophorectomy, or total abdominal hysterectomy and bilateral salpingo-oophorectomy (TAH/BSO) may be required. Simple resolution of the symptoms and the mass cannot be regarded as a cure. The critical questions remain. How will the episode have affected subsequent fertility, and will the patient be left with any residual disability?

Between 1953 and 1959 Collins and Jansen treated 174 presumptive cases of pelvic abscess (Table 16-1).[6] One hundred sixty-one responded to this approach. Nevertheless 113 subsequently required further surgery to deal with persistence of a painful pelvic mass, abnormal bleeding, or chronic pelvic pain.

One hundred thirty-seven consecutive cases of pelvic abscesses were treated by Franklin et al., who reported their findings in 1973.[7] One hundred twenty were treated conservatively. Twelve (10%) required definitive extirpative surgery during their initial hospital admission because of failure of the conservative approach. It was possible to follow 103 of these 120 for 2.5 to 8 years. Nineteen (16%), because of the presence of a persistent mass, pain, or abnormal bleeding, underwent a major operation. The effects on fertility were devastating. Only 10 of the 103 conceived. Two other studies from the 1960s and 1970s have confirmed these disappointing outcomes following conservative management of pelvic abscesses.[8,9]

It was hoped that the new-generation antimicrobials might produce better results. Landers and Sweet treated a group of patients with regimens that either did or did not contain clindamycin.[10] Of those 104 women who did not receive this medication, reduction in the size of the abscesses was noted in 38 (36.5%) at the time of discharge. In 39 of 84 (46%) patients seen in follow-up 2 to 4 weeks after discharge, further reduction of the size of the masses was noted. When clindamycin was included in the initial therapy, reduction in the size of the abscesses was noted in 43 of 63 (68%) women at the time of discharge. Fifty-eight women were available for long-term study. Of these, 31% had required further surgery.

Cefotaxime was given to 41 women in whom pelvic abscesses had complicated salpingitis.[11] All responded to the therapy, although it was necessary to add chloramphenicol to the treatment of two patients. The patients were followed for 31 to 43 months. The incidence of chronic pain and recurrent infection was low. Five women (12%) did require the performance of TAH/BSO for relief of a persistent pelvic mass, and one further patient underwent a unilateral salpingo-oophorectomy for the removal of a hydrosalpinx. Only six of 30 patients (20%) conceived.

Laparoscopy was used infrequently as the method of diagnosis in all of these studies, reliance being placed upon the clinical and ultrasonographic findings. Assuming the diagnoses to have been accurate, the outcome described would indicate that medical treatment alone for the patient who has developed a pelvic abscess is associated with pro-

Table 16-1. Results of medical therapy alone in PID

Study	No. of cases	No. of responders (%)	No. of responders requiring further surgery (%)	Comments
Collins and Jansen[6]	174	161 (93%)	113 (70%)	
Franklin et al.[7]	137	120 (88%)	12 (10%)	<10% of those followed 2.5-8 yr conceived
Landers and Sweet[10]	63	43 (68%)	Approx. 31%	Treatment included clindamycin
Hemsell et al.[11]	41	41(100%)	6 (15%)	Only 20% conceived

longed hospital stay (9 day average),[6] a high prevalence of adhesion formation, and a high rate of readmission and subsequent surgery. The future fertility of such patients must be considered to be poor.

Surgical treatment

Prior to the introduction of laparoscopic management of pelvic abscesses a number of surgical options were available, which included colpotomy drainage, percutaneous drainage, unilateral adnexectomy, and TAH/BSO.

Colpotomy. If the abscess pointed into the upper portion of the rectovaginal septum, it was drained through a posterior colpotomy. In 1976, Rubenstein et al. reported the results of 38 such procedures.[12] Four of these patients (11%) were required to undergo emergency TAH/BSO during the original hospital stay because of rapid progression of the infection following drainage. One patient underwent unilateral salpingo-oophorectomy and one a repeat colpotomy. The mean duration of hospital stay was 12.4 days, of which 7.7 were accounted for days following the original colpotomy. Subsequently, a further eight women underwent hysterectomy and salpingo-oophorectomy. Thus 37% of these patients treated with antibiotics and colpotomy ultimately required further surgical intervention. Eighteen women were followed for at least 1 year. Seven continued to have pelvic pain and only three conceived.

Rivlin has evaluated two groups of patients.[13,14] In the first study of 59 women treated by colpotomy, further surgery was carried out at the time of the admission on 13 and subsequently on a further 11. Only five of 40 potentially fertile women (12.5%) had successful pregnancies. In the second study of 348 colpotomies, there were 23 instances of diffuse peritoneal sepsis and six deaths.

Percutaneous drainage. The vaginal approach is being increasingly superseded by a percutaneous method of drainage. The results of a number of studies are still preliminary, none having long-term follow-up data. Two of the earlier studies reported successful treatment rates of 78% and 67% respectively.[15,16] Worthen and Gunning treated 35 patients.[17] Eleven cavities were successfully emptied in nine women by percutaneous catheter placement, a rate of 77%. Eighteen of 23 cavities were emptied by percutaneous aspiration in 19 women (94%). One of these women required surgical drainage. Technical difficulties precluded drainage in seven patients. Four of these women recovered following antibiotic treatment alone, and three required surgical drainage.

Radical treatment. The place of laparotomy to gain access to an unruptured pelvic abscess has always been controversial. Kaplan et al. advocated early TAH/BSO.[18] Between 1964 and 1966, 71 women in whom a presumptive diagnosis of pelvic abscess had been made were treated in this manner. Five received more than two units of blood. The rate of postoperative complications was high. Cuff abscesses occurred in three patients. There were seven superficial and one subfascial wound infections. There was one case of evisceration.

LAPAROSCOPIC MANAGEMENT OF PELVIC ABSCESS

Dellenbach et al., in 1972, were the first to propose laparoscopic management of pelvic abscesses.[19]

Others have reported satisfactory outcomes following such an approach.[5,20-22] These reports encouraged us to pursue these techniques,[2] which will now be described.

Preoperative preparation

The woman presenting with a history of significant lower abdominal or pelvic pain and clinical evidence of a suspected pelvic abscesses should be admitted and should undergo laparoscopy a soon as is reasonably possible. Such patients should be regarded as at high risk if they have a history of prior episodes of PID. The absence of fever and/or leukocytosis does not exclude the diagnosis.

Intravenous antibiotic therapy should be started as soon as the patient has been admitted. Laparoscopy should not be performed until at least 2 hours have elapsed from the time of first antibiotic administration to permit adequate blood levels to be attained. It has been our practice to give cefoxitin, 2 g, intravenously every 4 hours from the time of admission to the time of discharge. Administration of oral doxycycline, 100 mg twice daily, is started on the first postoperative day and continued for 10 days following discharge, which usually occurs on the second or third postoperative day. Clindamycin or metronidazole can be used as alternatives to cefoxitin.

Operative technique

The basic technique is similar to that used for most operative laparoscopies. A rapid flow insufflator is indispensable. A cannula should be attached to the cervix to be used both to manipulate the uterus and to perform chromopertubation if indicated. The laparoscope is inserted intraumbilically. The operating table is placed in 10° of Trendelenberg position. Two ancillary 5 mm lower quadrant punctures are made. One is sited suprapubically in the midline and the other lateral to the inferior epigastric vessels in the lower quadrant.

One portal is used to introduce the suction irrigation cannula, the other to accommodate a blunt probe or grasping forceps. The cannula and/or probe are used to mobilize omentum, small and large bowel, and any adhesions until the abscess has been identified and the cavity entered. All purulent fluid is aspirated. Specimens of this aspirate, exudates that have been excised, and material obtained from the tubal ostia are sent for bacteriologic evaluation.

Once the abscess cavity has been emptied, aquadissection is used to separate the omentum and bowel from the reproductive organs and to free completely any tubo-ovarian adhesions.

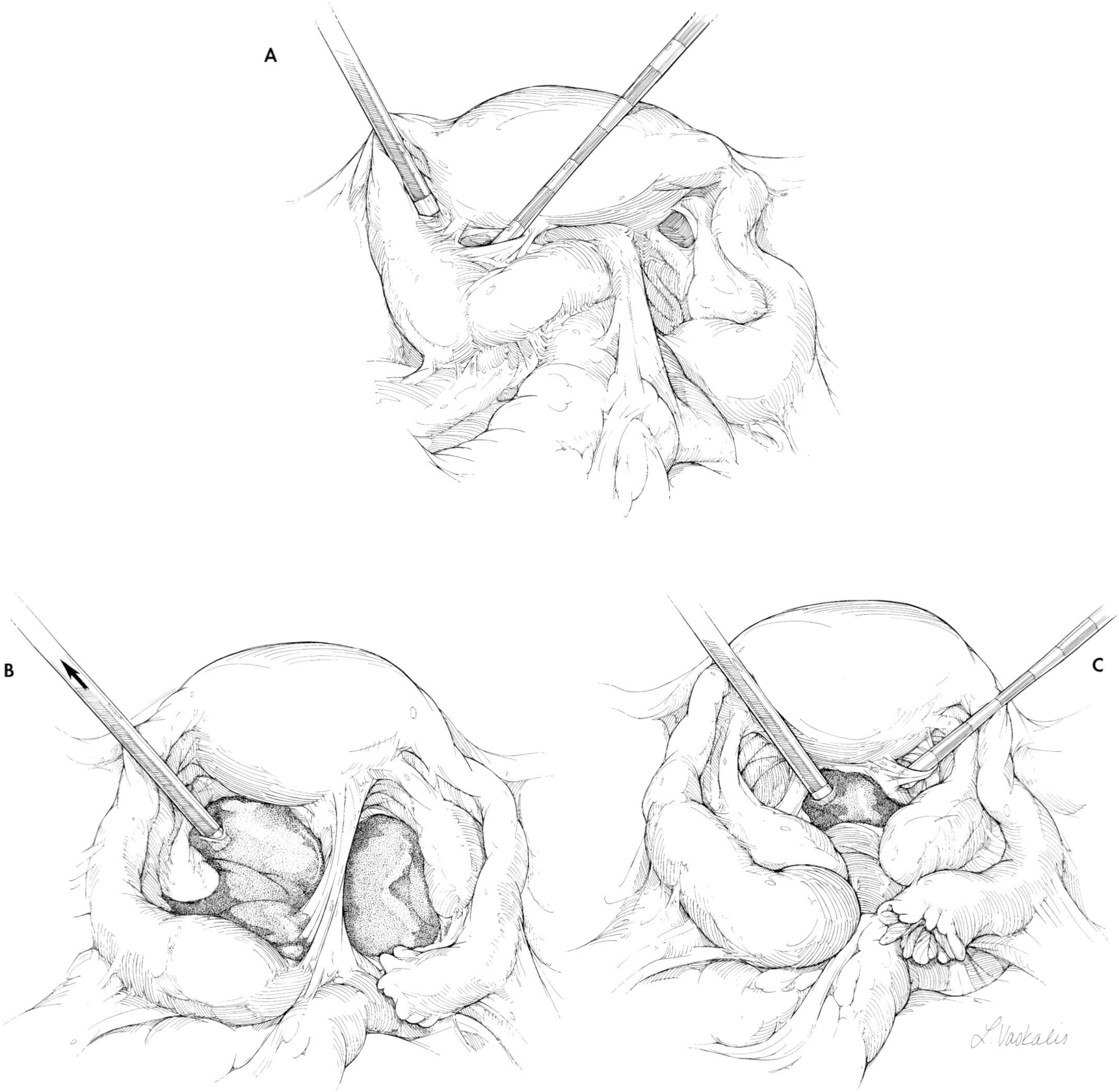

Fig. 16-1. Division of adhesions and drainage of pelvic abcess. **A,** Aquadissection and blunt dissection with both the irrigation-suction cannula and the probe. The probe is used to separate agglutinated organs and reach the abcess cavity. **B,** All pus is aspirated and necrotic tissue removed. **C,** The procedure is completed with copius lavage of both the pelvis and abdomen.

The tip of the irrigation cannula is worked between the loosely agglutinated tissues; a combination of blunt dissection with the tip and introduction of fluid under pressure will separate the tissues (Fig. 16-1, *A*). Counter traction is exerted with the probe or grasping forceps. Once this dissection has been completed and the agglutinated organs freed, the irrigation cannula is replaced with 5 mm biopsy forceps which are used to extract as much of the necrotic inflammatory exudate as possible, taking care not to damage vital structures (Fig. 16-1, *B*).

The ovary is frequently a part of the wall of the abscess. Furthermore, the inflammatory process can gain access to the interior of the ovary. When the dissection has been completed the surgeon may note a large gaping defect in the ovary (Fig. 16-1, *C*). Fortunately, after lavage the defects heal remarkably well and rarely bleed at the time of the surgery.

Once the dissection is complete the tubes are evaluated. The fimbria are gently elevated with 5 mm grasping forceps and a 3 mm forceps inserted into the ostia to tease apart any agglutination. Unless the 3 mm forceps are introduced through a cannula with a variable bore valve, it will be necessary to insert an adaptor to prevent gas leakage around the smaller instrument. If chromopertubation is attempted through the previously placed cervical cannula, no dye will be seen to pass in early cases. The edema of the tube causes a functional occlusion. If the abscess has been present for 1 week or more, tubal lavage may well demonstrate tubal patency or, on rare occasions, may dislodge inspissated material which can be seen to flow from the ostia.

One of the keys to success of the laparoscopic approach is the use of copious lavage. During an average procedure about 15 L of warmed Ringer's lactate will be used. The pelvis should be irrigated until the effluent is clear. Lavage of the upper abdomen is also important, as the use of the Trendelenberg position will inevitably have caused infectious material to flow cephalad. The suction cannula tip is placed in the upper abdomen and 1 L of fluid instilled on each side of the falciform ligament. The patient is then placed in the foot-down (Fowler's) position and as much of this fluid as possible removed.

Finally 2 L of Ringer's lactate is placed in the peritoneal cavity to permit the surgeon to carry out a final "underwater" examination of all the tissues (see Chapter 7) and confirm hemostasis. It is also to be hoped that this fluid will keep the tissues separate during the initial healing phase.

Vicryl 4-0 is used to close the fascia of the umbilical incision. The second and third punctures are loosely approximated with collodion, thus leaving a route of egress for the fluid that has been left in situ. Antibiotics and heparin are not used in the irrigation solution, nor are drains.

Our experience has shown that the earlier the surgery is performed the simpler it is to divide the adhesions before they have had a chance to become organized and fibrotic. Even chronic abscesses are amenable to careful blunt dissection and aquadissection.

Postoperative care

As soon as the patient has recovered from the anesthetic, she is encouraged to become ambulatory and is permitted to eat a diet as tolerated. It is unusual for her temperature to remain elevated after the second postoperative day. Antibiotics are given as follows: cefoxitin intravenously until discharge and doxycycline orally starting on the first postoperative day and continued for 10 days. The patient is examined 1 week after discharge.

Ruptured tubo-ovarian abscess

Prior to 1945 the mortality rate following ruptured tubo-ovarian abscesses was 90%. As surgeons became more willing to intervene, usually performing TAH/BSO, the rate dropped to 12% by 1954.[23] Others had similarly reported the reduction in mortality when early recourse was made to surgery.[24,25]

In an attempt to manage these patients without reliance on TAH/BSO, Rivlin and Hunt were more conservative.[26,27] Between 1972 and 1976, 113 patients with generalized peritonitis following abscess rupture were treated. Only four hysterectomies were performed. The approach of these authors was to attempt to remove the source of the sepsis while preserving the reproductive organs. The pus and necrotic material was removed and drains placed, through which continuous antibiotic containing lavage was maintained postoperatively. The mortality rate was 9%. Hormonal and menstrual function was preserved in 73.5% of patients and it was estimated that 42.5% had the potential to conceive in the future. Additional operative procedures became necessary in 17.5%.

The best treatment of any condition is prevention. Early laparoscopic intervention in cases of pelvic abscess will prevent rupture. If rupture has occurred laparoscopic management is possible. Reich has so managed one case of ruptured tubo-ovarian abscess and one case of diffuse fecal peritonitis that followed perforation of the rectosigmoid by an adenocarcinoma.

The first patient had been treated medically on three occasions over the preceding 3 months. During her final admission the pelvic abscess ruptured while she was receiving clindamycin-ampicillin-gentamycin therapy. Laparoscopy was performed during which all the purulent material was drained, the pelvic organs were freed, and the pelvic and abdominal cavities were extensively irrigated. Her immediate recovery was uneventful, and she has now been followed for 10 years without any recurrence of pain or abscess formation.

The 35-year-old woman with the perforating adenocarcinoma was less fortunate. Although use of a similar laparoscopic approach allowed her to recover from the fecal peritonitis her primary lesion proved to be inoperable when the laparotomy was performed 3 weeks later.

Results

Henri-Suchet et al. first used and reported a combined approach using antibiotic therapy and laparoscopic surgery (Table 16-2).[20] The diagnosis of acute PID was first confirmed laparoscopically in a continuous series of 569 women during the years 1974 to 1983. The laparoscopy was always performed within 24 hours of admission.

Fifty patients were found to harbor abscesses. In 32 of these, any friable adhesions were dissected free by using a blunt probe and any pus thus exposed removed by suction. The peritoneal cavity was cleansed by irrigation with normal saline containing antibiotics, either doxycycline or minocycline, and an antiseptic, noxythiolin. In the remaining 18 cases it was first necessary to mobilize the bowel from the pelvic organs by dividing chronic dense adhesions. In all these patients the adnexa were found to have formed complex masses in which it was impossible to identify the pyosalpinx and the ovary separately. The mass was punctured with a needle, copious pus aspirated, and the cavity flushed with the same irrigation mixture as previously described.

No permanent drain was left in any of the 50 women, and all were treated with intravenous antibiotics immediately after samples for bacteriologic assessment had been obtained. A wide range of different antibiotics was used including a cephalosporin, an aminoglycoside, cefotaximine, cetoperazone, tetracycline, and metronidazole. No immediate complications were recorded attributable to the laparoscopy. The adnexal mass disappeared within 3 to 4 days in 45 (90%) patients. Hospital stay was reduced from a range of 15 to 20 days prior to the use of laparoscopy to 6 to 8 days. Laparotomy was performed on the remaining five patients. Two underwent bilateral and two unilateral salpingo-oophorectomy. The remaining patient underwent a TAH/BSO.

Forty-four patients were followed. Six (13%) experienced persistent pelvic pain. Twenty-five had a second-look laparoscopy. The following findings were noted: no apparent residual disease, 12; unilateral adhesions, 5; and bilateral adhesions and tubal occlusion, 8. Of these eight patients, laparotomy was subsequently performed to relieve persistent pain in three and to attempt to restore fertility in five.

There are only limited data available by which to assess the North American experience. Adducci, in 1981, reported treating seven women by laparoscopically lysing the adhesions and placing colpotomy incisions under direct visualization to effect drainage.[21] In two more patients, in whom loops of bowel were adherent to the cul-de-sac, the pus was drained laparoscopically and the adhesions lysed. Penrose drains were placed transabdominally without recourse to laparotomy. The mean duration of hospital stay was 4 days, and the longest stay 7. No complications were reported and good resolution was noted at the time of follow-up.

Four women were treated by colpotomy, but laparoscopy was used to direct the placement of Penrose drains within the abscess cavity.[22] The drain was left in situ for 2 to 3 days, being held in place by a vaginal suture. Three of these women subsequently conceived. In another series of 13 women treated laparoscopically, 12 responded well.[5]

Reich has treated tubo-ovarian and pelvic abscesses in 40 women. These patients presented between December 1976 and December 1992. Two had laparotomies. One, who was diagnosed early in the study and treated by antibiotics alone, underwent TAH/BSO, and one was seen by the author during an intraoperative consultation after a laparotomy had been performed for suspected ruptured appendix. Thirty-eight were treated by a combination of antibiotics and laparoscopy. The lesions noted in these patients were as follows: unilateral tubo-ovarian abscesses, 20; bilateral tubo-ovarian abscesses, 14; diverticular abscesses, three; and postappendectomy abscess, one.

Since 1983 it has been our routine practice to lyse completely all adhesions and to debride extensively any necrotic exudate. The results have been encouraging. Thirty-seven patients had complete resolution of their abscesses. There were no complications attributable to the laparoscopy. Average operating time was 90 minutes, and the average post-laparoscopy length of stay was 4.1 days. Eight women who had a second-look laparoscopy were all found to have minimal residual adhesions.

Thirty-three of the thirty-four cases of tubo-ovarian ab-

Table 16-2. Results of medical therapy with laparoscopic surgery in PID

Study	No. of cases	No. of responders (%)	Comments
Henri-Suchet et al.[20]	50	45 (90%)	Only 44 patients followed; 8 (18%) required further surgery
Adducci[21]	7	7 (100%)	
Freistadt[22]	4	—	3 women conceived
Reich and McGlynn[2]	38	37 (97%)	

scess were successfully treated laparoscopically. The four cases of diverticular and appendiceal abscesses are not included here. The single failure occurred early in the series, the patient requiring TAH/BSO to treat persistent masses 1 month postlaparoscopy. Four of seven women who wished to conceive have had term deliveries. Two other patients did not wish to become pregnant but did so. One chose termination, the other aborted spontaneously in the first trimester.

There were no recurrences after 3 years' follow-up in the three patients who were treated for diverticular abscesses. Second-look laparoscopy in one of these revealed minimal adhesive disease.[2] One 10-year-old patient had developed a postappendicectomy abscess 18 days postoperatively. Despite antibiotic therapy and surgical drainage, she developed a peritoneal-vaginal fistula. Laparoscopy was carried out 5 days later, and the abscess drained. She was discharged on the third postlaparoscopy day, pain free and afebrile. She returned to full activity by the fifth day.[2]

Rationale for the laparoscopic approach

When pathogenic bacteria gain access to the peritoneal cavity, a number of defense mechanisms begin to work. Many of the microorganisms are absorbed by the lymphatics and transported through the diaphragm to the circulation to be dealt with by the systemic defense system. Within the peritoneal cavity, phagocytosis by both macrophages and leukocytes occurs. One important phenomenon is fibrin trapping.[28]

Although the fibrin traps the bacteria and initially contains the infection to prevent the systemic defences from being overwhelmed, the thick fibrin deposits represent an in situ barrier to neutrophil destruction. The end result is abscess formation. Once an abscess has formed with either 0.5 fibrin clots containing 2×10^8 *Eschericia coli* or normal saline containing the same number of the bacteria, the wall inhibits the effective penetration by antibiotics and the ability of the host organism to resolve the infection.

The role of fibrin has been studied by Ahrenholz and Simmons.[29] The peritoneal cavities of rats were inoculated with either 0.5% fibrin clots containing 2×10^8 *Eschericia coli* or normal saline containing the same number of the bacteria. Within 24 hours 100% of the rats that had not received the fibrin had died. None of the fibrin-treated animals had died, thus demonstrating the immediate protective effects of fibrin. Within 10 days 90% of the fibrin-treated animals were dead and all had developed intraperitoneal abscesses. A third group of rats had received sterile fibrin clots. Lysis of the material was complete within 1 to 2 weeks and no abscesses were noted. Both the size of the abscess and the likelihood of late death were related to the fibrin clot size but not to the concentration of fibrin in the clot. Some rats underwent operative debridement of the fibrin at 4 or 24 hours postinoculation. This approach completely eliminated the formation of abscesses in the surviving animals. It was concluded that while fibrin delays the onset of systemic sepsis it is integral to the formation of abscesses and that surgical removal of the fibrin decreased the formation of abscesses and of the incidence of peritonitis.

These observations have been confirmed in the human. Ninety-two patients who had advanced generalized bacterial peritonitis were treated by radical surgical debridement once the source of contamination had been eradicated.[30] All of the patients were critically ill. The surgery was tedious and prolonged (mean operating time, 3 hours). All of the patients survived.

The laparoscopic approach further substantiates these observations. The technique achieves the same end, namely, drainage of the abscess, lysis of all adhesions, and removal of inflammatory exudates. The extensive irrigation facilitates bacterial absorbtion into the bloodstream where antibiotics are more likely to be effective. Attention to detail must be meticulous during the division of adhesions and removal of the fibrinous exudates.

FINANCIAL IMPLICATIONS

The cost of treating the 1 million women annually who are diagnosed as suffering from acute PID exceeds 1 billion dollars.[31] Method et al., assuming that only 65% of these diagnoses are accurate, calculated that there would be no increased costs if laparoscopy were used to make a definite diagnosis, the savings accruing from the reduced hospital stays of those women who were incorrectly diagnosed by clinical means alone.[32]

A single case illustrates the cost effectiveness of laparoscopic treatment of a pelvic abscess. A patient with a painful pelvic mass was treated medically for 12 days. The diagnosis was confirmed laparoscopically but no attempt was made to drain the abscess. The total cost for this admission was $12,000. Nine days later she was readmitted and laparoscopic drainage and debridement was carried out. Because the adhesions had had time to become dense and organized the operating room time was prolonged. Despite the lengthy operating time the total cost for this second admission was $5642, half that of the previous admission.

CONCLUSIONS

Laparoscopy is the most accurate method of diagnosis of acute PID and provides access to obtain microbiologic specimens and to breakdown adhesions and separate agglutinated organs. If a patient is found to be suffering from a pelvic abscess or develops a pelvic abscess, the goals of treatment should be to effect a cure as rapidly as possible and to minimize any chronic effects, including persistent pelvic pain and infertility.

Laparoscopic drainage of the abscess cavity, debridement, adhesiolysis, and extensive lavage as described in this chapter, combined with the use of intravenous antibiotics, seem to hold out promise of being the optimal way to achieve these goals.

REFERENCES

1. Landers D, Sweet R: Current trends in the diagnosis and treatment of tubo-ovarian abscess. Am J Obstet Gynecol 151:1098, 1985.
2. Reich H, McGlynn F: Laparoscopic treatment of tubo-ovarian and pelvic abscess. J Reprod Med 32:747, 1987.
3. Simpson FF: The choice of time for operation for pelvic inflammation of tubal origin. Surg Gynecol Obstet 9:45, 1909.
4. Jacobson L, Westrom L: Objectivized diagnosis of acute pelvic inflammatory disease. Am J Obstet Gynecol 105:1088, 1969.
5. Binstock M, Muzsnai D, Apodaca L, et al: Laparoscopy in the diagnosis and treatment of pelvic inflammatory disease: a review and discussion. Int J Fertil 31:341, 1986.
6. Collins C, Jansen F: Treatment of pelvic abscess. Clin Obstet Gynecol 2:512, 1959.
7. Franklin E, Hevron J, Thompson J: Management of the pelvic abscess. Clin Obstet Gynecol 16:66, 1973.
8. Ginsburg D, Stern J, Hamond R, et al: Tubo-ovarian abscess: a retrospective review. Am J Obstet Gynecol 138:1055, 1980.
9. Hager WD: Follow-up of patients with tubo-ovarian abscess(es) in association with salpingitis. Obstet Gynecol 61:680, 1983.
10. Landers DV, Sweet RL: Tubo-ovarian abscess: contemporary approach to management. Rev Infect Dis 5:876, 1983.
11. Hemsell D, Santos-Ramos R, Cunningham G, et al: Cefotaxime treatment for women with community-acquired pelvic abscesses. Am J Obstet Gynecol 151:771, 1985.
12. Rubenstein P, Mishell D, Ledger W: Colpotomy drainage of pelvic abscess. Obstet Gynecol 48:142, 1976.
13. Rivlin M: Clinical outcome following vaginal drainage of pelvic abscess. Obstet Gynecol 61:169, 1983.
14. Rivlin M, Golan A, Darling M: Diffuse peritoneal sepsis associated with colpotomy drainage of pelvic abscesses. J Reprod Med 27:406, 1982.
15. Van Sonnenberg E, Wittich GR, Casola G: Percutaneous drainage of 50 pelvic abscesses; pitfalls and refinements. In ARRS Scientific Program, 1985.
16. Gerzof S, Johnson W, Robbins A, Nabseth D: Expanded criteria for percutaneous abscess drainage. Arch Surg 120:227, 1985.
17. Worthen N, Gunning J: Percutaneous drainage of pelvic abscesses: management of the tubo-ovarian abscess. J Ultrasound Med 5:551, 1986.
18. Kaplan A, Jacobs WM, Ehresman JB: Aggressive management of pelvic abscess. Am J Obstet Gynecol 98:482, 1967.
19. Dellenbach P, Muller P, Philippe E: Infections utero annexielles aigues. Encycl Med Chir Paris Gynecol 470:1410, 1972.
20. Henry-Suchet J, Soler A, Loffredo V: Laparoscopic treatment of tubo-ovarian abscesses. J Reprod Med 29:579, 1984.
21. Adducci JE: Laparoscopy in the diagnosis and treatment of pelvic inflammatory disease with abscess formation. Int Surg 66:359, 1981.
22. Freistadt H: The management of pelvic abscess by combined laparoscopy and colpotomy. Presented at the 14th Annual Meeting of the American Association of Gynecologic Laparoscopists, Anaheim, California, 1985.
23. Vermeeren J, TeLinde RW: Intra-abdominal rupture of pelvic abscesses. Am J Obstet Gynecol 68:402, 1954.
24. Pedowitz P, Bloomfield RD: Ruptured adnexal abscess (tubo-ovarian) with generalized peritonitis. Am J Obstet Gynecol 88:721, 1964.
25. Mickal A, Sellman AH: Management of tubo-ovarian abscess. Clin Obstet Gynecol 12:252, 1961.
26. Rivlin M, Hunt J: Surgical management of diffuse peritonitis complicating obstetric/gynecologic infections. Obstet Gynecol 67:652, 1986.
27. Rivlin M, Hunt JA: Ruptured tubo-ovarian abscess: is hysterectomy necessary? Obstet Gynecol 50:518, 1977.
28. Skau T, Nystrom P, Ohman L, Stendahl O: The kinetics of peritoneal clearance of *Escherichia coli* and *Bacteroides fragilis* and participating defense mechanisms. Arch Surg 121:1033, 1986.
29. Ahrenholz DH, Simmons RL: Fibrin in peritonitis. I. Beneficial and adverse effects of fibrin in experiment *E. coli* peritonitis. Surgery 88:41, 1980.
30. Hudspeth AS: Radical surgical débridement in the treatment of advanced generalized bacterial peritonitis. Arch Surg 110:1233, 1975.
31. Curran JW: Economic consequences of pelvic inflammatory disease in the United States. Am J Obstet Gynecol 138:848, 1980.
32. Method MW, Urnes PD, Neahring R, et al: Economic consideration in the use of laparoscopy for diagnosing pelvic inflammatory disease. J Reprod Med 32:759, 1987.

Chapter 17

OVARIAN SURGERY

The surgical management of endometriomas and ovarian cancers has been described elsewhere. This chapter will discuss laparoscopic surgery for other ovarian conditions and will deal with:

Cystic ovarian tumors
- Preoperative assessment
- Aspiration and fenestration
- Ovarian cystectomy
- Oophorectomy and adnexectomy

Torsion of the ovary
Paraovarian cysts
Polycystic ovarian syndrome (PCO)

CYSTIC OVARIAN TUMORS

Most cystic adnexal masses are benign. Since the introduction of ultrasound as a diagnostic method, ovarian cysts are being diagnosed with increasing frequency. When a cystic lesion of the ovary is detected a number of critical questions must be answered: Is the lesion a functional or neoplastic cyst? Is the lesion benign or malignant? The answer to this last question can be derived only with absolute accuracy from histologic examination of the cyst.

Preoperative assessment

The decision to treat the patient by observation, laparoscopy, or laparotomy will depend upon answering the questions that have just been posed.

Prior to the advent of ultrasound, a cyst was assumed to be benign and probably functional if it met certain clinical criteria. Lesions that were unilateral, cystic, regular in contour, freely mobile, and less than 5 cm in diameter in women in the premenopausal age group in whom were found no other clinical signs of malignancy that would include ascites, nodularity of the cul-de-sac, and leg edema satisfied these requirements. Differentiation between functional and neoplastic lesions in such cases was made by allowing time to elapse in the hope that the cyst would disappear spontaneously or could be made to disappear by suppressing the gonadotropins by administration of an oral contraceptive. Larger lesions that did not meet these clinical diagnostic criteria or failed to resolve had to be removed through a laparotomy incision.

More accurate assessment can now be made by a combination of the use of diagnostic ultrasonography, serum carcinoma antigen 125 (Ca 125) levels, and diagnostic laparoscopy.

Diagnostic ultrasound. Specific types of cysts may have specific ultrasonographic appearances. Dermoids vary. They may be seen to contain echogenic mural foci or structures that are identifiable as bone or teeth. Hemorrhagic cysts will contain internal echoes that can be focal or diffuse, the signals varying from low to high intensity. Their appearances will change over time and many will regress spontaneously.

Gray scale transvaginal ultrasonography has been used to differentiate benign from malignant lesions. Scoring systems have been devised based on the wall thickness, inner wall structure, characteristics of septa, and ecogenicity of the lesion.[1]

When the transvaginal ultrasonographic examination shows that the cyst is unilateral, less than 10 cm in diameter, has regular borders, and is unilocular it is likely to be benign (see the box on p. 190). Findings of bilateral masses, irregularity of the edges, multiple intracystic septa, papillae, solid areas, particularly if associated with matting of the bowel or ascites, are of more sinister significance. Herrmann et al.[2] using these strict criteria were accurate in their predictions in 96% of cases.

When the morphologic appearance and the derived scoring system is used alone, there is a degree of overlap between benign and malignant lesions. The additional use of

Characteristics of benign versus malignant cysts by ultrasonography

Benign	*Malignant*
Unilateral	Bilateral
Regular borders	Irregular borders
Unilocular	Multiple septa, papillae
<10 cm in diameter	Solid areas
	Ascites

color doppler provides a higher sensitivity and specificity in the differentiation of benign from malignant lesions. Fast-growing tumors contain neovascularization. Since these vessels contain little smooth muscle, they demonstrate a low resistance to blood flow. Thus the quantification of resistance to flow may be used in the differentiation of these lesions. Color doppler identifies vessels not visible in the gray scale and separates low and high resistance vessels. There is a highly significant difference in the presence of color flow which is noted more frequently in malignant tumors.[3] The resistance index (RI)

$$RI = \frac{\text{systolic peak} - \text{diastolic trough}}{\text{systolic peak}}$$

was significantly lower in malignant lesions,[3] as was the pulsatility index (PI)[4]

$$PI = \frac{\text{peak systolic flow velocity} - \text{end diastolic flow velocity}}{\text{mean flow velocity}}$$

Thus, the combination of morphologic parameters together with the RI and PI increase the sensitivity of differentiating between benign and malignant lesions. These parameters appear to be even more specific in postmenopausal women.

Serum Ca 125 levels. Serum carcinoma antigen 125 levels must be interpreted with caution. The cut point of the test is usually taken at 35 U/ml. Jacobs and Bast[5] compiled data from patients with stages 1 and 2 ovarian cancers. Only 50% of those with stage 1 and 90% with stage 2 had levels that exceeded the cut point, thus reliance on this assay alone would have resulted in misdiagnosis of many early ovarian cancers. The converse is also true. Levels of Ca-125 can be elevated in the presence of endometriosis, adenomyosis, fibroids, dermoid cysts, and acute and chronic salpingitis. While these remarks pertain to premenopausal women, the situation is more promising in the older woman. In the postmenopausal age group, Ca-125 values have been reported to have a specificity of 94%.[6]

Diagnostic laparoscopy. It should be possible to be fairly confident that a particular cyst is functional by using a combination of clinical examination and ultrasonography. Such lesions should be treated expectantly and the patient kept under review. In most centers, obviously cancerous tumors will be treated by laparotomy and combinations of adjunctive chemotherapy. Persistence of apparently functional cysts and the presence of a cystic mass that is believed to be neoplastic but benign constitute the indications for laparoscopic intervention.

The primary function of diagnostic laparoscopy in the patient with an apparently benign cystic mass is to refine the diagnosis. Occasionally visual indications that the cyst may indeed be malignant are found in such patients. The presence of excrescences on the surface of the ovary or peritoneum and ascites are usually the signs that the original diagnosis may have been incorrect. If such signs are encountered or the surgeon is concerned, any peritoneal fluid should be aspirated and cell washings should be obtained from the pelvis and upper abdomen. All of these samples should be sent for cytologic evaluation. Any excrescences should be sampled and the biopsy specimens sent for immediate frozen section examination.

The technique of endoscopic evaluation of the interior of a cyst will be described when the technical details of operative laparoscopy are discussed.

Laparoscopic management of cystic ovarian tumors

Laparoscopic surgical approaches to benign ovarian cysts include aspiration and fenestration, cystectomy, oophorectomy, or adnexectomy. These latter procedures can also be used to remove normal ovaries, for example, in cases of estrogen dependent breast cancer. All five techniques will be described.

General principles. Irrespective of the actual ovarian procedure a series of initial steps should first be completed. Once the pneumoperitoneum has been established, the principal trocar and cannula are inserted in the umbilicus and the laparoscope passed. Before the patient is placed in the Trendelenberg position, the upper abdomen undersurface of the diaphragm and liver are inspected, as is the entire parietal peritoneal surface and omentum. Any fluid is aspirated and any suspicious nodules are sampled using biopsy forceps, which are introduced through a secondary portal. The table is then placed in the head-down position, and the pelvic organs and particularly the ovarian tumors are inspected. It may be necessary to perform a preliminary adhesiolysis (see Chapter 7).

Mage et al.[7] have tabulated the contrasting laparoscopic appearances of both functional and neoplastic cysts. Five characteristics are compared (see the box on p.191). If the cyst is functional the ovarian ligament is likely to be of normal length, the cyst wall will be thin, the ovarian vessels scanty, and the fluid within the cyst will be saffron yellow in color. In contradistinction, if the cyst is neoplastic, the ligament is usually lengthened, the wall is thick, there are numerous surface vessels, and the fluid will be clear, dark brown or have the typical appearances associated with dermoid cysts. The fifth distinguishing characteristic is the appearance of the inner cyst wall, a finding that cannot be observed until the cyst has been opened.

Once the assessment has been made and the surgeon is

Characteristics of functional vs. neoplastic cysts

Functional	*Neoplastic*
Ovarian ligament is normal length	Ovarian ligament is lengthened
Cyst wall is thin	Cyst wall is thick
Few ovarian surface vessels	Numerous ovarian surface vessels
Cyst fluid is saffron yellow	Cyst fluid is clear, dark brown, or typical for dermoid

satisfied that the lesion is not malignant, the decision must be taken as to which procedure should be performed. It is a fundamental principle that in the premenopausal woman as much ovarian tissue as possible should be preserved[8] and oophorectomy or adnexectomy reserved for the postmenopausal woman or when more conservative measures prove to be impossible.

Most procedures can be carried out using a three-puncture technique. Cutting can be achieved with scissors or electrosurgical or laser energy. Dissection is effected with scissors, blunt forceps, laser energy, or with aquadissection. Hemostasis can be secured by ligatures, sutures, staples, or electrosurgery. Sutures and fibrin glue can be used to oppose cut ovarian surfaces. An irrigation suction system, aspirating needles, equipment for lavage, and, on occasion, a lapsac will be required.

Aspiration, cystoscopy, and fenestration. Simple aspiration with a needle is of little value as definitive treatment. It is innaccurate as a means of diagnosing malignancy, and the recurrence rate after simple aspiration is high. Partial aspiration of the cystic contents may aid in the diagnostic process, and may facilitate fenestration or excision of the cyst by reducing its volume and tension. Complete aspiration of the contents will be necessary if vizualization of the cystic cavity (cystoscopy) is desired; this will also facilitate removal of the cyst from the peritoneal cavity.

To effect simple aspiration, a special aspiration cannula with a needle-shaped extremity that can be introduced through one of the auxiliary portals is available. Alternatively, a long 16 to 20 gauge spinal needle is introduced with the stillet in place through the abdominal wall. Once the cystic cavity is entered the stillet is removed and a syringe affixed to the needle. The needle is introduced at the antimesovarial border at a site that subsequently will be included in any incision of the ovarian capsule. The contents are aspirated, collected, and sent for cytologic evaluation (Fig. 17-1). It may be necessary to stabilize the ovary either against the uterus or lateral pelvic wall or by grasping the ovarian ligament with atraumatic forceps. Examination of the aspirate is not an accurate method for the diagnosis of malignancy. In 10% to 65% of aspirates read as benign, malignancy is present.[9,10]

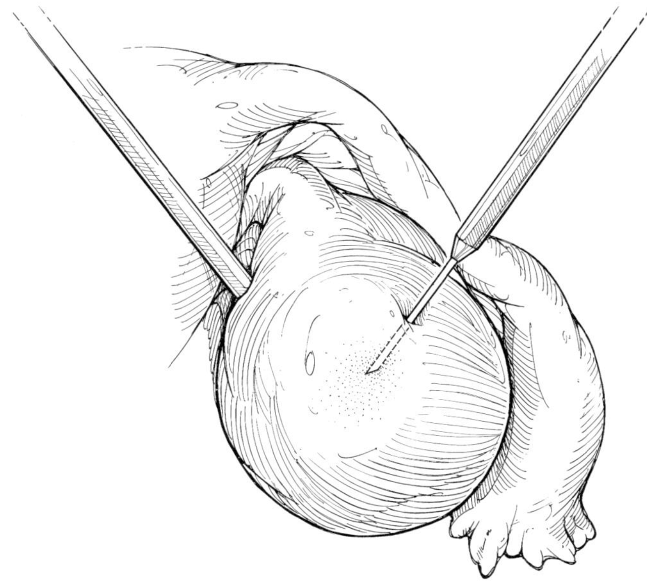

Fig. 17-1. Aspiration of cystic contents.

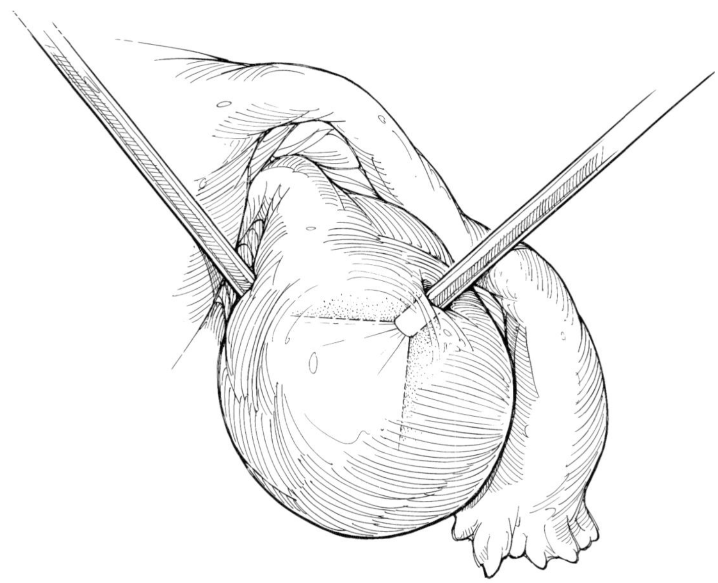

Fig. 17-2. Inspection of cystic cavity (cystoscopy).

To vizualize the cystic cavity it is necessary to fashion a small opening into the cyst. An incision of sufficient size to accommodate either the laparoscope itself or a rigid hysteroscope and its surrounding sheath is made using either scissors or an electrosurgical needle. The hysteroscope is introduced through one of the secondary portals (Fig. 17-2). When a hysteroscope is used, further aspiration of the cystic contents can be effected through its sheath as can the reinflation of the cyst by introducing a physiologic solution. When the laparoscope is used to inspect the cystic cavity, the cyst must be refilled prior to the insertion of the telescope. Upon thorough inspection, the smooth-appearing neoplastic cyst can often be immediately differentiated from the retina-like appearance of the functional cyst. If excrescences suggestive of malignancy are detected, biopsy specimens should be obtained for immediate frozen section examination.

If the cyst is functional and less than 5 cm in diameter, it can be fenestrated. A large elliptical window is cut in the overlying cortex and cyst wall and the excised tissue removed with grasping forceps (Fig. 17-3). Any bleeding vessels can be dealt with by spot desiccation.

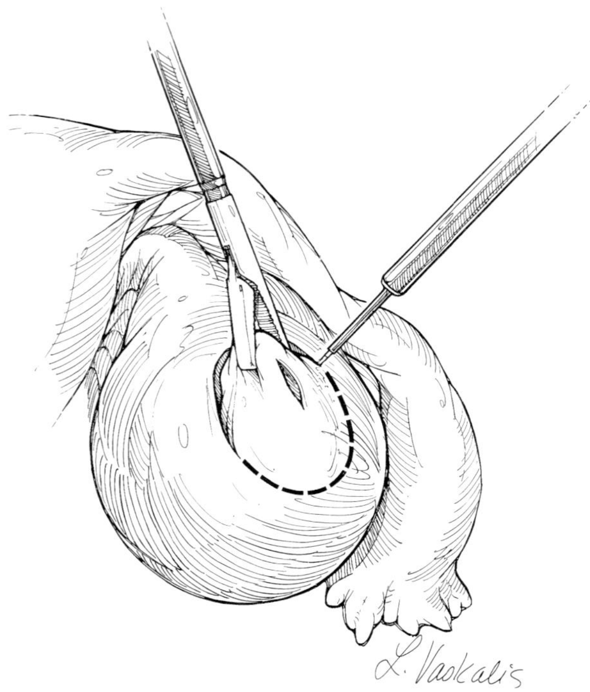

Fig. 17-3. Fenestration of functional cyst.

Once the procedure has been completed the cyst cavity and pelvis are thoroughly irrigated, the instruments removed, and the incisions closed.

Hasson[11] has treated 83 cysts of differing types in this fashion. Functional cysts did not recur. A 7 cm simple cyst did recur at 26 months. There were no intraoperative complications. The formation of adhesions was evaluated in 24 subsequent procedures. None was noted in 14 patients, a few in seven, and more extensive adhesive disease in three with recurrent endometriosis. This low rate of adhesion formation following fenestration has been reported by others.[12,13]

Ovarian cystectomy. Cystectomy refers to complete excision of the cyst. It can be argued that the cyst wall should be kept intact for as long as possible to facilitate dissection. This is indeed the case with either smaller 4 to 5 cm cysts that do not require that a cystoscopy be performed or with dermoid cysts that are best removed intact. Our experience with larger benign cysts has led us to prefer the controlled aspiration described above rather than uncontrolled spillage of the cystic contents that accompanies rupture of the cyst wall, a frequent occurence during cystectomy.

The initial steps are similar to those described for fenestration. Once the ovary has been entered the cut edges of the cortex and cyst wall are each firmly held with two pairs of 5 mm grasping forceps and the two structures are teased apart. It is often possible to develop the plane of dissection by using simple traction and counter traction with these two forceps (Fig. 17-4, *A*). Irrigation fluid introduced under pressure between the two layers (aquadissection) is a highly effective way of developing the tissue planes. The forceps

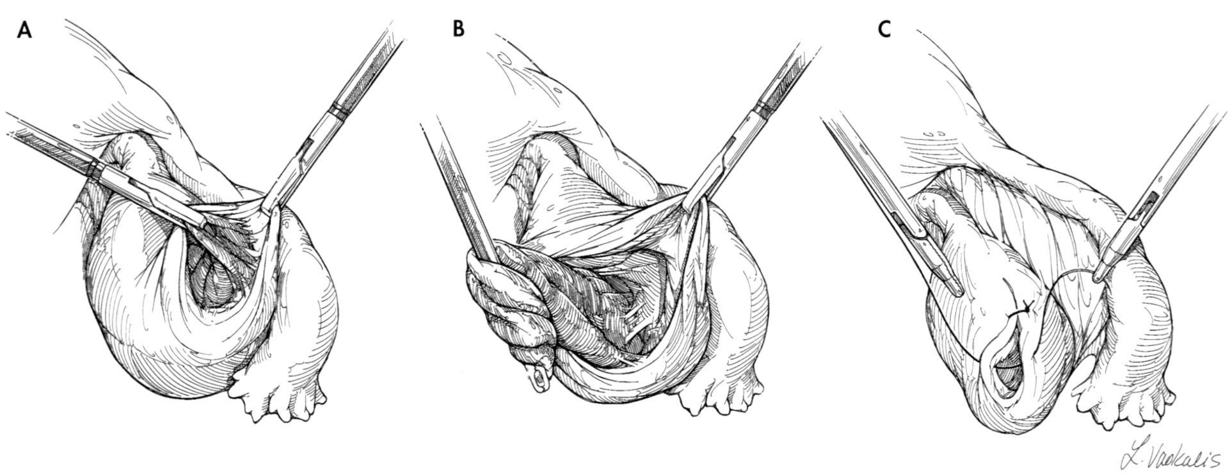

Fig. 17-4. Ovarian cystectomy after fenestration of the cyst. **A,** The cut edges of the ovarian cortex and cyst wall are each held and teased apart. **B,** The cyst wall may be striped off by twisting it around the grasping forceps. **C,** Apposing the edges of the ovary with two interrupted sutures.

which grasps the cyst wall may be twisted so that the cyst is stripped off as it is curled round the forceps (Fig. 17-4, *B*). Fibrous adhesions between the cyst and ovary or blood vessels in a similar position are electrodesiccated and cut with scissors or dealt with by using laser energy.

Once the cyst has been enucleated it can be removed from the abdominal cavity through the secondary or primary portals. If it is too large for removal in this fashion it can be parked in the cul-de sac or uterovesical pouch while the ovary is inspected. At this point any bleeding vessels should be coagulated. The ovarian edges frequently come together. The edges can be apposed with two or three interrupted 5-0 or 6-0 Vicryl sutures (Fig. 17-4, *C*). European surgeons frequently use fibrin glue to close the ovary.

If a large excised cystic remnant has been parked, it can now be dealt with, either by morcellation and removal piecemeal through one of the portals, or through an extended secondary incision or a colpotomy (see Chapter 7). The procedure is completed with copious lavage, the gas expelled, instruments removed, and the incisions closed. The removed tissue is sent for histologic examination.

Mage et al.[7] were able to treat 310 (86.6%) of 403 women with ovarian cysts by using laparoscopic techniques. Particularly encouraging was the finding that pseudomyxoma peritoneii did not occur following spillage of the contents of benign mucinous cystadenoma fluid.

It may be desirable to remove intact a cystic tumor of the ovary as is the case with teratomas. As indicated earlier, puncture and aspiration of cystic contents may be necessary to clarify its nature. Intact removal of a cyst is performed as follows: An initial small incision is made over the antihilar aspect of the affected ovary and continued down until the capsule of the cyst is reached (Fig. 17-5, *A*). A cleavage plane is established by using scissors between the ovarian cortex and the capsule of the cyst. The incision is enlarged sufficiently to permit removal of the cyst. The cut edge of the cortex is grasped with grasping forceps and retracted. Dissection of the cyst from the surrounding ovarian tissue is achieved by spreading the blades of the scissors and/or hydrodissection (Fig. 17-5, *B*). Fibrous adhesions between the cyst wall and the ovary are divided sharply. Blood vessels extending to the cyst, near the hilum of the ovary, are electrodesiccated and divided with scissors (or laser energy) (Fig. 17-5, *C*). Following total removal of the cyst, the excision site on the ovary is inspected and any bleeding vessels electrodesiccated using microbipolar forceps until complete hemostasis is obtained.

The intact cyst, depending on its size, may be removed intact or after aspirating all or part of its contents to reduce its size. Removal may be achieved either through a colpotomy incision or a small suprapubic midline incision by enlarging an auxillary puncture at the same site. An impermeable polythene sac (Endopouch), sufficiently large to accommodate the cyst, is introduced into the peritoneal cavity through this incision. The cyst is dropped into the sac, which is closed by pulling the drawstrings at the aperture of the sac (see Fig. 17-5, *D*). The drawstrings are delivered through the incision (either abdominal or culdotomy). If the cyst is too large to be removed intact, the bag is opened and the cyst drained under direct vision within the bag. This decompression permits removal of the bag, including the cyst, through a much smaller incision. Once the bag is removed the incision is closed. The remainder of the procedure, reconstruction of the ovary and pelvic lavage, have been described before.

Benign cystic teratomas (dermoid cysts). Dermoid cysts, benign cystic teratomas, account for about 13% of ovarian tumours. They are prone to undergoing torsion and may rupture producing a severe chemical peritonitis.[14] They may be malignant in about 1% to 3% of cases.[15]

Because of the concern about the potentially devastating effects of spillage of their contents, it was long believed that these tumors should not be removed laparoscopically. Semm[16] spoke about his experience in treating dermoid cysts using laparoscopic techniques. The cyst contents were allowed to drain into the cul-de-sac and thereafter the cyst walls stripped from the ovary. Nezhat et al.[17] reported seven such patients who were treated laparoscopically. Their technique was dependent on initial aspiration of the cystic contents. A 16 gauge needle was first inserted into the cyst and the cavity aspirated as much as possible. A 0.5 cm incision was made into the cyst to permit introduction of a suction aspiration cannula to irrigate and aspirate the remaining contents. The cyst wall was excised from the ovary and removed through the principal trocar.

Reich et al.[18] reported the intact removal of dermoid cysts from the abdominal cavity. Following excision from the ovary, the specimen was placed in the cul-de-sac. A culdotomy incision was made and the cyst pushed into the opening. The cystic contents were aspirated with a 14 gauge needle until the tumor had shrunk to a small enough size to be removed through the culdotomy incision. In the same report, in four cases (two cystectomies and two oophorectomies) the specimen was removed by placing it in an impermeable sac to prevent peritoneal contamination.

If a teratoma ruptures and spillage of its contents into the peritoneal cavity occurs, it is essential to remove all of these products to avoid a chemical peritonitis. This is achieved by copious lavage with warm lactated Ringer's solution. The lavage and suction is continued until the affluent is clear of fat globules and other debris.

While the optimum method of laparoscopic removal of dermoid cysts remains to be determined, the most important question to be resolved is whether or not spillage is of little consequence if lavage is sufficiently thorough. It is clear that such lesions can be dealt with safely by laparoscopic means.

Oophorectomy and adnexectomy. Oophorectomy and adnexectomy will be indicated in the younger woman if the ovary appears unsalvageable or the nature of the lesion de-

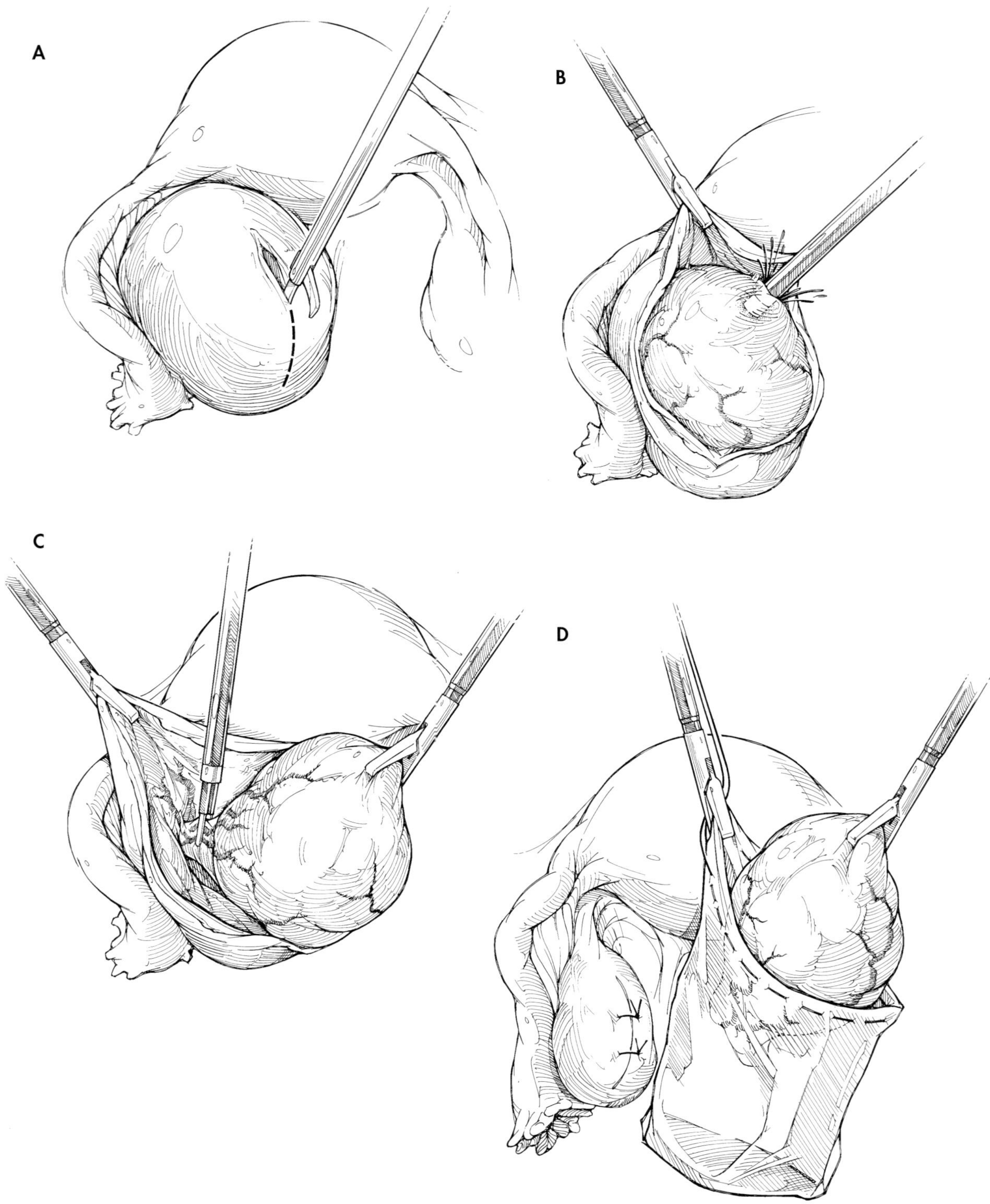

Fig. 17-5. Ovarian cystectomy with cyst intact. **A,** The ovarian cortex is incised at its antihilar aspect. **B,** A cleavage plane is established between the cortex and the capsule of the cyst. Dissection of the cyst is achieved by blunt and hydrodissection. **C,** The blood supply to the cyst is electrodesiccated. **D,** Removal of cyst in a polythene bag.

mands its removal, in cases of estrogen-dependent breast cancer, in rare cases of familial carcinoma of the ovary syndromes once child bearing has been completed, and in all postmenopausal women, unless the patient is concerned about the loss of her ovary. In this last situation she must be fully appraised of the risk of ovarian cancer existing in the ovarian mass or developing subsequently (box below).

Both oophorectomy and adnexectomy can be performed using one or a combination of the following techniques: ligatures, sutures, electrodessication, or staples. Irrespective of how the pedicle is dealt with, the specimen is removed through a colpotomy incision, a small suprapubic incision, or by morcellation.

Indication for oophorectomy and adnexectomy

- Ovary appears unsalvageable
- Nature of lesion warrants removal
- Patient has estrogen-dependent breast cancer
- Rare cases of familial carcinoma of the ovary
- In all postmenopausal women with a benign-appearing lesion

Oophorectomy. To perform an oophorectomy using ligatures the ovary is grasped and three successive Roeder loops are tied around the pedicle (meso-ovarium). Scissors are used to divide the pedicle distal to the last loop and the raw area remaining is coagulated[19] (Fig. 17-6).

If bipolar desiccation is used the ovary is elevated with grasping forceps. The mesovarium is grasped with bipolar forceps and the area between the blades desiccated. The desiccated tissue is divided with scissors. Sequential steps of desiccation and division are performed until the ovarian pedicle has been divided. We generally employ this particular method to perform oophorectomy.

Adnexectomy. If it is deemed necessary to remove the adnexa, the first step is always to identify the ureter. It is particularly vulnerable at the point at which it crosses the pelvic brim. On the left the sigmoid colon may be attached to the infundibulo pelvic ligament, in which case it will be necessary to dissect the sigmoid first.

Excision may be accomplished using electrodesiccation. While electrodesiccation of the utero-ovarian ligament may be achieved with either the unipolar or bipolar mode, it is more prudent to use the bipolar mode on the infundibulo pelvic ligament. Electrodesiccation will be more effective if the vessels in the infundibulo pelvic ligament are skeletonized. The adnexa is retracted appropriately. Successive steps of desiccation and transection with scissors will secure and divide the infundibulo pelvic and ovarian ligaments. This approach is slow and frequently requires repeat electrodesiccation because of bleeding. Furthermore, electrodesiccation generates smoke, which must be evacuated. Although we used this technique initially, we now prefer to use sutures or ligatures to secure the pedicles. Oelsner et

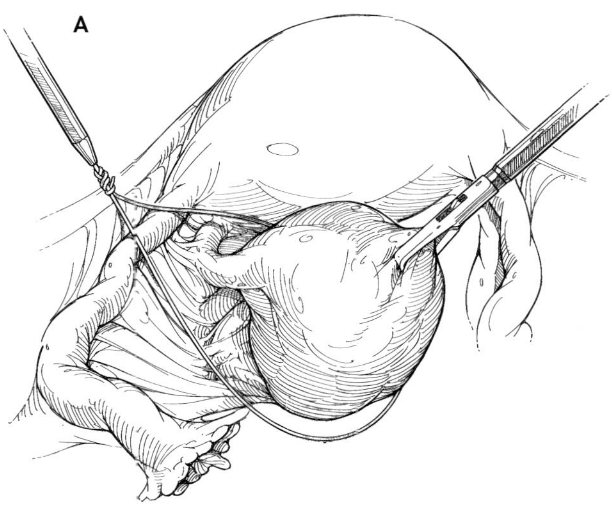

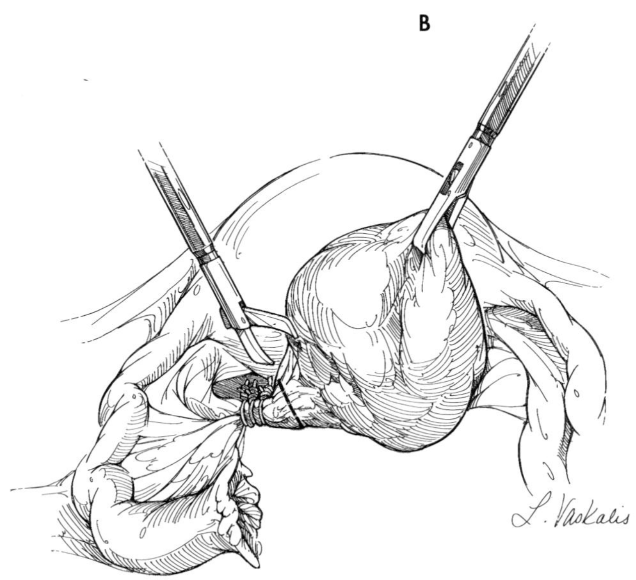

Fig. 17-6. A and **B,** Oophorectomy using Roeder loops to secure the mesoovarium.

al.[20] have reported successful performance of adnexectomy using the electrodesiccation technique in 30 patients with ovarian lesions that ranged in diameter from 3 to 12 cm. It is noteworthy that the average operating time was 90 minutes, with a range between 40 to 150 minutes.

When sutures or ligatures are used, the ureter is identified and the infundibulo pelvic ligament is secured first (Fig. 17-7, *A*). The second ligature encloses the proximal end of the tube and the utero-ovarian ligament. Both pedicles are now transected (Fig. 17-7, *B*). Any undivided tissue between these two pedicles may be electrodesiccated and divided. The area is thoroughly inspected and any minor bleeders electrodesiccated using microbipolar forceps.

Excision may also be achieved using stapling devices. However, in view of their width of 12 cm and the risk to the ureter, when this method is used it is absolutely necessary to ensure that the ureter is out of danger.

Results. The use of Roeder's loops for adnexectomies is somewhat crude, as the infundibulo pelvic ligament, utero-ovarian ligament, and tube must all be included in the ligature. As for oophorectomy three such loops are applied and scissors are used to divide the pedicle distal to the last loop.[19] Parker and Berek[21] reported 25 postmenopausal women predicted to have benign adnexal masses ranging from 3 to 9 cm. In 22 of these they were successful in performing an adnexectomy by laparoscopy using this technique. The operating times ranged from 20 to 180 minutes (mean, 73 minutes). There were two complications: one bladder injury and one sigmoid colon injury that required a laparotomy. Three patients had a laparotomy and included the preceding case, a patient in whom the frozen section of the biopsy specimen was inconclusive and one in whom the biopsy revealed metastatic carcinoma consistent with primary breast cancer.

TORSION OF THE OVARY

Torsion occurs when either a normal ovary (about 18% of cases[22]) or, more commonly, one containing a cyst twists on its pedicle. The presenting symptom is one of acute abdominal or pelvic pain (see Chapter 10). Although the diagnosis is frequently made preoperatively, recourse often has to be made to diagnostic laparoscopy to confirm or clarify the clinical picture. Once the definitive diagnosis has been made it must be decided whether or not the affected adnexa can be salvaged and what method of surgical access should be employed.

The degree of ischemic damage suffered by the adnexa is very much a function of the time elapsed from torsion to diagnosis. Clearly, early recourse should be made to laparoscopy if the diagnosis is suspected. Adnexectomy is indicated when the ovary is obviously necrotic or when the cause dictates removal of the adnexa. A laparoscopic adnexectomy can be performed as described above. Risk of embolization from the infarcted veins is small. Nonetheless, if an adnexectomy is projected, it is probably wise to refrain from untwisting the pedicle prior to securing it by ligation or other methods.

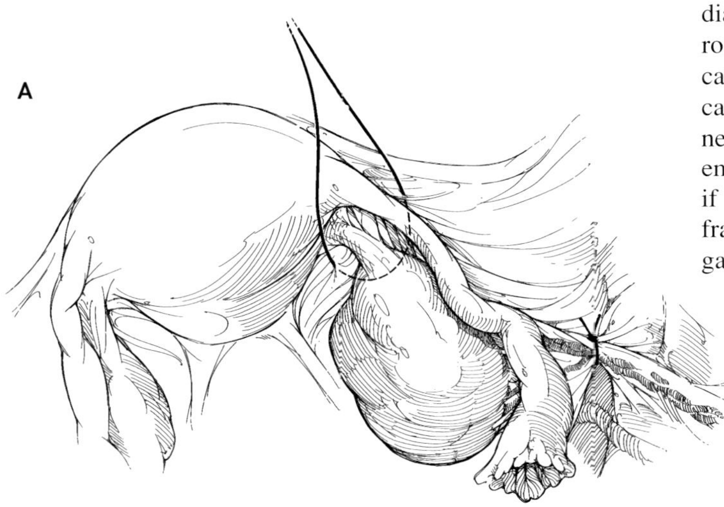

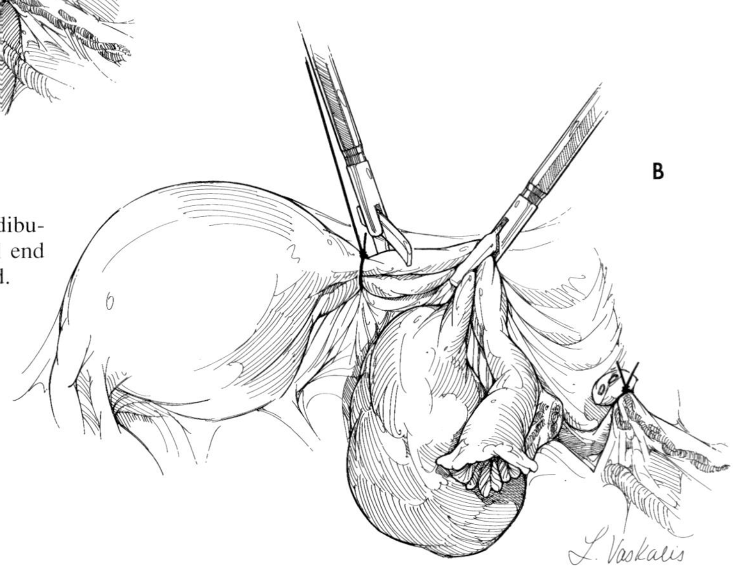

Fig. 17-7. Adnexectomy using suture ligatures. **A,** The infundibulopelvic ligament is secured. **B,** After securing the proximal end of the tube and the ovarian ligament the pedicles are divided.

If the surgeon is persuaded that the ovary can be salvaged, it is possible to do so laparoscopically. The ovary is inspected to determine if it contains a lesion. If a cyst is present, as is frequently the case, it can be fenestrated and drained or a cystectomy can be performed. The pedicle is then untwisted by turning the adnexa with atraumatic grasping forceps until the normal anatomic relationships have been restored. The ovary is observed to ensure that blood flow returns and that it assumes a more normal color. The ovarian ligament can be shortened by placement of a suture, but it is unclear if this is necessary. It can be expected that ovarian function will be restored, although risk remains that the adnexa may undergo retorsion at a later date.

Mage and co-workers reported 35 cases of adnexal torsion.[23] Torsion affected the whole adnexa in 25, the tube only in 9, and the ovary only in one case. The condition was treated conservatively in 27 patients with 1 subsequent recurrence. Of the 35 cases, the procedure was completed laparoscopically in 27 and laparotomy was performed in eight cases. With increasing experience in operative laparoscopy, it will be possible to treat most such cases laparoscopically and have recourse to a laparotomy only in rare circumstances.

Vancaillie and Schmidt[24] recommend that anticoagulant therapy be instituted using heparin 10,000 IU intravenously immediately followed by 7,500 IU subcutaneously twice daily for 10 days. However, there is no evidence to support the need for such treatment.

PARAOVARIAN CYSTS

Hydatid cysts of Morgagni may attain a considerable size. They usually have a narrow vascular pedicle (stalk), which attaches the cyst to the ampulla of the fallopian tube. It is possible to excise such cysts laparoscopically. It is imperative to ascertain that the mass is a hydatid cyst of Morgagni and to visualize its pedicle. The cyst is grasped with grasping forceps and retracted to expose the pedicle which in turn is grasped with a bipolar forceps and electrodesiccated. Replacing the bipolar forceps with laparoscopic scissors, the pedicle is divided along the line of coagulation. The scissors are replaced with an aspirating needle, the cyst is punctured, and its contents aspirated completely. This permits the excised deflated cyst to be removed through the ancillary or principal trocar.

Paraovarian cysts may be retroperitoneal. They can reach a considerable size and distort or stretch the adjacent fallopian tube. The peritoneum over the cyst is incised as far away from the fallopian tube (especially the fimbriated end) as possible, using scissors. The edge of the peritoneum is grasped with atraumatic grasping forceps and the cleavage plane between the peritoneum and the cyst identified and developed by spreading the blades of the scissors. Blunt dissection and/or hydrodissection is used to enucleate the cyst. It is useful to aspirate part of the cystic contents since otherwise the thin-walled cyst frequently ruptures during the dissection process. Aspiration is carried out with an aspirating needle introduced through one of the auxiliary portals (Fig. 17-8, *A*). The puncture or rupture site is grasped with grasping forceps to prevent complete evacuation of the

A

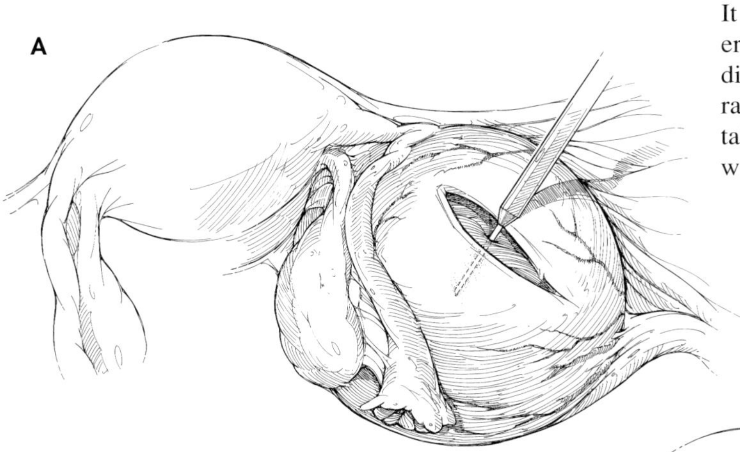

B

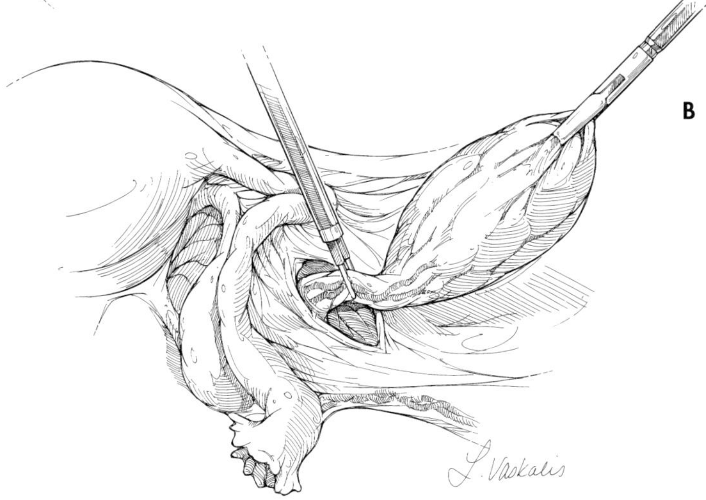

Fig. 17-8. Excision of retroperitoneal paraovarian cyst. **A,** The peritoneum over the cyst is incised away from the fimbriated end of the tube, and part of the cystic contents aspirated. **B,** After dissection of the cyst, its vascular pedicle is electrodesiccated prior to division.

cystic contents as presence of fluid in the cyst facilitates dissection and permits better appreciation of the landmarks. The vascular pedicle of the cyst, usually located close to the tube, is electrodesiccated and divided (Fig. 17-8, *B*). The contents of the enucleated cyst are aspirated and the cyst completely deflated. The deflated cyst is removed as described earlier. There is no need to close the peritoneal incision. The procedure is concluded with pelvic lavage. This is the technique we generally employ.

Herbert and co-workers described a variation of this technique in the two cases they have reported.[25] The peritoneal incision is kept small (1.5 cm to 2 cm). An aspiration needle is introduced through the incision and the cyst pierced. The cystic contents are aspirated and the cyst is incised. A grasper is then introduced into the cyst. The cystic lining is grasped and pulled through the peritoneal incision, to evert it, as it is stripped from the surrounding tissues. Once the pedicle of the cyst is reached, it is electrodesiccated and divided. After excision is complete, the inverted adventitial tissues are pushed back to their retroperitoneal location.

POLYCYSTIC OVARIAN SYNDROME

Polycystic ovarian syndrome (PCO) remains an ill understood disorder of ovulation characterized clinically by obesity, hirsutism, and oligoamenorrhea; biochemically by elevation of levels of androgenic hormones and an elevated luteinizing hormone (LH)/follicle-stimulating hormone (FSH) ratio; and morphologically by enlarged ovaries with thick shiny capsules containing multiple microcysts. Initially treatment was by wedge resection of the ovaries.[26] In more recent years medical induction of ovulation with a spectrum of agents has been the treatment of choice. Regrettably none of these approaches can always produce ovulation or the desired pregnancy. There has been a reawakening of interest in surgical treatment since the reintroduction of laparoscopic drilling of the ovarian cortex.[27] This procedure is carried out in an endeavour to induce ovulation and pregnancy in those women who are resistant to medical therapy or who, despite regularly demonstrated ovulation for a reasonable time, have not become pregnant.

Ovarian drilling or "ovarian electrocautery" is the creation of multiple openings through the ovarian capsule. This can be accomplished electrosurgically using a pointed monopolar electrode or with laser energy (CO_2, Nd:YAG, or KTP). Using instruments introduced through two auxiliary portals, each ovary is immobilized in turn and retracted out of harm's way. Depending on the size of the ovary 6 to 12 openings are drilled through the capsule. Each of these are approximately 3 mm in diameter and 3 to 4 mm in depth. Gjonness[27] performed the procedure in 62 patients with PCO resistant to clomiphene therapy. Fifty-seven of the 62 women (92%) thus treated ovulated within 3 months of the procedure. There were 35 patients who were involuntarily infertile because of PCO alone. Twenty-four of these (69%) became pregnant with no further treatment.

Greenblat and Casper[28] studied hormonal changes resulting from multiple electrosurgical punctate cauterization of the capsule of the ovaries in 6 PCO patients who failed to ovulate, despite increasing doses of clomiphene to a maximal dose of 150 mg/day and addition of human chorionic gonadotropin (5000 IU) on day 16, for at least three cycles. Six regularly cycling women undergoing either diagnostic laparoscopy or laparoscopic tubal ligation served as controls. In the patients with PCO, but not in controls, serum androstenedione, testosterone, estradiol, and LH significantly decreased to nadir levels on postoperative days 3 and 4. In contrast, FSH levels rose after the procedure. Of the six treated PCO women, five ovulated and four conceived. Similar results have been reported by others who used a similar or a modified technique.[29-31] These changes have been shown to persist for at least 8 weeks postoperatively.

Sumioki et al.[29] used a variation of the above described technique. They used a biopsy forceps equipped with unipolar electrical capability and obtained biopsies from six to 10 superficial follicles of 2 to 4 mm in diameter. The pieces of capsular tissue were removed and the biopsy site electrodesiccated to obtain hemostasis. The amount of tissue resected ranged from 0.2 g to 0.6 g of wet weight.

It has long been recognized that ovarian surgery can be associated with a high rate of occurrence of postoperative periadnexal adhesions. Gurgan et al.[32] performed second-look laparoscopy in 17 patients 3 to 4 weeks after ovarian capsule drilling by electrosurgery or Nd:YAG laser. Minimal adhesions were found in six, mild adhesions in another six, and moderate adhesions in two patients. Naether and Fischer[33] have recently reported the results of second look in 62 patients, all of whom previously had undergone electrosurgical ovarian capsule drilling. In 50 patients a second-look laparoscopy was performed, and caesarean section served as a second look in a further 12. A further subgroup of 30 women was studied; their ovarian procedures were complemented by extensive lavage and the creation of postoperative artificial ascites with saline. Adhesions were detected in 19.3% of the women who had undergone electrosurgical ovarian drilling alone, a rate that fell to 16.6% in the lavage/artificial ascites group. These rates were lower than those reported following laser drilling of the ovary.

The data resulting from ovarian capsule drilling is interesting and resembles findings that follow a wedge resection. The procedure is easy to perform and adds little morbidity to diagnostic laparoscopy. It appears to offer an additional therapeutic option to clomiphene citrate–resistant patients with PCO. In addition it may be argued that it offers the advantage of avoiding ovarian hyperstimulation that may be associated with gonadotropin therapy. However, in view of the potential for formation of ovarian adhesions, the procedure should be reserved to PCO patients who have not responded to an appropriate period of medical therapy.

CONCLUSIONS

Enthusiasm for dealing with ovarian lesions by laparoscopic means must not be permitted to compromise the safety of the patient. There are two major potential risks. One is the misdiagnosis and partial treatment of ovarian neoplasia, the other is the formation of postoperative periadnexal adhesions that might compromise the woman's reproductive potential.

We have been at pains to stress the need for accurate preoperative assessment based upon the fact that only women with benign ovarian lesions should undergo laparoscopic treatment. The need for thorough laparoscopic evaluation of the peritoneum, abdominal contents, any ascitic fluid, and the ovarian lesion itself cannot be overemphasized. If there is any doubt it is always safer to obtain specimens for immediate frozen section evaluation. There is no sin or shame in converting a laparoscopy to a laparotomy if such is in the patient's best interests. This advice is given primarily with respect to the woman who is known to have an ovarian lesion. It is no less pertinent if a suspicious ovarian mass is found unexpectedly when laparoscopy is being performed for some other indication.

While functional cysts can be fenestrated, all apparently benign neoplastic lesions should be excised *in toto* and sent for histologic scrutiny.

Despite observing all of these precautions surgeons have been disappointed when an apparently benign cyst, removed at the time of laparotomy, subsequently has been shown to be malignant. Laparoscopic removal of ovarian lesions confers no special protection from such an untoward event.

If it is immediately apparent at the time of laparoscopy either because of the appearance of the lesion or the results of the frozen section, or if the histologic evaluation of an apparently benign lesion detects the presence of malignancy, definitive staging and treatment must be carried out with immediacy.[34]

REFERENCES

1. Sassone AM, Timor-Tritsch IE, Artner A, et al: Transvaginal sonographic characterization of ovarian disease. Obstet Gynecol 78:70-6, 1991.
2. Herrmann U, Locher G, Goldhirsch A: Sonographic patterns of malignancy: prediction of malignancy. Obstet Gynecol 69:777, 1987.
3. Kurjak A, Schulman H, Sosic A, et al: Transvaginal ultrasound, color flow, and doppler waveform of the postmenopausal adnexal mass. Obstet Gynecol 80:917-21, 1992.
4. Timor-Tritsch IE, Lerner JP, Monteagudo A, Santos R: Transvaginal ultrasonographic characterization of ovarian masses by means of color flow-directed Doppler measurements and a morphologic scoring system. Am J Obstet Gynecol 168:909-13, 1993.
5. Jacobs I, Bast R: The CA-125 tumour associated antigen: A review of the literature. Hum Reprod 4:1, 1989.
6. Finkler N, Benacerrat B, Lavin F, et al: Comparison of serum CA-125, clinical impression, and ultrasound in the properative evaluation of ovarian masses. Obstet Gynecol 72:659, 1988.
7. Mage G, Canis M, Manhes H, et al: Laparoscopic management of adnexal cystic masses. J Gynecol Surg 6:71, 1990.
8. Maneschi F, Marasa L, Incandela S, et al: Ovarian cortex surrounding benign neoplasms: a histologic study. Am J Obstet Gynecol 169:388-93, 1993.
9. Kjellgren O, Angsrom T, Bergman F, et al: Fine needle aspiration biopsy in diagnosis and classification of ovarian carcinoma. Cancer 28:967, 1971.
10. Trope C: The preoperative diagnosis of malignancy of ovarian cysts. Neoplasia 28:117, 1981.
11. Hasson HM: Laparoscopic management of ovarian cysts. J Reprod Med 35:863-7, 1990.
12. Kleppinger RK: Ovarian cyst fenestration via laparoscopy. J Reprod Med 21:16, 1978.
13. Larsen JF, Pedersen OD, Gregersen E: Ovarian cyst fenestration via the laparoscope. Acta Obstet Gynecol Scand 65:539, 1986.
14. Caruso PA, Marsh MR, Minicowitz S, Karten G: An intense clinicopathologic study of 305 teratomas of the ovary. Cancer 27:343-8, 1971.
15. Woodruff JD, Protos P, Peterson WF: Ovarian teratoma. Am J Obstet Gynecol 102:702-15, 1968.
16. Semm K: AAGL 15th Annual Meeting, Orlando, Florida, November 19-23, 1986.
17. Nezhat C, Winer WK, Nezhat F: Laparoscopic removal of dermoid cysts. Obstet Gynecol 73:278, 1989.
18. Reich H, McGlynn F, Sekel L, Taylor P: Laparoscopic management of ovarian dermoid cysts. J Reprod Med 37:640-4, 1992.
19. Semm K: Operative manual for endoscopic abdominal surgery. Chicago, 1987, Year Book Med Pub.
20. Oelsner G, Admon D, Goldenberg M, et al: Laparoscopic adnexectomy in the management of benign-appearing ovarian masses. Gynecol Endoscop 2:25-8, 1993.
21. Parker WH, Berek JS: Management of selected cystic adnexal masses in postmenopausal women by operative laparoscopy: a pilot study. Am J Obstet Gynecol 163:1574-7, 1990.
22. Hibbard LT: Adnexal torsion. Am J Obstet Gynecol 152:456-61, 1985.
23. Mage G, Canis M, Manhes H, et al: Laparoscopic management of adnexal torsion. J Reprod Med 34:520-4, 1989.
24. Vancaillie T, Schmidt EH: Recovery of ovarian function after laparoscopic treatment of acute adnexal torsion. A case report. J Reprod Med 32:561-2, 1987.
25. Herbert CM III, Segars JH, Hill GA: A laparoscopic method for excision of large retroperitoneal paraovarian cysts. Obstet Gynecol 75:139, 1990.
26. Stein IF, Leventhal ML: Amenorrhea associated with bilateral polycystic ovaries. Am J Obstet Gynecol 29:181, 1935.
27. Gjönnaess H: Polycystic ovarian syndrome treated by ovarian electrocautery through the laparoscope. Fertil Steril 41:20, 1984.
28. Greenblatt E, Casper RF: Endocrine changes after laparoscopic ovarian cautery in polycystic ovarian syndrome. Am J Obstet Gynecol 156:279-85, 1987.
29. Sumioki H, Utsunomyiya T, Matsuoka K, et al: The effect of laparoscopic multiple punch resection of the ovary on hypothalamo-pituitary axis in polycystic ovary syndrome. Fertil Steril 50:567, 1988.
30. Armar NA, McGarrigle HHG, Honour J, et al: Laparoscopic ovarian diathermy in the management of anovulatory infertility in women with polycystic ovaries: endocrine changes and clinical outcome. Fertil Steril 53:45, 1990.
31. Sakata M, Tasaka K, Kurachi H, et al: Changes of bioactive luteinizing hormone after laparoscopic ovarian cautery in patients with polycystic ovarian syndrome. Fertil Steril 53:610, 1990.
32. Gürgan T, Kişnişçi, Yarali H, et al: Evaluation of adhesion formation after laparoscopic treatment of polycystic ovarian disease. Fertil Steril 56:1176-8, 1991.
33. Naether OGJ, Fischer R: Adhesion formation after laparoscopic electrocoagulation of the ovarian surface in polycystic ovary patients. Fertil Steril 60:95-8, 1993.
34. Maiman M, Seltzer V, Boyce J: Laparoscopic excision of ovarian neoplasms subsequently found to be malignant. Obstet Gynecol 77:563-565, 1991.

Chapter 18

ENDOMETRIOSIS

with
Camran Nezhat
Farr Nezhat

The clinical presentations of endometriosis (pain, infertility, and the presence of a pelvic mass and/or thickening and nodularity in the pouch of Douglas) and the use of laparoscopy for diagnosis have been described in Chapters 10 and 11. The condition can be managed expectantly, medically, or surgically. There are two surgical options: radical and conservative. This chapter will discuss the surgical options with particular reference to the use of operative laparoscopy.

Conservative surgery is rarely curative[1,2] but is the approach of choice for the woman who wishes to maintain her reproductive potential or her uterus and ovary(ies). The patient suffering with severe pain, in whom previous conservative measures have failed to give relief and childbearing is no longer an issue, should be offered radical surgery.

RADICAL SURGERY

Radical surgery refers to the removal of the uterus, ovaries, and all the endometriotic lesions. It remains the only definitive treatment. If one ovary is conserved, reasonable cure rates can be anticipated.[2-4] After 3 and 5 years of follow-up, however, recurrence of symptom rates of 13% and 40%, respectively, have been reported.[5] Henderson et al. studied 85 women.[6] Of those who had retained some ovarian tissue, 25% required further surgery as opposed to only 1.1% of those from whom the ovaries had been removed. The woman who has lost both ovaries will be estrogen deficient. Fortunately, estrogen replacement therapy seems to pose only a small risk of exacerbating the patient's symptoms.

Radical surgery can be performed through a laparotomy incision or by laparoscopy using techniques described here and in Chapter 22. In many of these cases the use of laparoscopy to free adhesions and obliterate the endometriosis may well spare the patient the increased discomfort and postoperative recovery time associated with a laparotomy. In advanced cases the procedure is frequently difficult. Dense fibrosis may make the dissection tedious and pose considerable hazards to the ureter, bowel and major blood vessels. There is no shame in abandoning the laparoscopic approach if the surgeon believes this will be in the best interest of the patient.

CONSERVATIVE SURGERY

Conservative surgery is cytoreductive, aiming as it does at removing or destroying the endometriotic lesions and any associated adhesions. The goal is to restore the normal anatomic relationships with a view to increasing the patient's chances of conception and/or obtaining relief from pain. Any woman who chooses the conservative approach must understand that the likelihood that she will require a further surgical intervention is of the order of 25%.[7] If she is fortunate enough to conceive this rate falls to 10%.[5,7] Any discussion of conservative surgery for endometriosis must consider certain general principles and the following:

- Surgery of the reproductive organs and surrounding peritoneum
  - Division and resection of adhesions
  - Excision or destruction of peritoneal implants
  - Restoration of the tubal and ovarian relationships
  - Management of ovarian lesions
  - Restoration of the cul-de-sac
  - Uterosacral ligament ablation or presacral neurectomy
- Surgery of the nonreproductive organs
  - Management of lesions of the genitourinary system
  - Management of lesions of the gastrointestinal system
  - Management of lesions of the diaphragm

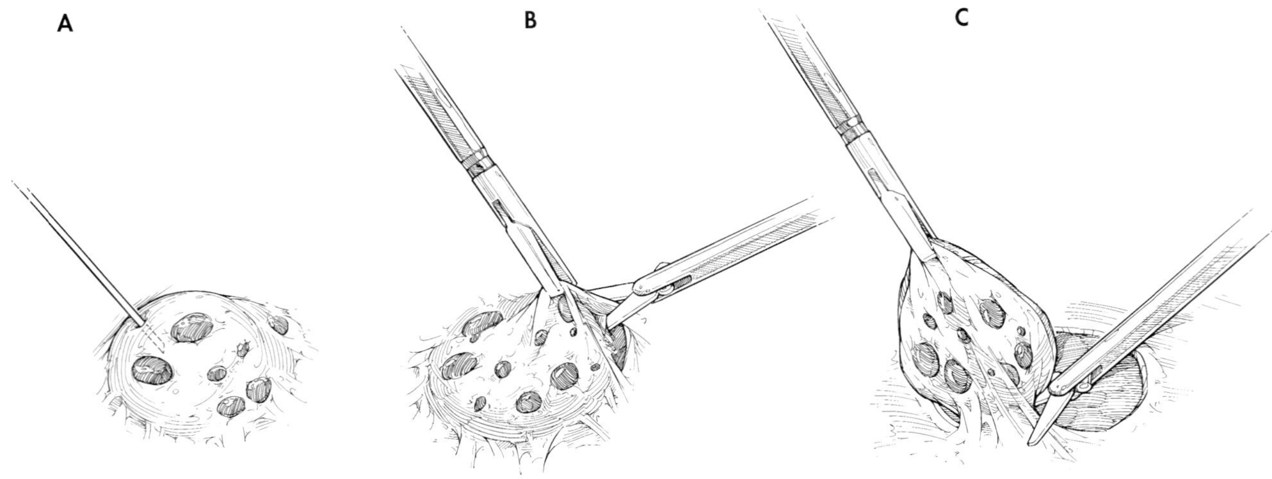

Fig. 18-1. Excisional biopsy of peritoneal implants. **A,** Injection of fluid under peritoneum. **B,** Elevation of lesion and surrounding peritoneum; initial incision. **C,** Lesion excised.

General principles

The goals of conservational surgery are to remove or destroy all implants, resect all adhesions, and restore the anatomic relationships. Every endeavour should be made to prevent recurrence of the endometriosis and re-formation or de novo formation of adhesions.

The procedure can be performed by using a variety of cutting instruments including mechanical (scissors) and electrical and laser energy. We believe that the carbon dioxide laser, especially the ultrapulse 5000L, offers certain advantages. The CO_2 laser beam does not obstruct the surgeon's view, and this laser will not penetrate water. This last property is particularly valuable if the CO_2 laser is used in conjunction with hydrodissection.[8] The fluid develops the tissue planes, and can be used as a backstop to protect sensitive tissues.

As described in Chapter 11, the final diagnosis of endometriosis is almost always made by laparoscopy. Despite the improvements in video technology, the diagnostic evaluation must commence with naked eye inspection, and the distal lens of the laparoscope almost in contact with the area under scrutiny. The gold standard is to take biopsy specimens from suspicious areas.

The biopsy technique is relatively simple. The lesion is elevated with grasping forceps. It may be advantageous to inject some Ringer's lactate beneath the peritoneal surface with a spinal needle to protect the underlying structures (Fig. 18-1, *A*). This step is particularly important when the CO_2 laser is being used. The peritoneum surrounding the lesion is incised with scissors or the laser (Fig. 18-1, *B*). The incised peritoneum on the side of the lesion is elevated with grasping forceps and the lesion is excised by using sharp and blunt dissection (Fig. 18-1, *C*). The specimen is removed. It is not usually necessary to control bleeding, but if such does occur the small vessels can be electrodesiccated.

Table 18-1. Histologic confirmation of endometriosis by its appearance at laparoscopy

Clinical appearance of endometriosis	Histologic confirmation rate of endometriosis (%)
Typical—dark, black	90[12,13]
White—opacified	81[14]
	91[13]
Red, flame-like	75[14]
	81[13]
Glandular lesions	67[14]
Subovarian adhesions	50[14]
Intraovarian cysts	48[15]
Yellow-brown patches	47[14]
Circular peritoneal defects	45[14]
	33[13]
Hemosiderin lesions	33[14]
Normal peritoneum	13-25[9-11]

Symptom recurrence is most likely when the disease is not completely obliterated. Recognition is hampered by the protean appearances of the disease and the probable existence of coexisting microscopic lesions in normal looking peritoneum.[9-14] Table 18-1 is derived from a number of studies that have correlated the surgical appearances of the lesions with the microscopic findings. These observations serve to underline the value of taking biopsy specimens.

The ovaries may contain unsuspected lesions. Candiani et al. identified small endometriomas in 48% of normal-appearing or slightly enlarged ovaries by placing a needle deep within the medulla of the ovary and aspirating[15] (Fig. 18-2). It has been estimated that the diagnosis of endometriosis is missed in 7% of patients and understaged in 50%.[12]

Once the laparoscopic diagnosis has been made, if the

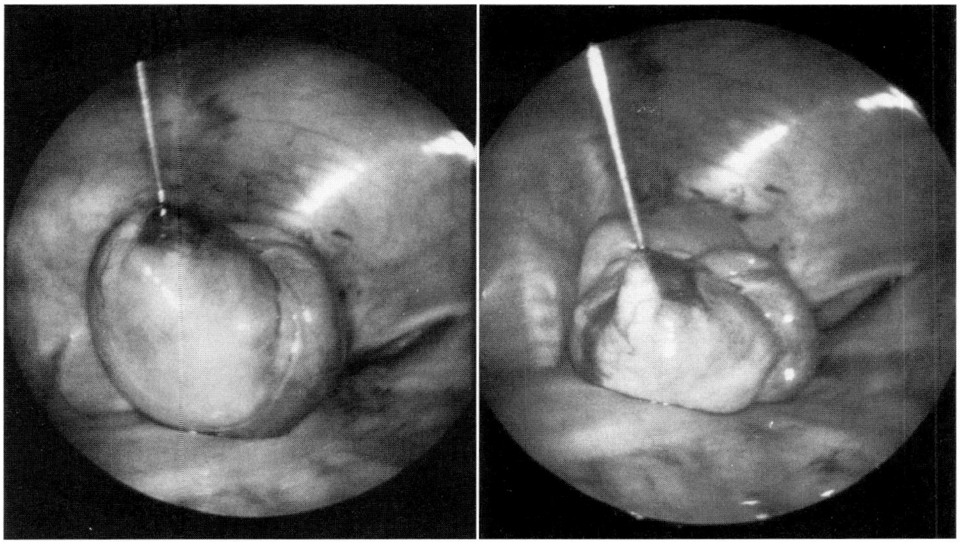

Fig. 18-2. **A** and **B,** Needle aspiration of the ovary.

surgeon works in a facility where a diagnostic procedure can immediately be converted to an operative one, the decision must be made whether or not to proceed to definitive surgery. Generally speaking, rAFS stages 1 and 2 lend themselves to this approach. When the disease is more severe it is usually advisable to proceed no further until the patient has had time to consider her options. It is also in these cases that preoperative suppression of the disease by using Danazol or one of the GNRH analogues may be advantageous.

Surgery of the reproductive organs and surrounding peritoneum

Division and resection of adhesions. In many cases it will first be necessary to perform a preliminary adhesiolysis. The technique has been described in Chapter 7. In cases of endometriosis every effort should be made to remove (rather than simply divide) adhesions and all fibrous tissue. They are often found to contain foci of glands and stroma. The adhesions associated with endometriosis frequently involve vital structures. Hydrodissection and the use of the ultra pulse CO_2 laser can greatly facilitate their dissection.

Excision or destruction of peritoneal implants. Peritoneal implants can be excised or ablated in situ. They must be completely eradicated. Superficial lesions up to 5 mm in diameter can be excised, electrodesiccated, or vaporized with the laser. It is preferrable to excise larger and infiltrating lesions. Excision is carried out, as described earlier for biopsy, using scissors or laser energy. Care is taken not to damage any surrounding structures. Any bleeding points are electrodesiccated with microbipolar forceps. Cutting in close proximity to vital structures should be done using scissors or the CO_2 laser.

Ablation of smaller lesions can be effected using bipolar current if the disease is superficial. Unipolar current is required if the lesion penetrates to any depth. The CO_2 laser, set at 3500 to 5500 watts/cm^2, can be used in a similar fashion. Larger lesions can be vaporized by using a combination of hydrodissection and the CO_2 laser. A small opening is made in the peritoneum with scissors or the laser. The suction irrigation cannula is introduced and fluid injected, thus partly dissecting the peritoneum and forming a backstop for the laser (Fig. 18-3, *A* and *B*). The laser is fired in a continuous mode and the lesion is ablated from the surface to its base. The appearance of normal retroperitoneal fat signals the end of the ablation. It will be necessary to remove the laser plume during this process.

It is important to use copious irrigation to remove any carbon particles from the site of ablation. If carbon is left it can be mistaken for recurrent endometriosis at the time of any subsequent laparoscopy. The tip of the suction-irrigation cannula is placed over the ablation sites and alternating lavage and suction is performed. Use of the superpulse/ultrapulse modes will result in more rapid vaporization and less carbon formation.

Restoration of tubal and ovarian relationships. When the surgery is being carried out to enhance fertility, it is very important to ensure that any distortion of the normal anatomic relationships between the tube and ovary be restored to normal or as nearly normal as is possible. Chromopertubation should be carried out to confirm that the tubes are patent.

In cases of advanced endometriosis the anatomic distortion may be severe. The ovary may be adherent in the fossa ovarica, to the back of the uterus or in the cul-de-sac. The tube and mesosalpinx may be adherent to the ovary, covering part of its surface. In addition there may be peritubal and periovarian adhesions. This ovarian entrapment inter-

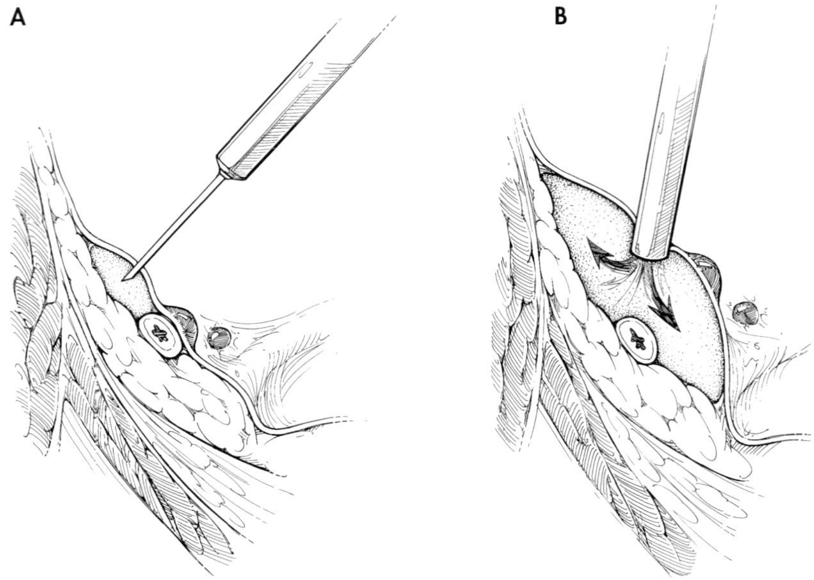

Fig. 18-3. Hydrodissection.

feres with ovulation and results in the formation of corpus luteum cysts. The condition also hampers oocyte pickup by the fimbria.[16] Although the tubes are usually patent, the fimbria may be agglutinated.

Adhesiolysis should be carried out in a systematic fashion, commencing in well-exposed areas and using hydro-, sharp, and blunt dissection as necessary. If the ovary or tube is adherent, as described earlier, they must be totally freed while making every effort to cause as little damage as possible to these structures and the surfaces to which they are adherent. It will now be necessary to remove all of the periovarian adhesions. Broad adhesions are divided on all sides and removed from the pelvis (see Chapter 7). When adhesiolysis is carried out with the CO_2 laser, the use of fluid as a backstop is particularly effective for dividing adhesions in the space between the tube and ovary. Fleshy or filmy adhesions on the surface of the ovary can be removed using sharp dissection. These can also be electrodesiccated or vaporized with the laser.

Management of ovarian lesions. Endometriosis of the ovary can exist as small superficial lesions or endometriomas of less than 2 cm in diameter, cysts of 2 to 5 cm in diameter and endometriomas that are greater than 5 cm.

In advanced cases there may be severe anatomical distortion. Ovarian entrapment results in the formation of corpus luteum cysts that may be difficult to differentiate from endometriomas. In such cases preoperative ovarian suppression largely eliminates the problem and prevents uneccessary ovarian dissection.

The smallest lesions can be electrodesiccated, laser ablated, or excised. All of the abnormal tissue must be destroyed or removed. Endometriomas of 2 to 5 cm can be excised as will shortly be described or the cyst can be fenestrated and the lining destroyed. Simple drainage or fenestration alone of such lesions will not effect a cure. Destruction of the cystic lining may be simpler to perform than ovarian cystectomy.[17-19] Brosens recommends that ovarian cystoscopy and, where necessary, biopsy be carried out as a preliminary step.[18] Once it has been determined that the cyst is not malignant, the lining can be destroyed to a depth of 3 to 4 mm by using either electrodesiccation or laser energy. Details of this procedure have been given in Chapter 17.

Larger cysts should be removed. The technique is the same as that described in Chapter 17. It should be noted that when endometriomas are being dissected, they may not be peeled off the healthy ovarian tissue with the same degree of ease as is the case with simple cysts. Hydrodissection between the cyst wall and the ovary may be helpful.[18,20] We have found that if the cyst is initially punctured, the contents aspirated, and the cyst rapidly re-expanded with the irrigation fluid at a pressure of 500 to 800 mm/Hg, which is then removed, this step, if repeated several times, may be all that is required to free the cyst wall.[21] On occasion sharp dissection will be required. Despite the surgeon's best endeavours to remove the entire cyst this may not be always possible. If such is the case, what tissue has been removed should be sent for histologic evaluation and the remaining parts of the cyst wall destroyed by electrodesiccation or with laser energy.

It is not often necessary to close the defect in the ovary.[22,23] If there is a very large raw area we will insert one or more sutures to appose the edges and reconstruct the ovary. Synthetic absorbable suture material, 5-0 to 6-0 gauge, is used. The sutures are placed in such a way as to ensure that the knot will remain buried within the ovary.

European surgeons frequently use fibrin glue (Tissucol) to close the defect.

In some cases of severe unilateral disease it may be necessary or beneficial to perform an oophorectomy on the affected side (see Chapter 17).

Restoration of the cul-de-sac. The cul-de-sac may be partly or totally obliterated, which is often a source of pain and may hinder oocyte pick-up by the fimbria. There is usually a great degree of anatomic disorganization involving the rectosigmoid, vaginal fornix, posterior aspects of the cervix and uterus, ureter, and major blood vessels.[24] There may be endometriosis of the rectovaginal septum. The bowel should be prepared pre-operatively in such cases.

Laparoscopic restoration of the cul-de-sac is not simple and should only be undertaken if surgical and/or urologic assistance is readily available, or by a surgeon who is familiar with the performance of surgery on the gastrointestinal and urinary tracts.

In many cases preliminary adhesiolysis will be required before the cul-de-sac can be approached. It will now be necessary to dissect the rectum from the back of the uterus and cervix and/or the uterosacral ligaments. An assistant stands between the patient's legs, manipulating the uterus with a previously placed cannula while performing a rectovaginal examination with the other hand. It may be necessary to use a rectal probe to facilitate identification of the rectum. In very difficult cases a sigmoidoscope may be used for the same purposes and to monitor for bowel perforation.

Dilute vasopressin solution, 5 to 10 ml, (10 units in 100 ml of lactated Ringer's) is injected with an 18-gauge laparoscopic needle into an adjacent uninvolved area of peritoneum. Access to the plane of dissection is gained by making an incision at this site with scissors or the CO_2 laser. Fluid is introduced under pressure to begin the dissection and by a combination of hydrodissection (Fig. 18-4, *A*), blunt dissection with the tip of the suction-irrigation cannula, and sharp dissection with the laser or scissors, the rectum is gradually separated from the back of the uterus, upper part of the back of the cervix (Fig. 18-4, *B* and *C*), and the uterosacral ligaments (Fig. 18-5). During the dissection, hemostasis is maintained by the injection of further amounts of the dilute vasopressin and/or by bipolar desiccation (Fig. 18-4, *C*). The uterosacral ligaments are very vital landmarks. If the surgeon can keep the dissection medial to these structures, the ureters and uterine vessels are relatively safe.

The dissection continues, the assistant helping to guide the surgeon until the rectum is entirely freed from the cervix and upper vagina. Once the rectum has been mobilized any endometriotic lesions on the rectum are excised or vaporised with the CO_2 laser. Involved areas may be fibrosed. Vaporisation or excision may result in perforation of the bowel. From time to time the cul-de-sac is filled with irrigation fluid and air insufflated into the rectum from below. The appearance of bubbles in the fluid will serve to identify any bowel perforation. Such perforations can be repaired with a single layer of interrupted 3-0 silk or 4-0 polydioxanone sutures (see later). It is unusual for endometriosis to penetrate the bowel mucosa. It often will involve the serosa and muscularis. If dissection has been deep within the muscularis, the bowel wall can be reinforced by placing interrupted 4-0 polydioxanone sutures.

Lesions in the rectovaginal septum are dissected out as the assistant palpates the affected site to ensure that complete removal has been achieved.[25] Once the surgeon is satisfied that the dissection has been completed, the pelvis is irrigated, the fluid aspirated, and then the pelvis is flooded with lactated Ringer's solution. Underwater observation will help in the identification of any residual disease or bleeding vessels which can be electrodesiccated.

No attempt is made to reperitonealize the raw surfaces of the rectum or cul-de-sac. It has been demonstrated that such attempts promote adhesion formation.[22,23,26,27]

Ablation of the uterosacral ligaments or presacral neurectomy. In cases of intractable pain, which has persisted despite the apparent destruction of all the endometriosis or in cases of severe pain, ablation of the uterosacral ligaments or presacral neurectomy have been advocated.[28-30] These procedures are described in detail in Chapter 20.

Surgery of the nonreproductive organs

It is not uncommon for other intra-abdominal or intrapelvic organs to be involved in the disease process. Endometriosis can affect the urinary system, gastrointestinal system, and, on rare occasions, may be found on the undersurface of the diaphragm. Lesions of these areas may be amenable to laparoscopic surgical management.

Genitourinary endometriosis. Ureteral involvement has been reported in 1% to 11% of women in whom a diagnosis of endometriosis has been confirmed.[31] It tends to be superficial but can be invasive on occasion and may even result in complete obstruction of the ureter. In most cases the diagnosis is made at the time of diagnostic laparoscopy for complaints of infertility or pain.

Bladder instability and decreased capacity that is unresponsive to conventional therapy may be due to endometriosis. Such a case has been reported.[32] The symptoms, which did not respond to parasympatholytic therapy, were corrected by surgical destruction of endometriosis of the bladder. Two years later, when the symptoms recurred, the patient was successfully treated with a course of Danazol. Invasive bladder involvement may be suspected clinically if there is a complaint of hematuria, particularly if it is temporally related to menstruation.

If there is reason to suspect genitourinary involvement preoperatively, urinalysis, measurement of the serum electrolytes, creatinine, and urea levels, ultrasonography of the kidneys, and intravenous pyelography should be performed. Cystoscopy is usually reserved for cases where there is evidence of recurrent hematuria.

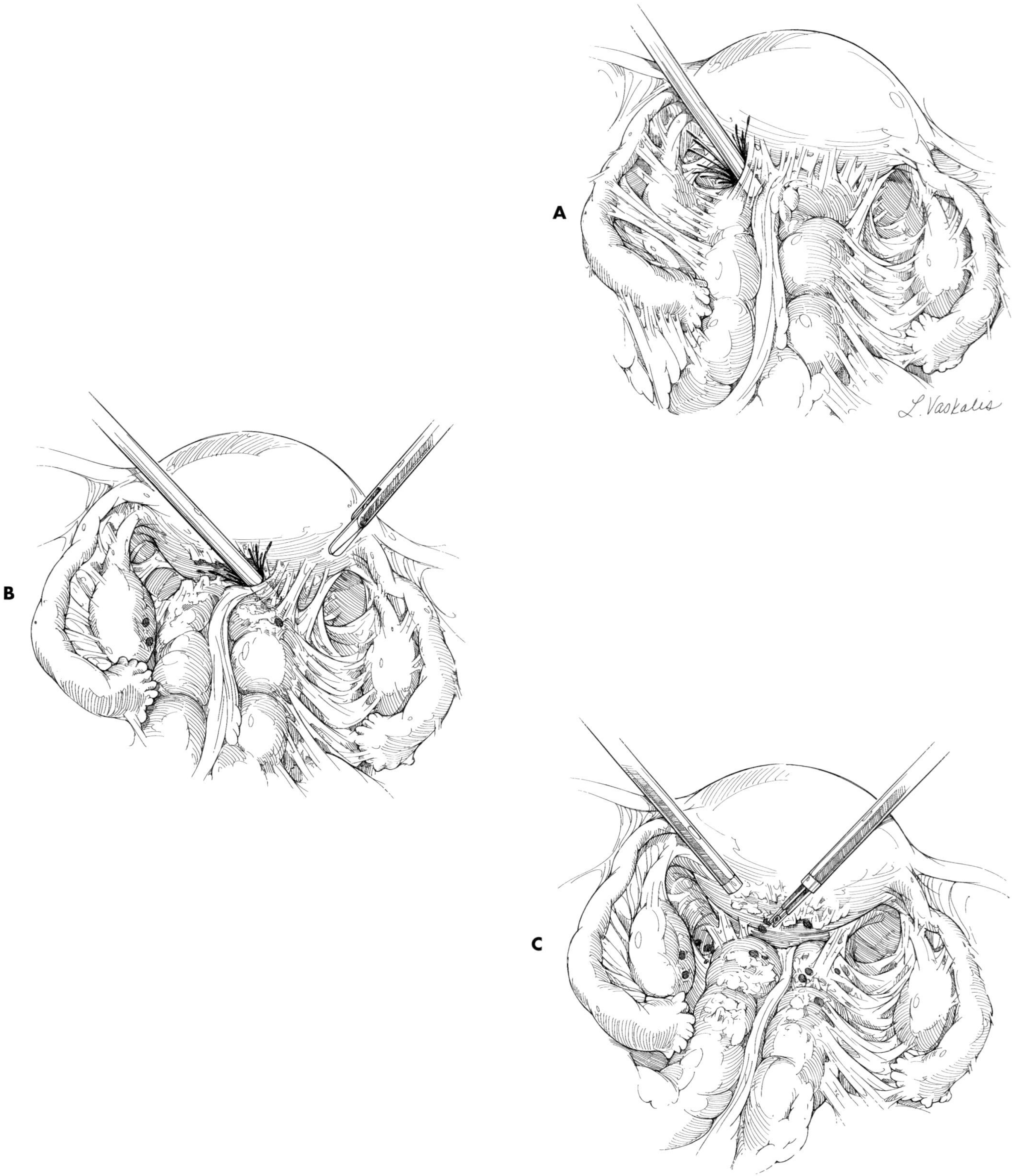

Fig. 18-4. Restoration of the anatomy of the obliterated cul de sac. **A,** Access is gained to the plane of dissection and hydrodissection commenced. **B** and **C,** The rectosigmoid is dissected from the back of the uterus and cervix using hydrodissection and sharp or laser dissection. Any bleeding vessels are electrodesiccated.

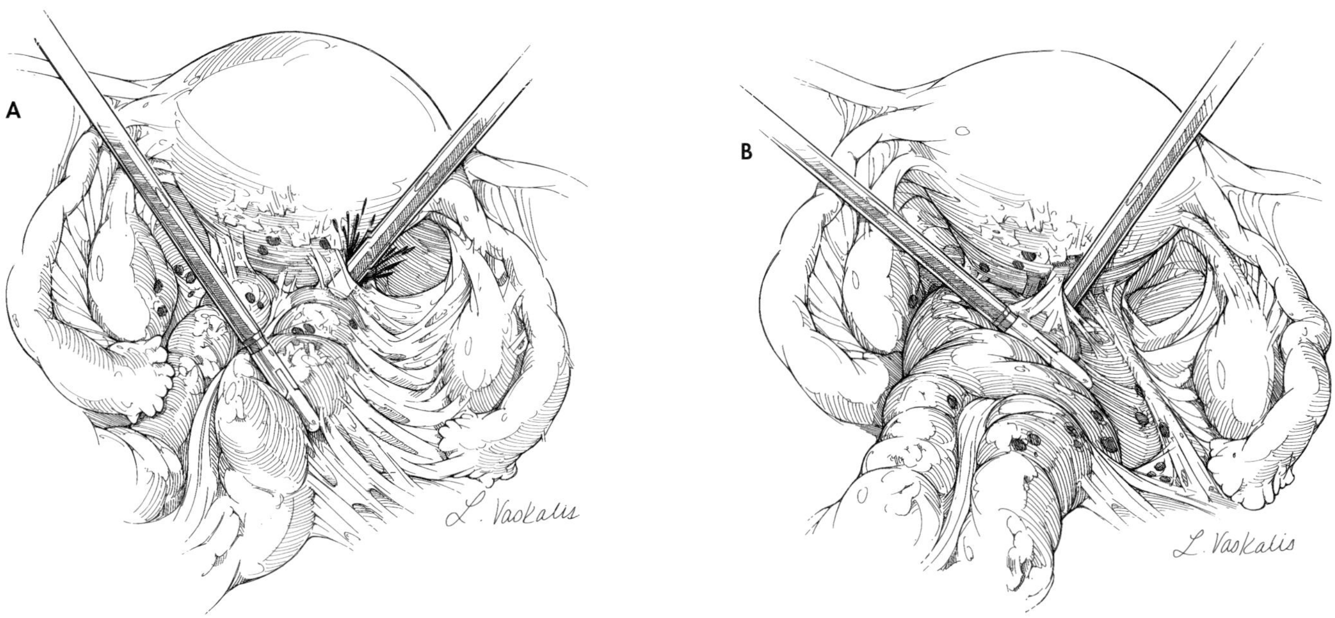

Fig. 18-5. Dissection of the rectum from the right uterosacral ligament and back of cervix. **A,** A small incision is made and the irrigation suction cannula introduced through this incision to start hydrodissection. **B,** The rectum has been dissected from the right uterosacral ligament and will be freed from the back of the cervix.

Surgery of the ureter. Hydrodissection has greatly simplified the laparoscopic management of superficial peritoneal implants that are sited over or in close proximity to the ureter. The first step is to inject about 20 to 30 ml of lactated Ringer's subperitoneally on the lateral pelvic wall. This will elevate the peritoneum. A 0.5 cm opening is made in the raised peritoneum, either with scissors or with the CO_2 laser. The incision should be made close to the pelvic brim. The suction irrigation cannula is inserted through this opening and about 100 ml of irrigation fluid is injected along the course of the ureter. The pressure should be set at 200 mm Hg. The fluid will surround the ureter and displace it posteriorly, usually leaving the peritoneal implant accessible to excision or laser vaporisation. The fluid also provides a backstop for the laser. The implant together with a margin of approximately 1 cm of healthy-appearing peritoneum should be excised or vaporized in a circular fashion. It is preferrable to excise lesions which are larger than 2 to 3 mm. To excise the lesion, once the incision has been made, grasping forceps are used to pull the tissue away from the ureter.

Implants that are firmly embedded, with scarring to the subperitoneal connective tissues, can be more difficult to remove, but, once again, hydrodissection can often be used to tunnel beneath the lesion and thus protect the ureter when vaporizing or excising the endometriosis. Following excision or vaporization, the area should be irrigated copiously, both to remove all carbon particles and to expose any bleeding vessels that can be spot desiccated.

Fortunately cases of partial or complete ureteral obstruction due to endometriosis are rare and have been managed by resection of the obstruction, access having been gained through a laparotomy incision. Nezhat et al. have treated four such patients by laparoscopic means.

The first case was reported in 1992.[33] The patient was a 36-year-old woman in whom a diagnosis of ureteric obstruction due to endometriosis had been made at the time of an earlier laparoscopy. She had refused to have a laparotomy and a nephrostomy tube had been inserted 4 years previously. A 3 to 4 cm fibrotic nodule was identified laparoscopically. It was sited 4 cm above the bladder, in a position that corresponded to that which had been observed by using radioimaging techniques. Attempts to place a ureteric catheter were unsuccessful. The ureter was mobilized, divided above and below the lesion, and the obstructed portion removed. Indigo carmine was injected intravenously and could be seen to be flowing from the proximal end of the ureter. An end-to-end anastomosis was performed over a ureteric catheter. The procedure lasted for 117 minutes, during which an estimated blood loss of less than 100 ml occurred. The patient was discharged on the first postoperative day. An external stent was left in situ for 4 weeks and was then replaced by an internal stent which remained in place for a further month. The recovery was uneventful and a postoperative intravenous pyelogram confirmed that renal function was normal. The follow-up of the four such

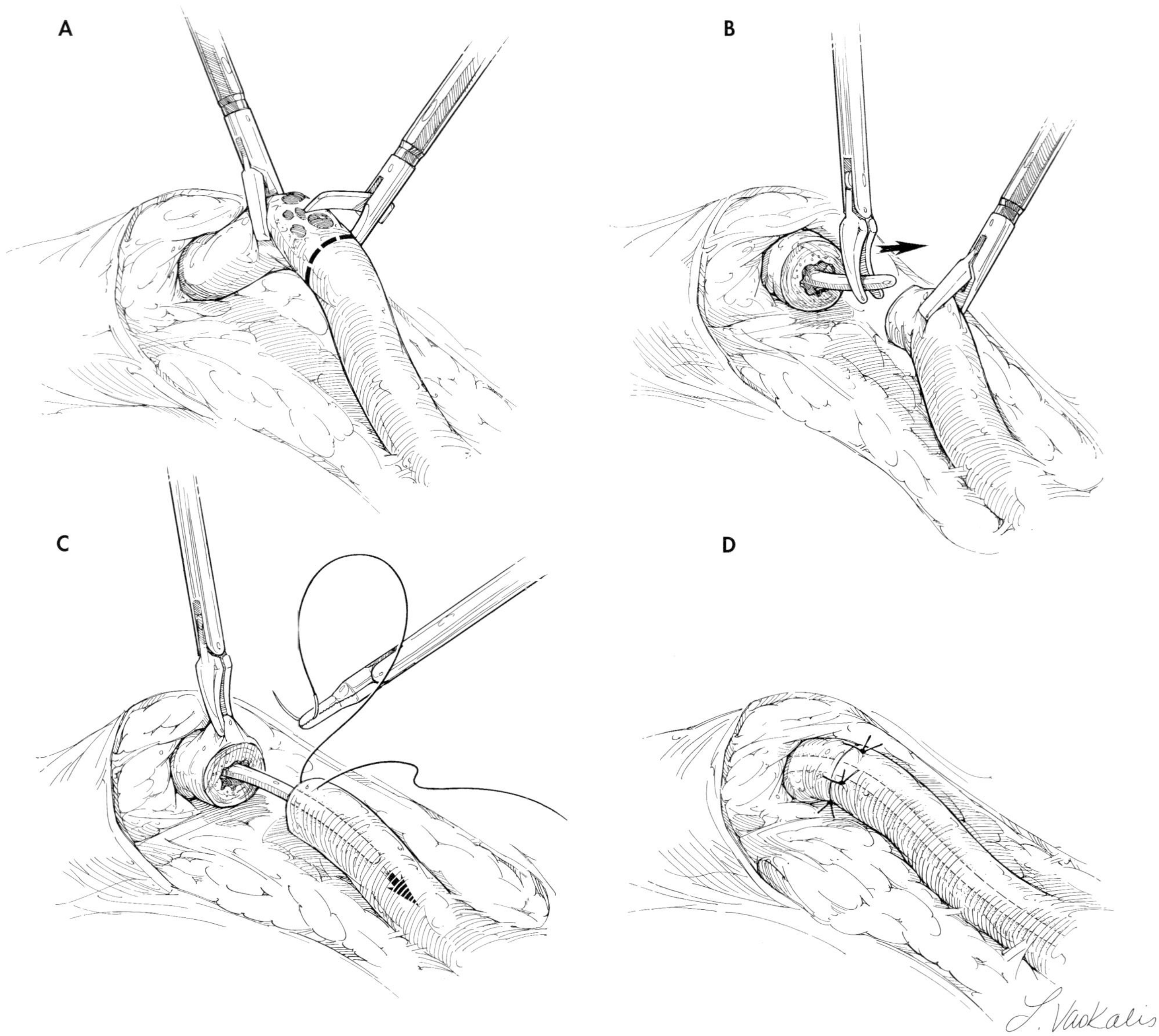

Fig. 18-6. Excision of the occluded segment of the ureter and end-to-end anastomosis. **A,** The ureter is dissected and the occluded area grasped. The ureter is transected above the site of occlusion. **B** and **C,** The occluded, diseased segment of ureter is excised and grasping forceps are used to manipulate the previously placed ureteric catheter into the upper ureteric lumen. **D,** The cut edges of the ureter are approximated with four sutures of 4.0 polydioxanone placed at cardial points.

cases treated by Nezhat et al. ranges from 1 to 3 years. All patients are well and normal renal function and ureteral patency has been confirmed.

Technique. The retroperitoneal space is entered at the pelvic brim as described above. By using a combination of hydrodissection and cutting, the ureter is mobilized and the affected region of the ureter exposed. A no. 7 French ureteric catheter is inserted under cystoscopic guidance. This catheter helps to identify the distal site of occlusion and acts as a stent for the anastomosis. The ureter is divided above and below the affected section which is excised (Fig. 18-6, *A*). Grasping forceps are used to maneuver the ureteric catheter into the proximal ureter (Fig. 18-6, *B* and *C*) and on into the renal pelvis. The healthy segments of the ureter are approximated with four 4-0 polydioxanone sutures which are placed at cardinal points (6, 12, 9, and 3 o'clock) (Fig. 18-6, *D*).

Surgery of the bladder. Endometriosis of the bladder wall is uncommon.[32] The lesions are usually superficial. When invasive they usually penetrate the muscularis but spare the mucosa. Rarely they may infiltrate the full thickness of the bladder wall. They can be dealt with by laparoscopic means.

Superficial lesions can be treated by excision, electrodesiccation, or laser vaporization as for other peritoneal implants. Fluid may be injected between the serosa and muscularis with a spinal needle or laparoscopic needle tip cannula to elevate the lesion and also provide a backstop when the CO_2 laser is used. Small superficial lesions can be electrodesiccated or vaporized with the laser. To excise endometriotic lesions, a circumferential incision is made in the serosa around the nodule including a margin of healthy peritoneum. The peritoneum on the side of the lesion is grasped with grasping forceps and elevated. The affected tissue is excised from the underlying structures using sharp and blunt dissection. Small vessels may need to be electrodesiccated. This approach can also be used when the muscularis is involved. It will be necessary to excise the affected muscularis and close the defect (see below). Residual disease can be treated with postoperative ovarian suppression.[32]

If the entire thickness of the bladder wall has been infiltrated by endometriosis it is necessary to excise the affected section of the bladder wall and reconstruct the defect.[34] A cystoscopy is performed, and when necessary ureteric catheters are inserted to facilitate the identification of the ureters. Grasping forceps are used to elevate the affected portion of the bladder wall, which is excised using the CO_2 laser or scissors (Fig. 18-7, *A* and *B*). The excision lines should be placed 5 mm beyond the limits of the nodule. The specimen is removed from the peritoneal cavity and sent for histologic examination. The interior of the bladder is then distended with CO_2 and the laparoscope inserted through the defect in the bladder wall so that the ureteral openings and bladder mucosa can be evaluated. The incision is closed with a continuous or interrupted 4-0 polydioxanone sutures (Fig. 18-7, *C*). These sutures include all tissue layers and are tied extracorporeally or intracorporeally (see Chapter 7). The bladder is distended with methylene blue or indigo carmine solution and observed laparoscopically to ensure that the suture line is watertight. A Foley catheter is left in the bladder. It is removed after 10 to 14 days if a cystogram demonstrates bladder integrity.

Nezhat et al. have treated four women and Gomel one woman in this fashion. The operating times were approximately 35 minutes and average estimated blood loss was 150 ml. All patients were discharged on the first postoperative day. Trimethopterin and sulphamethoxazole were given for 2 weeks. Follow-up of 10 to 13 months has shown that all patients are well and none are experiencing hematuria.

Gastrointestinal endometriosis. The gastrointestinal tract is involved in 3% to 37% of woman with endometriosis.[35,36] The rectosigmoid is most commonly affected. Clinical presentations vary from the asymptomatic where the disease is noted at the time of laparoscopy or laparotomy to one of complete intestinal obstruction. The presence of intestinal endometriosis should be suspected in any woman of child bearing age who presents with gastrointestinal symptoms and a prior history of known endometriosis or intestinal stricture in the absence of an intraluminal mass.[37] Cyclical rectal bleeding is a rare presentation and occurs when the lesion infiltrates the bowel mucosa. Because, in addition to the rectosigmoid, the uterosacral ligaments and rectovaginal septum are often involved in the disease process, the patient may complain of low abdominal pain, back pain, dysmenorrhea, and dyspareunia. She may experience diarrhea, constipation, and tenesmus. Radiographic studies that suggest constriction of the bowel, proctoscopy, and colonoscopy may provide helpful clues but are rarely diagnostic.[38] Occasionally microscopic examination of a biopsy of the bowel mucosa may reveal the presence of endometrial tissue.[39] Laparoscopy is the best method of diagnosis.

The implants can occur at any location from the small bowel to the anal canal. The rectum and sigmoid colon are most commonly affected and involved in 76% of such cases. The appendix and cecum are involved in 18% and 5%, respectively.[37] The cul-de-sac may be completely obliterated (see earlier).

Medical treatment rarely yields satisfactory long-term results. Surgical intervention will usually be required. Small lesions of the appendix can be laser vaporized, but, as many appendical lesions can be detected only by palpation, a case can be made for performing routine appendectomy (see Chapter 23) for patients with severe endometriosis.

Infiltrating bowel lesions may be dealt with by full-thickness resection of the affected area of the colon wall and reconstruction of the defect. This approach has been shown to be safe, carry a low morbidity rate, and give satisfactory symptomatic relief.[40] Circumferential bowel lesions will require a bowel resection and anastomosis. These procedures can be effected by laparoscopic means. A pre-

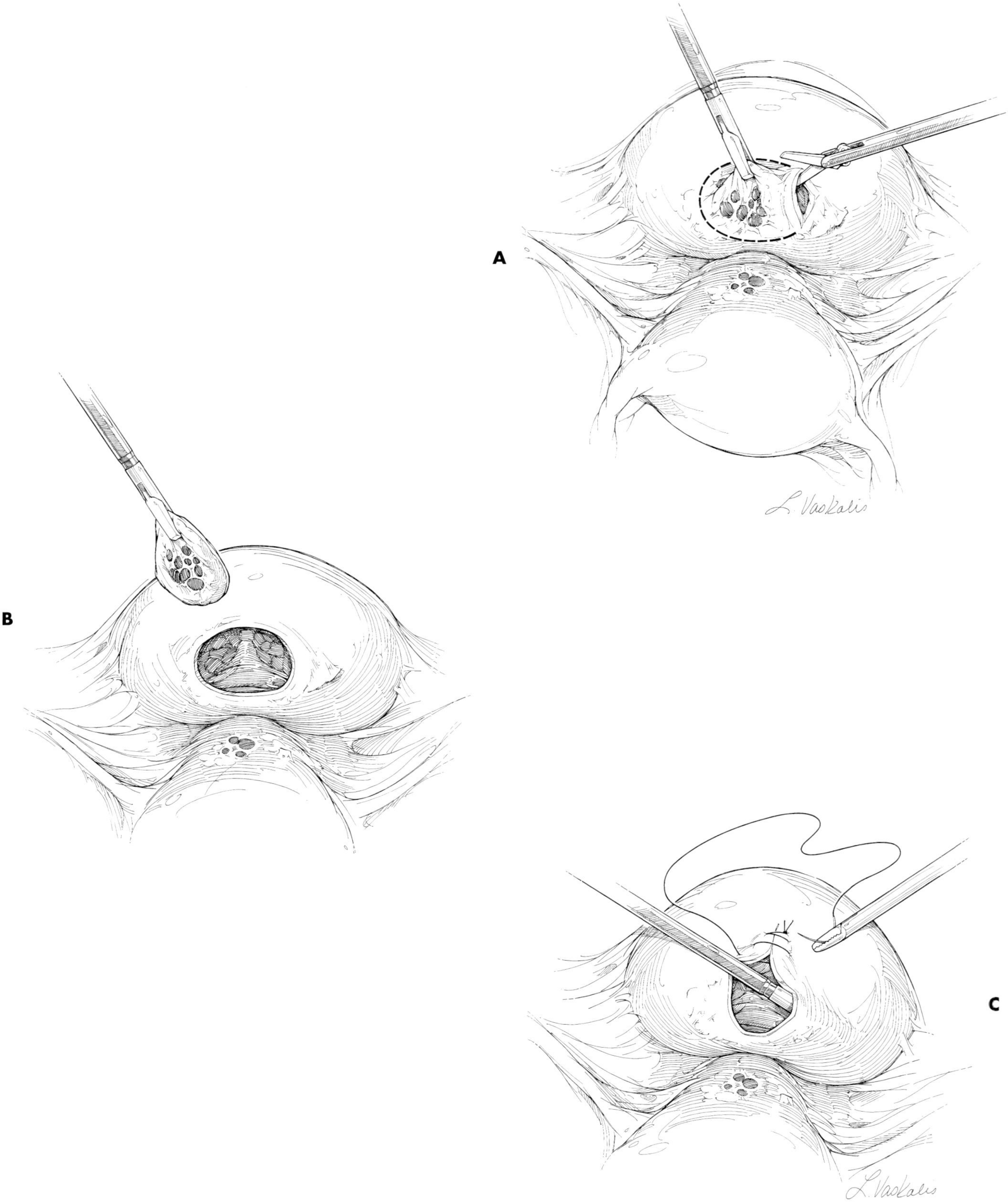

Fig. 18-7. Excision of lesion infiltrating the full thickness of the bladder wall. **A,** The lesion in the dome of the bladder is grasped and a circumferential incision made. **B**, The involved section of bladder wall is excised. **C**, The defect is repaired.

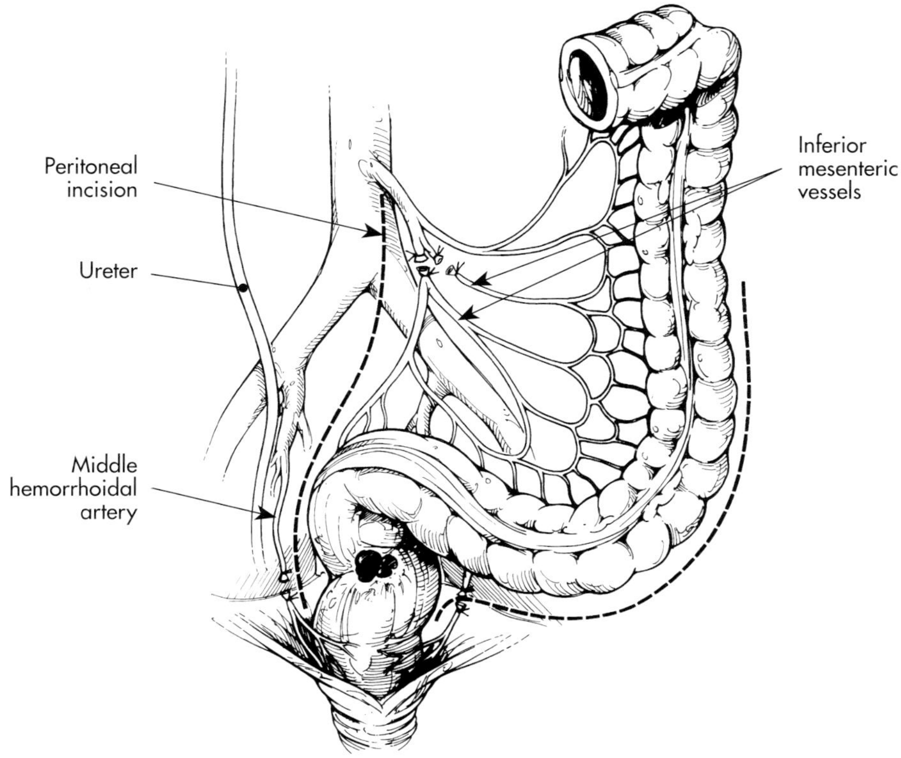

Fig. 18-8. Mobilization of the rectosigmoid.

operative full bowel preparation forms an integral part of such procedures.

To resect endometriosis of the large bowel three ancillary portals are used, with one being sited in the midline and one in each iliac fossa. There are three steps to the procedure; mobilization of the lower colon, transanal prolapse of the bowel segments, and resection-anastomosis. The operation is essentially that performed by laparotomy, the role of laparoscopy being to provide access for the mobilization step.[25,41]

To mobilize the lower colon and rectum the lateral rectal pedicles are electrodesiccated and divided and the presacral space entered. Dissection proceeds to the level of the levatores ani. Descending branches of the inferior mesenteric vessels are electrodesiccated and cut (Fig. 18-8). Anterior rectal lesions are treated differently from circumferential lesions.

Excision of anterior rectal lesion. If an anterior lesion is present, once the lower colon and rectum have been mobilized, the rectum is prolapsed through the anal canal until the lesion has been exteriorized. The affected portion of the anterior rectal wall is placed in the jaws of a stapling device (RL30 or RL60—Ethicon) (Fig. 18-9, *A*). When the device is fired the diseased section of the anterior wall is excised and the first layer of the repair accomplished (Fig. 18-9, *B*). The site is reinforced with interrupted 2-0 polyglactin sutures.

Excision of circumferential lesion. Circumferential lesions are dealt with by excision of the affected segment and end-to-end anastomosis. The rectum is laparoscopically transected cephalad to the lesion (Fig. 18-10, *A*). Babcock forceps introduced through the anal canal, grasp the cephalad limb of bowel, and pull it through the caudad rectal stump to the exterior. A 2-0 polypropylene purse string suture is inserted around the periphery of the cut edge, the anvil of a 29 or 33 ILS stapler (Ethicon) (see Fig. 18-11) is inserted into the bowel and the purse string tightened and tied around the anvil (Fig. 18-10, *B* and *C*). The cephalad rectum and the enclosed anvil are replaced in the pelvis.

The caudad limb of the rectum that harbors the diseased segment is prolapsed, using Babcock forceps introduced through the anus. The diseased segment is stapled with an RL60 device (Ethicon) proximal to lesion and the diseased segment excised (Fig. 18-10, *D* and *E*). The ILS stapler is placed against the closed rectal stump and used to push this stump into the abdomen (Fig. 18-10, *F*). The trocar of the ILS stapler penetrates the closed rectal stump. The assistant holds this part of the stapler steady while the surgeon uses laparoscopic grasping forceps to maneuver the anvil over the trocar (Fig. 18-10, *G*). When the ILS stapling device is locked by traction from below, the cephalad and caudad rectal stumps are brought into apposition. The stapler is fired, restoring rectal patency and completing the anastomosis (Fig. 18-10, *H*).

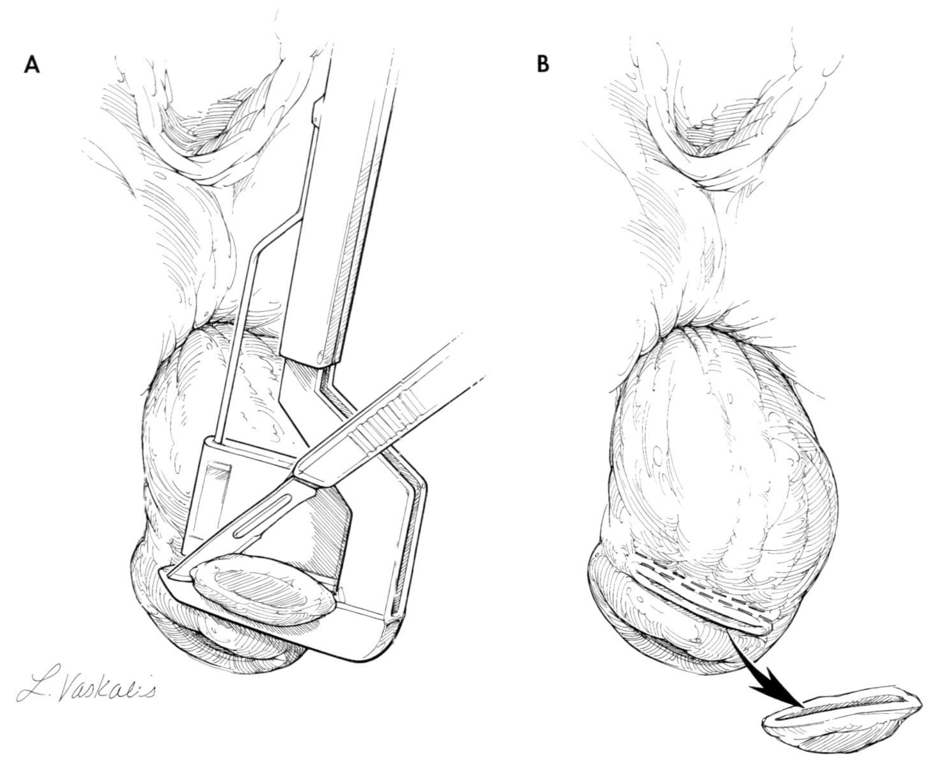

Fig. 18-9. Excision and repair of infiltrating lesion of the anterior rectal wall. **A** and **B**, The rectum is prolapsed and an automatic stapling device used to excise the lesion and repair the defect.

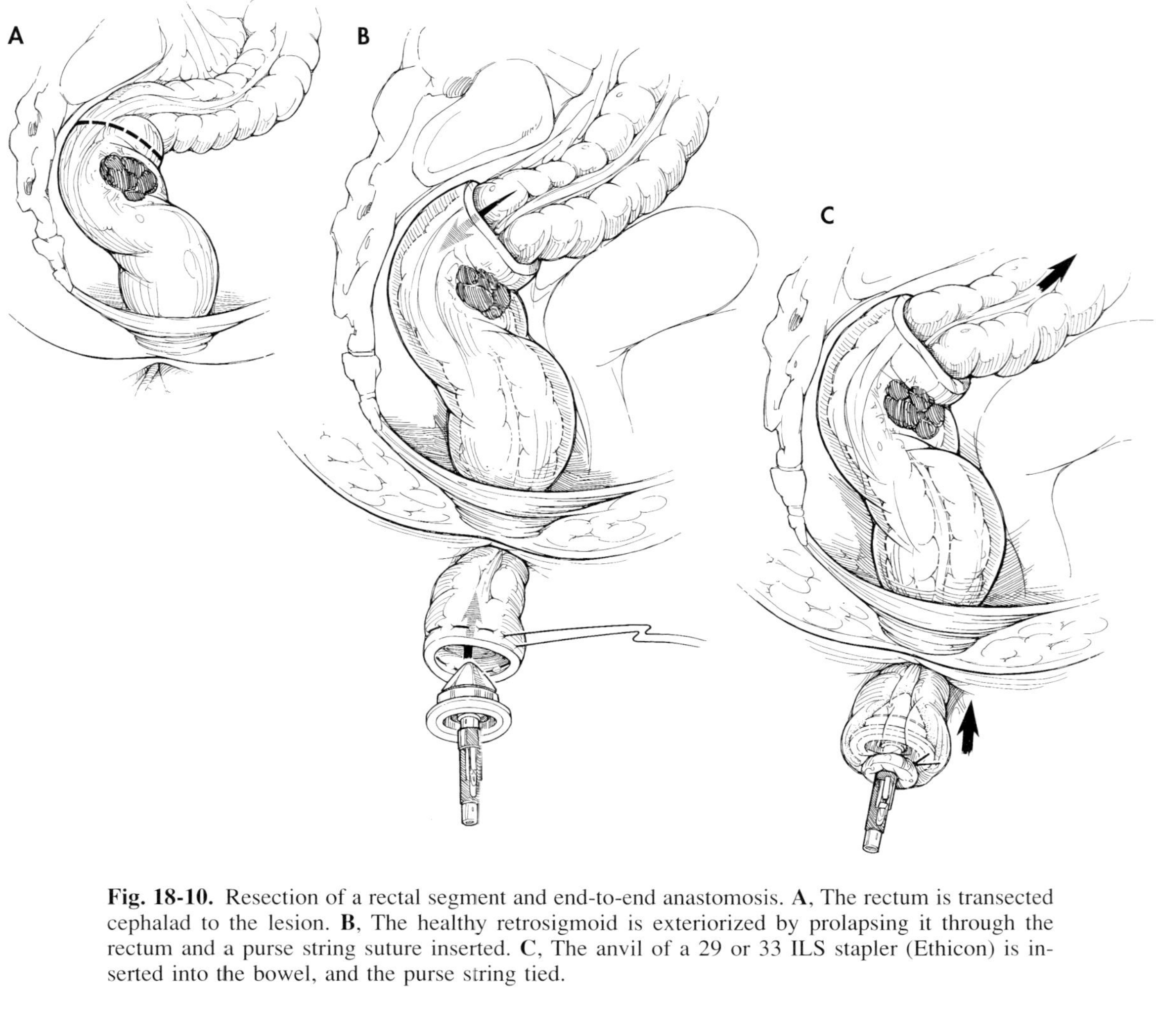

Fig. 18-10. Resection of a rectal segment and end-to-end anastomosis. **A**, The rectum is transected cephalad to the lesion. **B**, The healthy retrosigmoid is exteriorized by prolapsing it through the rectum and a purse string suture inserted. **C**, The anvil of a 29 or 33 ILS stapler (Ethicon) is inserted into the bowel, and the purse string tied.

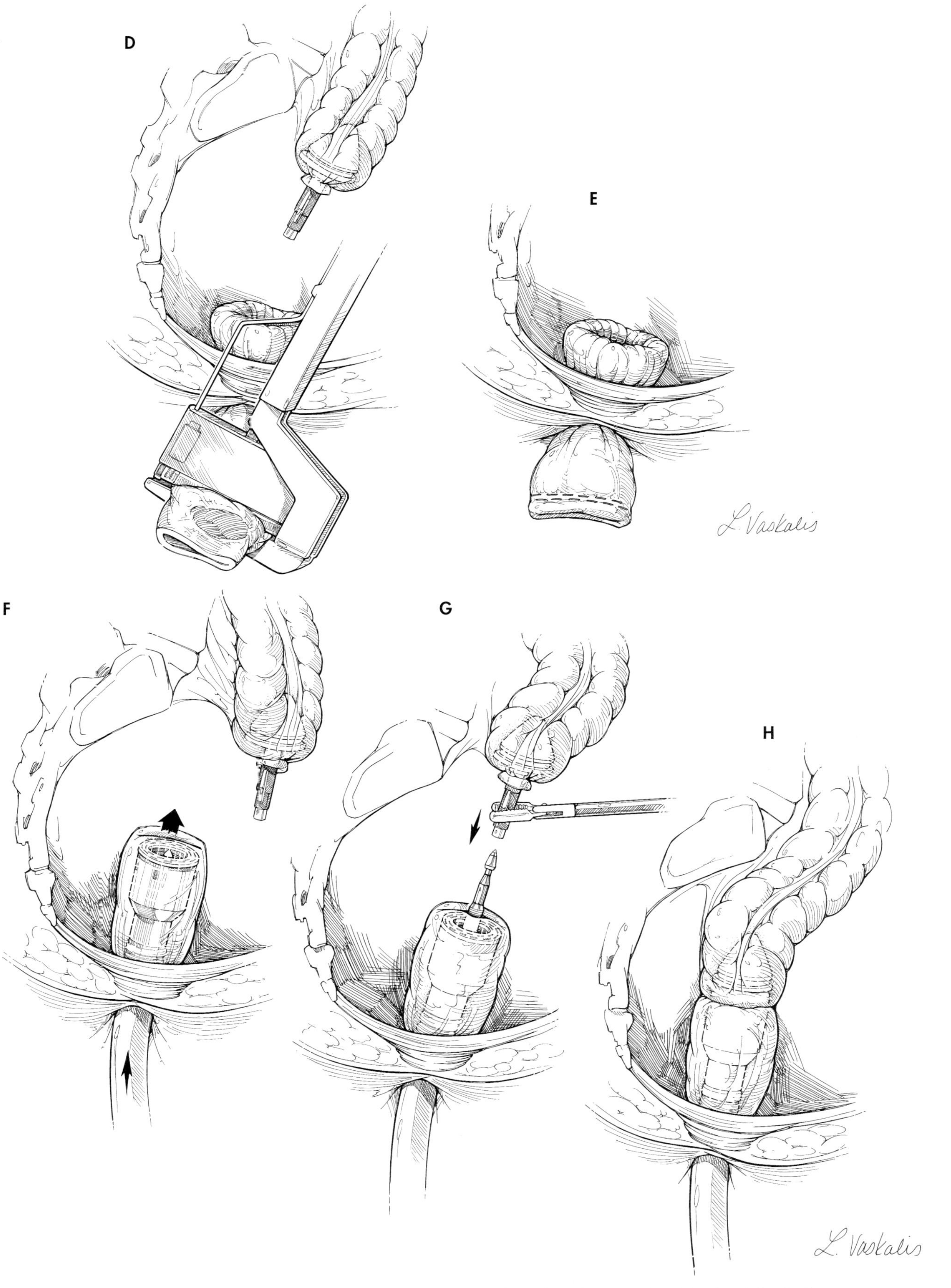

Fig. 18-10, cont'd. D and **E,** The healthy rectosigmoid and anvil are replaced in the abdominal cavity. The distal rectum is prolapsed and stapled between healthy tissue and the lesion. The diseased segment is thus excised. **F**, The ILS stapler is placed into the closed rectal stump and used to push the stump into the abdominal cavity. **G**, The trocar of the stapling device penetrates the rectal stump. Laparoscopic grasping forceps are used to maneuuver the anvil over the trocar. **H**, The ends of the two segments of bowel are brought together and the stapling device fired to complete the anastomosis.

Once these steps have been completed a series of further steps are taken, irrespective of the type of resection. A proctoscope is passed to permit inspection of the internal site of anastomosis to confirm structural integrity and that there is no bleeding. The pelvis is flooded with irrigation fluid and air is insufflated into the rectum. If air is seen to leak, 2-0 polyglactin sutures can be placed to close the defect.

Excision of anterior colonic lesion. Excision of the affected portion of the colonic wall and reconstruction of the defect has been shown to be effective for treating infiltrating localized lesions.[42] This approach is simpler to perform and less extensive than segmental bowel resection and anastomosis. The lesion is evaluated visually and by palpation with the tip of the suction irrigator to delineate the extent of involvement. Low lesions can also be palpated by digital rectal examination. Sigmoidoscopy is also used for this purpose.

The ureters are identified, and the lateral aspects of the colon are mobilized. Mobilization is carried out by a combination of hydrodissection and laser division of tissue. This step can be performed with scissors. The colon is separated from the adjacent organs.

Grasping forceps are applied to the affected portion of the bowel wall to elevate and steady it. An incision is made through the full thickness of the bowel wall to encircle the lesion completely with a margin of healthy tissue (Fig. 18-12, *A*). The excised tissue can be removed either through one of the laparoscopic portals or preferably by introducing polyp forceps through the anus and pulling the specimen out by that route (Fig. 18-12, *B*).

Two traction sutures are applied, one in the middle of each of the lateral margins of the wound, and brought out through the portals in the iliac fossae. Traction on these sutures will transform the incision, which is usually in the longitudinal axis of the bowel, into a transverse incision (Fig. 18-12, *C*). The bowel is repaired by placing several interrupted sutures that incorporate the full thickness of the wall. Closure is effected in the transverse axis to minimize the risk of subsequent stricture (Fig. 18-12, *D*). The sutures are placed at 0.4 to 0.6 cm intervals. A straight or curved needle carrying 0 polyglactin or polydioxanone sutures is used and the knots are tied intra or extracorporeally. Once the defect in the bowel is closed, copious lavage is performed and the pelvis flooded with the irrigation solution. The procedure is concluded, as before by using a sigmoidoscope to identify any bleeding or lack of tissue integrity. The traction sutures, which up to this point serve a useful function as retractors, are removed.

Endometriosis of the diaphragm

Endometriosis of the diaphragm is rare. In centers that deal with a very large number of patients with endometriosis such lesions are identified in under 1% of cases. Since most of these cases are asymptomatic, identification of such lesions requires a thorough examination of the under surface of the diaphragm, which is more easily effected by laparoscopy than by laparotomy. The prevalence of symptomatic lesions is eight in 4,875. The symptoms included pleuritic, shoulder, or upper abdominal pain which occurs in conjunction with the menses.

Laparoscopic removal of such lesions is hazardous, as the phrenic nerves, lungs, and heart may all be at risk of injury. All other treatment options should be fully explored before recourse to surgery. A course of medical suppressive therapy may be all that is required, and cure is almost assured if radical treatment of pelvic endometriosis is undertaken. If fertility is still an issue and symptoms have not responded to medical therapy, laparoscopic intervention may be justified.

The laparoscope is introduced intraumbilicaly and three ancillary portals are placed in the upper quadrant, in a fashion akin to that used for cholecystectomy. Two expandable retracting probes or closed grasping forceps are used to retract the liver and expose the operative field. Lesions are removed by a combination of hydrodissection, excision, or laser vaporization. Should a diaphragmatic defect appear it can be repaired with interrupted 4-0 polydioxanone sutures.

While the patient is still under aesthesia, the pharynx, larynx, trachea, and proximal main bronchi should be evaluated by a cardiopulmonary consultant. Pulmonary endometriosis may co-exist.

Results

Surgery of the reproductive organs. It is difficult to compare the relative values of the two methods of access by which endometriosis can be treated surgically. Tentative conclusions can be drawn from observations of adhesion formation following either approach for conditions other than endometriosis. Uncontrolled clinical series can be compared, but no firm conclusions can be drawn from these data. Outcomes following laparoscopic techniques described in this chapter can be discussed.

Postoperative de-novo adhesions and reformation of adhesions following standardized injury and adhesiolysis have been evaluated in animal models at the times of laparoscopy and laparotomy.[43-45] Whereas some of these animal studies reported better outcomes associated with laparoscopy, others reported no difference. Lundorff et al. prospectively randomized a group of 105 women with ectopic pregnancies to one of the two approaches. The patients were stratified by age and risk factors.[46] Second-look laparoscopy showed that significantly more adhesions had formed in the laparotomy group compared to those treated by laparoscopy.

Table 18-2 is a comparison of published case series.[17,47-58] Because the groups are so heterogeneous it is not possible to say with any authority which approach is superior for the management of rAFS stages 2 and 3 endometriosis. Chong et al. compared the outcomes when one

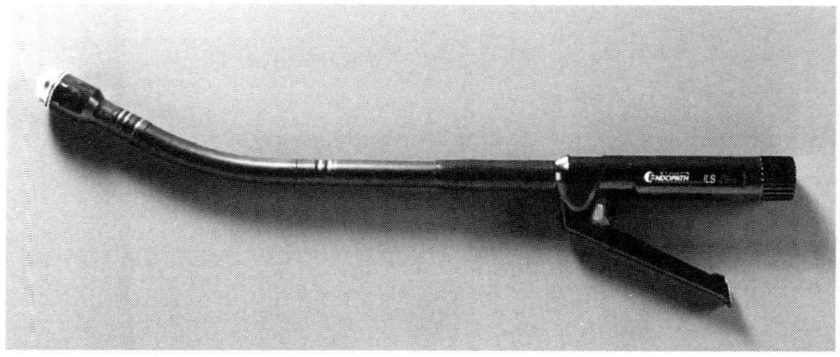

Fig. 18-11. The ILS stapler from Ethicon Endosurgery.

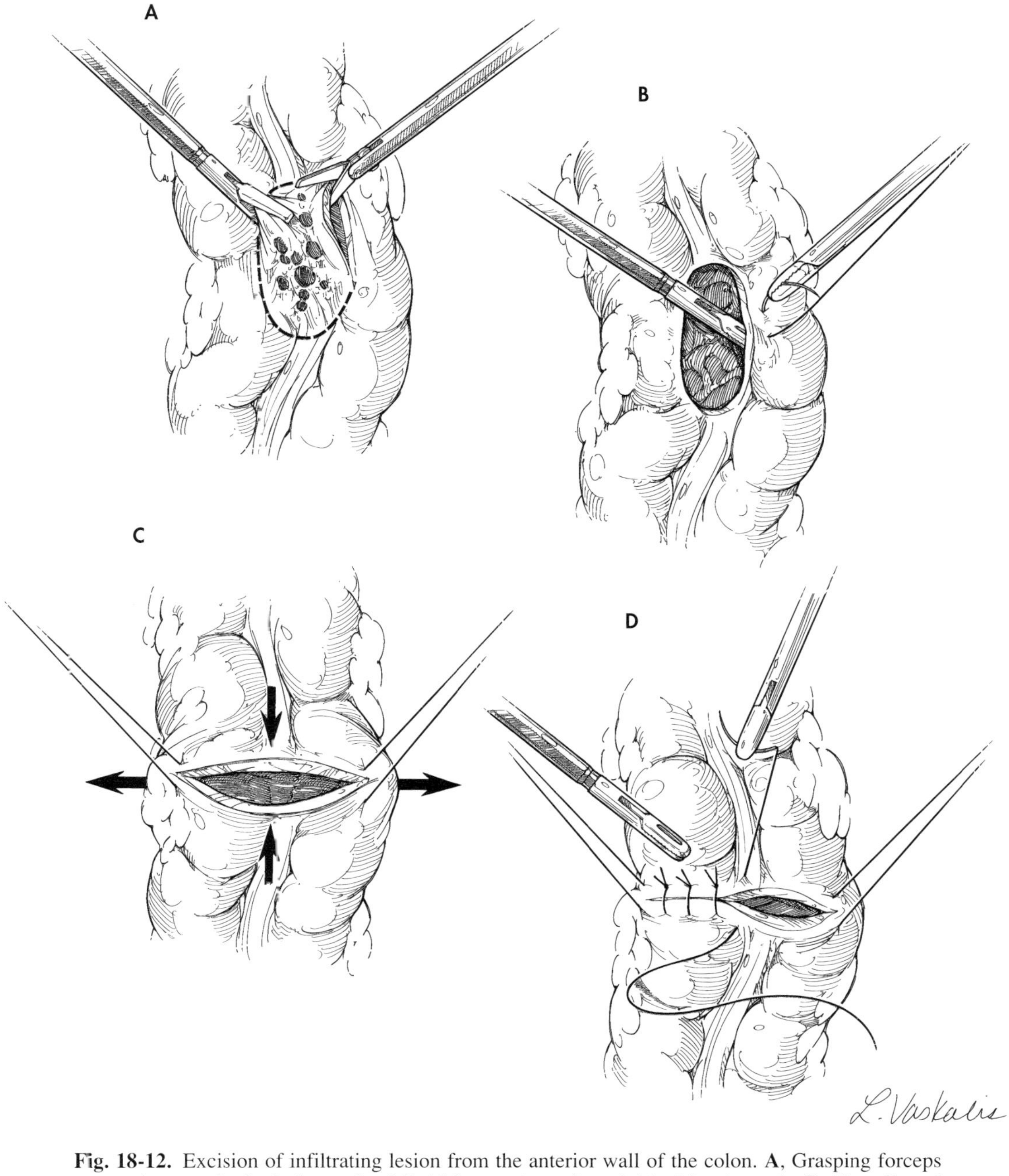

Fig. 18-12. Excision of infiltrating lesion from the anterior wall of the colon. **A**, Grasping forceps are used to steady the lesion and a full thickness circumferential incision is made. **B**, The affected segment of bowel wall is removed. **C**, Stay sutures are placed at the edges of the incision and traction applied to realign the axis of the incision. **D**, Interrupted sutures are placed to close the incision transversely.

Table 18-2. Number of patients (N) and pregnancy rates (%) following conservative surgery for endometriosis by laparotomy or laparoscopy

	Mild		Moderate*		Severe	
	N	%	N	%	N	%
Laparotomy						
Buttram[58]	88	69.3%	50	45.0%	68	47.1%
Rock et al.[47]	45	62.0%	88	54.0%	81	48.1%
Rantala et al.[48]	44	59.1%	39	56.0%	46	30.1%
Gordts et al.[49]	20	40.0%	99	42.4%	47	35.1%
Olive and Lee[50]	11	45.0%	43	51.2%	34	29.4%
Chong et al.[51]	0		0		13	53.8%
Fayez et al.[17]	0		0		42	36.0%
Adamson et al.[52]					52	34.6%
Total	208	61.3%	319	49.9%	393	39.1%
Laparoscopy						
Feste[53]	47	51.6%	6	66.3%	5	40.1%
Martin[54]	27	25.9%	19	15.8%	4	25.2%
Nezhat[55]	24	75.1%	51	62.7%	27	44.4%
Olive et al.[56]	59	36.6%	48	35.4%	21	54.4%
Nezhat et al.[57]	39	71.8%	153	68.6%	51	68.6%
Chong et al[51]	0		0		11	54.5%
Fayez et al.[17]	0		0		106	58.0%
Adamson et al.[52]	0		0		48	37.5%
Total	196	50.3%	277	58.1%	272	57.2%

*Stages 2 and 3, rAFS classification.

surgeon skilled in laser microsurgery (Chong) and one in laser laparoscopy (Luciano) operated on two groups of women with disease of comparable severity.[51] Similar pregnancy rates were recorded by both surgeons.

Surgery to restore obliteration of the cul-de-sac is not without risk of bowel perforation. When nodular endometrial lesions were removed from the rectosigmoid in 356 patients, bowel was entered in 23.[59] A one-layer repair was immediately performed. There were no immediate or long-term adverse sequelae.

Complete dissection of the rectovaginal space was performed in 185 women.[60] The procedures lasted from 55 to 245 minutes. Only ten patients were not discharged within 24 hours. Among these ten patients there were nine who suffered bowel perforation and one who required segmental bowel resection. Follow-up data for 1 to 5 years was available from 174 women. Moderate to complete pain relief had been obtained by 162 (93%). Thirteen had undergone a second procedure and four a third. Twelve (7%) were experiencing pain that had worsened.

Surgery of the nonreproductive organs. Ureteric anastomosis has been performed on four patients. Follow-up of 1 to 3 years has been satisfactory. Similarly, five women have undergone partial resection of the bladder. No intraoperative or immediately postoperative complications were noted. Ten to 13 months of follow-up have shown that all five women are doing well and none have had recurrence of symptoms.

Segmental bowel resection for circumferential lesions has been performed 16 times.[61] In one patient the operation had to be completed by laparotomy. No other short- or long-term complications were recorded. Partial resection has been performed in 32 women.[42] The lesions measured from 4 to 10 cm. There were no complications postoperatively or at the 24-month follow-up.

Diaphragmatic lesions have been treated in eight patients. No immediate complications were recorded. Follow-up has been for 6 to 36 months. Six patients are doing well. One experienced no pain relief and one had the symptoms return 1 year postoperatively.

FUTURE DEVELOPMENTS

The question of which is the best of the currently available means of access can be answered only by prospective comparative studies. It must be acknowledged that the time taken for some cases of extensive dissection can be very long. It is possible that technologic advances may overtake both laparotomy and laparoscopy before large enough comparative studies have been completed.

Tiny endoscopes of about 1 mm in diameter may permit diagnosis to be made simply. It is possible that combinations of microendoscopes and photodynamic therapy may revolutionize the treatment of endometriosis. It has already been demonstrated in animal models that dihydro porphyrin ether (DHE) is selectively taken up by endometrial tissue. When tissues that have been so treated are treated with low-energy argon laser, only the tissues that have absorbed the DHE are destroyed.[62]

REFERENCES

1. Ranney BR: Endometriosis III: Complete operations. *Am J Obstet Gynecol* 109:1137, 1971.
2. Wilson EA: Surgical therapy for endometriosis. *Clin Obstet Gynecol* 31:857, 1988.
3. Betts WJ, Buttram CVJ: A plan for managing endometriosis. *Contemp Ob/Gyn* 15:121, 1980.
4. Ranney BR: Endometriosis: Conservative operations. *Am J Obstet Gynecol* 107:743, 1970.
5. Wheeler JH, Malinak LR: Recurrent endometriosis: incidence, management, and prognosis. *Am J Obstet Gynecol* 146:247, 1983.
6. Henderson AF, Studd JWW, Watson N: A retrospective study of estrogen replacement therapy following hysterectomy for the treatment of endometriosis. In Shaw RW, editor: *Advances in Reproductive Endocrinology,* Vol 1. Endometriosis. Carnforth, Lancs, Parthenon, 11:131, 1989.
7. Schenken SR, Malinak RL: Reoperation after initial treatment of endometriosis with conservative surgery. *Am J Obstet Gynecol* 131:416, 1978.
8. Nezhat C, Nezhat FR: Safe laser endoscopic excision or vaporization of peritoneal endometriosis. *Fertil Steril* 52:149, 1989.
9. Murphy AA, Green WR, Bobbie D, et al: Unsuspected endometriosis documented by scanning electron microsurgery in visually normal peritoneum. *Fertil Steril* 46:522, 1986.
10. Nezhat F, Allan JC, Nezhat C, et al: Nonvisualized endometriosis at laparoscopy. *Int J Fertil* 36:340, 1991.
11. Vasquez G, Cornille F, Brosens IA: Peritoneal endometriosis: Scanning electron microscopy and histology of minimal pelvic endometriotic lesions. *Fertil Steril* 42:696, 1984.
12. Martin DC, Hubert GD, Vander-Zwaag R, et al: Laparoscopic appearances of pelvic endometriosis. *Fertil Steril* 51:63, 1989.
13. Stripling MC, Martin DC, Chatman DL, et al: Subtle appearance of pelvic endometriosis. *Fertil Steril* 49:427, 1988.
14. Jansen R, Russell P: Nonpigmented endometriosis: clinical, laparoscopic, and pathological definition. *Am J Obstet Gynecol* 155:1154, 1986.
15. Candiani GB, Vercelli P, Fedele L: Laparoscopic ovarian puncture to correct staging of endometriosis. *Fertil Steril* 53:984, 1990.
16. Luciano AA, Marana R, Krakta S, et al: Ovarian function after incision of the ovary by scalpel, CO_2 laser and microelectrode. *Fertil Steril* 56:349, 1991.
17. Fayez JA, Collazo LM: Comparison between laparotomy and operative laparoscopy in the treatment of moderate and severe endometriosis. *Int J Fertil* 35:272, 1990.
18. Brosens I, Puttemansi: Double optic laparoscopy. *Ballieres Clin Obstet Gynecol* 3:595, 1989.
19. Keye WR, Hansen LW, Astin M, et al: Argon laser therapy of endometriosis: a review of 92 consecutive patients. *Fertil Steril* 47:208, 1987.
20. Nezhat C, Winer W, Cooper J, et al: Endoscopic infertility surgery, *J Reprod Med* 34:127, 1989.
21. Nezhat F, Nezhat C, Allan CJ, et al: A clinical and histologic classification of endometriomas: implications for a mechanism of pathogenesis. *J Reprod Med* 37:771-776, 1992.
22. Marana R, Luciano AA, Muzii L, et al: Reproductive outcome after ovarian surgery: suturing versus nonsuturing of the ovarian cortex. *J Gynecol Surg* 7:155, 1991.
23. Nezhat C, Nezhat F: Postoperative adhesion formation after ovarian cystectomy with and without ovarian reconstruction. Abstract O-012 47th Annual meeting of the American Fertility Society, Orlando, Florida, October 21-24, 1991.
24. Nezhat C, Nezhat F, Ambroze W, Pennington E: Laparoscopic repair of small bowel, colon, and rectal endometriosis: a report of twenty-six cases. *Surg Endosc* 7:88-9, 1993.
25. Nezhat C, Pennington E, Nezhat F, Silfen SL: Laparoscopically assisted anterior rectal wall resection and reanastomosis for deeply infiltrating endometriosis. *Surg Laparosc Endosc* 1:2:106-8, 1991.
26. Brumsted JR, Deaton J, Lavigne E, et al: Postoperative adhesion formation after ovarian wedge resection with and without ovarian reconstruction in the rabbit. *Fertil Steril* 53:723, 1990.
27. Ellis H: The cause and prevention of postoperative intraperitoneal adhesions. *Surg Gynecol Obstet* 133:497, 1971.
28. Black WT: Use of presacral sympathectomy in the treatment of dysmenorrhea: a second look after twenty-five years. *Am J Obstet Gynecol* 89:16, 1964.
29. Lee RB, Stone K, Magelssen D, et al: Presacral neurectomy for chronic pelvic pain. *Obstet Gynecol* 68:517, 1986.
30. Tjaden B, Schlaff WD, Kimball A, et al: The efficacy of presacral neurectomy for the relief of midline dysmenorrhea. *Obstet Gynecol* 76:89, 1990.
31. Stanley EK, Utz DC, Dockerty MB: Clinically significant endometriosis of the urinary tract. *Surg Gynec et Obstet* 120:491, 1965.
32. Goldstein MS, Brodman ML: Cystometric evaluation of vesical endometriosis before and after hormonal or surgical treatment. *Mt. Sinai J Med* 57:109, 1990.
33. Nezhat C, Nezhat F, Green G: Laparoscopic treatment of obstructed ureter due to endometriosis by resection and ureteroureterostomy: a case report. *J Urol* 148:659, 1992.
34. Nezhat C, Nezhat F: Laparoscopic segmental bladder resection for endometriosis: a report of two cases. *Obstet Gynecol* 81:882, 1993.
35. Jenkinson EL, Brown WH: Endometriosis: A study of 117 cases with special reference to constricting lesions of the rectum and sigmoid colon. *JAMA* 122:349, 1943.
36. Samper ER, Sagle GW, Hand AM: Colonic endometriosis, its clinical spectrum. *South Med J* 77:912, 1984.
37. Prystowsky JB, Stryker SJ, Ujiki GT, et al: Gastrointestinal endometriosis: incidence and indications for resection. *Arch Surg* 7:855-8, 1988.
38. Ponka JL, Brush BE, Hodgkinson CP: Colorectal endometriosis. *Dis Colon Rectum* 16:490, 1973.
39. Meyers WC, Kelvin FM, Jones RS: Diagnosis and surgical treatment of colonic endometriosis. *Arch Surg* 114:169-175, 1979.
40. Coronado C, Franklin RR, Lotze EC, et al: Surgical treatment of symptomatic colorectal endometriosis. *Fertil Steril* 3:411, 1990.
41. Nezhat C, Nezhat F, Pennington E: Laparoscopic proctectomy for infiltrating endometriosis of the rectum. *Fertil Steril* 57:1129, 1992.
42. Nezhat C, Nezhat F, Pennington E, Nezhat CH: Laparoscopic partial colon resection and reanastomosis for deeply infiltrative endometriosis. *Surg Endosc* (Accepted for publication.)
43. Filmar S, Gomel V, McComb P: Operative laparoscopy versus open abdominal surgery: a comparative study on postoperative adhesion formation in the rat model. *Fertil Steril* 48:486-490, 1987.
44. Luciano AA, Maier DB, Nulsen ZC et al: A comparative study of postoperative adhesion formation following laser surgery by laparoscopy versus laparotomy in the rabbit model. *Obstet Gynecol* 74:220, 1989.
45. Maier DB, Klock A, Nulsen J et al: Laser laparoscopy vs laparotomy in lysis of dense and incidental pelvic adhesions. *J Reprod Med* 37:965, 1992.
46. Lundorff P, Hahlin M, Kallfelt B et al: Adhesion formation after laparoscopic surgery in ectopic pregnancy: A randomized trial versus laparotomy. *Fertil Steril* 55:91-915, 1991.
47. Rock JA, Guzick DS, Sengoo C et al: The conservative surgical treatment of endometriosis: Evaluation of pregnancy successes with respect to the extent of disease as categorized using contemporary classification systems. *Fertil Steril* 35:131, 1981.
48. Rantala ML, Kahanpaa KV, Koskimies AL et al: Fertility prognosis after surgical treatment of pelvic endometriosis. *Acta Obstet Gynecol Scand* 62:11, 1983.

49. Gordts S, Boeckx W, Brosens I: Microsurgery of endometriosis in infertile patients. *Fertil Steril* 42:520, 1984.
50. Olive DL, Lee KL: Analysis of sequential treatment protocols for endometriosis-associated infertility. *Am J Obstet Gynecol* 154:613, 1986.
51. Chong AP, Luciano AA, O'Shaughnessy AM: Laser laparoscopy versus laparotomy in the treatment of infertility patients with severe endometriosis. *J Gynecol Surg* 6:179, 1990.
52. Adamson DG, Subak LL, Pasta DJ, et al: Comparison of CO_2 laser laparoscopy with laparotomy for the treatment of endometriomata. *Fertil Steril* 57:965, 1992.
53. Feste JR: Laser laparoscopy: a new modality. *J Reprod Med* 30:413, 1985.
54. Martin DC: CO_2 laser laparoscopy for the treatment of endometriosis associated with infertility. *J Reprod Med* 30:409, 1985.
55. Nezhat C, Crowgey S, Nezhat F: Surgical treatment of endometriosis via laser laparoscopy. *Fertil Steril* 45:778, 1986.
56. Olive DL, Martin DC: Treatment of endometriosis associated infertility with CO_2 laser laparoscopy: The use of 1- and 2-parameter exponential models. *Fertil Steril* 48:18, 1987.
57. Nezhat C, Growgey S, Nezhat F: Videolaseroscopy for the treatment of endometriosis associated with infertility. *Fertil Steril* 51:123, 1989.
58. Buttram VC: Surgical treatment of endometriosis in the infertile female: a modified approach. *Fertil Steril* 32:635-40, 1979.
59. Nezhat C, Silfen SL, Nezhat F, et al: Surgery for endometriosis. *Curr Opin Obstet Gynecol* 3:385, 1991.
60. Nezhat C, Nezhat F, Pennington E: Laparoscopic treatment of lower colorectal and infiltrative rectovaginal septum endometriosis by the technique of videolaseroscopy. *Br J Obstet Gynaecol* 99:664-667, 1992.
61. Nezhat F, Nezhat C, Pennington E, Ambroze W: Laparoscopic segmental resection for infiltrating endometriosis of the rectosigmoid colon: a preliminary report. *Surg Laparosc Endosc* 2:212-216, 1992.
62. Manyak MJ, Nelson LM, Solomon D, Russo A, et al: Photodynamic therapy of rabbit endometrial implants: a model treatment of endometriosis. *Fertil Steril* 52:140, 1989.

Chapter 19

MYOMECTOMY

Alan G. Gordon

The advent of endoscopic surgery in the 1980s heralded the first significant change in the treatment of uterine fibroids since the introduction some 50 years previously of myomectomy as an alternative to hysterectomy.

ABDOMINAL MYOMECTOMY

The first report of successful myomectomy was in 1845.[1] In 1931 Bonney published his description of the principles of myomectomy and hysterectomy that he had been performing for the previous 20 years.[2] In his monograph published in 1946 he reported 806 myomectomies with only nine deaths, a mortality rate of 1.1%.[3] Only two of the deaths occurred in his last 400 cases. By the end of the 1950s surgical treatment of myomas had been accepted by most gynecologists. Myomectomy was performed if preservation of fertility was desired, otherwise hysterectomy was recommended. The goals of myomectomy should be the return of normal menstrual function, uterine morphology, and the enhancement of fertility achieved by an operation that keeps blood loss and tissue trauma to a minimum.

Surgical technique

The uterine incisions were planned to minimize potential adhesion formation. Incisions were placed on the anterior uterine wall and as many fibroids as possible were removed through a single approach. Fibroids situated on the posterior uterine wall were removed through a fundal hood incision to prevent the formation of adhesions between loops of bowel and uterus.

At the completion of the operation the uterus was carefully palpated to ensure that all the fibroids had been removed. Accurate repair of the uterine defect using nonreactive sutures was considered mandatory. Some surgeons also used fibrin glue of "Tissuecol" to prevent adhesion formation.[4] Recently the use of microsurgical techniques has been advocated to minimize postoperative adhesions. The value of using lasers to perform abdominal myomectomy is debatable. Maheux[5] reported no advantage but others[6-8] believed that there was less blood loss, less adhesion formation, and better pregnancy rates.

Results

The results of conventional myomectomy for infertility are impressive. About 20% to 59% of patients will conceive postmyomectomy[9] and 75% of them will do so in the first year after surgery.[10] These figures, while encouraging, are taken from series in which the patients served as their own controls. The question, "How many would have conceived without surgery?" remains unanswered (see Chapter 27). The ability to remove fibroids of any size, number, and location has ensured the continued popularity of the procedure.

Laparoscopic management of fibroids, especially in the infertile patient, must be considered against the background of the results of conventional surgery. It is a tribute to Bonney that the practice of abdominal surgery was standardized for so long. It remains to be seen if endoscopic treatment is destined to stand alongside abdominal myomectomy as a standard technique or eventually become an historic relic.

It must be added that although these figures are impressive and that many of these patients had long-standing infertility, myomectomy for infertility has never been submitted to the rigorous scrutiny of a randomized prospective study.

The development of endoscopic surgery has provided an opportunity to reassess the surgical management of uterine fibroids. The choice of treatment depends on the relationship of the fibroid to the uterus, whether it is submucous, interstitial, or subserous, its size, and the number of fibroids present.

Hysteroscopic surgery

Hysteroscopic surgery has developed in the past decade and its value in treating fibroids that impinge upon the uterine cavity is widely accepted. Submucous fibroid up to 2.5 cm in diameter that may be associated with infertility, early pregnancy loss, and menstrual disturbance may be treated easily by hysteroscopic resection[11-12] or ablation with neodymium:yttrium aluminum garnet (Nd:YAG) laser.[13] Larger fibroids or those with a greater intramural component may be treated with drugs to diminish their volume and then excised with a resectoscope loop or ablated with Nd:YAG laser in one or two stages. The results of the treatment of menorrhagia and infertility are impressive.[14]

PRINCIPLES OF LAPAROSCOPIC MYOMECTOMY

Subserous or intramural fibroids may be treated by a laparoscopic approach, although this has not attained the wide acceptance of hysteroscopic myomectomy. Small subserous fibroids do not require removal. Larger ones close to the intramural segment of the fallopian tube are difficult to remove laparoscopically without the risk of damage to the tube. Repair of the myometrium following removal of deeply situated fibroids is difficult and requires considerable manual dexterity. There may also be technical difficulty in removing broad ligament fibroids because of their proximity to the ureter and uterine vessels. The size and number of the fibroids limit the performance of laparoscopic surgery.

Advantages and disadvantages of laparoscopic surgery

The advantages of laparoscopic surgery are well recognized. The hospital stay is shorter than that for laparotomy. Most patients may be discharged within 1 to 2 days of surgery and many on the same evening. The recovery period is also shorter and normal activities should be resumed within 1 to 2 weeks. There is also considerably less postoperative pain. There are fewer postoperative complications such as ileus and the sequelae of venous stasis.

The disadvantages must be also considered. A different and possibly greater degree of skill is required. The number of instruments and the angles with which they may be used to approach the operation site are limited by the number and position of the secondary portals. It is not possible to be flexible in planning the incision sites or to remove multiple fibroids through a single approach. The instruments are long. The surgeon's hands are far removed from the tips of the forceps. This limits the ability to perform fine and delicate movements and to use very fine sutures. Operating time is frequently longer. With experience, most myomectomies can be completed in 2 hours or less, but this is approximately twice as long as that for myomectomy by laparotomy. Although it is believed that laparoscopic surgery is followed by less formation of new adhesions than conventional surgery, the difficulty of obtaining accurate apposition of the edges of the uterine wound following myomectomy may produce more adhesions, especially on the posterior uterine wall. Infertility initially associated with fibroids may become obstructive infertility.

Indications and contraindications to myomectomy

Myomectomy is the preferred treatment for the patient with large or symptomatic fibroids who wishes to retain her potential fertility or does not wish to lose her uterus. The most common indications for laparoscopic myomectomy are a pelvic mass, infertility, pelvic pain, abnormal bleeding, and the coincidental presence of severe endometriosis.[15] Large fibroids may produce pressure symptoms on the bladder, ureter, or, less commonly, bowel. Fibroids may seriously complicate a pregnancy with pain, bleeding, abnormal presentation and placentation, premature labor, infection, or degeneration of the fibroid.[5] The occurrence of any of these complications in a previous pregnancy may be an indication for myomectomy.

Nonetheless, the technique is limited by the number, size, and location of the tumors. Numerous (four or more over 3 cm in diameter) or voluminous (over 10 cm in mean diameter) fibroids are contraindications to laparoscopic surgery.[16] Fibroids with a mean diameter of over 4 cm should be treated medically prior to surgery to reduce size and vascularity. Laparoscopic myomectomy is suitable only for subserous fibroids and those intramural fibroids to which access can be easily gained without entering the uterine cavity. Deep intramural fibroids are difficult and tedious to remove laparoscopically and there is little justification for operating by this means if surgery is likely to take several hours to perform. It is also technically difficult to remove intraligamentous fibroids because of the potential risks of damage to the ureter and uterine artery and hematoma formation.

Preoperative assessment

Presenting symptoms. Fibroids are one of the most common tumors found in the pelvis. Although most are asymptomatic, about 20% to 50% of patients present with a variety of symptoms, which include menorrhagia, pelvic pain, infertility, increased fetal loss, or the recognition of an abdominal mass.[17] While polypoid or submucous fibroids are nearly always associated with menorrhagia, many patients with subserous and interstitial fibroids also present with heavy bleeding.[18]

Noninvasive investigations. A detailed clinical history should be taken and a general physical and gynecologic examination performed. The diagnosis may be suspected by history and palpation of a pelvic tumor, or the fibroid may be discovered during an examination carried out for other reasons. It is important to be aware of the number of fi-

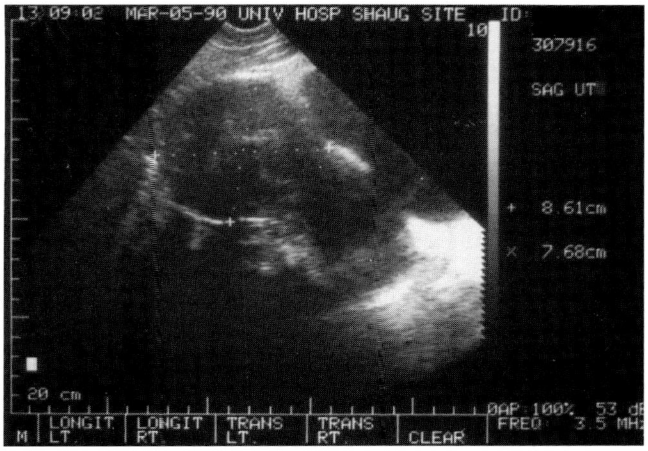

Fig. 19-1. Ultrasonography permits detection and measurement of uterine fibroids.

broids, their size, and their relationship to the uterus, its cavity, and the fallopian tubes. Fibroids can be detected and measured by transabdominal or transvaginal ultrasonography (Fig. 19-1) but magnetic resonance imaging (MRI) is more sensitive and specific[19] (Fig. 19-2). Magnetic resonance imaging is better than other methods to define the relationship of fibroids to the fallopian tube. There are not sufficient data available at present to assess the value of MRI in detecting sarcomatous changes in myomas.

Hysterosalpingography. If the patient is infertile or wishes to preserve potential fertility, hysterosalpingography (HSG) should be performed. As well as identifying the presence of any submucous fibroid, it will also determine whether or not the cavity is being distorted by an intramural lesion. In addition, the state of the fallopian tubes will be revealed (see Chapter 9).

Hysteroscopy. Preoperative hysteroscopy should be performed in those patients who have not had an HSG and selectively in those in whom the HSG has identified a uterine filling defect. If submucus fibroids are present, they should be treated at the same time as the interstitial or subserous fibroids.

MEDICAL TREATMENT

Conservative medical treatment was attempted in the 1950s for fibroids if they were small and the symptoms were mild.[20] The use of iron and blood transfusion was suggested. Testosterone had been reported to reduce the size of the tumor and the induction of a radiation menopause was included among the therapeutic options. The pharmaceutical preparations then available were relatively ineffective, so little progress was made until the last decade. Modern drug regimens make it possible to reduce the size of those rare fibroids that impinge on the intramural segment of the tube. This may restore patency for long enough to allow conception to occur. Reduction of the size and vascularity of the tumor may also allow conservative endoscopic surgery to be used in cases in which the fibroids would otherwise be considered too large.

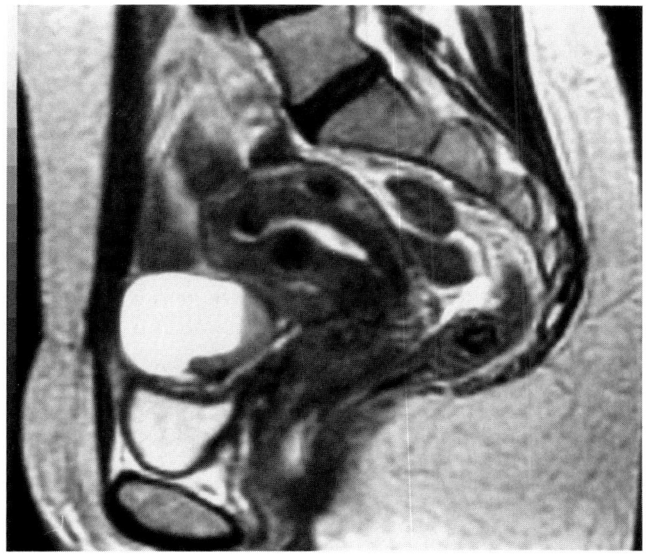

Fig. 19-2. Magnetic resonnance imaging (MRI) is the most sensitive and specific method by which to assess fibroids.

A number of hormonal preparations have been used. There has been little benefit from prostaglandin synthesase inhibitors, progesterone, or oral contraceptives. Danazol, which has been useful in inducing oligomenorrhoea in dysfunctional uterine bleeding, appears to have little effect on the size of the fibroids, although menorrhagia is improved as a result of endometrial atrophy.

Agonist therapy

The most useful group of drugs appears to be the gonadotrophin-releasing hormone (GnRH) agonist analogs. These induce a hypoestrogenic state and decrease the size of the fibroid. The fibroid shrinks rapidly during the first 3 months of treatment with little further reduction thereafter. Regrowth to pretreatment size occurs within 3 months of discontinuing treatment in parallel with the return of ovarian function.[21] The shrinkage of fibroids during treatment with GnRH analogs and the reduction of blood flow demonstrated by Doppler ultrasound[22] has suggested a role as a preoperative adjunct to surgery. A marked reduction of blood loss has been observed during both myomectomy[23] and hysterectomy.[24] However, there have been anecdotal reports of difficulty in dissecting the fibroid out of its pseudocapsule following treatment with the analogs. The prevention of uterine bleeding during myomectomy appears to be more important when the fibroid is greater than 4 cm in mean diameter.[15]

The analogs cannot be administered orally because they are inactivated by gastric peptidase. They may be given by nasal spray, subcutaneous injection, intramuscular depot injections, or implants. The implants are given at monthly intervals into the abdominal subcutaneous fat. Injection is followed by a rise in serum gonadotrophin levels and an increased concentration of sex steroids for several days followed by suppression of the pituitary-ovarian axis and the induction of a pseudomenopausal state. If treatment is commenced in the follicular phase of the cycle there may be unopposed estrogen secretion and a withdrawal bleed 10 to 14 days later. If begun in the luteal phase, normal menstruation occurs and there is no withdrawal bleed in the subsequent cycle. Almost all patients will experience some menopausal symptoms and, if treatment is prolonged over 6 months, there is danger of osteoporosis developing.[25]

Treatment with GnRH analog preoperatively reduces the uterine and fibroid size and also the perioperative blood loss. Injections of a depot preparation should be given at monthly intervals for 3 months to patients with fibroids with a mean diameter greater than 4 cm. Most patients are amenorrhoeic during therapy but resume normal menstrual function shortly after treatment is discontinued.

TECHNIQUE OF LAPAROSCOPIC MYOMECTOMY

Subserous fibroids

Myomectomy using the laparoscope as a means of access was described by Semm and Mettler[26] in 1980. They removed pedunculated subserous fibroids (Fig. 19-3, *A*). The pedicle was coagulated with endotherm forceps and the fibroid twisted off (Fig. 19-3, *C*). Additional hemostasis was achieved with the endotherm point coagulator. Small fibroids were removed through an 11 mm cannula after morcellation with a tissue punch. Larger ones were removed through a posterior colpotomy incision.

Many North American centers do not use the endotherm equipment. The pedicle of the myoma can be desiccated with bipolar or unipolar current (Fig. 19-3, *B*). The pedicle is more cleanly dealt with by sharp division with scissors rather than avulsion by twisting (Fig. 19-3, *D*). The fibroid is removed piecemeal after morcellation using a morcellator (Fig. 19-4) of 15 mm or 20 mm diameter. Alternate removal methods are discussed later.

Intramural fibroids

Removal of larger and more deeply situated fibroids has been described in recent years.[15,16,27-29] In addition to the standard instruments for operative laparoscopy, 5 and 11 mm toothed grasping forceps, a 5 mm myomectomy drill, 5 mm scissors, a flushing cannula, needle holder, and suture equipment are required. An electrosurgical unit with both monopolar and bipolar capabilities must be available even if the surgeon elects to use laser surgery.

The patient should be placed in a modified lithotomy position with the thighs flexed to 5 degrees to 10 degrees. Trendelenberg tilt is required to allow the bowel to be lifted out of the pelvis. Laparoscopy is performed through a standard intraumbilical incision using a 10 mm laparoscope and video camera. Two secondary trocars and cannulas are inserted lateral to the deep inferior epigastric arteries and slightly higher than usual. A third trocar and cannula is inserted in the midline at a level dependent on the size of the fibroid. The larger the fibroid, the higher the insertion of the third cannula. Blood loss may be decreased and the operation facilitated by injection of a vasoconstrictive agent into the myometrium around the fibroid. This is achieved by passing a long spinal needle directly through the abdominal wall. Depending on the size of the fibroid, 5 to 10 ml of a 1 U in 20 cc of normal saline solution of Vasopressin is usually sufficient to provide hemostasis.

A vertical incision is made with a monopolar pointed knife or hook electrode or laser in the uterine wall and through the pseudocapsule of the fibroid at the apex of the dome of the tumor (Fig. 19-5, *A*). The characteristic pearl white appearance of the fibroid will appear. The incision may extend into the surface of the tumor. The striking differences between healthy myometrium and the whorls of fibromyomatous tissue facilitate identification of the plane of dissection. The myoma may then be fixed with the 5 mm grasping forceps or the myomectomy drill.

Igarashi has recently advanced cogent arguments for why a horizontal incision will result in less bleeding. The arteries and arterioles in the myometrium run not vertically but almost transversely and as such are most susceptible to division by a vertical incision[30] (Fig. 19-6).

Dissection is carried out by traction on the fibroid and countertraction on the uterus and division with the unipolar scissors, or laser (Fig. 19-5, *B*). Vessels in the connective tissue bridges between the fibroid and uterus should be identified and desiccated with bipolar or unipolar current before sectioning. Occasionally hydrodissection may aid the separation of the fibroid from the uterus. The pelvis is rinsed and cleaned with copious warm Ringer's lactate solution during the operation. The vascular pedicle of the fibroid must be recognized and desiccated before section and removal of the tumor from the uterus (Fig. 19-5, *C*). The fibroid is then stored in the pouch of Douglas pending the eventual removal from the abdomen.

Complete hemostasis must be achieved in the fibroid bed before closing the uterine defect. This may be obtained by lavage with Ringer's lactate solution at 40° Celsius, monopolar or bipolar electrocoagulation, or a combination of all three. Deep defects should be closed with interrupted sutures of polyglactin 0 or 2-0 (Vicryl, Ethicon) swaged on a curved needle. The technique of laparoscopic suturing with a curved needle is difficult to acquire because the rotatory movement of the needle requires considerable manual dexterity. The curved needle may be inserted alongside a 5 mm cannula[31,32] or through a 10 mm cannula (see Chapter 7).

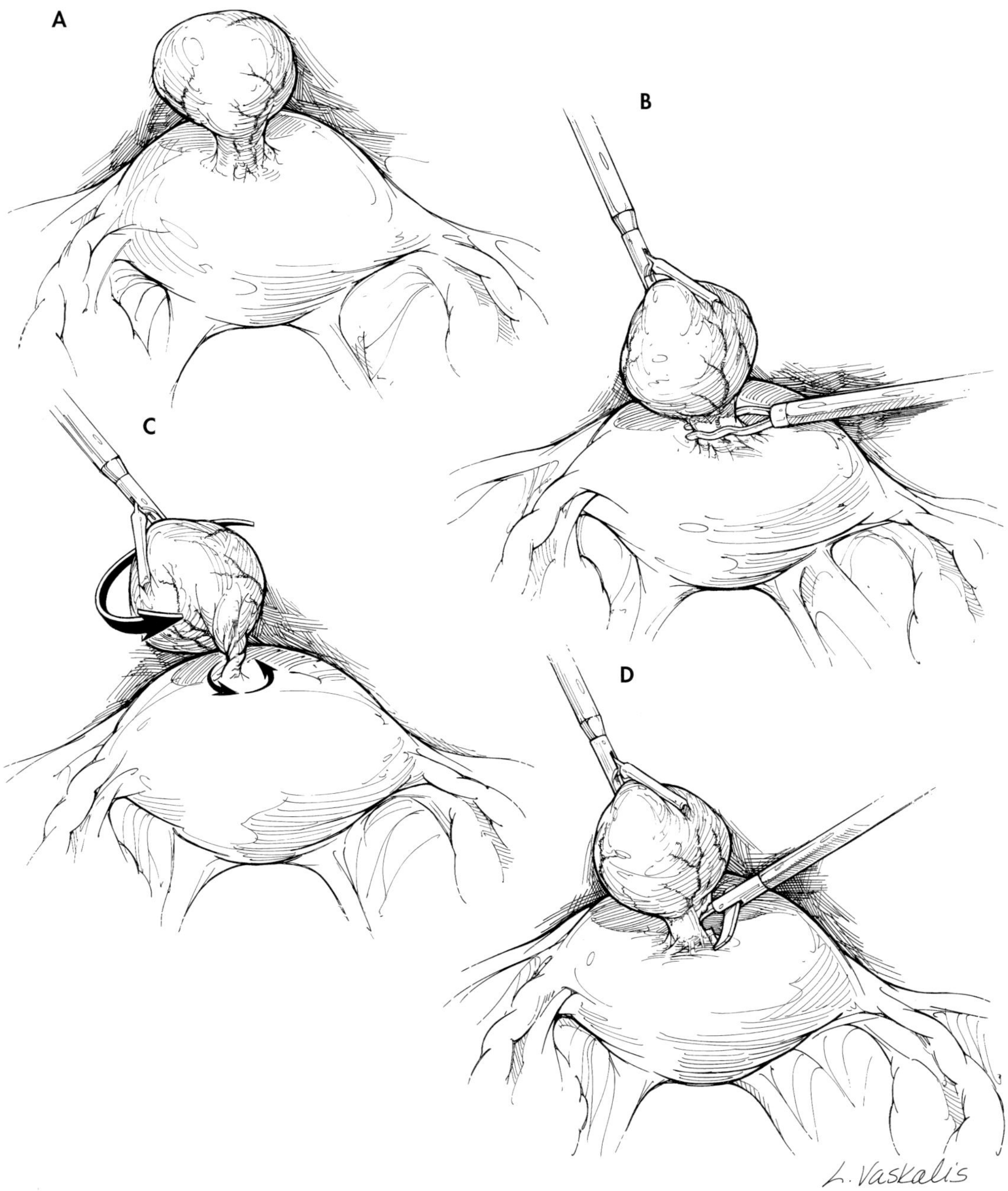

Fig. 19-3. Excision of subserous fibroid. **A,** Subserous fibroid. **B,** The pedicle is electrodesiccated with bipolar current. **C,** The myoma is removed by twisting it with strong grasping forceps. **D,** The desiccated pedicle is transected.

The serosa is then sutured with interrupted or continuous 3/0 polyglactin on a straight or ski needle to bring the edges together (Fig. 19-5, *D*). It is almost impossible to suture laparoscopically with the same precision as that by open laparotomy using magnification because the laparoscopic instruments are long and the fine movements integral to microsurgery are difficult to reproduce (see Chapter 15).

Removal of the fibroid from the abdominal cavity

The fibroid should next be removed from the abdomen. Although some surgeons leave it to undergo avascular necrosis tucked behind the colon, this does pose some risk of revascularization and the formation of a parasitic fibroid. Morcellation of a large fibroid by a tissue punch is tedious and time consuming and this technique is falling into dis-

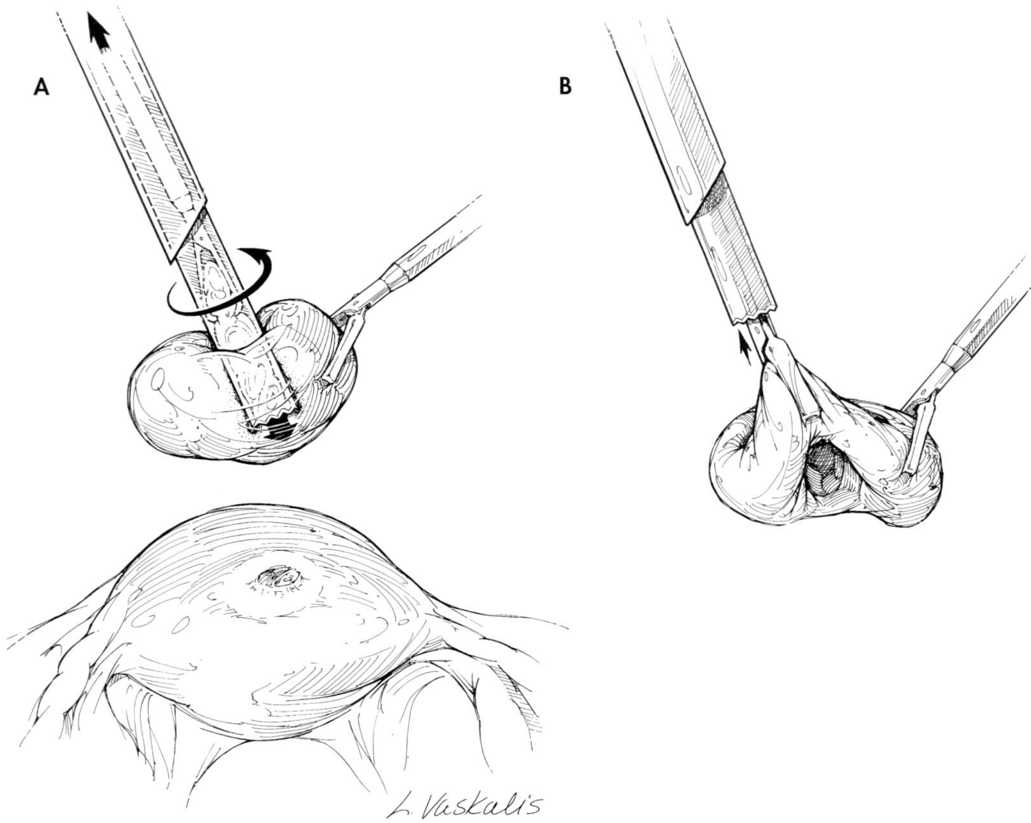

Fig. 19-4. Removal of the fibroid from the abdomen. **A,** The myoma is morcelated. **B,** The myoma is removed piecemeal along the cannula of the morcellator.

use. Newer morcellators are more effective (see Fig. 19-4) and motorized versions are now available.

Small fibroids may be removed through a 10 mm cannula. Fibroids up to 5 cm in diameter may be removed by the "orange-peel technique."[29] The fibroid is held at opposing poles by toothed forceps and converted into narrow strips with the use of sharp scissors (Fig. 19-7, *A* and *B*). The pieces of tissue may then be removed from the abdomen through an 11 mm cannula (Fig. 19-7, *C*). This approach is also time consuming.

Alternatively, the fibroid may be removed from the abdomen by enlarging one of the suprapubic incisions.[16] The myoma is held with forceps and brought against the abdominal wound to provide an air-tight seal, which prevents loss of the pneumoperitoneum. A small blade is passed through the wound and used to morcellate the fibroid under laparoscopic control (Fig. 19-8). The pieces may then be removed through the incision.

A third method of removal is to make a transverse or cruciate incision in the posterior vaginal fornix. The fibroid is pressed against the anterior wall of the pouch of Douglas below the cervix and moved from side to side by the laparoscopic surgeon. At the same time a second surgeon working between the patient's legs passes a speculum and identifies the fibroid by its movements. It is then safe to incise the posterior vaginal wall and expose the fibroid. It is easy to remove quite large tumors because the elasticity of the vagina enables the passage of masses that are at least twice the size of the incision. Larger tumors may need to be cut into two or more smaller pieces to effect removal. The vaginal incision is then closed by an interrupted or purse string suture inserted vaginally and thorough pelvic lavage carried out laparoscopically to ensure that hemostasis is complete (see Chapter 7).

A posterior wall fibroid may be removed through a colpotomy incision after preparing it laparoscopically. Adhesions and/or endometriosis, if present, are dealt with to allow the uterus to be retroverted and the fibroid to be brought into the pouch of Douglas. An incision is then made in the posterior vaginal wall and the myomectomy completed through the colpotomy incision.[33]

Gomel has used a combined laparoscopy, minilaparotomy approach for large intramural fibroids. During the laparoscopic step of the procedure the myoma(s) is excised.

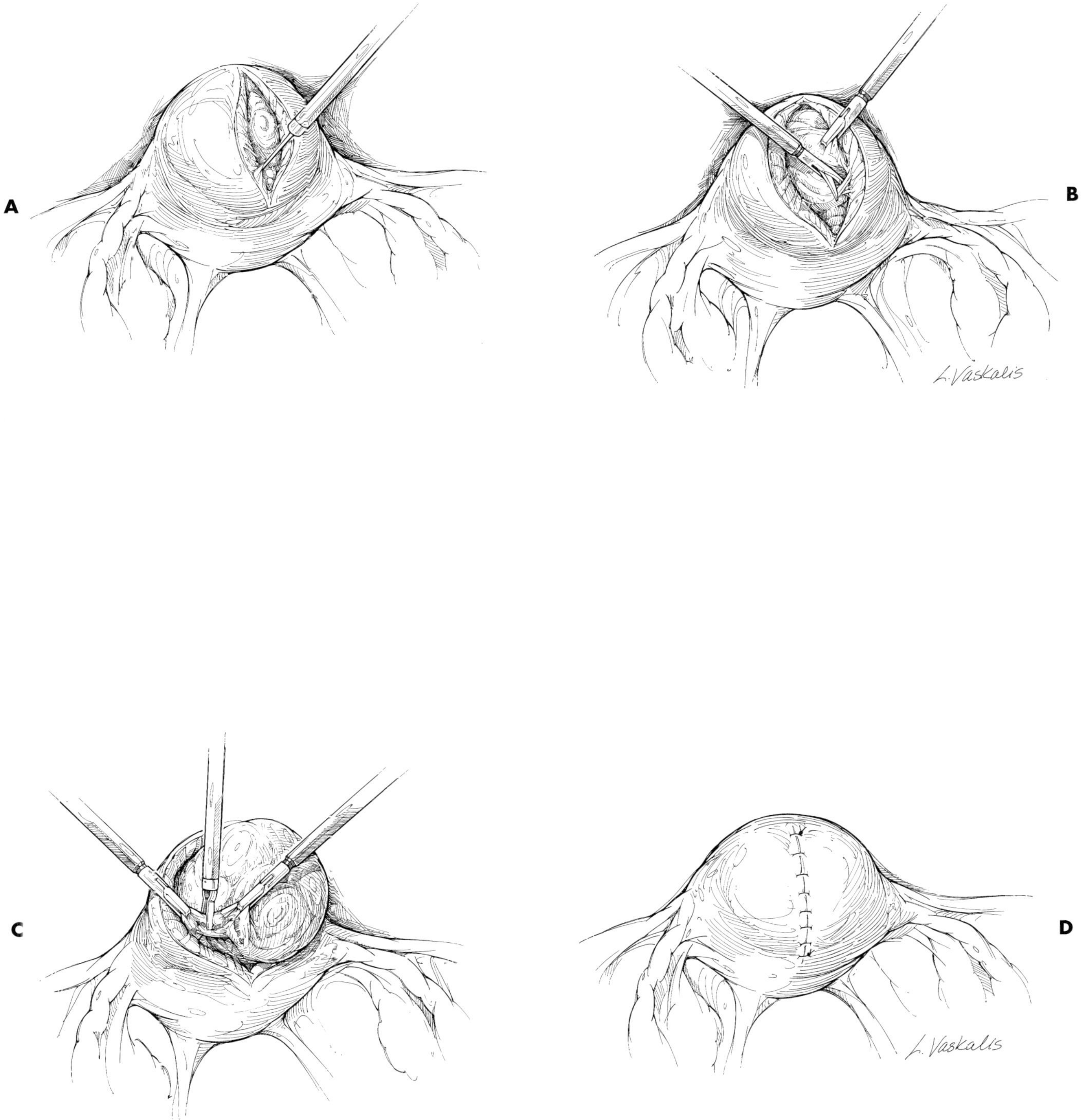

Fig. 19-5. Excision of intramural fibroid. **A,** A vertical incision is made in the uterine wall and through the pseudocapsule of the fibroid at the apex of the dome of the tumor. **B,** The fibroid is dissected by traction on the fibroid. **C,** The vascular pedicle of the tumor is desiccated before transection. **D,** After approximation of the myometrium the serosa is joined with continuous 3-0 polyglactin suture.

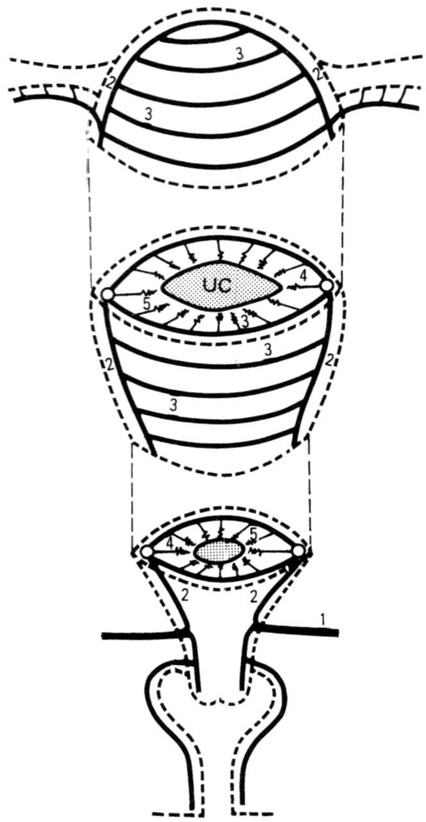

Fig. 19-6. Scheme of arterial vasculature of the uterus. *1*, Uterine arteries. *2*, Ascending branches of uterine arteries. *3*, Arcuate arteries. *4*, Radial arterioles. *5*, Spiral arterioles (*uc*, uterine cavity). (From Igarashi M. Fertil Steril 59:1331, 1993. Published with permission.)

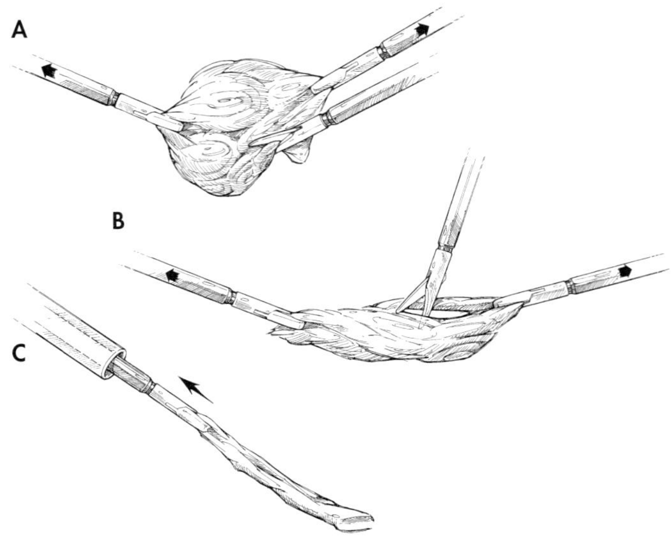

Fig. 19-7. The "orange-peel technique" to remove tissue from the abdomen. **A** and **B,** The fibroid is held at opposing poles by toothed forceps and cut into narrow strips with sharp scissors. **C,** The strips of tissue are removed through an 11 mm cannula.

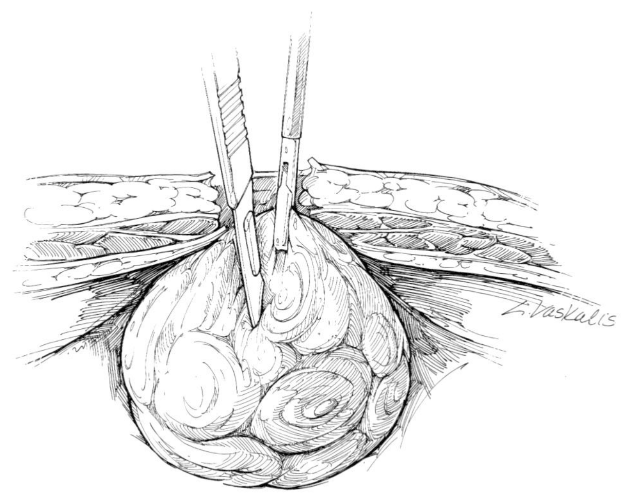

Fig. 19-8. Removal of fibroid from abdomen through an enlarged suprapubic portal. The myoma is held with forceps and brought against the incision and morcellated using a scalpel passed through the same incision.

The subsequent minilaparotomy (see Chapter 15) permits removal of the myoma(s) from the peritoneal cavity and effective closure of the uterine defect.

Myolysis

The Nd:YAG laser has been used to coagulate and reduce symptomatic subserous and intramural fibroids of up to 10 cm in diameter.[34] Preoperative depot leuprolide was given for 2 to 6 months, which resulted in 40% to 60% shrinkage of the fibroid. The laser was used at 50 watts of power with a 500 μ fiber to drill the fibroid at multiple concentric sites. Because the Nd:YAG laser has a coagulating effect with a 5 mm diameter, a 5 cm fibroid requires 10 punctures per diameter. Thus 75 to 100 punctures were performed for a 5 cm myoma. Follow-up for 6 to 14 months has revealed no recurrence.

Leaving a large number of necrotic punctures in the uterine surface could stimulate adhesion formation. Second-look laparoscopies were performed in seven of 20 women who had undergone myolysis.[35] In all seven, dense fibrous adhesions were noted between the necrosed myoma and small bowel and/or omentum.

Myolysis holds a certain appeal, permitting as it does the surgeon to dispense with the time-consuming and technically difficult aspects of laparoscopic myomectomy. There is no need to dissect, suture, or repair the uterus. There is no specimen to remove, which is often the most time-consuming step. However, the apparent ability of myolysis to stimulate dense adhesion formation would suggest that this procedure should not be carried out in a woman who wishes to preserve reproductive potential. This procedure is new, promising, and requires rigorous evaluation before wide clinical applications.

Intraoperative complications

The intraoperative complications of laparoscopic myomectomy are the same as those for any advanced laparoscopic operation. They include failure to complete the procedure because of multiple fibroids or adhesions, primary hemorrhage, and damage to the bowel, especially when there are adhesions, or to the ureter in cases of broad ligament fibroids.

Postoperative course

Recurrence of fibroids. The estimated risk of recurrence of fibroids depends on the number of fibroids present, follow-up examinations by ultra sonography, and the duration of follow-up. Most series report a recurrence rate of about 15% but, in a series of 622 cases reported from Milan using ultrasound to assess the uterus at follow-up examination, the cumulative 10-year recurrence rate was 27%, which increased with time. There was no association with age and there were fewer recurrences when there was a single fibroid and in the patients who had a subsequent pregnancy.[36]

Healing. Small superficial myomas are easily removed and the surface coagulated. Treatment of the uterine defect after removal of multiple fibroids or deeply situated fibroids may be effected by coagulation or suturing. Coagulation leads to the formation of more granulation tissue and resultant weakness of the uterine wall. Suturing produces better healing but more adhesions. Suturing is difficult and time consuming. Failure to appose the serosal edges accurately results in the formation of adhesions between the uterus and loops of bowel. Second-look laparoscopy (SLL) has shown varying results. Hasson[29] found 46% had moderate to extensive adhesions, although some of them were present at the original operation. Dubuisson[16] found adhesions in only one of six cases when SLL was carried out. Nehzat[28] found a greater prevalence of new adhesion formation when sutures were used and if the myoma was on the posterior uterine wall. However, if deep fibroids were removed without suturing there was an indentation on the uterine wall, the depth of which was proportional to the size of the fibroid. Thus suturing resulted in better healing but more adhesion formation.

Fertility. There has been no long-term follow-up of patients with infertility. Dubuisson[16] reported 21 patients who had undergone myomectomy for infertility with a follow-up between 12 and 20 months. There have been two normal deliveries and one spontaneous abortion without scar dehiscence. Hasson[29] noted that 12 of 17 patients with infertility conceived; six of them became pregnant within 6 months of surgery. There were no obstetric complications associated with the myomectomy.

Dehiscence. There has been one report of uterine dehiscence following laparoscopic myomectomy.[37] Dehiscence is a well-recognized although uncommon complication of abdominal myomectomy. It might be expected that the risk with laparoscopic myomectomy would be greater. A number of factors may contribute to wound dehiscence. It is more difficult to repair the myometrium accurately. Most surgeons place just enough interrupted sutures to approximate the uterine serosa and obtain hemostasis. It may be difficult to know whether or not the uterine cavity has been entered, although the instillation of methylene blue in cases of deep fibroids would help. The use of electrocoagulation to obtain hemostasis may contribute to tissue destruction and defective healing.

CONCLUSIONS

Myomectomy by laparoscopy is technically feasible, but does feasibility equate with good practice? The "gold standard" is still laparotomy and myomectomy using microsurgical principles, especially when fertility is at stake. To be acceptable, laparoscopic surgery must prove to give equally good results and be preferable by a significant number of surgeons.

If the fibroid is small, the operation may not be necessary. If the fibroids are large, multiple, or situated deep in the myometrium, the procedure is difficult. Multiple large fibroids, which are more likely to cause symptoms, are more difficult to excise, are associated with more bleeding, and are more difficult to remove from the abdominal cavity. Myomectomy may be facilitated by pretreatment with GnRH agonists, but reconstruction of the uterine defect is never easy. The inability of the surgeon to suture the serosa as accurately as with microsurgical techniques may be detrimental to fertility. Finally, the integrity of the uterine scar must give cause for concern when fertility is desired. All of these factors cast doubt on the value of laparoscopic myomectomy.

A minilaparotomy or a combined laparoscopy-minilaparotomy approach permits the surgeon to overcome these drawbacks and is preferable in selected cases.

REFERENCES

1. Atlee WL: Case of successful extirpation of a fibrous tumor of the peritoneal surface on the uterus by the large peritoneal section. *Am J of Med Sci* 9:309-335, 1845.
2. Bonney V: The technique and end results of myomectomy. *Lancet* 220:171, 1931.
3. Bonney V: The Technical Minutiae of Extended Myomectomy and Ovarian Cystectomy. London, 1946, Cassell.
4. Benagiano G, Morino A, Primiero FM: Fibroids: overview of current and future treatment options. *Br J Obstet Gynaecol* 99 (Suppl 7) 18-22, 1992.
5. Maheux R: Treatment of uterine leiomyomata: past, present and future. In Genazzani AR, Petraglia F, Volpe A, editors: Progress in Gynecology and Obstetrics. Carnforth, 1990, Parthenon Publishing Group.
6. Reyniak JV, Corenthal L: Microsurgical laser technique for abdominal myomectomy. *Microsurgery* 8:92-98, 1987.

7. Starks GC: CO_2 laser myomectomy in an infertile population. *J Reprod Med* 30:184-186, 1988.
8. March CM: Update: laser surgery. *Endocrinol Fertil Forum* 9:1-5, 1989.
9. Seoud MA-F, Patterson R, Muasher SJ, Coddington CC: Effect of myomas or prior myomectomy on in vitro fertilization performance. *JARGE* 9:217-221, 1992.
10. DeCherney AH: The effects of leiomyomata on fertility. *Obstet Gynaecol Forum* 4:3-5, 1990.
11. Norment WB, Sikes H, Berry F, Bird I: Hysteroscopy. *Surg Clin North Am* 37:1377-1386, 1957.
12. Neuwirth RS: A new technique for and additional experience with hysteroscopic resection of submucous fibroids. *Am J Obstet Gynaecol* 131:91-94, 1978.
13. Donnez J, Gillerot S, Bourgonjon D, et al: *Fertil Steril* 54:999-1003, 1990.
14. Gordon AG: Endoscopic surgery. In Shaw RW, editor: Uterine Fibroids: Time for review. Carnforth, 1992, Parthenon Publishing Group.
15. Dubuisson JB, Lecuru F, Foulot H, et al: Myomectomy by laparoscopy: a preliminary report of 43 cases. *Fertil Steril* 56:827-830, 1991.
16. Dubuisson JB, Lecuru F, Foulot H, et al: Gonadotrophin-releasing hormone agonist and laparoscopic myomectomy. *Clin Ther* 14:51-55, 1992.
17. Buttram VC, Reiter RC: Uterine leiomyomata: etiology, symptomatology and management. *Fertil Steril* 36:433-435, 1992.
18. Fraser IS: Hysteroscopy and laparoscopy in women with menorrhagia. *Am J Obstet Gynecol* 162:1264-1269, 1992.
19. Mitchell DG: Benign disease of the uterus and ovaries, applications of magnetic resonance imaging. *Radiol Clin North Am* 30:777-787, 1992.
20. Baird D: Combined Textbook of Obstetrics and Gynaecology. Edinburgh, 1957, Livingstone.
21. West CP, Lumsden MA, Lawson S, et al: Shrinkage of uterine fibroids during therapy with LHRH agonist (Zoladex): a luteinizing hormone–releasing hormone agonist administered as a monthly subcutaneous depot. *Fertil Steril* 48:45-51, 1989.
22. Matta WHM, Stabile I, Shaw RW, Campbell S: Doppler assessment of uterine blood flow change in patients with fibroids receiving the gonadotrophin-releasing hormone agonist buserelin. *Fertil Steril* 49:1083-1085, 1988.
23. Shaw RW: Mechanism of LHRH analogue action in uterine fibroids. *Hormone Res* 32:150-153, 1988.
24. Lumsden MA, West CP, Baird DT: Goserelin therapy before surgery for uterine fibroids. *Lancet* 1:36-37, 1987.
25. Vollenhoven BJ, Lawrence AS, Healy DL: Uterine fibroids: a clinical review. *Br J Obstet Gynaecol* 97:285-298, 1990.
26. Semm K, Mettler L: Technical progress in pelvic surgery via laparoscopy. *Am J Obst Gynecol* 138:121-127, 1980.
27. Daniell JF, Gourley LD: Laparoscopic treatment of clinically significant symptomatic uterine fibroids. *J Gynecol Surg* 7:37-40, 1991.
28. Nehzat C, Nehzat F, Silfen SL, et al: Laparoscopic myomectomy. *Intl J Fertil* 36:275-280, 1991.
29. Hasson HM, Rotman C, Rana N, et al: Laparoscopic myomectomy. *Obst Gynecol* 80:884-888, 1992.
30. Igarashi M: Letter to Editor. *Fertil Steril* 59:1331, 1993.
31. Reich H, Clarke HC, Sekel L: A simple method for ligating in operative laparoscopy with straight and curved needles. *Obstet Gynecol* 79:143-147, 1992.
32. Gordon AG, Taylor PJ: Practical Laparoscopy. Oxford, 1993, Blackwell Scientific Publications.
33. McLucas B: Myomectomy via colpotomy with laparoscopic assistance. Presented at Biennial Meeting of the International Society for Gynecologic Endoscopy, Barcelona, October, 1991.
34. Goldfarb HA: Nd:Yag laser laparoscopic coagulation of symptomatic myomas. *J Reprod Med* 37:636-638, 1992.
35. Nisolle M, Smets M, Malvaux V, et al: Laparoscopic myolysis with the Nd:Yag laser. *J Gynecol Surg* 9:95-99, 1993.
36. Candiani GB, Fedele L, Parazzini F, Villa L: Risk of recurrence after myomectomy. *Br J Obstet Gynaecol* 98:385-389, 1991.
37. Harris WJ: Uterine dehiscence following laparoscopic myomectomy. *Obstet Gynecol* 80:545-546, 1992.

Chapter 20

ABLATION OF THE UTEROSACRAL LIGAMENTS AND PRESACRAL NEURECTOMY

James F. Daniell
Bryan R. Kurtz

Dysmenorrhoea, pain associated with menstruation, is a common and, on occasion, an incapacitating complaint. Its surgical management by presacral neurectomy dates back to the end of the nineteenth century. In extreme cases a laparotomy would be performed and the hypogastric plexus divided. Black has reviewed reports of almost 10,000 patients who were so treated between 1936 and 1963.[1] Following presacral neurectomy, pain relief was experienced by 83% of those with primary and 72% of those with secondary dysmenorrhoea.

Surgical therapy of dysmenorrhea fell out of favor in the early 1960s when advances were made in medical management. The introduction of nonsteroidal antiinflammatory medications, oral contraceptives, as well as ovarian suppressive therapy with Danazol or gonadotropin-releasing hormone agonists led to a more conservative approach. Alternative treatment has been sought for those patients in whom medical treatment failed.[2,3]

In 1972, Frangenheim described performing laparoscopic segmental ablation of the uterosacral ligaments to treat pelvic pain.[4] There was concern about the risk of bleeding. In 1987, Lichten and Bombard reported their experiences with laparoscopic ablation of the uterosacral nerves in cases of primary dysmenorrhea.[5] More recently, presacral neurectomy has been carried out laparoscopically.[6,7] These procedures can be performed in an outpatient setting, allowing the patient to recover and return rapidly to full activities.

This chapter will describe the surgical anatomy and the background and procedures of both laparoscopic uterosacral nerve ablation (LUNA) and presacral neurectomy.

SURGICAL ANATOMY

The female pelvis is supplied by the autonomic nervous system (see also Chapter 10). The sympathetic components of the pelvic plexus originate from the upper segments of the lumbar cord and from the lower thoracic segments, reaching the pelvic plexus by way of the superior hypogastric plexus. This plexus divides over the middle of the first sacral vertebrae to form the right and left inferior hypogastric nerves. These pass downward and laterally near the sacral end of each uterosacral ligament and then forward over the lateral aspect of the rectal ampulla and upper vagina. In this vicinity, they are known as the pelvic or inferior hypogastric plexuses.

Each pelvic plexus consists of a large complex of nerve fibers and numerous minute ganglia spread over an area of 2 or 3 cm. They represent the focal point of distribution for the nerves to the uterus. They also receive branches from the sacral ganglia of the sympathetic trunk and parasympathetic fibers from the second, third, and fourth sacral spinal nerves. Each pelvic plexus is then subdivided into secondary plexuses, which follow the course of the visceral branches of the hypogastric vessels. These include the rectal plexus (to the rectum), the uterovaginal plexus (to the inner aspect of the fallopian tubes, uterus, vagina, and erectile tissues of the vestibular bulb), and the vesical plexus (to the bladder). The uterine nerves are intimately associated with the uterosacral ligaments, with a supply of small ganglia around the area of attachment of the ligaments to the cervix. In the uterus, the nerves accompany the blood vessels through the entire musculature to the basal layer of the mucosa.

It has long been understood that the sensory nerve supply for the cervix differs from that of the uterine fundus. Afferent impulses from the uterine fundus enter the cord at the eleventh and twelfth thoracic nerves. On the other hand, afferent impulses from the cervix, vagina, and perineum enter at the second, third, and fourth sacral nerves. Bilateral paravertebral blocks at T-11 and T-12 relieve fundal pain of patients in labor but do not relieve the associated backache and pelvic ache.[8] This is controlled by anesthetizing the sacral nerves by caudal blockade.

As early as 1948, Ingersoll and Meigs noted that backache was often unrelieved by presacral neurectomy.[9] They concluded that the afferent nerve supply from the lower part of the uterus and cervix must pass outward through some other afferent rather than the presacral plexus. This impression was further confirmed by the inability to dilate the cervix subsequent to presacral neurectomy without causing pain, although the fundus could be curetted painlessly. In 1952, White noted that stimulation of the cervix or distention of the bladder and rectum after presacral neurectomy still produced characteristic discomfort that could completely be eliminated by sacral block or by interruption by disease or injury of the lower sacral nerves.[10]

The ovarian plexuses are composed of a mesh of nerve fibers arising from the intermesenteric or renal plexus at the point of origin of the ovarian artery. They accompany the ovarian vessels to supply the ovaries, the outer aspects of the fallopian tubes, and the broad ligaments. Some of the nerves for the ovarian plexus communicate with fibers of the uterine plexus within the folds of the broad ligaments.

In his excellent discourse on paracervical uterine denervation by transection of the uterosacral ligaments, Doyle described in great detail the anatomic relationship of the nerve supply to the pelvis.[11] He concluded that, except for some of the nerve supply that travels through the communication to the ovarian plexus, the majority of nerves can be transected in the terminal 2.5 cm within the uterosacral ligaments. He felt that since both types of neurovascular and neuromuscular fibers pass through the same area, the procedure would leave the uterus in a state of autonomic balance rather than set up a state of autonomic imbalance as probably follows a presacral type of denervation. Furthermore, by transecting the nerves distal to separation of the pelvic plexus into the rectal, uterovaginal, and vesical plexuses, there is less chance of causing impairment of bladder or bowel function.

When discussing transection of the presacral nerve or uterosacral ligaments, anatomic relationships are of extreme importance. Fig. 20-1 depicts the anatomic relationships in the presacral space. Beneath the peritoneum at the level of the bifurcation of the aorta, the superior hypogastric plexus is found embedded in loose areolar tissue, overlying the middle sacral vessels and the bodies of the fourth and fifth lumbar vertebrae. The plexus usually consists of two or three incompletely fused trunks. In some patients, however, a single nerve is present. Fine nerve strands pass from the lumbar sympathetic ganglia beneath the common iliac vessels to the presacral nerve. When performed following laparotomy, presacral neurectomy involves dissection of a 2 to 4 cm segment of tissue overlying the sacral periosteum, starting at the sacral prominence and proceeding caudad. The lateral boundaries of dissection are usually described as the ureter on the right and the inferior mesenteric artery on the left.

Fig. 20-2 depicts the anatomic relationships of the uterosacral ligaments. They are true musculofascial ligaments that run from the upper part of the cervix to the sides of the sacrum. They enter their insertions at the uterus by merging with the adjacent posterior aspect of the cardinal ligaments.

At about the level of the ischial spine, the ureter turns and runs forward and medially beneath the broad ligament just above the uterosacral ligament. Especially in thin patients, the course of the ureter is easily seen underlying the peritoneum. At a point approximately 2 cm lateral to the cervix, the ureter enters the canal through the cardinal ligament just below the uterine artery and vein. The uterine vessels enter the organ at the level of the internal cervical os. Pulsations can often be seen just above the insertion of the uterosacral ligament. Generally loose areolar tissue underlies the uterosacral ligaments. However, there can be some small thin-walled veins on the medial aspect.

LAPAROSCOPIC UTEROSACRAL NERVE ABLATION (LUNA)

Background

Interruption of the uterosacral nerves was first performed by Ruggi in 1899.[12] The following year, Jellett described transection of the top of the vagina, drawing of the uterosacral ligaments forward and attaching them to the anterior aspect of the cervix to cure retroversion of the uterus.[13] He believed the relief of pain was due to the correction of the retroverted uterus. Several European gynecologists subsequently described techniques for the treatment of dysmenorrhea, performed either vaginally or abdominally, in which the uterosacral ligaments were interrupted. At the same time, presacral neurectomy was also popularized. In his landmark article in 1955, Doyle studied the results of vaginal or abdominal transection of the uterosacral nerves for the treatment of dysmenorrhea. He found that over 70% of patients had relief from pain.[11]

Although uterosacral ligament transection fell out of favor with the advances in medical management, the expansion in the use of laparoscopy has led to a revival of the procedure. In 1985 Feste, using the CO_2 laser to effect seg-

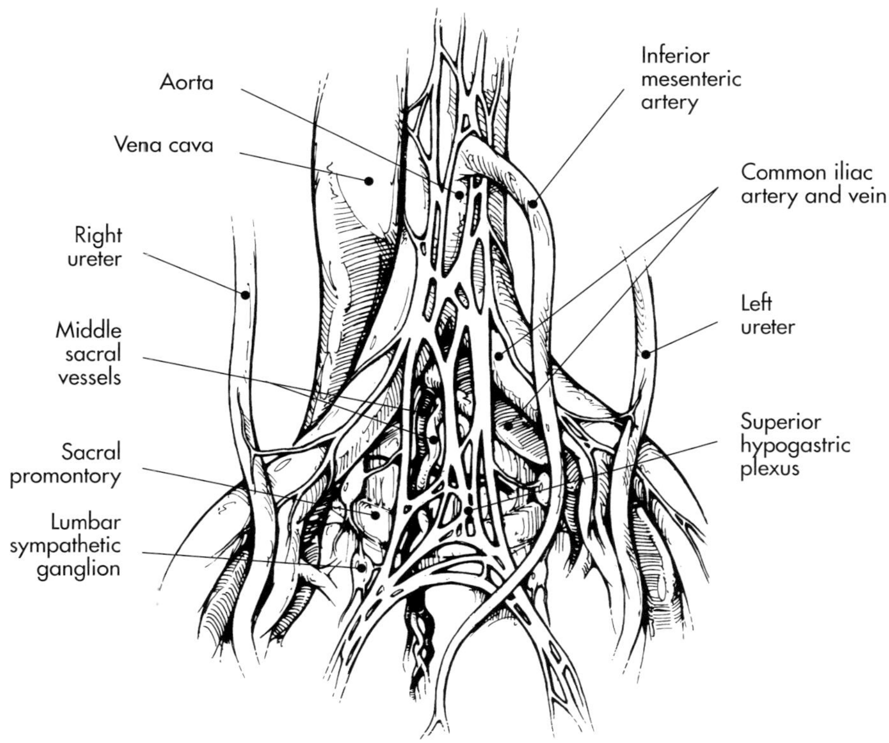

Fig. 20-1. Anatomic relationships in the presacral space. The superior hypogastric plexus overlies the middle sacral vessels and the bodies of the fourth and fifth lumbar vertebrae.

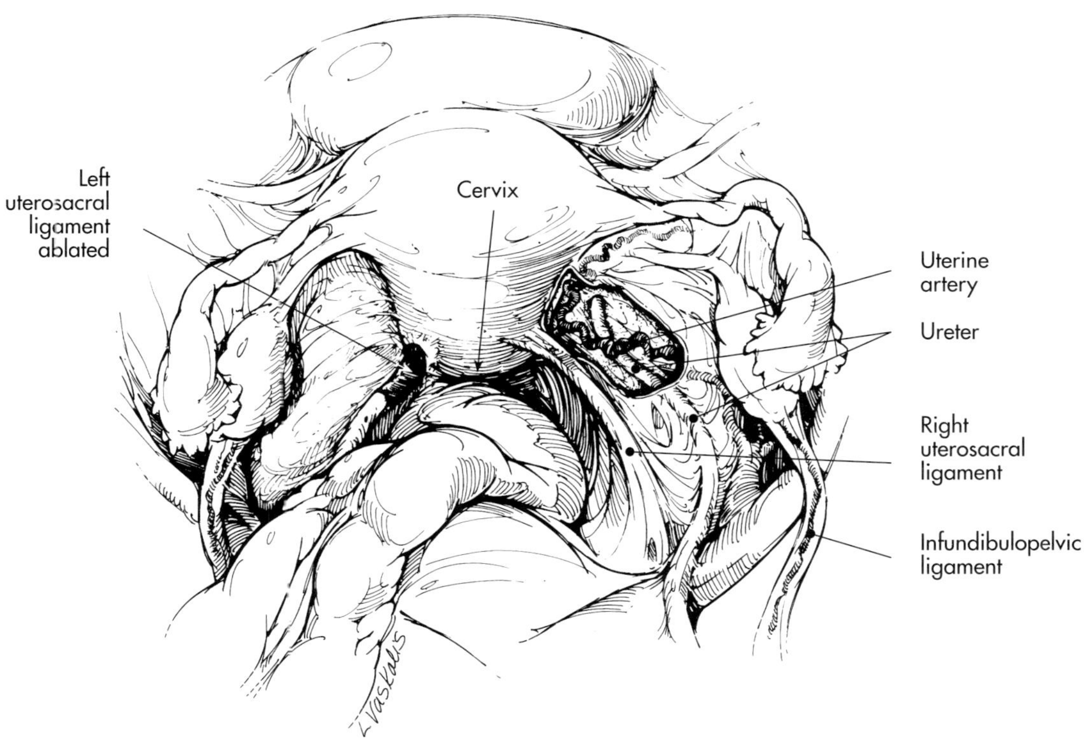

Fig. 20-2. Anatomic relationships of the uterosacral ligaments. The left uterosacral ligament has been segmentally ablated.

Table 20-1. Laparoscopic uterosacral nerve ablation (LUNA) results with KTP laser (6-month follow-up)[17]

Diagnosis	Patients	Postoperative result		
		Worse	Same	Improved
Endometriosis	80	3 (4%)	17 (21%)	60 (75%)
1° Dysmenorrhea	20	2 (10%)	6 (30%)	12 (60%)
Total	100	5 (5%)	23 (23%)	72 (72%)

mental ablation of the uterosacral ligaments, described an improvement rate of approximately 70% in 42 patients, with primary or endometriosis related dysmenorrhea.[14] In a controlled double-blind study using electrocoagulation, Lichten and Bombard reported significant relief of menstrual pain in nine of eleven patients who had a LUNA procedure, compared with no relief in ten patients who underwent diagnostic laparoscopy alone. These observations were made 3 months postoperatively. At 12 months only five remained pain free.[5] Lichten later used the CO_2 laser and demonstrated significant relief of dysmenorrhea in 60% of patients.[15] In 1989, Sutton demonstrated an 86% improvement rate in 100 women with endometriosis and 73% in 26 women with primary dysmenorrhea.[16] Using the KTP laser, Daniell achieved a 75% improvement rate in 80 patients with endometriosis and a 60% improvement rate in 20 patients with primary dysmenorrhea (Table 20-1).[17]

Procedure

Adequate visualization is of utmost importance. The patient should be placed in steep Trendelenburg position to allow the sigmoid colon to fall out of the pelvis. Manipulation of the cervix and uterus is important to allow for proper definition of the ligaments. A uterine cannula is placed through the cervix and secured to a tenaculum on the anterior lip. By pushing the cervix inward and upward, the ligaments will be tented up and better defined. The course of the ureter should be traced out and the area of insertion of the uterine artery into the lateral cervix should be noted.

Occasionally, in the presence of endometriosis, the posterior cul-de-sac will be distorted. Even with tension on the cervix, the uterosacral ligaments may not be clearly definable. We inform our patients preoperatively that we will attempt to cut the ligaments as completely as possible within the realm of safety. They must understand beforehand that the result may be incomplete transection or that the procedure may be discontinued.

The ligaments can be divided using the CO_2 laser, fiberoptic lasers (especially the KTP), bipolar desiccation, and transection with scissors or unipolar current.

Recently, the argon beam coagulator (ABC) has become available for laparoscopic use (Fig. 20-3). The ABC provides conventional unipolar fulguration through a plume of argon gas. Electrosurgical energy is directed to the tissue using a nontouch technique. There is minimal or no smoke production. This allows for excellent visualization during the procedure. The depth of penetration of the electrosurgical effect is minimal, as the energy is evenly distributed over a relatively large surface. These physical attributes cause rapid fulguration with limited depth penetration. Since spring of 1992, we have preferred to use the ABC routinely for transection of the uterosacral ligaments. While it is not a cutting instrument, if proper tension is applied to the uterosacral ligaments the fibers will separate bloodlessly. We are in the process of accumulating the data to assess the efficacy of this new energy source. Our initial experience with the ABC for LUNA has been excellent. We have yet to encounter bleeding or other complications.

Irrespective of the energy source used, the goal is complete transection of the uterosacral ligaments. As described by Doyle, the majority of the nerve fibers can be transected in the proximal 2 cm of the uterosacral ligament.[11] If endometriosis is found to be present on the uterosacral ligament, we will often transect distally (on the "brain" side) to the implants to interrupt the afferent nerve fibers. Transection is carried down until the loose areolar tissue is seen. Occasionally, there can be an artery on the medial aspect of the uterosacral ligament, as well as some large thin-walled veins. Care should be taken either to avoid the vessels or to allow for their complete occlusion prior to transection.

Complications

Few complications have been formally reported following LUNA. However, in the United States there have been two deaths of which we are aware from postoperative bleeding from the divided uterosacral ligaments. Apparently the surgeons were unfamiliar with the poor hemostatic property of the CO_2 lasers that were used.

Lateral spread of electricity may jeopardize the ureter if bipolar or unipolar current is used. We know of one incident of delayed fistula formation following ureteric injury in a case treated by bipolar current and scissor transection of the ligaments.

To avoid such complications it is imperative to identify the course of the ureter. Keeping the bowel out of the way and ensuring adequate ventilation of the smoke produced

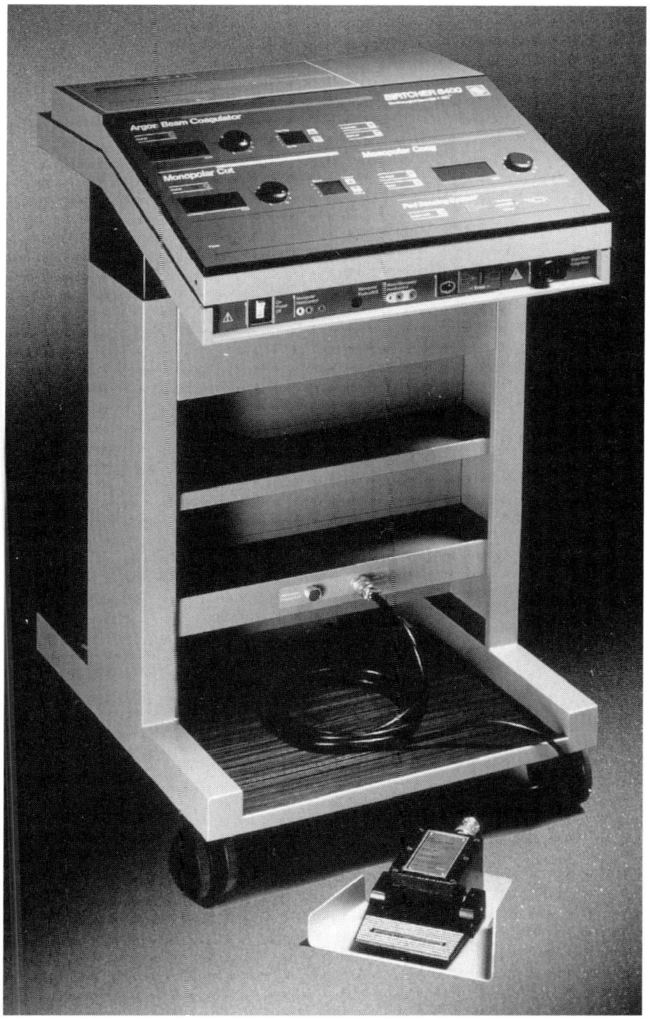

Fig. 20-3. Electrosurgical generator with argon beam coagulator; Birtcher Medical Systems Model 6400. (Courtesy Birtcher Medical Systems.)

by laser or electrosurgical energy are important to ensure adequate visualization. An energy source that will desiccate vessels should be available if it becomes necessary to secure hemostasis.

There have also been reports of uterine prolapse in young women following the LUNA procedure.[18]

PRESACRAL NEURECTOMY

Background

Black's 1964 review of presacral neurectomy for the treatment of pelvic pain that was unresponsive to medical therapy included 9,937 cases.[1] Over 2,500 of these were taken from the world literature, representing procedures performed between 1936 and 1963. Over 7,300 of the cases were analyzed from information provided by a questionnaire that he had sent to colleagues. He also included 43 of his own patients in the study. He found that 83% of patients with primary dysmenorrhea and 72% of patients with secondary dysmenorrhea experienced relief of pain following presacral neurectomy. Those patients reported long-lasting relief over a 10-year period of follow-up. Garcia and David reported relief of dysmenorrhea in 97% of patients and dyspareunia in 74% of patients in a study of 35 women who underwent conservative surgery and presacral neurectomy for pelvic endometriosis.[19]

In 1980, Polan and DeCherney reviewed 20 cases of presacral neurectomy in patients who had endometriosis or pelvic inflammatory disease (PID). They found that 75% of the patients with either PID or endometriosis had significant relief of pain following presacral neurectomy compared with only 26% of a control group with pelvic pain and infertility, but neither endometriosis nor PID, who underwent a laparotomy only without presacral neurectomy.[20]

Candiani et al. conducted a randomized controlled study of conservative surgery alone versus conservative surgery plus presacral neurectomy in 71 patients with endometriosis and midline dysmenorrhea. They were unable to demonstrate any significant difference in postoperative pain scores.[21] In the 35 women who underwent neurectomy, pain developed or worsened in 13 and urinary urgency developed in three. They concluded that neurectomy should not be a routine procedure in women with endometriosis.

Laparoscopic presacral neurectomy was initially described by Perez.[6] He used a vertical peritoneal incision initially using bipolar forceps to desiccate the superior and inferior trunks and sharp dissection to resect a segment of the nerve. In later cases he used a combination of bipolar current and Nd:YAG laser with a contact tip to resect the segment. He demonstrated a significant reduction in postoperative pain scores in 25 women who underwent operative laparoscopy for endometriosis, at which time a presacral neurectomy was performed. Five of the patients had adnexal pain, and four of these continued to experience at least 70% of their original adnexal discomfort. One patient obtained complete relief by taking oral contraceptives. Twenty-four of the patients were followed for at least 6 months, and none reported a worsening in the postoperative pain score. One of these 25 patients required laparotomy for control of retroperitoneal bleeding.

Procedure

Adequate visualization is essential to avoid potential complications. Perez initially described inserting a laparoscope suprapubically to view the sacral promontory.[6] The peritoneum overlying the sacral promontory was elevated and the retroperitoneal space was injected with a dilute vasopressin solution. The peritoneum was then incised parallel to the long axis of the sigmoid colon. The incision was extended cephalad to just below the bifurcation of the aorta. The great vessels and the ureter on the right were then identified as were the inferior mesenteric artery and superior hemorrhoidal vessels on the left. The underlying tissue was then dissected bluntly. The presacral tissue was identified and grasped. Dissection continued caudad to isolate the inferior hypogastric plexus from its underlying tissue. A segment of the nerve was then isolated with suture, bipolar desiccation, or with Nd:YAG laser. If the middle sacral vessels were in close proximity, they were ligated with endoloop sutures. In Perez's initial paper, he had to ligate the superior hemorrhoidal vessel in one patient. A 2 to 3 cm segment of nerve was excised, and the peritoneal edges were usually left open.

Technique using the argon beam coagulator

The vasculature poses the greatest difficulty in dissection of the presacral space. We have recently been using the argon beam coagulator to achieve hemostasis and transect the presacral tissues. We use a four-puncture technique siting the laparoscope in the umbilicus. The three 5 mm ancillary portals are sited as follows, one suprapubically in the midline and one each in the lower quadrants. Our initial technique was different from the one we currently use. We retracted the sigmoid mesocolon to the left lateral position to expose the sacral promontory, using a forceps introduced through the left lower quadrant portal. The peritoneum was incised transversely with a unipolar needle electrode. The retroperitoneal fat was dissected with aqua dissection and with scissors to expose vessels and nerves. If a large middle sacral vessel was encountered, it was occluded with bipolar current. The exposed presacral nerves were destroyed using either the KTP laser or bipolar current and divided with scissors.

The drawbacks to this technique were bleeding, distortion of the anatomic relationships as a result of aqua dissection, and prolonged operating time. These drawbacks led us to develop our current technique using the argon beam coagulator (ABC) (Fig. 20-3; see also Chapter 4).

Three 5 mm ancillary portals are placed as described earlier. A forceps is introduced through each of the lower quadrant portals. The cannula of the ABC is inserted through the suprapubic portal. The sigmoid colon is retracted to the left with the forceps introduced through the left portal, exposing the sacral promontory. The peritoneum above the promontory is retracted cephalad using the forceps introduced through the right portal. The major vessels and ureter are easily visible on the right side. Using the ABC (with 80 watts power and an argon flow of 4 L/minute) the peritoneum over the promontory is fulgurated in a transverse manner. The fulguration extends laterally to about 1 cm from the vessels on the right to the mesentery of the sigmoid on the left, taking care not to damage the mesenteric vessels. Division of the peritoneal layer occurs because of a combination of the fulguration and the concomitant retraction. Fulguration is continued down to the periosteum through the underlying layers of fat, vessels, and nerves. It is essential to keep the argon beam perpendicular to the sacrum to avoid deflection of the electron stream off the bone and onto vital structures.

This approach we believe is superior and safer than our earlier technique. Because of the mesentery on the left side, it can often be difficult to define the lateral edges of the dissection. This is especially true when there is a great amount of fatty tissue in the presacral space. With the ABC technique we do not isolate and remove a segment of nerves to confirm that the nervous tissue was transected. Such a step would increase operating time and the risk of bleeding and is not necessary since transection of all presacral tissue down to the periosteum is directly observed.

Results. Table 20-2 documents our preliminary data using the argon beam coagulator for presacral neurectomy compared to our initial technique, which was similar to that described by Perez, using bipolar energy and dissection of the nerves. There was one major complication that involved operative injury to the left common iliac vein. In this case, however, the argon beam coagulator was directed tangentially through a right lateral portal; thus the beam was deflected onto the left vein. Since that time, we have been directing the ABC through the suprapubic portal and there have not been any further complications. Of the 15 patients

Table 20-2. Results of presacral neurectomy[22]

	ABC fulguration technique	Bipolar desiccation and section technique
No. of cases	15	17
Average age	31.1 years	27.7 years
Average OR time	64 min	92 min
Average blood loss	11.0 cc*	13.0 cc
Complications	1†	0
Improved	11 (73%)	12 (70%)
Same	3	2
Worse	1	2

*Not including complication.
†Laceration of left common iliac vein.

in the study, 85% reported subsequent improvement in their dysmenorrhea during a minimum of 3 months' follow-up.

CONCLUSION

The management of intractable dysmenorrhea and chronic pelvic pain is not simple, as has been noted in Chapter 10. Although older studies, and indeed our recent work, would suggest that surgical interruption of the nerve supply to the pelvic viscera may be beneficial to some patients, this conclusion can be fully substantiated only when further randomized prospective studies have been performed.

Laparoscopic surgery is less invasive than laparotomy and interruption of the uterosacral ligaments less difficult to perform and less risky than presacral neurectomy. We reserve presacral neurectomy for patients who have had an adequate transection of the uterosacral ligaments but have continued to experience pelvic pain and dysmenorrhea. More long-term data, however, are needed to ascertain the true benefits of both of these procedures.

REFERENCES

1. Black WT Jr: Use of presacral sympathectomy in the treatment of dysmenorrhea: a second look after 25 years. *Am J Obstet Gynecol* 89:17, 1964.
2. Dawood YM: Premenstrual syndrome and dysmenorrhea. Baltimore, 1985, Urban & Schwarzenberg.
3. Henzl MR: Dysmenorrhea: achievements and challenge. *Sex Med Today* 9:8, 1985.
4. Frangenheim H: Laparoscopy and culdoscopy in gynecology. Stuttgart, 1972, G. Thieme.
5. Lichten EM, Bombard J: Surgical treatment of primary dysmenorrhea with laparoscopic uterine nerve ablation. *J Reprod Med* 32:37, 1987.
6. Perez J: Laparoscopic presacral neurectomy: results of the first 25 cases. *J Reprod Med* 35:625, 1990.
7. Perry CP, Azziz R: Laparoscopic uterine nerve ablation, presacral neurectomy and appendectomy. In Azziz, Murphy, editors: Practical Manual of Operative Laparoscopy and Hysteroscopy. New York, 1992, Springer-Verlag.
8. Cleland JGP: Paravertebral anaesthesia in obstetrics: experimental and clinical basis. *Surg Gynecol Obst* 57:51, 1933.
9. Ingersoll FM, Meigs JV: Presacral neurectomy for dysmenorrhea. *N Engl J Med* 238:357, 1948.
10. White JC: Conduction of visceral pain. *N Engl J Med* 246:686, 1952.
11. Doyle JB: Paracervical uterine denervation by transection of the cervical plexus for the relief of dysmenorrhea. *Am J Obstet Gynecol* 70:11, 1955.
12. Ruggi J, Crossen HS, editors: Gynecology. St. Louis, 1915, CV Mosby.
13. Jellet H: Short Practice of Gynecology, London, 1900, Churchill.
14. Feste JR: Laser laparoscopy, a new modality. *J Reprod Med* 30:413, 1985.
15. Lichten EL: Three years experience with L.U.N.A.: Outpatient laser laparoscopic treatment of dysmenorrhea. *Am J Gynecol Health* 3:144, 1989.
16. Sutton CJ: Laser laparoscopic uterine nerve ablation. In Donnez J, editor: Operative Laser Laparoscopy and Hysteroscopy. Brussels, 1989, Nauwelaerts Publishers.
17. Daniell JF: Laser laparoscopy using the KTP laser. In McLaughlin D, Ed. Lasers in Gynecology. Philadelphia, 1991, JB Lippincott.
18. Good MC, Copas PR, Doody MC: Uterine prolapse after laparoscopic uterosacral transection. *J Rep Med*
19. Garcia CR, David SS: Pelvic endometriosis: infertility and pelvic pain. *Am J Obstet Gynecol* 129:740, 1977.
20. Polan ML, DeCherney A: Presacral neurectomy for pelvic pain in infertility. *Fertil Steril* 34:557, 1980.
21. Candiani GB, Fedele L, Vercellini P, et al: Presacral neurectomy for the treatment of pelvic pain associated with endometriosis: a controlled study. *Am J Obstet Gynecol* 167:100-103, 1992.
22. Daniell JF, Kurtz BR, Gurley LD, Lalonde CJ: Laparoscopic presacral neurectomy versus neurotomy: use of the argon beam coagulator compared to conventional technique. *J Gynecol Surg*. (in press.)

Chapter 21

UTERINE DISPLACEMENTS

The indications for surgical correction of uterine retroversion are limited. Third-degree uterine prolapse is usually treated by vaginal surgery. In correctly selected patients there is a place for both laparoscopic ventrosuspension and ventrofixation. This chapter will describe these techniques.

UTERINE RETROVERSION

Retroversion, posterior displacement of the uterus, may either be a normal anatomic variant or may be the result of a number of pathologic processes. In the former situation it is usually symptomless but may be associated with a complaint of deep dyspareunia. When the patient is examined the uterus will be noted to be lying posteriorally but will be freely mobile. Gentle bimanual compression may reproduce the same sensations of pain in those patients who suffer from deep dyspareunia. In this case it is reasonable to assume that the uterine position may be the causative factor, but it must be remembered that the complaint may be due to impalpable endometriosis.

If the uterus is immobile but of normal configuration, it is probably that either endometriosis or chronic pelvic inflammatory changes are present. On occasions a fibroid uterus may be retroverted. It is difficult to tell whether the fibroid(s) have arisen in a previously retroverted organ or whether the weight of the fibroid(s) has caused the displacement of the uterus.

If the retroversion is an accompaniment of some other disease, treatment should be directed toward the disease rather than the uterine displacement; although it may be decided to correct the uterine position as part of the overall surgical management. It is rarely necessary to do anything for the patient with a mobile retroversion unless there is a complaint of deep dyspareunia that is believed to be directly attributable to the retroversion.

At one time designing a variation on the theme of surgical correction was a sure route to medical immortality with an eponymous procedure being attributed to its inventor. As many as 200 such operations were described.[1] Today, if it is decided that surgical replacement is indicated either in an attempt to cure deep dyspareunia or as part of the management of a specific intrapelvic lesions, ventrosuspension can be effected laparoscopically using variations of the Gilliam or Webster-Baldy techniques.

Surgical technique

The patient is anesthetized, positioned, and draped. It is important to insert a uterine cannula, to manipulate the uterus, to test for tubal patency when indicated, and, before the final sutures are tied, to ensure that tubal integrity has not been compromised. Once the pneumoperitoneum is created and the laparoscope inserted, the patient is placed in the Trendelenberg position.

Modified Gilliam suspension. Regardless of whether the ventrosuspension is to be the primary procedure or part of a more extensive operation, the first ancillary puncture should not be made in the midline but rather in one or other flank at the site where one round ligament will be sutured to the sheath of the rectus abdominis. This insertion should be made 5 to 6 cm from the midline and 3 cm above the inguinal ligament. The blunt probe is inserted and a thorough pelvic survey carried out. If suspension will be feasible the skin incision is extended to a length of 2 to 3 cm and the underlying aponeurosis exposed.

It will now be necessary to make a second ancillary puncture to begin the suspension, to introduce the instruments required to deal with any unsuspected endometriosis that has been discovered, or to carry out the planned laparoscopic surgery. The second 5 mm trocar and cannula are inserted through a 2 to 3 cm skin incision that is placed in the contralateral flank, in a position which corresponds to that of the other ancillary portal.

If any procedures are to be undertaken they are usually

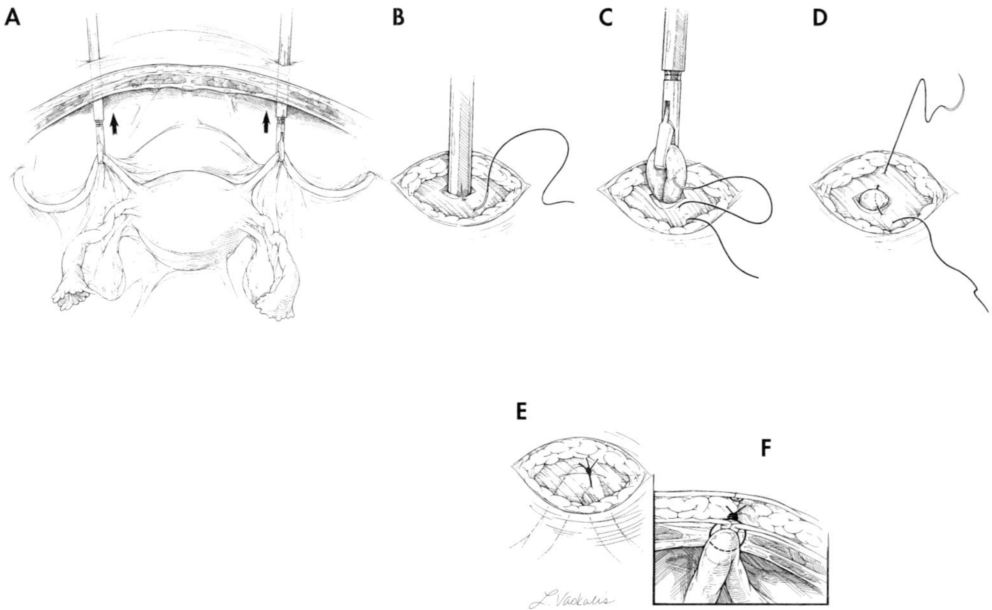

Fig. 21-1. Modified Gilliam suspension. *A,* Grasping forceps are introduced through both ancillary portals (placed in the flanks), and the round ligaments grasped approximately 4 cm lateral to their insertion into the uterus. *B,* The 2 to 3 cm skin incision made at the site of the ancillary portals permits the dissection of the adipose tissue from the fascia. The ligament is sutured to the rectus sheath. A nonabsorbable suture is passed through the fascia cranial to the cannula. *C,* The ligament is withdrawn through the cannula track and the needle passed through the ligament. D, The needle is now passed through the fascia caudad to the cannula track. *E* and *F,* The suture is tied and cut and the skin incision closed.

completed before beginning the suspension, although on occasion it may be advantageous to fix the uterus in anteversion to facilitate access to structures deep within the pouch of Douglas. The uterus is brought into a position of anteversion by manipulating the uterine cannula, and tubal patency is confirmed by chromopertubation. A grasping forceps is introduced through each of the lateral cannulas and the round ligaments seized at a point about 3 to 4 cm lateral to their insertions into the uterus (Fig. 21-1, *A*). The forceps, enclosed ligaments, and cannulas are withdrawn through the abdominal wall. The patient is returned to the supine position and the pneumoperitoneum allowed to escape. It will still be possible to view the uterus with the laparoscope as the tension on the ligaments is adjusted to place the fundus in a satisfactory position. The ligaments are sutured to the external aspect of the rectus sheath with nonabsorbable material. The suture should take one fascial edge (Fig. 21-1, *B*), go through the center of the ligament (Fig. 21-1, *C*), and include the other fascial edge (Fig. 21-1, *D*). Placing the suture in this fashion will not encircle the ligament and compromise its blood supply. The suture is tied and cut (Fig. 21-1, *E* and *F*).

The abdomen is now partially reinflated so that the uterus and tubes can be observed. Chromopertubation is repeated to confirm that the tubes are patent. The round ligaments are inspected to ensure that there are no gaps between the suspension site and the ligaments through which bowel might potentially herniate and strangulate. If these conditions are not satisfied it may be necessary to reposition the round ligaments. It is for this reason that the defects in the rectus sheath were left open.

Once the surgeon is satisfied that there has been minimal distortion of the pelvic architecture, the gas is once again expelled and the telescope and primary trocar are removed. The defects in the rectus sheath are sutured and the three skin incisions closed. This technique is essentially that described by Steptoe.[2]

Injection of 0.25% bupivicaine (Marcaine) or 0.5% lidocaine (Xylocaine) mixed in 1:200000 epinephrine solution into the fascia and skin of the puncture sites before closure will greatly reduce the need for postoperative analgesia.

Modified Webster-Baldy suspension. The ancillary portals are made in the right and left lower quadrants. Using the uterine cannula, the uterus is anteverted and displaced laterally to the left to expose the right broad ligament. Grasping forceps are introduced through the left portal and used to elevate the right tube and ovary to expose

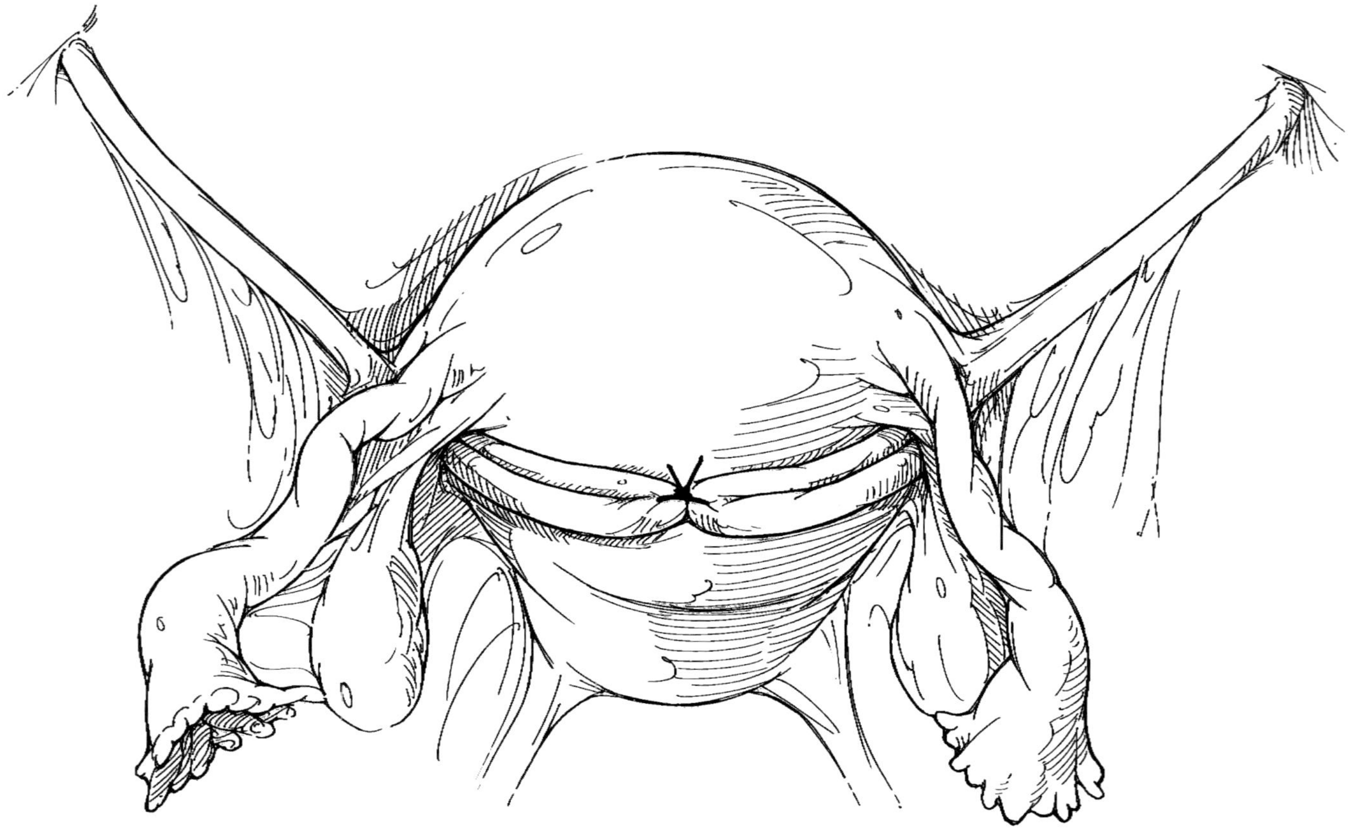

Fig. 21-2. Modified Webster Baldy suspension.

the posterior leaf of the broad ligament. Pointed grasping forceps are introduced through the other portal and guided to an avascular area of the broad ligament approximately 2 cm below the ovarian ligament and close to the lateral wall of the uterus. Blunt dissection with these forceps is used to create an opening in the broad ligament through which the forceps are passed.

The round ligament is seized with the other pair of forceps approximately 5 to 6 cm from its attachment to the uterus and brought down to the now open jaws of the pointed forceps. The latter is used to pull the round ligament through the opening in the broad ligament. The uterus is manipulated so that it lies in the sagittal plane and the loop of round ligament is manipulated with both pairs of forceps so that the knuckle lies in the midline of the posterior wall of the uterus at the same level as the opening in the broad ligament. The knuckle of round ligament is grasped and steadied with one set of grasping forceps. The other pair of grasping forceps is removed. A curved needle bearing 2/0 mersilene suture is introduced as described in Chapter 7. The needle holder is introduced through this portal and the needle is grasped. The suture is placed in the apex of the knuckle of the ligament and a bite is taken in the midline of the posterior wall of the uterus. The suture is tied to anchor the ligament.

The needle is parked temporarily. The uterus is manipulated to the right side and the left round ligament dealt with in a similar fashion. Once the left ligament has been brought into apposition to the right round ligament at the back of the uterus, the needle is retrieved and passed through the knuckle of the left ligament. Chromopertubation is performed to ensure that tubal patency has not been compromised. The knot is now tied fixing the round ligaments in close approximation with each other and the back of the uterus (Fig. 21-2). This technique is time consuming and carries some risk of causing bleeding from the vessels of the broad ligament.

Three stitch technique. Gargiulo[3] has described a simplified "three stitch technique," which apposes the uterosacral ligaments behind the uterus and shortens the round ligaments by hitching them to the fundus of the uterus (Fig. 21-3). Each round ligament is picked up in turn 3 cm to 5 cm from its uterine insertion with a nonabsorbable suture. The stitch is passed through the anterior wall of the uterus and tied. The uterus is manipulated with the uterine cannula to the anteverted position in the midline. The next step is to approximate the uterosacral ligaments directly behind the cervix. The ureters are identified and the third stitch taken through both uterosacral ligaments 5 cm from their uterine insertions. Care is taken to avoid the ureters. The suture is tied and cut. Obviously, the needle is removed from the peritoneal cavity.

Gargiulo reported 22 cases using this technique. Symptoms disappeared in 19 and were significantly reduced in three of 22 women who underwent the three stitch technique.[3]

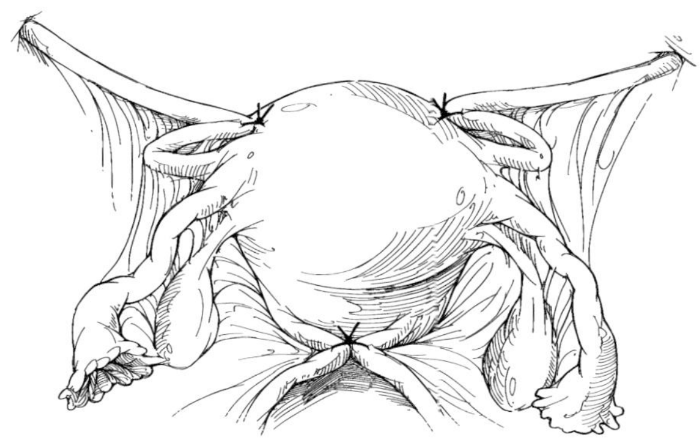

Fig. 21-3. Gargiulo's "three stitch technique" for uterine suspension.

UTERINE PROLAPSE

Third-degree uterine prolapse is usually treated by vaginal surgery. In some elderly patients with third-degree prolapse there may be a considerable degree of ulceration, infection, and discomfort. In such women vaginal surgery is difficult. The postoperative course tends to be stormy and prolonged. In 1970 Kapandji described a laparoscopic technique of uteroligamentous fixation.[4] Laparoscopy was performed under general anesthesia and a uterine cannula was used to elevate the uterus until it was in contact with the anterior abdominal wall. At this location a 1.5 to 2 cm incision was made through the skin and subcutaneous fat only. The fat was dissected from the intact fascia in all directions. A curved Bonney-Reverdin needle was directed through this incision under laparoscopic guidance and passed from the anterior to the posterior surface of the uterine fundus in the midline. A second straight Bonney Reverdin needle was inserted 1 cm above the first. The free end of the absorbable suture was picked up by the second needle and disengaged from the first. Both needles were withdrawn. The suture was held in artery forceps. The same technique was used to place additional sutures in the uterine fundus and round ligaments (Fig. 21-4). The knots were tied above the intact fascia and the skin incision closed.

We have no experience with this technique, nor have we seen any subsequent publications describing its use. As ventro fixation of the uterus by laparotomy still has a small place in gynecologic practice, it seemed worthwhile to de-

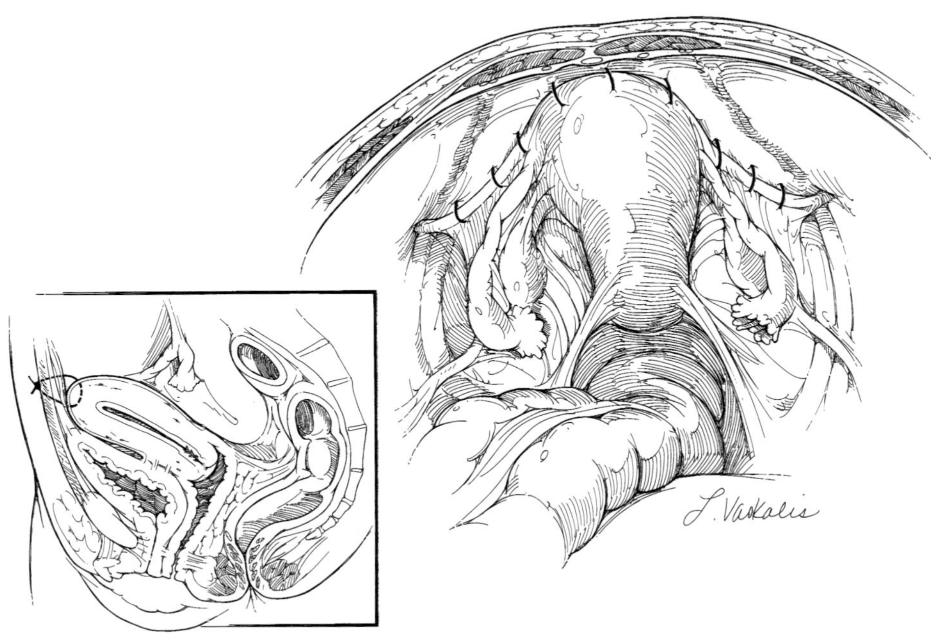

Fig. 21-4. Kapandji's technique of uteroligamentous fixation for uterine prolapse.

scribe a laparoscopic approach for the benefit of those readers who might encounter a patient in whom its use could be of value.

CONCLUSION

For a small number of patients remarkable relief of symptoms can be obtained from a properly performed uterine suspension. For an even smaller number ventrofixation may be indicated. Neither is particularly difficult to perform laparoscopically, and it would seem that if there are true indications the patients can be spared postoperative pain and can return more rapidly to their normal activities.

REFERENCES

1. Jeffcoate TNA: Other displacements of the uterus. In Jeffcoate TNA, Principles of Gynaecology. ed 3. London, 1967, Butterworths.
2. Stepoe PC: Laparoscopy in Gynaecology. Edinburgh 1967, Livingstone.
3. Gargiulo T: Hysteropexis by laparoscopic access. Personal communication.
4. Kapandji M: L'hystero-ligamentopexie laparoscopique des prolapsus du troisieme degre. Gyn Obst (Paris) 69:551-560, 1970.

Chapter 22

HYSTERECTOMY

Hysterectomy is the second most common major surgical procedure (after cesarean section) performed in the United States.[1] Approximately 600,000 hysterectomies are currently performed annually.[2] There are very significant regional and international variations in the hysterectomy rates.[2-5]

Technical and medical advances (IV therapy, antibiotics, blood transfusion) over the past 50 years markedly improved the safety and efficacy of hysterectomy. Owing to these advances the mortality rate decreased significantly to approximately one per 1,000.[6,7] During the same period the rate of hysterectomy increased sharply in the U.S. There were 725,000 hysterectomies performed in 1975.[6] Hysterectomy remained the most frequently performed major surgical procedure until 1981 when it fell to second position due to the increasing rates of birth by cesarean section. It is noteworthy that more than 37% of women have had a hysterectomy before they reach 60 years of age.[6] There has been a decline in the rate of hysterectomy along with other major gynecologic operations since the mid 1970s. This decline has been the result of changing attitudes on the part of women and gynecologists and the development of alternative management options.

INDICATIONS FOR HYSTERECTOMY

The major indications for hysterectomy include one or more of the following: leiomyomata uteri, endometriosis, uterine prolapse, endometrial hyperplasia, and gynecologic malignancy. Other indications are responsible for 15% to 21% of hysterectomies and include disorders of menstruation, pelvic infection, ovarian tumors, and complication of pregnancy.[6,8,9]

Hysterectomy was most frequently performed (33.5%) when a diagnosis of uterine fibroids had been made. Other common indications were endometriosis (18.9% of hysterectomies), uterine prolapse (17.2%), genital cancer (10.8%), and endometrial hyperplasia (5.6%).[6,8,9]

Indications for hysterectomy

- Leiomyomata uteri
- Endometriosis
- Uterine prolapse
- Endometrial hyperplasia
- Gynecologic malignancy
- Disorders of menstruation
- Pelvic infection
- Ovarian tumors
- Complications of pregnancy

It is evident that hysterectomy for genital malignancy is a potentially life-saving procedure. However, this represents a minority of cases and the vast majority are performed to improve the quality of life by correcting a deformity that interferes with function (large uterine fibroids, uterine prolapse) and/or relieve suffering (pain, endometriosis, dysfunctional uterine bleeding). In the absence of clear objective criteria defining these indications, especially the latter group, the appropriateness of the indication must be individualized in each case. Improved laboratory and other diagnostic methods such as ultrasonography, computed tomography, magnetic resonance imaging, endometrial biopsy or curettage, laparoscopy, and hysteroscopy facilitate this task.

It is essential to determine that the symptoms are of uterine origin and that hysterectomy will most probably alleviate them. Alternative nonsurgical and more conservative surgical methods must be discussed together with the patient who must participate in the decision-making process. This participation by the woman is especially important since the loss of the uterus has an important psychologic effect in some women and may lead to subsequent psychosexual dysfunction.[10,11] Such manifestations appear to be related to hormonal, psychologic, social, and cultural factors.[12,13]

RECENT DEVELOPMENTS

The past decade has been a time during which alternative treatment methods for conditions that represent indications for hysterectomy have been developed. These advances have been paralleled by an increased awareness and knowledge of hysterectomy by women and a reluctance to submit to this operation. Lay publications have played an important role in this regard. These factors are producing a decline in the rate of hysterectomy.

While leiomyomata uteri are the most common indication for hysterectomy, only a small fraction of the large percentage of women who have fibroids should require the procedure. Excessive bleeding and, less frequently, pain or pressure symptoms (urinary or rectal) from large leiomyoma may be valid indications. Myomectomy represents the treatment of choice for women who wish to retain their fertility potential. Preoperative use of a 3 month course of GnRH analogs significantly decreases the volume of the fibroids and thus facilitates the procedure.[15,16] In addition, the amenorrhea associated with the course of treatment permits, if necessary, the patient to restore the hemoglobin level to normal and to store autologous blood for the procedure.

In patients with uterine fibroids, menorrhagia is frequently associated with submucous tumours. Hysteroscopy permits both the diagnosis and excision of many of these myomas, often resulting in alleviation of the symptoms even in the presence of other fibroids of intramural or submucous location.[17,18]

A surgical technique introduced recently for treatment of symptomatic leiomyomas is laparoscopic coagulation of the tumors (myolysis). This technique is designed to replace myomectomy by significantly reducing the size of the tumor. Myolysis should be reserved for patients who are not desirous of retaining their fertility. The patient is treated with a 3-month course of GnRH analogs to reduce the size of the fibroids. The presence of submucous myomas is ruled out by diagnostic hysteroscopy performed during the course of medical treatment. At the subsequent laparoscopy each fibroid is coagulated using Nd:YAG laser at 50 watts of power in the following manner. The myoma is pierced with a 600 μ fiber and laser energy applied. The entire myoma is coagulated by repeated drilling and ablation at concentric sites. Since the coagulation effect of the Nd:YAG laser has a 5 mm diameter, a 5 cm myoma requires 10 punctures per diameter and a total of approximately 75 to 100 punctures for complete coagulation of the tumor. A steerable probe permits puncture of the myoma at right angles when it is located anteriorly or posteriorly. The procedure appears to be effective in the long term and is promising. If submucous myomas are present these are treated hysteroscopically at the same time.[19] Myolysis appears to cause significant postoperative adhesions as noted at the time of second-look laparoscopy[20] and thus must be reserved for those women with symptomatic myomas who are not interested in retaining fertility (see Chapter 19).

Endometriosis has been responsible for an increasing number of hysterectomies.[6,8] Medical treatment with old and new agents (progestins, Danazol, GnRH agonists) are often effective in relieving symptoms such as dysmenorrhea, dyspareunia, and dyschezia.[21-23] Conservative surgical treatment of endometriosis alone or in combination with medical treatment represents another option. Many such procedures can be performed laparoscopically[24] (see Chapter 18).

Endometrial ablation provides a therapeutic alternative for the patient with dysfunctional uterine bleeding or menorrhagia in the absence of pelvic lesions.[25-27]

Treatment of endometrial hyperplasia with progestins and in situ carcinoma of the cervix by laser vaporization or electrosurgical excision with a wire loop have proved successful alternatives to hysterectomy.

TYPES OF HYSTERECTOMY

The place of radical hysterectomy and the role of laparoscopy in oncologic cases will be discussed in Chapter 25. This chapter will be confined to a discussion of hysterectomy for benign gynecologic disease.

Once it has been decided that the uterus should be removed it is the responsibility of the surgeon to offer the patient the method that is most likely to effect a cure. In addition, the method chosen should be the one with the lowest mortality and morbidity rates, cause the patient the least postoperative discomfort, and allow her to return to her usual activities as rapidly as possible.

The uterus and cervix can be removed by the abdominal or vaginal routes (total hysterectomy). Although the uterus, cervix, and adnexae (total hysterectomy and bilateral salpingo-oophorectomy) can be excised vaginally it is often technically easier to do so abdominally. The cervix can be left in situ and the uterus and, if necessary, the adnexae can be removed abdominally (subtotal hysterectomy). Of these procedures, vaginal hysterectomy has the lowest rate of mortality and morbidity, causes the least postoperative discomfort, and is associated with the most rapid return to normal activity.

Whereas 50% or more of hysterectomies are performed by the vaginal route in centers experienced with this approach,[28,29] less than one third of all hysterectomies in the U.S. are done by this method.[30] Decreasing numbers of such procedures in training programs are likely to diminish the experience of new gynecologists with vaginal surgery and further increase the rate of abdominal hysterectomies.

Few subtotal hysterectomies are performed currently since total hysterectomy is considered to be the standard of practice except in rare situations in which removal of the cervix would pose a significant risk to the patient. The main purpose for the removal of the cervix is prophylaxis against cancer in this organ.

Subtotal hysterectomy is experiencing some resurgence and may indeed have a place in selected patients. Because of the advantages attributed to this approach, the issue is under current debate. The alleged advantages include prompt ambulation, less postoperative discomfort and morbidity, better vaginal support, decreased overall morbidity, and avoidance of sexual dysfunction.[31-36]

TOTAL LAPAROSCOPIC HYSTERECTOMY AND LAPAROSCOPICALLY ASSISTED HYSTERECTOMY

The first report of laparoscopic hysterectomy was by Reich et al. in 1989.[37] Since the initial publication of this report, many series of laparoscopic hysterectomy have appeared.[34-36, 38-47]

Laparoscopic hysterectomy should not be undertaken in place of vaginal hysterectomy but rather as an alternative approach to abdominal hysterectomy. The relative contraindications to vaginal hysterectomy are endometriosis, prior pelvic surgery, adhesive disease, adnexal lesions, limited uterine mobility, and uterine enlargement. Laparoscopic evaluation alone may demonstrate absence of such relative contraindications and permit the surgeon to carry out the hysterectomy conventionally by the vaginal route.[48] In the presence of one or more of the earlier cited conditions a laparoscopic hysterectomy may replace the abdominal procedure.

The laparoscopic approach may be of assistance in other circumstances. For example, in a case in which a vaginal hysterectomy appears feasible but in addition removal of the ovaries is indicated it may be difficult to achieve this portion of the procedure by the vaginal route. The difficulty may arise either because the ovaries lie high in the pelvis, there is a narrow vaginal access, and/or because of limited surgical expertise. The laparoscopic approach under such circumstances may render a challenging vaginal hysterectomy easier to perform.

From the foregoing it is clear that, when a total hysterectomy is performed with laparoscopic assistance, the steps of the procedure that are performed laparoscopically or through the vagina may vary. These variations have led to arbitrary classifications. These include *total laparoscopic hysterectomy,* which is complete excision by laparoscopy of the uterus from its attachments. The vaginal cuff in this case may be repaired laparoscopically or vaginally. Some authors have made the distinction between *total laparoscopic hysterectomy* and *laparoscopically assisted hysterectomy* on the basis of whether or not the uterine arteries were ligated laparoscopically or vaginally. *Laparoscopically assisted vaginal hysterectomy* refers to those cases in which a portion of the procedure is performed vaginally. *Laparoscopic subtotal hysterectomy* refers to the removal of the uterus only, the cervix being left in place and the stump closed laparoscopically.[43,49] More complex classifications have been proposed recently, on the basis of which steps of the procedures are performed by laparoscopy or by the vaginal route.[50,51] There is obviously no practical value to such classifications but they may have a role for clinical research purposes.

Relative Contraindications to Vaginal Hysterectomy

- Endometriosis
- Prior pelvic surgery
- Adhesions
- Adnexal lesions
- Limited uterine mobility
- Uterine enlargement

There are aspects of the laparoscopic surgical technique that are common to all of the variations. These common aspects will be described first and details of each particular technique later.

Preoperative preparation

The evening before the surgery the rectosigmoid should be cleansed by either an enema or an oral electrolyte bowel preparation such as Go-Lytely. An intravenous drip is started an hour before the operation and a single dose of antibiotic, usually a cephalosporin, is administered prophylactically.

Once in the operating room, the patient is anesthesitized and placed in the modified lithotomy position. Great care is taken to ensure that no vessels or nerves of the legs are being compressed. The choice of stirrups is important, since these should allow for changing the position of the patient's legs with ease to accommodate both the laparoscopic and the vaginal steps of the operation. While for most laparoscopic procedures knee braces or Lloyd-Davis type stirrups are employed, these are difficult to adjust intraoperatively. Stirrups that hold the foot and ankle are preferable since they can be easily adjusted.

The abdomen and perineum are washed and draped. The bladder is catheterized with a Foley catheter, which is left in place. A careful bimanual pelvic examination is performed, assessing the size, shape, and mobility of the uterus. When indicated, as with patients who have had a prior cesarean section, 60 ml of methylene blue or indigo carmine solution is instilled in the bladder and the catheter clamped.

This step facilitates recognition of any unexpected entry into the bladder. Some surgeons insert ureteral catheters to facilitate identification of the ureters. A rigid cannula is placed in the cervix to permit manipulation of the uterus from below. The Valtchev mobilizer is well suited for this purpose.

Insertion of the laparoscope and laparoscopic survey

The laparoscope is inserted intraumbilically. A suprapubic midline portal of entry is established and a probe or blunt atraumatic forceps is introduced. A thorough survey of the upper and lower abdomen is performed before the patient is placed in the Trendelenberg position. The bowel is manipulated from the pelvis and the pelvic contents assessed. Based on this assessment, two further portals will be inserted, one in the right and one in the left lower quadrants at about the McBurney points. The height of these ancillary puncture sites will depend upon the size of the uterus or any adnexal mass if one is present. The caliber will be determined by that of the instruments to be used. Short ancillary cannulas that can be secured in place greatly facilitate the procedure as nonsecurable cannulas can slip from the abdominal wall during the operation as instruments are removed and reinserted. These self-securing cannula have the additional advantage of preventing the formation of abdominal wall emphysema that may occur when large volumes of carbon dioxide are being insufflated and cannulas slip out. Once the ancillary portals have been established, the operation either proceeds directly or it may be necessary to deal with additional lesions prior to undertaking the hysterectomy.

Treatment of additional lesions

Often additional lesions will be noted, which may include adhesions, subserous myomata, or areas of endometriosis. It may be necessary or more practical to deal with these lesions first. Adhesiolysis and/or excision of a large subserous myoma may improve visibility and facilitate performance of the remainder of the procedure. It may be preferable to ablate and/or excise endometriotic lesions at the beginning of the operation. The steps involved in dealing with these conditions have been described in the appropriate chapters and will not be redescribed here.

If unilateral or bilateral salpingo-oophorectomy is to form part of the procedure, removal of the adnexa may precede or follow the excision of the uterus. The choice will depend upon the findings and the preference of the surgeon.

Technique of total laparoscopic hysterectomy

Total laparoscopic hysterectomy is performed by following a series of steps that are essentially the same as those used in performing an abdominal hysterectomy. These steps, the sequence of which may vary depending on the circumstances of each case, are:

1. Identification and/or dissection of the ureters.
2. Securing and dividing the round ligaments.
3. Securing and dividing the infundibulopelvic or the ovarian ligaments.
4. Downward dissection of the bladder.
5. Securing and dividing the uterine vessels.
6. Securing the cardinal and uterosacral ligaments.
7. Entry into the vaginal fornices and excision of the cervix.
8. Removal of the specimen.
9. Vault support and vault closure.
10. Final laparoscopic inspection.
11. Removal of the laparoscopic equipment and closure of the abdominal incisions.

Each of these steps will now be described in detail.

There is no standard approach to securing the pedicles. Ligatures, sutures, desiccation, and stapling devices have all been used. Although the ideal pedicle securing technique has yet to be developed, at present we favor a combination of electrodesiccation, ligating, and suture-ligating (see Chapter 7).

Step 1: Identification and/or dissection of the ureters. The course of the ureters must be identified and, when conditions mandate, the ureters dissected at the start of the procedure. The retroperitoneal edema and suppression of the peristaltic activity of the ureters that occurs during the operation renders their identification difficult if undertaken later during the procedure. If complete dissection of the ureter is not necessary the most vulnerable segment should be exposed. The peritoneum over the ureters is incised with scissors near the site at which the ureter crosses the uterine vessels (Fig. 22-1, *A*). The scissors are introduced through this incision and spread. The peritoneal incision is then extended downward for a total length of about 2 cm (Fig. 22-1, *B*), and the medial aspect of the ureter is exposed (Fig. 22-1, *C*).

Step 2: Securing and dividing the round ligaments. To secure and divide the left round ligament, the left ovarian ligament is grasped using a strong self-locking forceps introduced from the opposite side. The uterus is pulled to the right. The round ligament is grasped with a bipolar or unipolar forceps 2 to 3 cm distal to its uterine insertion and desiccated for a length of about 1.5 cm (Fig. 22-2, *A*). This desiccated area is then divided with scissors introduced through the midline ancillary puncture site. The visceral peritoneum is incised parallel to the uterus and the incision is then curved medially to the midline above the bladder. This commences the development of the U-shaped bladder flap (Fig. 22-2, *B*). The clear area in the upper broad ligament is identified (Fig. 22-2, *C*). The same procedure will be carried out on the opposite side. But, to limit changes of instruments and to speed the procedure, the next step is performed on the ipsilateral side before switching to the other side.

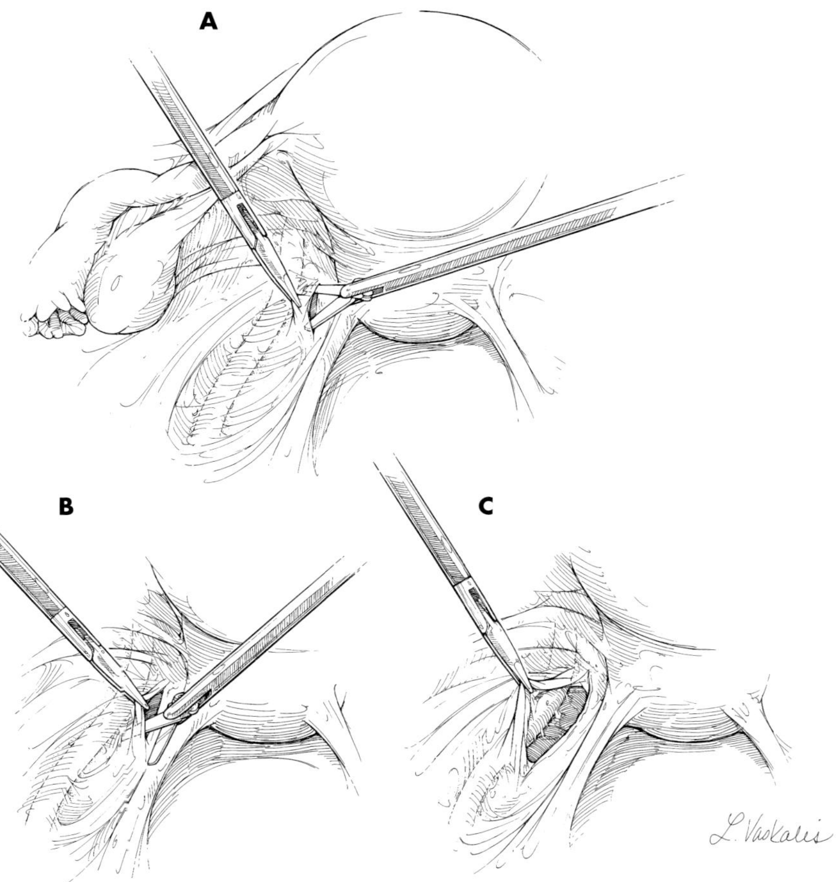

Fig. 22-1. Identification of the ureter. **A,** The trajectory of the ureter is identified. The peritoneum is grasped medial to the ureter, near the site where it crosses the uterine vessels, and incised. **B,** The incision is enlarged for about 2 cm. **C,** The medial aspect of the ureter is exposed.

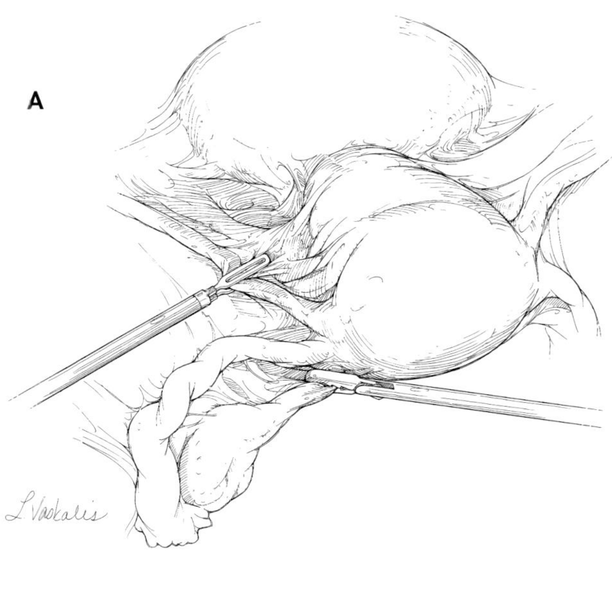

Fig. 22-2. Securing and dividing the round ligament. **A,** The ovarian ligament is grasped and the uterus retracted. The round ligament is desiccated with bipolar or unipolar current.

Continued.

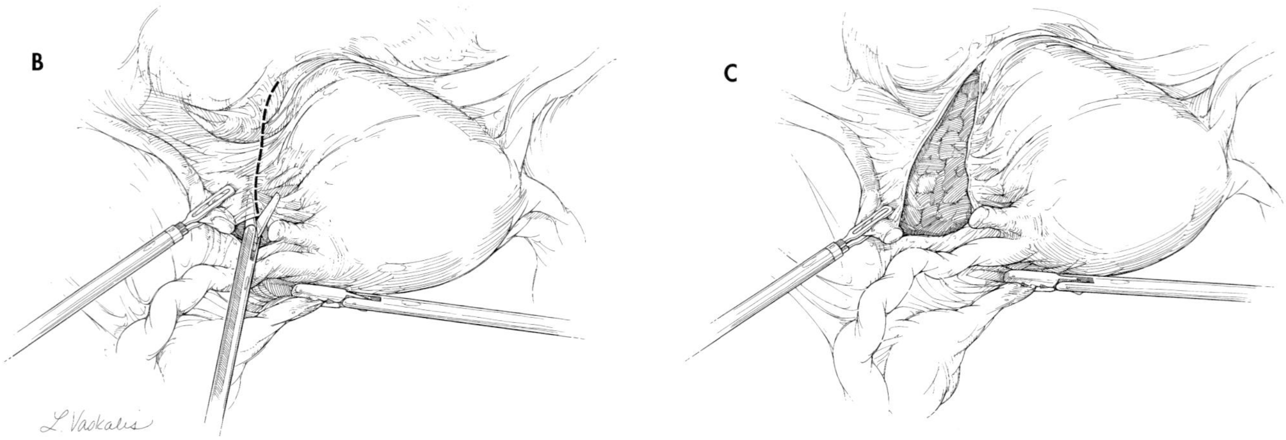

Fig. 22-2, cont'd. B, The round ligament is divided over the desiccated area. Development of the bladder flap commences with incision of the visceral peritoneum, parallel to the uterus. **C,** The clear area in the upper broad ligament is exposed.

Step 3: Securing and dividing the infundibulopelvic or the ovarian ligaments. If a salpingo-oophorectomy forms part of the procedure, the infundibulopelvic ligament is secured down to the clear area in the upper broad ligament. Care must be taken to avoid the ureter in the process. This is especially important when a stapling device is used to occlude the infundibulopelvic ligament, since this instrument has a width of 12 mm. To secure the left infundibulopelvic ligament, the operating instrument is introduced through the left portal. The uterus is pulled to the opposite side with the self-locking forceps grasping the left ovarian ligament. On the left side, exposure of the infundibulopelvic ligament may necessitate release of the peritoneal reflection of the sigmoid. On occasion it may be necessary to grasp and retract the ovary (instead of the ovarian ligament) to the contralateral side to achieve proper exposure of the infundibulopelvic ligament. The infundibulopelvic ligament is secured and divided (Fig. 22-3).

If the ovary is to remain in place, the ovarian ligament and the proximal tube are secured down to the clear area in the broad ligament and divided.

Backflow from the pedicles is not an issue when a stapling device or electrodesiccation is employed. However, if suturing is used it will be necessary to place an additional medial suture prior to the division of the pedicles. Alternatively, the medial side of the pedicle may be grasped with a strong self-locking grasping forceps with monopolar capability, and after the division of the pedicle the medial side is electrodessicated.

When the ovary is to be conserved and a stapling device used, it is possible to secure both the round and ovarian ligaments in one step. The two structures are grasped down to the clear zone in the broad ligament with the stapling device, which in turn is locked in place and fired.

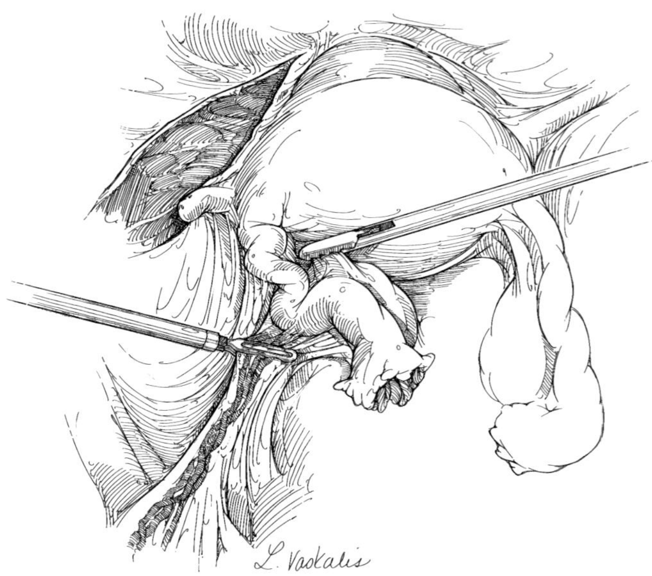

Fig. 22-3. Securing and dividing the infundibulopelvic ligament.

These steps are repeated on the opposite side, and development of the bladder flap completed.

Step 4: Downward dissection of the bladder. The U-shaped incision over the visceral peritoneum having been completed (Fig. 22-4, *A*), the peritoneum above the bladder is elevated with a grasping forceps and the bladder is dissected from the uterus downward and laterally (Fig. 22-4, *B*). This can be achieved by hydrodissection and/or by sharp and blunt dissection. Hemostasis of the bladder pillars and other bleeding points is achieved by electrodesiccation (Fig. 22-4, *C*). The dissection of the bladder is continued until

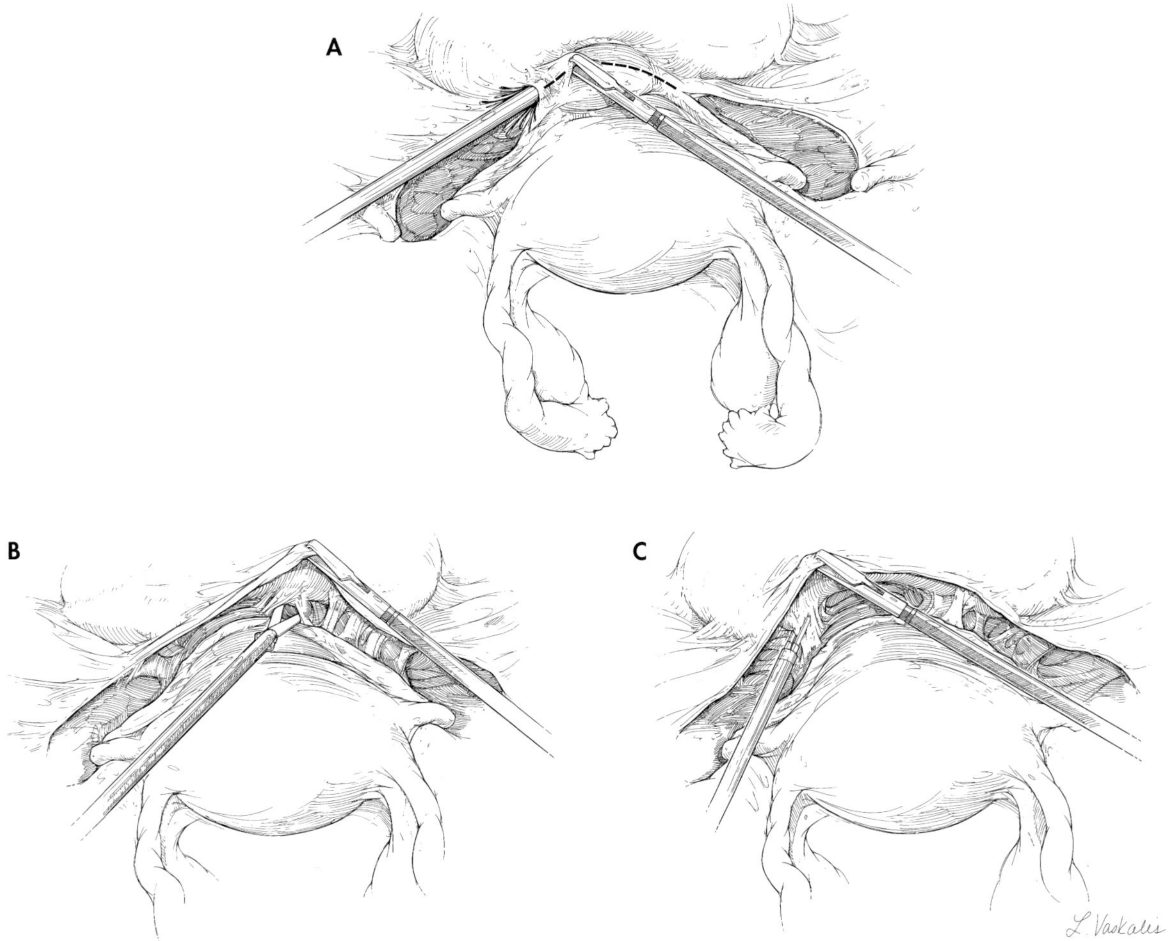

Fig. 22-4. Dissection of the bladder. **A,** Development of the bladder flap with hydrodissection. **B,** The peritoneum is elevated and the bladder is dissected from the uterus. **C,** Hemostasis of the bladder pillars is achieved by electrodesiccation.

the anterior vaginal wall is reached. This dissection will be more difficult if the bladder has been previously dissected as, for example, at the time of cesarean section. Identification of the anterior vaginal fornix is facilitated by placement of a damp sponge held in a sponge forceps, which is now introduced through the vagina and thus adequacy of the bladder dissection confirmed.

Step 5: Securing and dividing the uterine vessels. The posterior peritoneal leaf of one broad ligament is incised with scissors parallel to the uterus, downward to the level of the uterosacral ligament (Fig. 22-5, *A*). This step is repeated on the opposite side.

Connective tissue between the previously exposed ureter and the uterine vessels is dissected. The uterine vessels are skeletonized, secured, and divided (Fig. 22-5, *B*). When, as we prefer, sutures are used to secure the uterine vessels, suturing the vessels on both sides of the uterus, before sectioning them, will significantly reduce the backflow from the uterus, thus obviating the need to doubly suture-ligate each pedicle.

Step 6: Securing the cardinal and uterosacral ligaments. The cardinal ligament is exposed by positioning the uterine manipulator and retraction of the uterus to the contralateral side using the upper grasping forceps. The ligament is secured adjacent to the cervix and divided (Fig. 22-6, *A*). The procedure is repeated on the opposite side.

The remaining attachments of the uterus are now its circumferential attachment to the vaginal vault and the uterosacral ligaments. The uterosacral ligaments are exposed, one at a time, by manipulation of the uterine cannula; they are secured and divided (Fig. 22-6, *B*). Securing these ligaments with suture ligatures permits the use of the same suture to attach them to the vaginal vault for support purposes. If this technique is to be used the suture is not cut and the needle parked temporarily in the cul-de-sac.

Step 7: Entry into the vaginal fornices. The posterior vaginal fornix may be entered either prior to or after the division of the uterosacral ligaments (Fig. 22-6, *B*). To enter the posterior vaginal fornix the uterus is anteverted by manipulation of the uterine cannula. A wet gauze held in a

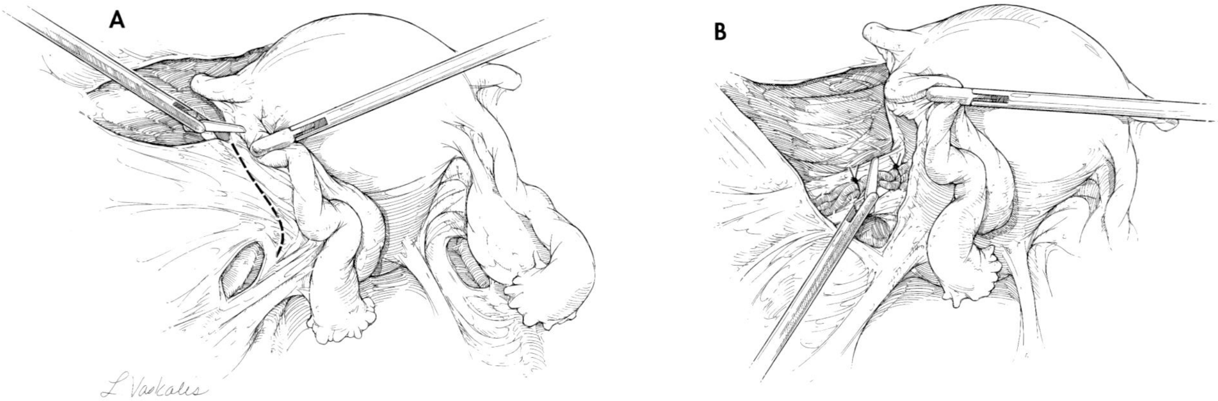

Fig. 22-5. Securing and dividing the uterine vessels. **A,** The posterior leaf of the broad ligament is incised downward, parallel to the uterus, and the uterine vessels are skeletonized. **B,** The uterine vessels are secured and divided.

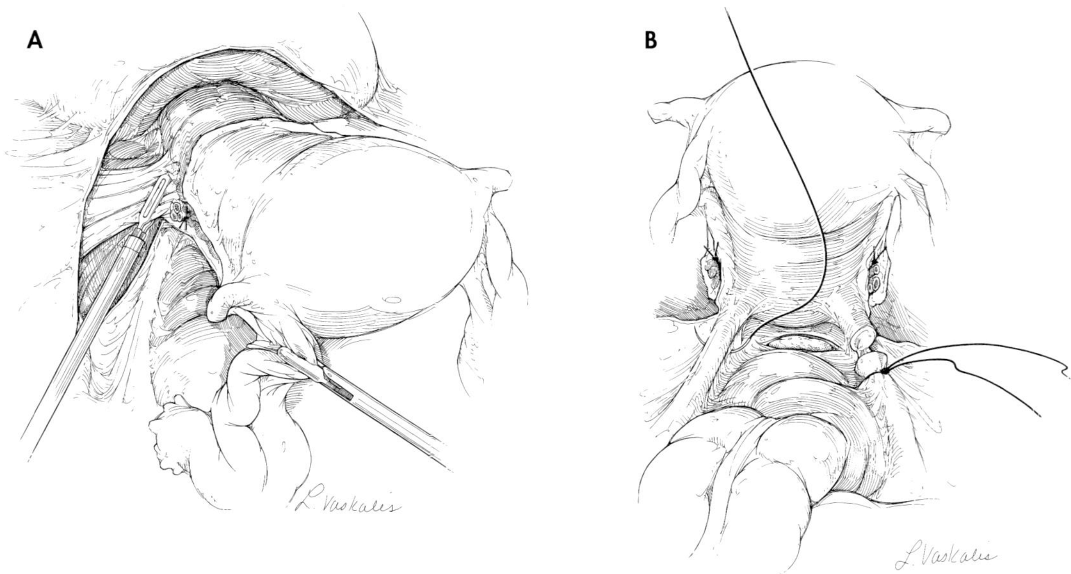

Fig. 22-6. Securing the cardinal and uterosacral ligaments. **A,** Securing the cardinal ligament. **B,** Securing the uterosacral ligament.

ring forceps is introduced into the posterior vaginal fornix to assist in the identification of the site of incision and to prevent loss of the pneumoperitoneum. The fornix is entered electrosurgically close to the cervicovaginal junction (Fig. 22-6, *B*). The anterior fornix is entered in a similar fashion using a wet sponge as a backstop (Fig. 22-7, *A*). The incision is then extended along the circumference of the cervix, over the lateral fornices continuing to use the wet sponge as a backstop (Fig. 22-7, *B*). The uterus is now totally free.

Step 8: Removal of the uterus. The uterus is removed vaginally. When the uterus is too large, morcellation may be necessary. Leaving the whole uterus or a portion of it (when morcellation is necessary) in the vagina will prevent subsequent deflation of the pneumoperitoneum. Alternatively, a large wet sponge may be used for the same purpose.

Step 9: Vault support and vault closure. This step may be performed either laparoscopically or through the vagina. The vaginal approach, which will be described later, is usu-

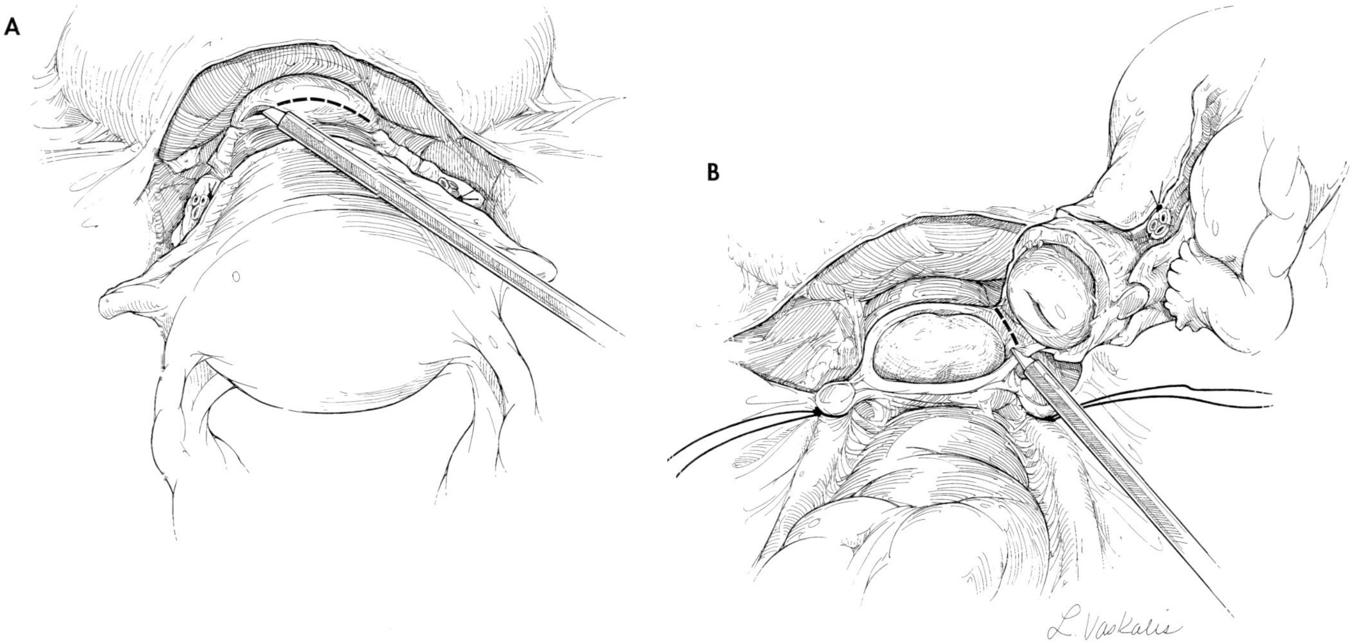

Fig. 22-7. Entry into the vaginal fornices and incision of the vaginal vault. **A,** The anterior vaginal fornix is entered. **B,** The vaginal vault is incised along the circumference of the cervix.

ally faster. Circumstances may necessitate laparoscopic closure, which will now be discussed.

The left uterosacral ligament is elevated with a grasping forceps and a suture is placed through this ligament. The left posterolateral aspect of the vagina is elevated. The needle is introduced through the wall of the vagina into the lumen of the vagina. The needle is then turned backward toward the pouch of Douglas and reintroduced through the vaginal wall on the left. The suture is tied around the uterosacral ligament. The same step is repeated on the opposite side. If the uterosacral ligaments were secured with suture ligatures (see above), the same sutures may be used to join the uterosacral ligaments to the posterolateral aspects of the vaginal vault (Fig. 22-8, *A*).

The edges of the vagina, including the overlying pubocervical fascia, are approximated with a continuous suture. Closure is frequently effected in the sagittal plane (Fig. 22-8, *B*). The peritoneum is usually left unsutured.

Step 10: Final laparoscopic inspection. The pelvis and abdominal cavity are thoroughly irrigated with lactated Ringer's solution. It is necessary to elevate the head of the operating table while aspirating to bring into the pelvis any fluid that has accumulated in the paracolic gutters. Once the irrigation fluid is clear, the pressure of the pneumoperitoneum is reduced and the operative site and each pedicle are inspected to ensure presence of good hemostasis. Any bleeding points are electrodesiccated using a microbipolar forceps.

We tend to leave some 200 ml of irrigation solution in the pelvis, although some advocate leaving as much as 2 L in the periteonal cavity.[50]

Step 11: Removal of the laparoscopic equipment and closure of abdominal incisions. The ancillary cannulas are removed and the peritoneal aspect of each one is examined through the laparoscope to ensure that there is no bleeding. Only then is the gas expelled and the laparoscope and the principal cannula removed. It is usually sufficient to approximate the edges of the smaller (5 mm) incisions with Steristrips after applying tincture of benzoin to the adjacent skin. With larger incisions (8 mm or greater) the facia should be closed with single or figure eight 0 vicryl suture(s). The skin edges may be approximated with steristrips (see Chapter 7).

Laparoscopically assisted vaginal hysterectomy

The laparoscopic portion of the procedure may be limited to the treatment of any associated lesions, and may include division of adhesions, excision and/or ablation of endometriotic lesions; or excision of an ovarian cyst when the ovary(ies) are to be preserved. The hysterectomy is then performed by the vaginal route. In a recently published classification system this has been termed "laparoscopically directed preparation for vaginal hysterectomy."[51]

The laparoscopic approach to each step of the procedure was described in the immediately preceding section. Depending on the circumstances many of these steps may be performed vaginally.

When bilateral or unilateral oophorectomy forms part of

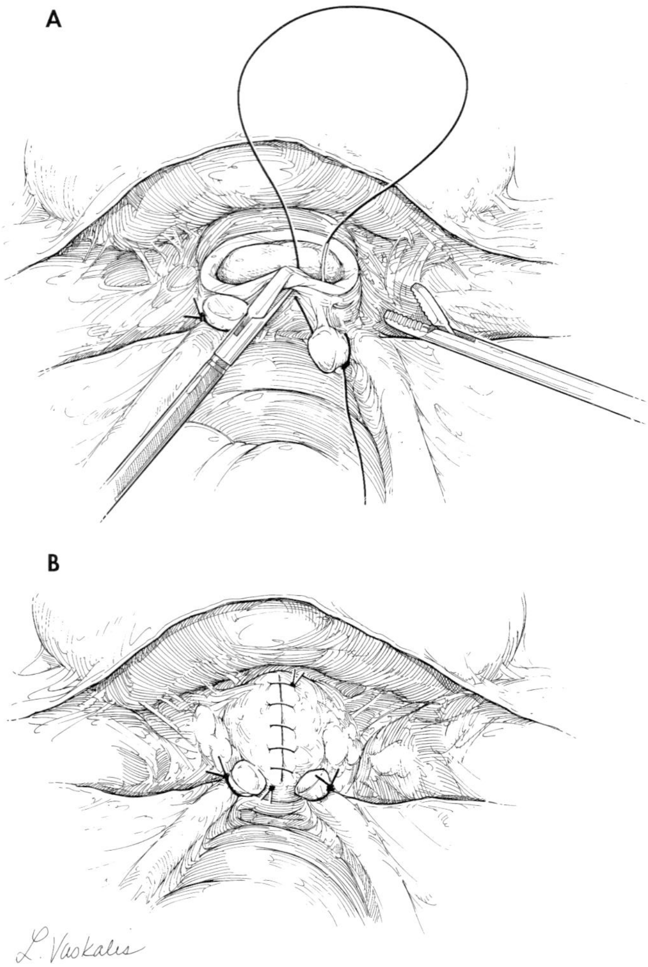

Fig. 22-8. Vault support and vault closure. **A,** The uterosacral ligament is sutured to the vaginal vault. **B,** The vaginal vault is closed, usually, in the sagital plane.

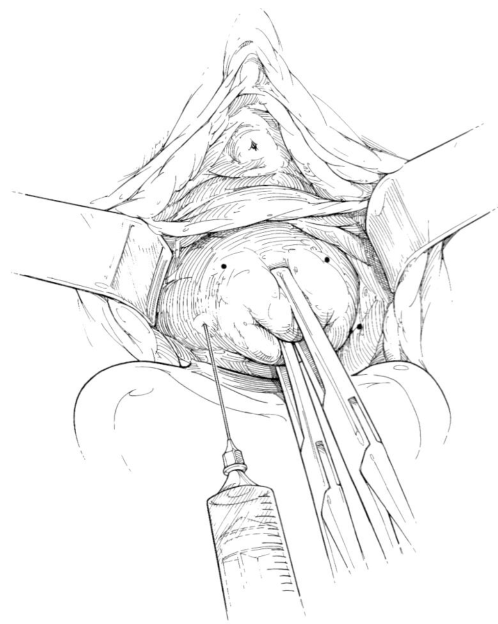

Fig. 22-9. LAVH: Injection of local anesthetic into the paracervical tissues.

the procedure, the laparoscopic portion may be limited to securing and dividing the infundibulopelvic ligament(s) or completion of the salpingo-oophorectomy. Alternatively any of the previously described successive steps from 1 to 5 inclusive may be performed laparoscopically.

When a portion of the procedure is performed vaginally the anterior and posterior vaginal fornices may be entered laparoscopically as described earlier or the lower part of the procedure performed totally by the vaginal route as will now be described.

Repositioning of the patient and preparation for the vaginal portion of the procedure. The stirrups are repositioned to accommodate the vaginal portion of the operation. A weighed speculum is inserted into the vagina. The uterine cannula is removed and either one or two tenacula applied to the cervix. The tenacula are pulled downward to expose the cervix and upper vagina. The exposure is enhanced with the use of vaginal retractors. Infiltration of 20 ml of 0.5% lidocaine (Xylocaine) or 0.25% bupivacaine (Marcaine) in epinephrine (1:200,000) solution will decrease blood loss considerably during the procedure. This is particularly important in premenopausal women who have a greater tendency to bleed. In those instances when the use of epinephrine is contraindicated, local anesthetic diluted in normal saline solution is used. Before injecting the solution the surgeon must ascertain that the needle is not within a vessel. The solution is injected into the paracervical tissues and not into the cervical body itself (Fig. 22-9). A subsequent pause of a few mintues will permit dissemination of the solution.

Circumferential incision of the vaginal vault. The incision around the cervix should be appropriately placed (neither too low nor too high) and commence posteriorly at the level of the base of the cul-de-sac. The incision is carried around the cervix in a circumferential fashion along a grooved depression of the rugae of the upper vagina and through the full thickness of the epithelium (Fig. 22-10).

Entering the pouch of Douglas and the vesicouterine pouch. Two Allis forceps are applied to the lateral edges of the incised posterior vaginal epithelium. Pulling these

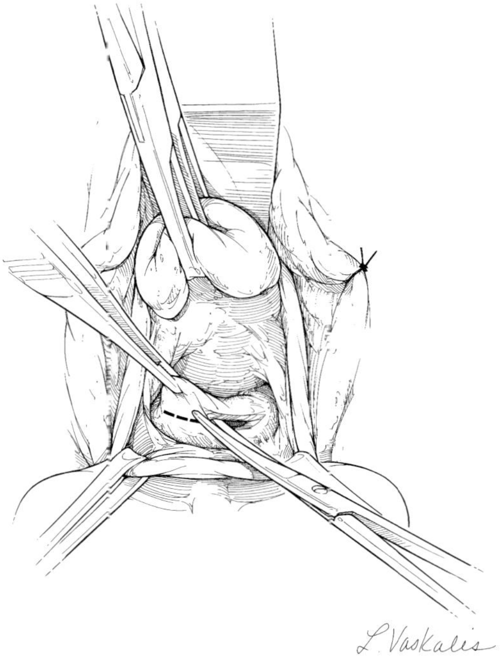

Fig. 22-10. LAVH: The cervical epithelium is incised in a circumferential manner and the peritoneum of the pouch of Douglas exposed and entered.

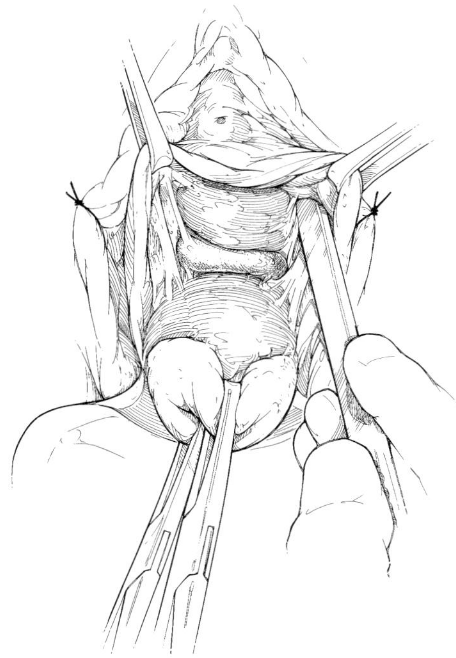

Fig. 22-11. LAVH: The bladder is dissected from the cervix and the peritoneum of the vesicouterine pouch is exposed and entered.

forceps downward and the cervix upward with the attached tenacula will expose the peritoneum of the pouch of Douglas (Fig. 22-10). The peritoneum is grasped with a pair of dressing forceps and incised to open the peritoneal cavity. It is important to deflate completely the peritoneal cavity before this last step, otherwise any blood or irrigation fluid accumulated in the pelvis will escape and spray the surgeon.

The uterosacral ligaments can be secured and divided at this point or after entering the vesicouterine pouch.

Anteriorly the incised vaginal epithelium is grasped with two Allis forceps and freed from the cervix by upward dissection. It will now be necessary to dissect the bladder from the cervix. This is accomplished largely by sharp dissection using Mayo scissors, while the cervix is pulled downward by the assistant. The curved tips of the scissors are pointed toward the cervix and spread while pressure with them is maintained against the cervix. Repeating this step along the appropriate plane, the dissection is carried upward until the vesicouterine fold of the peritoneum is reached. During this dissection the scalpel handle can be also used as a blunt dissector (Fig. 22-11). Active bleeding points are either electrodesiccated or ligated. The bladder pillars are identified and electrodesiccated or ligated near their cervical attachment and divided.

Exposure of the periteonal fold between the bladder and the cervix is facilitated by downward retraction of the cervix and upward retraction of the bladder with a vaginal retractor. The peritoneum is grasped and incised. This opening is enlarged. By introducing the index fingers of both hands into the incision and pushing laterally the ureters are displaced out of harm's way.

Division of uterosacral and cardinal ligaments. Each uterosacral ligament is exposed by pulling the cervix upward and to the contralateral side. The ligament is clamped with a Rogers clamp and transected (Fig. 22-12). A suture ligature is applied and the ligament is transfixed before the suture is tied. This suture is kept long and held with a Kelly clamp for later identification. The contralateral uterosacral ligament is treated in a similar fashion. Once both of the uterosacral ligaments have been divided the uterus will descend further.

The next steps are the identification, clamping, division, and suturing of the cardinal ligaments. This step is facilitated by the use of an anterior vaginal retractor, which is introduced into the vesicouterine pouch and the replacement of the weighed speculum, the tip of which is introduced into the cul-de-sac. The uterus is retracted to the contralateral side, one ligament is clamped, divided, and suture ligatured, and the suture is cut short. The same step is repeated on the opposite side.

Ligation and division of the uterine vessels. At this point it will be easy to identify the uterine vessels, especially if the remainder of the upper pedicles have all been dealt with laparoscopically. Retracting the uterus to the contralateral side, each uterine artery is clamped close to the cervix, divided between the clamp, and the cervix and su

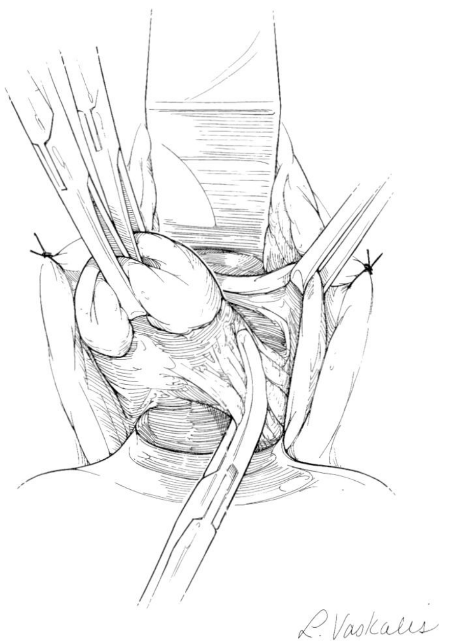

Fig. 22-12. LAVH: The uterosacral ligament is exposed, clamped, divided, and ligatured.

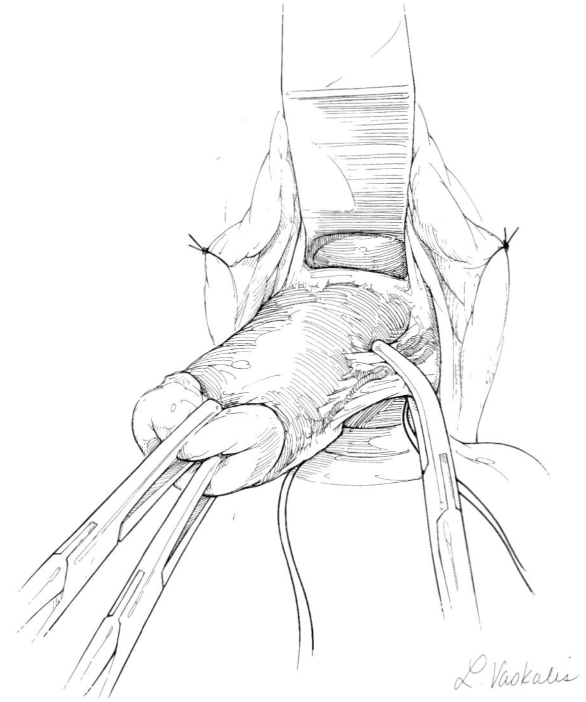

Fig. 22-13. LAVH: Ligation and division of uterine vessels.

ture ligatured (Fig. 22-13). Alternatively the uterine vessels are primarily suture ligatured and divided between the ligature and the uterus.

Removal of the specimen. The uterus and cervix, which are now free from all of their attachments, can now be easily removed through the vagina. In most instances it will be possible to remove the specimen intact, however, hemisection or morcellation may be required with larger specimens (see Chapter 7). In the case of hemisection the cervix is grasped with two tenacula placed at the 3 o'clock and 9 o'clock positions (Fig. 22-14, *A*) and the specimen divided in two portions, along the sagittal plane, using a sharp scalpel blade (Fig. 22-14, *B*).

Vault support and vault closure. The uterosacral ligaments are joined to the posterior vaginal vault at the 4 o'clock and 8 o'clock position to achieve vault support (Fig. 22-15). This may be accomplished with the initial suture that secured the uterosacral ligaments by incorporating the full thickness of the vaginal wall and retying the suture. Alternatively a new suture is used and both the full thickness of the uterosacral ligament and that of the vaginal wall is included in the suture, which is then tied.

It is essential to search for evidence of an enterocele. If present the enterocele sac is completely dissected from the surrounding connective tissue with sharp and blunt dissection. The redundant peritoneum is excised. The posterior peritoneum is closed high at the level of the reflection from the anterior surface of the rectum. This suture incorporates the peritoneum of the uterosacral ligament on one side, the posterior peritoneum, which is taken in small bites, and the peritoneum on the uterosacral ligament on the opposite side. If it is the intention of the surgeon to close the peritoneum with a purse string suture, the suture placed on the posterior peritoneum is held until the application and tying of the second suture, which is posteriorly placed above the previous suture.

The vagina is closed in the sagittal plane with a continuous interlocked suture that incorporates the full thickness of the wall. Closure in the sagittal plane increases the vaginal length by 2 to 3 cm.[52]

Final laparoscopic inspection and closure. Once the vaginal vault is closed, the final laparoscopic inspection is carried out. The peritoneal cavity is reinflated and the pelvis is thoroughly irrigated. The intraperitoneal gas pressure is lowered to reduce the tamponade effect and the operative site inspected to ensure that there is proper hemostasis. The laparoscopic instruments are removed, the abdominal cavity deflated, and the incisions closed.

Laparoscopic subtotal (supracervical) hysterectomy

Laparoscopic subtotal hysterectomy is designed to conserve the cervix, irrespective of whether or not oophorectomy is performed.

From a technical standpoint the procedure is the same as that for total laparoscopic hysterectomy up to and including step 5 of the procedure.

Step 5 of the procedure refers to the securing and divi-

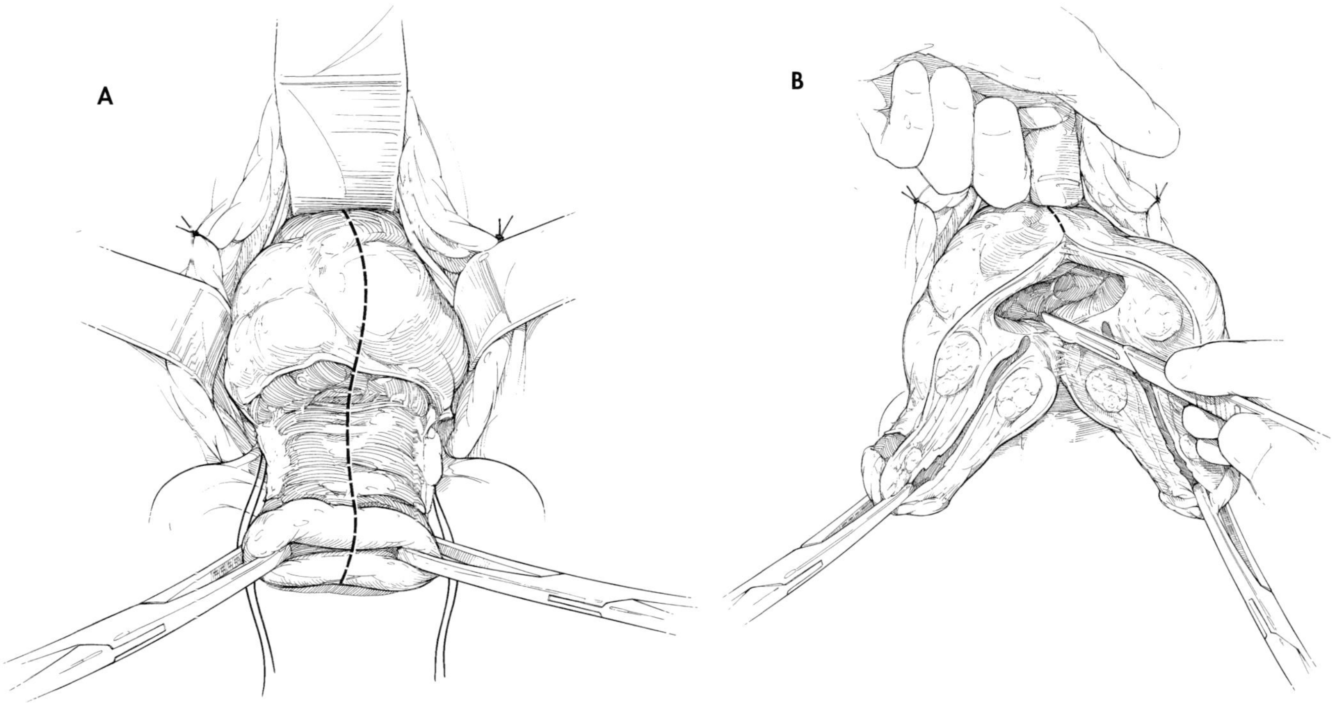

Fig. 22-14. LAVH: Hemisection of the uterus. **A,** The cervix is grasped with tenacula placed at 3 o'clock and 9 o'clock positions. **B,** The uterus is divided into two portions along the sagital plane.

sion of the uterine vessels. While most authors secure and divide the uterine vessels,[34] there are those who simply identify and occlude only the ascending branches of these vessels.[53,54] The subsequent steps of the procedure are as follows.

Resection of the corpus uteri from the cervix. This step is usually accomplished using a unipolar knife or pointed electrode, which in addition to transection permits hemostasis to be obtained on the cervical aspect of the cut surface.

If closure of the cervix is anticipated, excision of the uterus from the cervix in a conical fashion by angling the circumferential incision toward the vagina will facilitate the approximation of the edges of the remaining cervical body.

Positioning the uterus appropriately, with the aid of the manipulator and with a grasping forceps introduced through one of the ancilliary portals, will facilitate this step. The excised uterus is placed out of the operative field for later removal.

Cervical closure and peritoneal approximation. The cervix may be closed by approximation of the edges with a continuous or interrupted suture(s) placed laparoscopically. Most authors avoid this step and simply approximate the peritoneum. The peritoneal edges are approximated over the cervix with a continuous vicryl 2-0 suture.

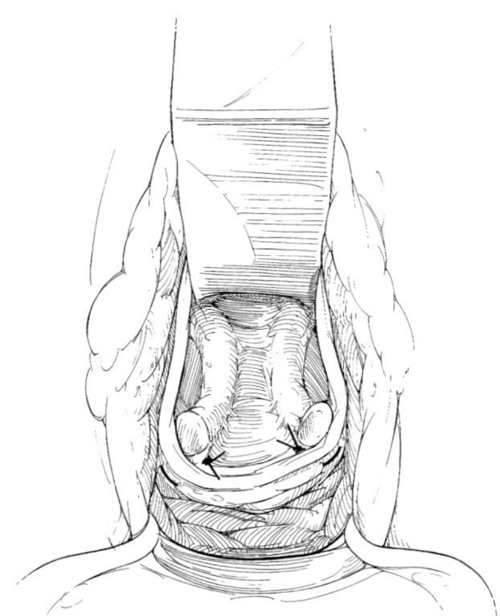

Fig. 22-15. LAVH: Vault support is obtained by joining the utero-sacral ligaments to the posterior vaginal wall at 4 o'clock and 8 o'clock position.

Removal of the uterus. The uterus must be removed from the peritoneal cavity. This is achieved using one of the following approaches:

1. Through a colpotomy incision. A colpotomy incision (usually vertical) is made and the uterus is removed intact or morcellated through the vagina.[34]

2. Through a minilaparotomy incision. A 10 mm cannula is introduced through the midline suprapubic ancilliary portal. The specimen is grasped with a strong-toothed grasping forceps introduced through this cannula. The skin incision is enlarged on both sides of the cannula. The fascia is identified and incised. The recti muscles are separated in the midline and the peritoneal defect is enlarged. Assisted by the instrument to which it is attached, the specimen is removed or morcellation carried out on the partly exteriorized specimen.[53]

3. Morcellation using a no. 11 scalpel blade and piecemeal removal. An 11 scalpel blade can be attached to a scalpel handle modified for laparoscopic use. This instrument is introduced through an appropriately sized cannula. The specimen is cut into longitudinal strips that will pass through the largest portal in use.

4. Piecemeal removal after laparoscopic morcellation. The specimen can be morcellated using a good laparoscopic morcellator and removed piecemeal. Improved manual morcellators are now available and motorized versions are under current production. One of the recently introduced devices is the Semm, serrated edged macromorcellator (Wisap, Tomball R, TX). This instrument is available in 11 mm, 15 mm, and 20 mm shaft diameters and obviously requires preliminary insertion of an appropriately sized cannula to permit its introduction into the peritoneal cavity. The specimen is grasped either with a claw-shaped forceps or a myoma drill (that possesses a tip like a cork screw) introduced within the cylindrical morcellator. The latter has a cylindrical shaft with a serrated cutting edge. Rotation of this shaft while pulling on the forceps or the drill will excise a cylindrical portion of the specimen, which remains within the morcellator and is then removed. By repeating the same step the specimen is removed piecemeal. Morcellation of large specimens may be tedious and fairly time consuming. Improved motorized devices facilitate this task (see Chapters 7 and 19).

The final two steps of the procedure are the same as those in total laparoscopic hysterectomy and include final laparoscopic inspection and removal of the laparoscopic equipment and closure of the abdominal incisions.

Auxiliary cervical procedures. One of the major drawbacks of subtotal hysterectomy is the potential for developing carcinoma of the cervix. To obviate this risk, procedures to ablate or remove the endocervical lining and the transformation zone have been proposed. These include: removal of the cervical transformation zone using an electrosurgical wire loop,[34] electrosurgical ablation of the endocervical lining,[53] and cylindrical excision of the inner portion of the cervical body. The first two procedures can be performed after the excision of the uterus from the cervix.

The third approach is advocated by Semm, who produced an instrument, the calibrated uterine resection tool (CURT), designed to core out the inner portion of the cervix (Fig. 22-16). This instrument is composed of four parts: (1) a central rod of 5 mm in diameter with a conical tip, (2) a guiding cylinder, with centimeter markings, that supports, (3) a serrated edged cutting cylinder placed over the second piece, and (4) a hand grip that is attached to the distal blunt end of the morcellator. The use of this instrument with a summary of the subtotal hysterectomy technique used by Semm follows.

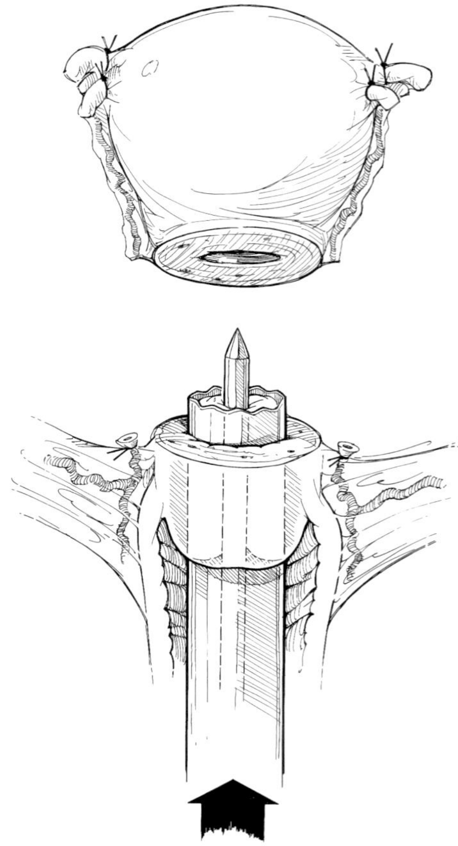

Fig. 22-16. Subtotal hysterectomy: Excision of the inner portion of the cervical body (after completion of subtotal hysterectomy) with Semm's calibrated uterine resection tool (CURT).

Semm's technique. The central rod of the CURT instrument is used as a uterine manipulator in the following manner. Vaginal tenacula are applied to the lateral aspects of the cervix. The central rod is introduced through the cervical canal, past the internal os into the cavity of the uterus, which is brought into an axial position by laparoscopic manipulation. The rod is advanced and the fundus of the uterus pierced in the midline (Fig. 22-17). The rod is affixed to the handles of the tenacula by a special clamp placed at the distal end of the rod.

The subtotal hysterectomy is carried out by securing the pedicles principally with ligatures and/or Roeder loops. The

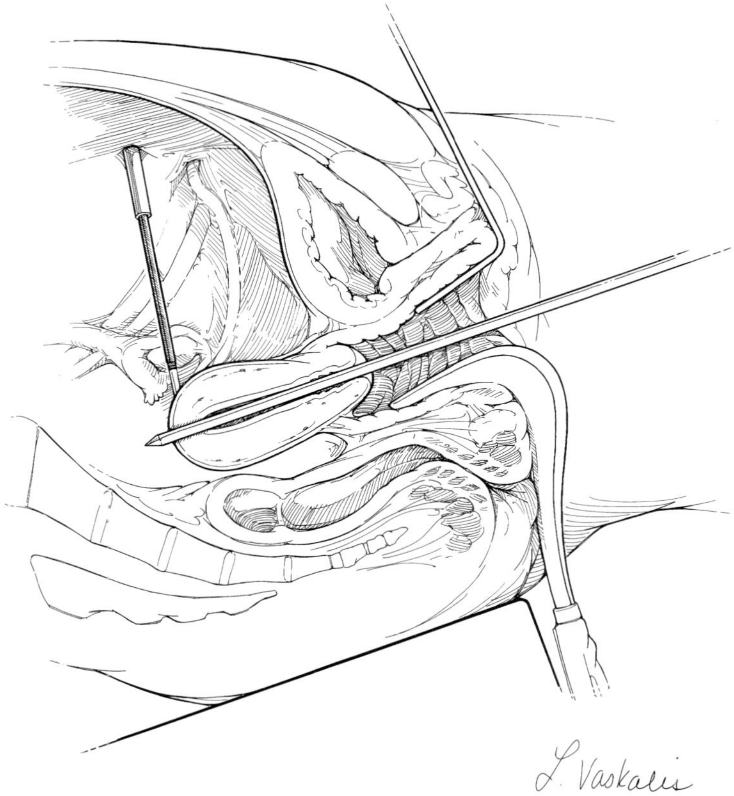

Fig. 22-17. Semm's subtotal hysterectomy technique. The central rod of the CURT instrument is advanced and the uterine fundus pierced in the midline.

excision is carried down to, but not including, the uterine vessels.

Coring out the cervix may be performed either before or after the uterine corpus is amputated from the cervix. At the outset, pericervical tissues are infiltrated with 10 ml of dilute vasopressin solution (5 U diluted in 100 ml) at both 3 o'clock and 9 o'clock positions. The central rod is dislodged from the tenacula. The clamp stabilizing the rod is removed. The assembled serrated edged cutting cylinder is passed over the rod from below and the cutting edge brought into contact with the cervix. The cutting cylinder comes in diameters of 11 ml, 15 ml, and 24 ml to accommodate variations in cervical calibre. Excision is accomplished by clockwise rotation of the serrated edged cylinder with a hand grip (Fig. 22-18). As the cutting tube is rotated and advanced, centimeter markings are revealed on the guiding cylinder, which remains static against the exocervix. The centimeter markings demonstrate the distance cored out. The assistant performs the coring procedure while the surgeon observes through the laparoscope. As the cutting edge is advanced it reaches the uterine fundus, which is also cored out, at which point the serrated edge protrudes into the peritoneal cavity. The morecellator is slightly withdrawn to return the tip back into the uterine cavity.

A Roeder loop is placed around the upper third to the cervix and tightened after ensuring that the bladder, which had been previously dissected off the cervix, is out of the way. Next, while the uterus is held cephalad and the assistant slowly removes the CURT device enclosing the cored cervical tissue, the Roeder loop is tightened further to close the cervical opening and ligate the ascending branches of the uterine arteries which are also incorporated within this loop (Fig. 22-19, *A*). Two additional Roeder loops are applied around the upper third of the cervix. They are tightened and each reinforced by the placement of a further knot. These ligatures effectively close the cervical stump. The fundus is then amputated from the cervix above the Roeder loops (Fig. 22-19, *B*). The periphery of the cored area in the cervix is electrodesiccated or endocoagulated from below for additional hemostasis.

The endocervical tissue may be cored out after the amputation of the uterus. This is preferable if the uterus is enlarged and/or the cavity distorted. In this instance the ascending branches of the uterine vessels must be ligated before excision of the uterine corpus. The cervix is then cored out as previously described (see Fig. 22-16). The edges of the upper cervix are approximated by laparoscopic suturing. Reperitonealization is performed after either approach and a Robinson drain is left in the pelvis at the close of the procedure.[54]

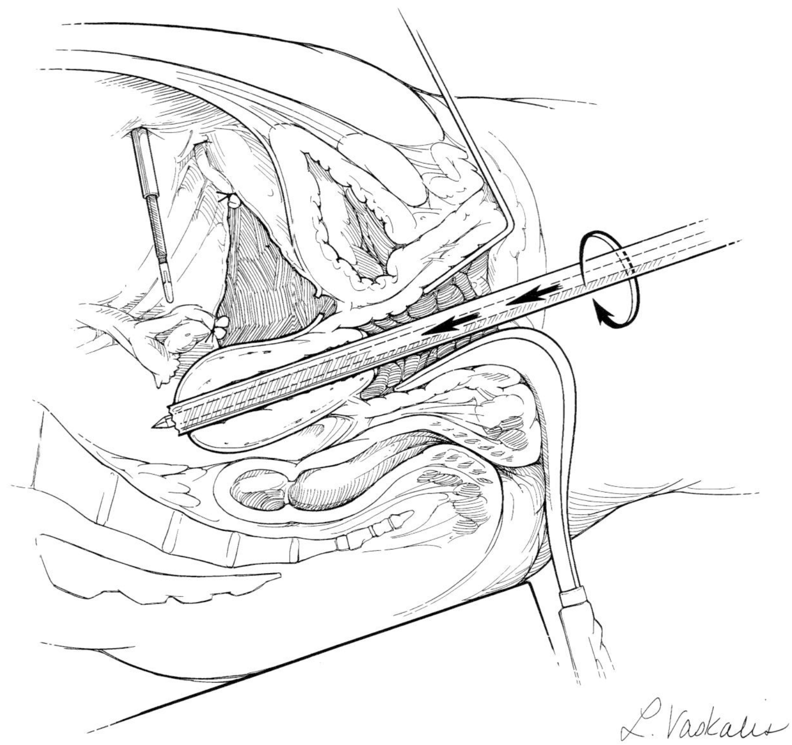

Fig. 22-18. Semm's subtotal hysterectomy technique. Excision of the inner portion of the cervical body is accomplished by clockwise rotation of the cutting cylinder in the CURT instrument.

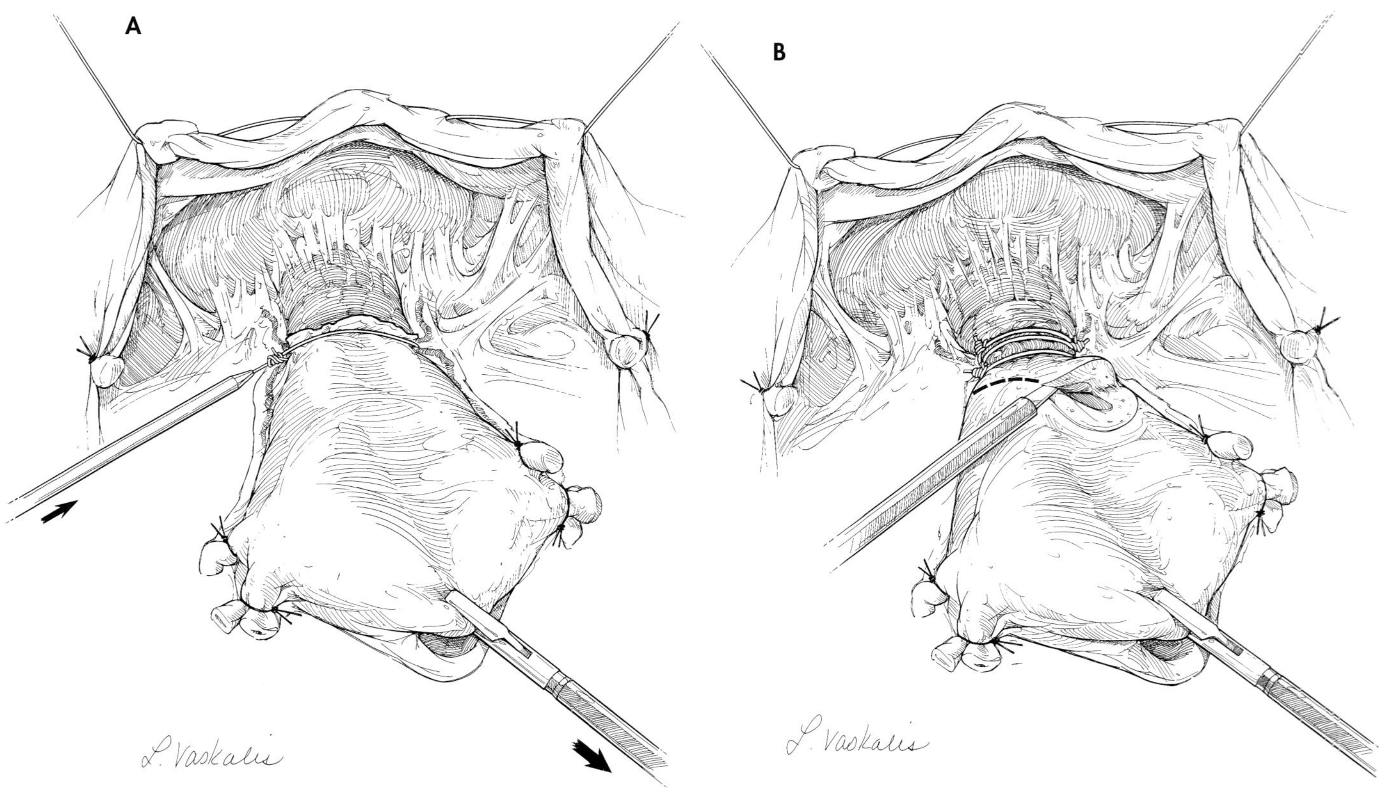

Fig. 22-19. Semm's subtotal hysterectomy technique. **A,** Once the upper uterine pedicles have been secured Roeder loops are placed around the upper third of the cervix and tightened as the CURT device is removed. **B,** Once three Roeder loops are placed around the cervix and tightened, the fundus is amputated from the cervix above the ligatures.

RESULTS

Laparoscopic hysterectomy should not replace vaginal hysterectomy, which is a safe and effective procedure. In a well-designed randomized prospective study, Summitt et al.[55] compared outpatient laparoscopic assisted vaginal hysterectomy (LAVH) with standard outpatient vaginal hysterectomy (VH). Fifty-six women scheduled for vaginal hysterectomy were randomly assigned to either LAVH (n = 29) or a standard VH (n = 27). The criteria used to decide upon the vaginal route were: (1) uterine size no larger than 16 gestational weeks, (2) presence of uterine mobility, and (3) a pubic arch of at least 90 degrees. The presence of preoperative pelvic pain, the need for oophorectomy, or a history of previous pelvic surgery did not influence the decision to use a vaginal approach. Exclusion criteria were few and legitimate.

There were no differences between the two groups with regard to age, gravidity, parity, in preoperative indications, and previous operations. All of the procedures, including unilateral or bilateral oophorectomy when indicated, were completed without incident. The mean operating time was significantly longer for the LAVH group, 120 minutes, versus 65 minutes for vaginal hysterectomy. Those in the LAVH group required more pain medication and had a lower postoperative hematocrit. Although the differences were statistically significant, it did not appear to make a clinical difference in the postoperative course. In addition, the mean hospital charges for the LAVH group were significantly higher ($7,905 versus $4,891) (see Chapter 27).

In an earlier study, 20 women who had indication for abdominal hysterectomy (with or without salpingo-oophorectomy) were assigned alternatively either to total abdominal hysterectomy (TAH) or LAVH.[38] This study demonstrated a longer operating time with LAVH compared to TAH (160 minutes versus 102 minutes). However the ten patients in the LAVH group had shorter hospital stays (2.4 versus 4.4 days) and more rapid recuperation (3 weeks versus 5 weeks). It is interesting that this study, which compared LAVH versus TAH, excluded uteri larger than 14 weeks' gestational size, whereas the previous study included those up to 16 weeks' gestational size. This clearly demonstrates that a significant overlap exists in the indications for abdominal and vaginal hysterectomy and undoubtedly that this will also be the case with laparoscopic hysterectomy.

COMPLICATIONS

The complication rates associated with abdominal and vaginal hysterectomy have been clearly established by the evaluation of large numbers of cases.[56] As laparoscopic hysterectomy and its many variants are new procedures, such large numbers are not available for analysis. Several small series have been published.[40,43,46,50,57,58] The smallest of these described the results[58] of 55 and the largest 215 cases.[40] The rates of major complications ranged from approximately 5% to 10%. The most common complications were damage to the urinary tract involving either the bladder or the ureter, postoperative febrile mobility, and hemorrhage. The bleeding was due either to failure to secure the uterine vessels or trauma to the inferior epigastric vessels. Prior bladder dissection, as in cesarean section, seemed to increase the risk of bladder injury. Bowel injuries have also been reported.

It would appear that the reported incidence of major complications of laparoscopic hysterectomy is relatively low. Unfortunately, major complications do occur that are not formally reported. We are aware of a number of such cases. Recently we have been asked to review the case records of a woman in whom both ureters were occluded and transected. Automatic staples had been used to secure the uterine vessels. Preoperative use of ureteric catheters had failed to protect the ureters.

CONCLUSIONS

Vaginal hysterectomy, where feasible, carries a lower rate of complication and more rapid return to normal activity than abdominal hysterectomy. It still remains to be shown that laparoscopic hysterectomy offers any great advantage to vaginal hysterectomy.

It can be shown that it is to the patient's advantage if a procedure that would have to have been performed abdominally can be completed vaginally with laparoscopic assistance.

That laparoscopic hysterectomy is technically feasible is no longer in doubt. This chapter has described the technical details of many variants of laparoscopic hysterectomy technique. It is to be hoped that by critical assessment of these techniques in properly conducted studies those which are demonstrably superior will enter routine practice and those of little value will be discarded.

REFERENCES

1. Pokras R: Hysterectomy: past, present and future. *Stat Bull Metrop Insur Co.* 70:12, 1989.
2. Graves EJ: National hospital discharge survey: annual summary, 1990. National Center for Health Statistics, *Vital Health Stat Series* 13, No. 112, 1992.
3. Roos NP: Hysterectomy: variations in rates across small areas and across physicians' practices. *Am J Public Health* 74:327, 1984.
4. McPherson K, Strong PM, Epstein A, et al: Regional variations in the use of common surgical procedures: within and between England and Wales, Canada and the United States of America. *Soc Sci Med* 15a:273, 1981.
5. McPherson K, Clifford P, Wennberg JE, et al: Small area variations in the use of discretionary surgery: an international comparison between New England, England and Norway. *N Engl J Med* 307:1310, 1982.
6. Hysterectomies in the United States, 1965-84. *Vital Health Stat* (13), 1988.
7. Pokras R, Hufnegal VG: Hysterectomies in the United States, 1965-84. *Vital Health Stat* 13;l1987.
8. Pokras R, Hufnagel VG: Hysterectomy in the United States, 1964-84. *Am J Public Health* 78:852, 1988.

9. Nichols DH: In Nichol DH, editor: Some technical points and indications for hysterectomy in gynecologic and obstetric surgery. St. Louis, 1993, Mosby–Yearbook.
10. Sloan D: The emotional and psychosexual aspects of hysterectomy. *Am J Obstet Gynecol* 1312:598, 1978.
11. Richards DH: Depression after hysterectomy. *Lancet* 2:430, 1973.
12. Dennerstein L, Wood C, Burrows GD: Sexual response following hysterectomy and oophorectomy. *Obstet Gynecol* 49:92, 1977.
13. Zussman L, Zussman S, Sunley R, et al: Sexual response after hysterectomy-oophorectomy: recent studies and reconsideration of psychogenesis. *Am J Obstet Gynecol* 140:725, 1981.
14. Friedman AJ, Hoffman DI, Comite F, et al: Treatment of leiomyomata uteri with leuprolide acetate depot: A double-blind, placebo-controlled, multicenter study. *Obstet Gynecol* 77:720-725, 1991.
15. Derman SG, Rehnstrom J, Neuwirth RS: The long-term effectivenss of hysteroscopic treatment of menorrhagia and leiomyomas. *Obstet Gynecol* 77:591-594, 1991.
16. Friedman AJ, Rein MS, Harrison-Atlas D, et al: A randomized, placebo-controlled, double-blind study evaluating leuprolide acetate depot treatment before myomectomy. *Fertil Steril* 52:728-733, 1989.
17. Loffer FD: Removal of large symptomatic intrauterine growths by the hysteroscopic resectoscope. *Obstet Gynecol* 76:836-840, 1990.
18. Corson SL, Brooks PG: Resectoscopic myomectomy. *Fertil Steril* 55:1041-1044, 1991.
19. Goldfarb HA: Nd:YAG laser laparoscopic coagulation of symptomatic myomas. *J Reprod Med* 37:636-638, 1992.
20. Nisolle M, Smets M, Malvaux V, et al: Laparoscopic myolysis with the Nd:YAG laser. *J Gynecol Surg* 9:95-99, 1993.
21. Wheeler JM, Knittle JD, Miller JD: Depot leuprolife versus danazol in treatment of women with symptomatic endometriosis. *Am J Obstet Gynecol* 167:1367-1371, 1992.
22. Waller KG, Shaw RW: Gonadotropin-releasing hormone analogues for the treatment of endometriosis: long-term follow-up. *Fertil Steril* 59:511-515, 1993.
23. Fedele L, Bianchi S, Bocciolone L, et al: Buserelin acetate in the treatment of pelvic pain associated with minimal and mild endometriosis: a controlled study. *Fertil Steril* 59:516-521, 1993.
24. Gomel V: Operative laparoscopy: time for acceptance. *Fertil Steril* 52:1-11, 1989.
25. Derman SG, Rehnstrom J, Neuwirth RS: The long-term effectiveness of hysteroscopic treatment of menorrhagia and leiomyomas. *Obstet Gynecol* 77:591-594, 1991.
26. Magos AL, Baumann R, Lockwood GM, Turnbull AC: Experience with the first 250 endometrial resections for menorrhagia. *Lancet* 337:1074-1078, 1991.
27. Serden SP, Brooks PG: Treatment of abnormal uterine bleeding with the gynecologic resectoscope. *J Reprod Med* 36:697-699, 1991.
28. Copenhaver EH: Hysterectomy: vaginal versus abdominal. *Surg Clin North Am* 45:751-763, 1965.
29. Gitsch G, Berger E, Tatra G: Trends in thirty years of vaginal hysterectomy. *Surg Gynecol Obstet* 172:207-210, 1991.
30. Ranney B: Decreasing numbers for vaginal hysterectomy and plasty. *South Dakota J Med* 43:7-12, 1990.
31. Kilkku P: Supravaginal uterine amputation vs. hysterectomy—Effects on coital frequency and dyspareunia. *Acta Obstet Gynecol Scand* 62:141-145, 1983.
32. Kilkku P, Grönroos M, Hirvonen T, Rauramo L: Supravaginal uterine amputation vs hysterectomy—Effects on libido and organsm. *Acta Obstet Gynecol Scand* 62:147-152, 1983.
33. Kilkku P, Grönroos M, Rauramo L: Supravaginal uterine amputation with preoperative electrocoagulation of endocervical mucosa—Description of the method. *Acta Obstet Gynecol Scand* 64:175-177, 1985.
34. Donnez J, Nisolle M: Laparoscopic supracervial (subtotal) hysterectomy (LASH). *J Gynecol Surg* 9:91-94, 1993.
35. Pelosi MA, Pelosi III MA: Laparoscopic supracervical hysterectomy using a single-umbilical puncture (mini laparoscopy). *J Rep Med* 37:777-784, 1992.
36. Schwartz RO: Laparoscopic supracervical hysterectomy versus vaginal assisted. 1-16, 1993.
37. Reich H, DeCaprio J, McGlynn F: Laparoscopic hysterectomy. *J Gynecol Surg* 5:213-216, 1989.
38. Nezhat F, Nezhat C, Gordon S, Wilkins E: Laparoscopic versus abdominal hysterectomy. *J Rep Med* 37:247-250, 1992.
39. Liu CY: Laparoscopic hysterectomy. *J Rep Med* 37:351-354, 1992.
40. Liu CY: Laparoscopic hysterectomy—Report of 215 cases. *Gynecol Endo* 1:73-77, 1992.
41. Padial JG, Sotolongo J, Casey MJ, et al: Laparoscopy-assisted vaginal hysterectomy: report of seventy-five consecutive cases. *J Gynecol Surg* 8:81-85, 1992.
42. Boike GM, Elfstrand EP, DelPriore G, et al: Laparoscopically assisted vaginal hysterectomy in a university hospital: report of 82 cases and comparison with abdominal and vaginal hysterectomy. *Am J Obstet Gynecol* 168:1690-1701, 1993.
43. Phipps JH, John M, Hassanaien M, Saeed M: Laparoscopic and laparoscopically assisted vaginal hysterectomy: a series of 114 cases. *Gyn Endo* 2:7-12, 1993.
44. Daniell JF, Kurtz BR, McTavish G, et al: Laparoscopically assisted vaginal hysterectomy—The initial Nashville, Tennessee, experience. *J Rep Med* 38:537-542, 1993.
45. Davis GD, Wolgamott G, Moon J: Laparoscopically assisted vaginal hysterectomy as definitive therapy for stage III and IV endometriosis. *J Rep Med* 38:577-581, 1993.
46. Lee C-L, Soong Y-K: Laparoscopic hysterectomy with the Endo GIA 30 stapler. *J Rep Med* 38:582-586, 1993.
47. Howard FM, Sanchez R: A comparison of laparoscopically assisted vaginal hysterectomy and abdominal hysterectomy. *J Gyn Surg* 9:83-90, 1993.
48. Kovac SR, Cruikshank SH, Retto HF: Laparoscopy-Assisted vaginal hysterectomy. *J Gyn Surg* 6:185-193, 1990.
49. Nezhat C, Nezhat F, Nezhat C: Operative laparoscopy (minimally invasive surgery) state of the art. *J Gynecol Surg* 8:111-134, 1992.
50. Reich H, McGlynn F, Sekel L: Total laparoscopic hysterectomy. *Gynecol Endo* 2:59-63, 1993.
51. Munro MG, Parker WH: A classification system for laparoscopic hysterectomy. *Obstet Gynecol* 82:624-9, 1993.
52. Nichols DH: Vaginal hysterectomy. In: Nichols Dh, editor. Gynecologic and Obstetric Surgery. St. Louis, 1993, Mosby–Yearbook.
53. Hasson HM, Rotman C, Rana N, Asakura H: Experience with laparoscopic hysterectomy. *J Am Assoc Gynecol Lapar* 1:1-11, 1993.
54. Semm K: Intrafascial hysterectomy. Munich 1993, Wisap.
55. Summitt RL, Stovall TG, Lipscomb GH, Ling FW: Randomized comparison of laparoscopy-assisted vaginal hysterectomy with standard vaginal hysterectomy in an outpatient setting. *Obstet Gynecol* 80:895-901, 1992.
56. Dicker RC, Greenspan JR, Strauss LT, et al: Complications of abdominal and vaginal hysterectomy among women of reproductive age in the United States. *Am J Obstet Gynecol* 144:841-8, 1982.
57. Hourcabie JA, Bruhat M-A: One hundred and three cases of laparoscopic hysterectomy using endo-GA staples and a device for presenting the vaginal fornices. *Gynecol Endo* 2:65-72, 1993.
58. Schwartz RO: Complications of laparoscopic hysterectomy. *Obstet Gynecol* 81:1002-4, 1993.

Chapter 23

APPENDECTOMY

Although appendectomy is usually performed by general surgeons, it is not unusual for gynecologists to discover an inflamed appendix when a diagnostic laparoscopy has been undertaken for a woman with acute lower abdominal pain. Laparoscopic appendectomy is a procedure of intermediate difficulty and it would seem reasonable that gynecologists, while making every endeavour to make the diagnosis preoperatively and seeking the appropriate consultation, should be able, if circumstances dictate, to remove the appendix.

SURGICAL ANATOMY

The appendix is an organ that is found only in the great apes, the human, and the wombat. It is an elongated diverticulum of the cecum which is richly endowed with lymphoid tissue. It is normally 7.5 to 10 cm in length, but specimens of up to 30 cm have been recorded.

It receives its blood supply from the appendicular artery, which is a branch of the lower division of the ileocecal artery. An accessory appendicular artery may be present in almost 50% of patients. The major vessel enters the mesoappendix a short distance from the base of the appendix (Fig. 23-1). The appendicular vein drains into the ileocolic vein.

The position of the organ is extremely variable. Up to 70% will be retrocecal, with the remainder lying primarily in front of the large bowel. Although it is usually found in the right iliac fossa, in maldescent of the cecum or advanced pregnancy the appendix can be sited in the right hypochondrium. The rare, (one in 3,500) condition of situs inversus will place the organ in the left iliac fossa.

SYMPTOMS AND SIGNS OF APPENDICITIS

Acute appendicitis occurs most frequently between the ages of 20 and 30. It is of particular significance to the woman who wishes to bear children. Rupture of an inflamed organ or even transmigration of microorganisms through the appendicular wall can set up a purulent peritonitis that can most adversely affect the fallopian tubes and adnexa, causing postinflammatory scarring and adhesion formation. If for no other reason every attempt should be made to make the diagnosis early.

The clinical onset may be gradual or acute. In the former case the patient will experience generalized abdominal pain, followed shortly afterward by vomiting. Nausea and anorexia are frequently associated. As time passes the pulse rate and body temperature increase. Within 24 hours of the onset of the symptoms the pain will have become localized to the right iliac fossa. In more acute cases colic, usually centered at the umbilicus, is the presenting symptom. Vomiting and localization of the pain to the right iliac fossa is more rapid.

When the patient is examined, she will be flushed, warm, and may have marked halitosis. The abdomen will be tender, with the tenderness most marked in the right iliac fossa. Guarding and rebound tenderness may be elicited. Gynecologists tend to move next to the pelvic examination. Marked tenderness may be noted in the right fornix if the appendix is lying in the pelvis. Rectal examination may elicit the same signs.

All of these symptoms and signs can be very similar to those found in association with acute pelvic inflammatory disease (PID). A moderate leucocytosis will be found in both disorders. Ultrasound may be of some help. If the appendix is easily visualized and clearly distended, a diagnosis of appendicitis is more likely. Consultation with a general surgeon should be sought if the gynecologist is sufficiently suspicious of the diagnosis. If there remains doubt the final diagnosis may be made by recourse to laparoscopy (see Chapter 10). In women the false positive rate for acute appendicitis is 39%.[1] The use of diagnostic laparoscopy can reduce the normal appendectomy rate to 1%.[2]

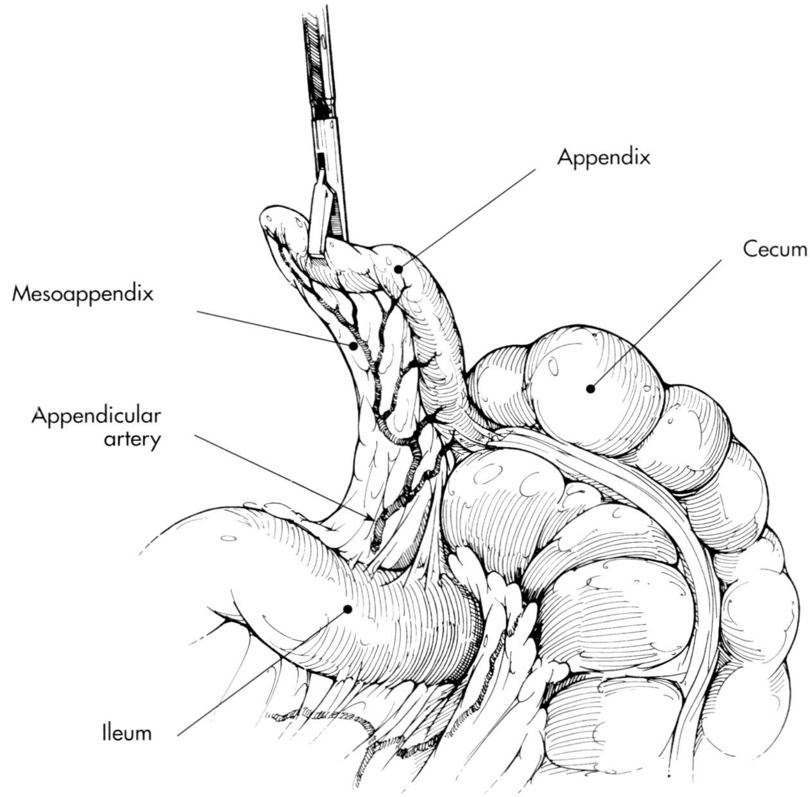

Fig. 23-1. Surgical anatomy of the appendix.

ROLE OF LAPAROSCOPY

The principal trocar, cannula, and telescope are introduced intraumbilically. A second puncture is made suprapubically in the midline with a 5 mm cannula through which a blunt probe or an atraumatic, blunt-tipped grasping forceps is introduced. After inspection of the upper abdomen, the patient is placed in the deep Trendelenberg position and bowel manipulated out of the way. A complete survey is performed and the genital organs are inspected (Chapter 5). Even if the fallopian tubes are obviously inflamed, the appendix should be visualized. It is usually easy to identify the ascending colon and by following it caudad to find the cecum. Gentle manipulation of the cecum will usually display the appendix. It is important to be sure to observe the entire organ from its base up to its tip (see Chapter 10).

If the diagnosis is clearly one of acute PID, nothing further need be done to the appendix if this organ is grossly normal. If the tubes are healthy, the appendix should be removed, even if it appears grossly to be normal. A significant number of such appendices will be shown to be acutely inflamed when submitted to histologic examination. If the appendix is removed, the patient must be so informed. Should she present again in the future with abdominal pain, the classical McBurney incision which shows the physician that appendicitis does not form part of the differential diagnosis will not be present.

Once a decision has been taken to remove the appendix, the removal may be carried out either by laparoscopically assisted appendectomy or by intracorporeal (laparoscopic) appendectomy. Each will be described.

Laparoscopically assisted appendectomy

This procedure is somewhat akin to laparoscopically assisted vaginal hysterectomy. The organ is freed from its attachments laparoscopically and the operation completed on the body surface.

A 10 mm trocar and cannula (to accommodate the introduction of sutures and permit removal of the specimen) is inserted in the right iliac fossa, as directly over the appendix as is consistent with safe avoidance of parietal vessels and the intraabdominal structures. Unless a special cannula is used, a reducer is placed in the 10 mm cannula to prevent gas loss when instruments of smaller caliber are used. Grasping forceps are introduced through this cannula and used to draw the appendix within the cannula. The mesoappendix is now under tension and the inflamed organ sequestered from the peritoneal cavity. Bipolar grasping forceps (5 mm) are introduced through the other ancillary cannula (placed suprapubically in the midline) and used to desiccate the mesentery of the appendix, 0.5 to 1 cm distal to the ileocecal junction (Fig. 23-2, *A*). The desiccated area is divided. This involves exchanging scissors for the coagu-

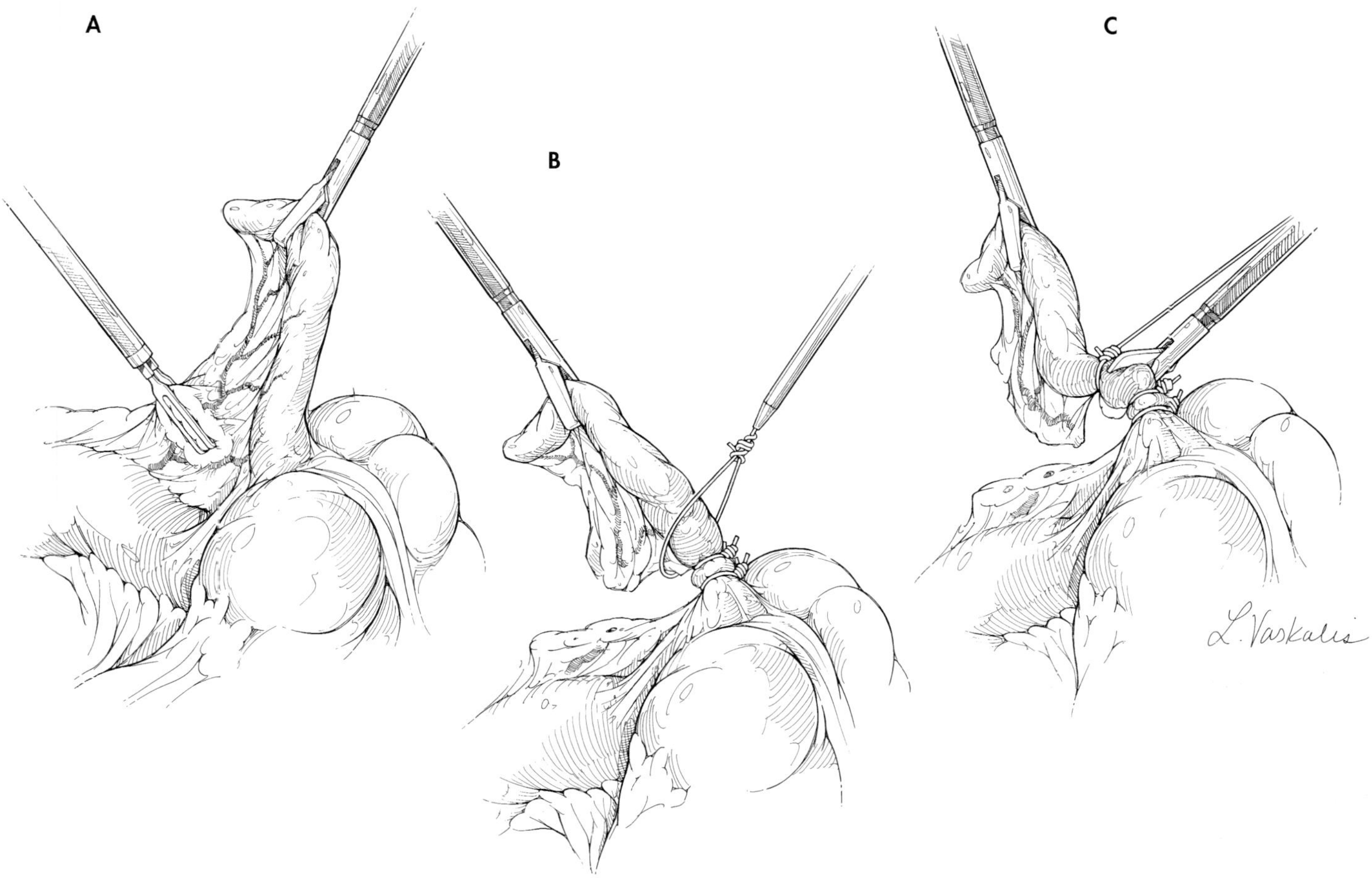

Fig. 23-2. Appendectomy. *A*, Desiccation of the mesentery of the appendix. *B*, Ligation of the base of the appendix. *C*, Division of the base of the appendix.

lating forceps. Alternatively a third ancillary 5 mm portal can be introduced in the left iliac fossa, or scissors with coagulating capability can be used. Dissection stops before the base of the appendicular artery is reached. If deemed necessary, the divided mesoappendix can be ligated with an endoloop or suture. It is very rare for a properly coagulated mesoappendix to bleed.

The 10 mm cannula is withdrawn, along with the forceps that are holding the appendix, until the surface of the cecum has been exteriorized. It will be necessary first to deflate the peritoneal cavity to shorten the distance between the cecum and abdominal wall. It is simple now to clamp the appendix and appendicular artery, doubly ligate the proximal stump and vessels, and excise the organ. It is a matter of personal preference whether or not the stump is buried.

The cecum is returned to the abdominal cavity. The abdomen is reinflated and the cecum gently pulled back into position using 5 mm bowel forceps. The operative site is irrigated and a final check made to confirm that there is no bleeding. The instruments are removed and the incisions sutured.

Intracorporeal (laparoscopic) appendectomy

Two 5 mm ancillary portals are placed, one over the McBurney's point and the other suprapubically in the midline. Mobilization of the appendix is performed as described above.

Once the mesosalpinx has been dissected (Fig. 23-2, *A*) a series of three endoloops are introduced through the 5 mm cannula. Each in turn is placed over the base of the appendix and tightened (Fig. 23-2, *B*). Alternatively three simple ligatures as described in Chapter 7 can be used in place of Roeder loops. Sufficient space must be left between the two proximal and the distal ligatures to permit transection of the appendix. The loop introducer is replaced with scissors and the appendix severed between the ligature that is most distal from the cecum and the other two (Fig. 23-2, *C*). The appendix is removed through the principal cannula. This is accomplished by introducing a 5 mm laparoscope through

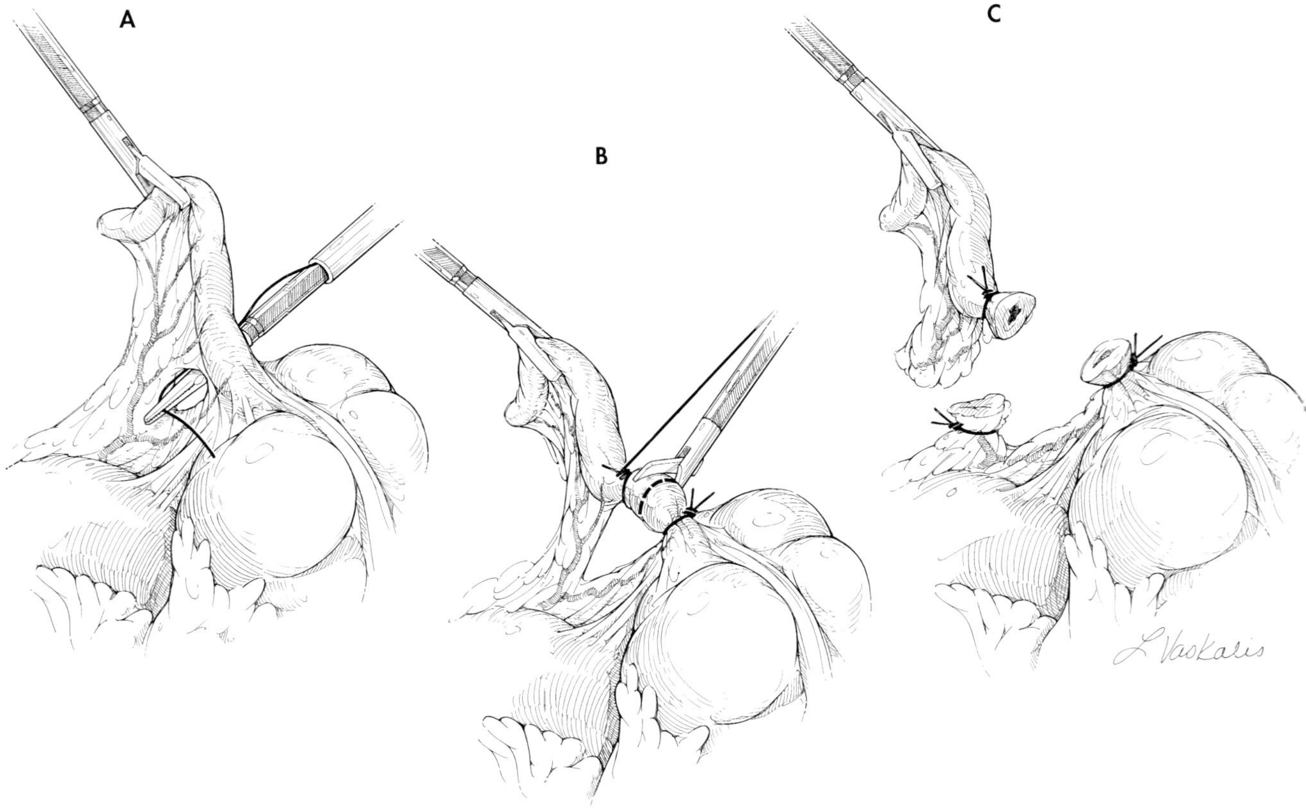

Fig. 23-3. Appendectomy. *A*, An opening is fashioned in the mesentery near the base of the appendix and a ligature is introduced through this opening. *B*, The ligatures are tied and the base of the appendix transected with scissors between the ligatures. *C*, The mesoappendix is ligatured and divided distal to the ligature.

one of the ancillary cannulae, removing the umbilically placed laparoscope and introducing a grasping forceps through the same portal.

The other intracorporeal approach resembles that practiced by laparotomy. The appendix is grasped near its tip and put on a stretch as described earlier. Using a pair of pointed grasping forceps, introduced through the second ancillary portal, the mesentery is pierced close to the base of the appendix. This hole is enlarged by opening the jaws of the forceps, which are then used to crush the base of the appendix. A 00 Vicryl ligature is introduced into the peritoneal cavity and manipulated through the opening in the mesoappendix and pulled around the crushed base of the appendix (Fig. 23-3, *A*). The suture is tied (see Chapter 7) and cut. A similar ligature is applied distal to the first and cut long. Scissors are used to transect the base of the appendix between the two ligatures (Fig. 23-3, *B*). The mesentery of the appendix is similarly ligated near the base and cut distal to the suture and divided (Fig. 23-3, *C*). The excised appendix is removed.

To bury the appendiceal stump is now concidered of dubious value and many surgeons no longer practice it routinely.[3] However, if the surgeon wishes to do so a 2-0 or 3-0 Vicryl suture on a gastrointestinal type needle is introduced into the peritoneal cavity (see Chapter 7) and manipulated with a laparoscopic needle holder, which is passed through one of the 5 mm cannulae. The stump of the appendix is buried by placing a figure 8 or a purse string suture through the serosa and superficial muscularis of the cecum. This suture is tied and cut. The pelvis is irrigated. The pneumoperitoneum is released and the instruments removed. The abdominal incisions are closed.

Unusual circumstances

If the appendix is not sufficiently mobile, it may be necessary to divide the reflection of the peritoneum in the right pericolic gutter to free both the cecum and a portion of the ascending colon. This step frequently is required if the organ is retrocecal. Just as with traditional surgery, a retrograde approach to appendectomy may be necessary. The base of the appendix is isolated from the mesoappendix by blunt dissection. Because the tip is at this time inaccessible, ligation of the appendix must first be carried out. This is accomplished by introducing two or three ligatures and manipulating them to encircle the base of the appendix as described above. These are tied either intra- or extracorporeally. The appendix is now divided between the proximal and distal ligatures. The appendix is grasped and dissected from the mesoappendix from the base toward its tip.

RESULTS

In a study from Denmark[4] 60 women aged 15 to 56 years with clinical signs of acute appendicitis were randomized into two groups of 30. Patients in the first group underwent immediate appendectomy. For those in the other group a diagnostic laparoscopy was first performed. Appendectomy was undertaken when acute appendicitis was confirmed and when the diagnosis of acute appendicitis could not be excluded, as when the appendix could not be visualized. Patients with signs of diffuse peritonitis and with more than two previous lower abdominal operations were excluded. Unnecessary appendectomies were performed in 11 women in the first group (immediate appendectomy) and in two among those submitted to initial diagnostic laparoscopy. In both of the latter two cases the appendix could not be visualized at laparoscopy. Although the appendix could not be visualized in a further three patients in the laparoscopy group, acute appendicitis was found at open operation. The initial laparoscopy was not associated with any increase in morbidity. Patients with a normal appendix were frequently found to have other lesions, often of gynecologic nature. This study demonstrates the value of laparoscopy as a diagnostic tool in women with clinical signs of acute appendicitis.

In a nonrandomized recent study[5] patients undergoing laparoscopic appendectomy ($n = 53$) were compared to those in whom the traditional approach was used ($n = 103$). Incidental appendectomies and those with perforated appendicitis were excluded. The patient sample was derived from four Nashville, Tennessee, hospitals during a period of 6 months. The age, race, and sex distributions were similar in the two groups. It is of interest that the laparoscopic approach was attempted in 61 patients but had to be converted to an open procedure in seven. One patient was excluded because the appendix had perforated. Although a variety of techniques was used to perform the appendectomy laparoscopically, the specimen was always placed in a condom or a laparoscopic bag (Endopouch) prior to its removal. In this study the mean operating time was significantly higher in the laparoscopy group (98.6 ± 5.3 minutes vs. 61.2 ± 2.6 minutes, $p < 0.01$). There were seven wound infections in the traditional appendectomy group, all in patients with acute appendicitis and none in the laparoscopy group. This difference was attributed to their use of a bag for the removal of the appendix from the peritoneal cavity in the laparoscopy group. However in the laparoscopy group one patient had a pelvic abscess that was drained percutaneously ten days postoperatively.

The largest case series of laparoscopic appendectomy is that of Pier and co-workers.[6] Of the 997 patients presenting with typical signs and symptoms of acute appendicitis, 64 had conventional appendectomy and the laparoscopic approach was attempted in 933. The procedure was converted to open surgery in 18 (2%, mostly in the initial phase of the trial period). Appendectomy was successfully carried out in 915. The patient's ages ranged from 2 to 86 years, 57% were female and the remainder males. Histologic examination of the extracted appendix revealed that 12% had no evidence of inflammation, 13% were labeled as subacute, and 5% were recurrent or peracute. Acute appendicitis was noted in 70% of the cases. Of the appendices removed, 84 were phlegmonous, 15 were gangrenous, and 15 were perforated. There were several complications, the most severe of which was postoperative abscess formation that occurred in two cases (0.2%) of perforated and phlegmonous appendices. Both of these patients required a subsequent laparotomy.

In a well-designed prospective study 62 consecutive patients with symptoms and signs of acute appendicitis were randomized to either laparoscopy ($n = 30$) or open surgery ($n = 32$) and cared for by a single surgeon.[7] Laparoscopic appendectomy was performed by securing the vessels in the mesoappendix electrosurgically and the base with Roeder loops, as described in this chapter. Open appendectomy was performed using a transverse muscle-splitting incision. The two groups were comparable in age and sex. Among the 30 patients in the laparoscopy group, 27 appeared to have an inflammed appendix, which was removed successfully in 25. In two patients, one because of gross fecal contamination from a perforated appendix and one with an inflammatory mass, early decision was made to convert the appendectomy to an open procedure. In the three patients (all under age 25) with a normal-appearing appendix, the structure was left in situ. Pathologic examination revealed 23 of 25 appendices removed to be inflamed. All 32 patients in the laparotomy graoup had the appendix removed. Pathologic examination revealed acute inflammation in 29. The median operating time for the laparoscopy group was 61 minutes (range, 20 to 130) vs. 51 minutes (range, 15 to 100) for the open group, which was not statistically significant. The median length of stay was two days (mean, 2.5) after laparoscopy and three days (mean, 3.8) after open appendectomy. Four complications occurred in the open group (wound infection, 1; urinary retention, 2; prolonged paralytic ileus, 1). In the laparoscopy group two patients were readmitted to the hospital for nonspecific lower abdominal pain, which resolved spontaneously. The period of bed rest, duration of pain, return to employment, and return to full fitness were all less in the laparoscopy group.

CONCLUSIONS

Laparoscopic appendectomy is a procedure that should be part of the surgical repertoire of any gynecologic surgeon. However, it must be remarked that many of our surgical colleagues are still uncertain whether or not laparoscopic appendectomy offers any real advantage over removal of the appendix through a small gridiron incision.

The diagnosis of acute appendicitis is often in doubt and may require that diagnostic laparoscopy be performed. If such has been the case there is a certain logic to completing the extirpation laparoscopically.

REFERENCES

1. Paterson-Brown S, Thompson J, Eckersley J, et al: Which patients with suspected appendicitis should undergo laparoscopy? *Br Med J* 296:1363-4, 1988.
2. Leape L, Ramenofsky M: Laparoscopy for questionable appendicitis. *Ann Surg* 191:410-3, 1980.
3. Street D, Bodai B, Owens L, et al: *Arch Surg* 123:689-690, 1988.
4. Olsen JB, Myrén, Haahr PE: Randomized study of the value of laparoscopy before appendicectomy. *Br J Surg* 80:922-923, 1993.
5. Richards W, Watson D, Lynch G, et al: A review of the results of laparoscopic versus open appendectomy. *Surg Gynecol Obstet* 177:473-480, 1993.
6. Pier A, Götz F, Bacher C, Ibald R: Laparoscopic appendectomy. *World J Surg* 17:29-33, 1993.
7. Atwood SEA, Hill ADK, Murphy PG, et al: A prospective randomized trial of laparoscopic versus open appendectomy. *Surgery* 112:497-501, 1992.

Chapter 24

UROGYNECOLOGIC PROCEDURES

Thierry G. Vancaillie

Urogynecology can be defined as a medical subspecialty that deals with the female pelvic floor Expressions such as "laparoscopic treatment of genuine stress urinary incontinence" are misleading because they imply that laparoscopy is a form of treatment. It is not. Laparoscopy simply provides access to the anatomic area of interest, nothing more.

The main issue is whether there is a need for abdominal access to the pelvic floor. Does the vagina not provide sufficient access? I do not believe that there is a satisfactory answer to this question. A philosophical answer is that a combined abdominal and vaginal approach for surgical correction of the pelvic floor is not necessarily a "fundamental mistake" or "illogical" as some may argue. Rather the best surgical approach is the one that provides optimal exposure and access needed to reach the anatomic elements. Furthermore, I am not opposed to applying techniques that obviate the need for a dual approach, provided they are effective. These theoretic considerations cannot be supported at present by hard data. It appears that vaginal procedures have been introduced to eliminate the need for abdominal access with the objective of reducing postoperative morbidity. Procedures that I consider optimal for particular aspects of correction of pelvic floor relaxation, such as urethropexy and enterocele repair, should however, be performed by the abdominal route. To avoid the morbidity of dissection of the abdominal wall, the scalpel can be replaced by laparoscopy. The reduction in postoperative morbidity resulting from the use of laparoscopic techniques contributes significantly to the applicability of abdominal procedures for pelvic floor reconstruction.

Urinary incontinence is one of the most common problems for women in general, and postmenopausal women in particular. Thirty-eight percent of women over the age of 60 experience some form of urinary incontinence. More than half of the women residing in nursing homes or other institutions suffer from one or other form of urinary incontinence.[1] Physicians are increasingly confronted with elderly patients seeking treatment to achieve a better quality of life. Incontinence in elderly patients presents rarely as uncomplicated stress or urgency. It is necessary to become familiar with a number of therapeutic options other than surgery, such as biofeedback, electrostimulation, physiotherapy, and behavioral intervention. Surgery is only one of many steps in the treatment of pelvic floor relaxation.

ANATOMY RELATED TO PELVIC FLOOR SUPPORT

Bladder

There are no well-defined ligamentary suspensory structures that hold the bladder in place (see Fig. 24-1). This gives the bladder its characteristic distensibility. Fibrous attachments run from the posterior rectus muscle to the anterior wall of the bladder. The so called bladder "pillars" are extensions of the endopelvic fascia covering the anterior vagina. They provide some support for the base of the bladder, although most rigidity is provided by the vagina itself. The base of the bladder, resting on the upper half of the vagina, is actually the weak spot of the pelvic floor. Defects in this region are the most difficult to repair, due to the lack of muscular or ligamentary tissues.

Urethra

The urethra runs above the endopelvic fascia of the middle third of the vagina, from which it can be dissected with relative ease. When the urethra reaches the lower third of the vagina, it becomes incorporated into the vaginal wall and surrounding fascial and muscular tissue. Dissection of the urethra at this level is not feasible. It is also here that the so-called "pubourethral" ligaments can be identified. These ligaments enclose the urethra and anterior vaginal wall and then project, fanlike, toward the pubic bone anteriorly and toward the obturator muscle laterally. The dominance of the pubic component versus the obturator component is variable from patient to patient. Whether the configuration of the ligament plays a role in the development of incontinence is unknown. Robert Zacharin[2] was the first to identify the importance of this ligament in the pathophysiology of urinary incontinence. He was also the first correctly to include the ligament within the surgical repair procedure.

Vagina

The upper third of the vagina, mainly the posterior fornix, is free of attachments in the area corresponding to the cul de sac. The lateral aspects of the vagina are intimately connected to the ligamentary complex of the cardinal and uterosacral ligaments, the so-called paracolpos, in continuation with and inseparable from the parametrium.

The middle third of the vagina is well supported, since this is the main site of insertion of the cardinal (Mackenrodts) ligament. This fascial tissue originates along the pelvic brim on both sides and funnels down to blend with the endopelvic fascia. More distinct structures that are integral parts of the endopelvic fascia are the cardinal and uterosacral ligaments. Both ligaments are attached to the lower uterine segment and the middle third of the vagina. The cardinal ligament complex, visualized in a craniocaudad direction, looks like a large wing, attaching the cervicovaginal complex to the pelvic side wall. The cardinal ligament complex is quite voluminous, as it occupies the space between the levator muscle plate and the parietal peritoneum. In the sagittal plane the ligament is fan shaped, similar to the pubourethral ligament.

The lower third of the vagina is attached along the lateral walls to the levator muscle posteriorly and the obturator muscle anteriorly. The anterior and posterior vaginal walls of the lower third have no actual attachments but are supported by fascial tissue which may be considered part of the endopelvic fascia complex. These fascial structures are called Denonvillier's fascia of the rectovaginal septum and the vesicovaginal fascia.

Cul-de-sac

The anatomy of the cul-de-sac is poorly delineated, but it is the space between the rectum and the vagina forming the bottom of the pelvis. Little is known about the normal length of the rectovaginal septum and the normal depth of the cul-de-sac. How can a deep cul-de-sac and an enterocele be differentiated? Some years ago, I attempted to quantify the depth of the "normal" cul-de-sac in patients undergoing laparoscopy for tubal sterilization. Soon it became apparent that this was an impossible task, due to lack of well-defined anatomic reference points.

The cul-de-sac is bordered by the vagina in front and the rectum behind. The lateral walls are formed by the insertions of the endopelvic fascia onto the lateral walls of the rectum. Thickenings of the fascia form the uterosacral ligaments. When a laparoscopy is performed, the normal cul-de-sac will have a typical funnel-like appearance with a triangular base. The base is formed by the two uterosacral ligaments that join at the level of the uterine cervix or vaginal cuff. These insertions describe a typical inverted V.

In the presence of an enterocele, the insertions of the uterosacral ligaments separate and the base of the cul-de-sac acquires the shape of a horseshoe. The position of the uterosacral ligaments mirrors the change that has happened to the levator muscles. Widening of the arch formed by the uterosacral ligaments is paired with a separation of the crura levatores. This is important from the point of view of recontruction since both the crura and the ligaments must be approximated to treat an enterocele.

The diagnosis of an enterocele is usually made by examining the patient's posterior vaginal wall and/or the cul-de-sac under stress conditions compared with the resting position. An enterocele is a hernia and will enlarge under stress, whereas a deep but normal cul-de-sac will not vary when intra-abdominal pressure is increased. This is the only possible differential diagnostic test.

Rectum

The main attachments of the rectum to the pelvis are the levator muscles. There are some fibrous attachments to the endopelvic fascia at the level of the cul-de-sac, which some call the "rectal pillars," analogous to similar fibrous structures supporting the bladder. Additional fibrous attachments connect the rectum to the sacrum and coccyx through the median raphe.

PATHOPHYSIOLOGY OF STRESS INCONTINENCE

Genuine stress incontinence occurs when insufficient resistance counteracts an increase in intra-abdominal pressure. This lack of resistance results from a combination of weak muscles and a defect in the relationship between the urethra and the surrounding pelvic structures.

In the upright position, the intra-abdominal force is mainly vectored toward the promontory and hollow of the sacrum, bony structures that are fortunately solid and absorb a great amount of pressure. However, because the abdomen is a fluid-filled cavity, the force vectors will reflect and transmit pressure to all sides. This pressure will, under normal anatomic circumstances, help maintain closure of the urethra (closing pressure). When urethral detachment occurs, the force vector, which helped close the urethra, becomes less and less effective. Contraction of the sphincters is sufficient in some cases to prevent incontinence, especially if the patient is able to anticipate the intra-abdominal pressure increase.

The occurrence of stress incontinence is the result of a disequilibrium between the intra-abdominal pressure, the intravesical pressure, and the closing pressure. The intravesical pressure depends on the volume of urine the bladder contains and the transmission of force from the abdomen. The intravesical volume is in itself not a major contributor to intravesical pressure. However, a distended bladder will have to absorb more force that is transmitted from the abdomen. Filling of the bladder will adversely affect its ability to withstand increased pressures.

The pathophysiology of pelvic floor relaxation is a combination of genetic predisposition and environmental factors, such as childbearing, obesity, chronic cough, lack of exercise, and hormone depletion. Moschcovitz expressed the theory that all clinical forms of pelvic floor relaxation begin with weakness of the cul-de-sac.[3] Based on this hypothesis, the mainstay of repair was obliteration of the cul-de-sac. Nichols describes four different types of enterocele: congenital, pulsion, traction, or iatrogenic. They may occur singly or in combination.[4]

Analogous to inguinal hernias, the pathophysiology of pelvic floor relaxation can be described as follows. An initial event, either inborn weakness, trauma, or both, causes a rent in the supportive fascial structure of the pelvis. This weakness is gradually aggravated by traction or pulsion over the ensuing years, resulting in herniation. Depending on the location of the defect, the hernia will contain bladder, rectum, small bowel, and/or omentum. It is important to locate the different defects during thorough clinical examination prior to embarking on a surgical repair. Defects of the supportive structures of the pelvis are evaluated under resting and straining conditions. Although awkward, ideally the patient should be examined in the upright position.

All herniation of the pelvis results in lateralization of the support structures. Both the cardinal ligament complex and the levatores are gradually displaced toward the pelvic side wall, widening the distance between the crura levatores. This space is then occupied by the hernia. However, lateral defects can occur simultaneously. Lateral defects are more common in the anterior compartment of the pelvis involving the lower anterior vagina, whereas the midline defect is more prevalent in the posterior compartment of the pelvis, involving the cul-de-sac and posterior wall of the vagina. Different combinations are common.

In the presence of a large enterocele combined with a cystocele, stress urinary incontinence may be masked. Under these anatomic conditions, the upper urethra is kinked, which leads to continence through compression of the upper urethra by the base of the bladder itself during times of increased intra-abdominal pressure. Correction of the enterocele may then reveal the occult incontinence. Only careful evaluation of the anatomy, with or without the assistance of a pessary and vaginal ultrasonography, will provide the examiner with the necessary information to prevent postoperative incontinence.

EVALUATION OF STRESS INCONTINENCE

The mainstay of investigation of a patient with urinary incontinence or pelvic floor relaxation is the interview. Many clinicians find it helpful to follow a set questionnaire to avoid forgetting important questions. The interview of the patient with urinary incontinence yields diagnostic, but not pathognomonic, information for stress incontinence. Further clinical tests are aimed at determining confounding factors such as urgency and intrinsic urethral pathology, the so called "type three" stress incontinence.

The next important step is the physical examination of the patient. The physical examination will determine which defects of the pelvic floor exist and their extent. The surgeon must evaluate the patient thoroughly, as the examination will determine the extent of the surgery.

When examining the pelvic floor of a patient complaining of relaxation, convention divides the region into three anatomic compartments: anterior, posterior, and middle. This subdivision is artificial but has the merit of forcing the examiner to evaluate the entire pelvis. The anterior compartment corresponds to the anterior vaginal wall and relates to urethro- and cystocele; the posterior compartment corresponds to the posterior vaginal wall and relates to recto- and enterocele; the middle compartment relates to vaginal vault prolapse. The most common confusion is between a true vault prolapse and an enterocele. A careful examiner should be able to differentiate both entities by clinical evaluation alone. I believe that a true vaginal vault prolapse is rare.

In addition to the anatomic division of the pelvic floor, a "functional" division should be considered. Three "functional compartments" can be differentiated: the muscular compartment, the fascial compartment, and, finally, the vascular compartment. Each one of these needs to be addressed appropriately and is probably equally important for the long-term resolution of pelvic floor relaxation. Zacharin vehemently defends the position that the levator muscle complex is the main active mechanism of support of the pelvic floor.[2] He argues that Chinese women demonstrate a lack of pelvic floor relaxation because they have a well-developed levator plate. They maintain excellent muscle tone because of their cultural habit of "squatting." There is certainly much truth in this statement. The lesson to learn is that re-education of the pelvic floor muscles is part of the treatment of pelvic floor relaxation. All patients cannot be converted into "squatters," but a number of exercises and biofeedback mechanisms exist that will improve pelvic floor muscle tone. Approximation of the crura levatores during rectocele and enterocele repair does not make the muscles stronger. Only regular physical exercises will influence muscle strength.

The vascular compartment of the pelvis is most influenced by the hormonal status of the patient. Hormone replacement in amounts sufficient to foster epithelial maturation of the vagina is an integral part of the treatment of pelvic floor relaxation.

The third and last compartment is the fascial, which is the only one that is addressed by a surgical procedure. Even approximation of the levator plates is part of reconstructing the fascial structure of the pelvis, which consists of reinforcing natural fascia with scar tissue!

Additional tests are performed to learn more about the patient's condition. These tests have in common that they either provoke a symptom or imitate the results of the surgery, thereby providing prognostic information. The following tests are helpful in confirming the presence of stress incontinence. They are aimed at reproducing or arresting hypermobility of the bladder neck. Obviously these tests have a predictive value inasmuch as they mimic the mechanical impact of the corrective surgical procedure.

The Q-tip test aims at reproducing and quantifying the hypermobility of the urethra and bladder neck. A Q-tip is introduced into the urethra up to the level of the bladder neck. The patient is asked to strain or cough. The upward movement of the Q-tip can then be observed and quantified. There is no clear correlation between the severity of the hypermobility and the occurrence of incontinence. However there is no possibility of correcting stress incontinence with a simple urethropexy operation without the presence of hypermobility. Surgery provides correction of a mechanical problem.

In the Bonney test, two Q-tips or other rigid instruments are introduced into the vagina and held laterally to the urethra along the upper third of its course. The Q-tips are loosely held in place and the patient is again asked to strain or cough. If the hypermobility of the urethra is reduced and there is no involuntary loss of urine, then the test is said to be positive. This test reproduces the effect of surgical immobilization of the urethra on the occurrence of stress incontinence. The combination of the simple Q-tip and Bonney tests is quite effective in confirming the presence of stress urinary incontinence and in predicting a positive outcome of the corrective procedure.

In the presence of atypical symptomatology and inconclusive physical examination, a cystometrogram and possibly cystoscopy are indicated. These tests are aimed at detecting concomitant lesions that complicate the clinical presentation. In addition, patients who have been previously operated upon for incontinence are also subjected to a complete urodynamic evaluation. The principal objective of a cystometrogram is to detect detrusor instability and urethral disease. The presence of urgency incontinence is not necessarily a containdication to surgery. However, it will warn the physician and the patient that the surgery may not cure all of the symptoms. Neurologic disorders secondary to spine injuries, multiple sclerosis, diabetes, and other systemic conditions will not be considered in this chapter.

SURGICAL CORRECTION

Contraindications

Contraindications include the contraindications related to laparoscopy and surgery in general and those related to the correction of incontinence. Contraindications to laparoscopy are discussed in Chapter 6. In a patient who has had multiple previous abdominal operations in the pelvic area, it may be wise to gain access to the space of Retzius by the preperitoneal route.

There are also contraindications to surgery itself, including systemic conditions that would jeopardize the patient's life (e.g., low cardiac output, severe emphysema).

Contraindications of the correction of incontinence are related to intrinsic urethral disease. These patients have stress incontinence, but immobilization of the urethra will not result in cure. Without going into detail, it may be said that patients presenting with intrinsic urethral disease are best treated with a sling procedure, if surgery is indicated at all.

Indications

The indications for laparoscopic treatment of stress urinary incontinence are the same as those for conventional surgical treatment. There are no specific indications for the choice of the route of access. I believe that laparoscopic surgery is less traumatic than surgery performed by laparotomy. This has been shown extensively in other surgical procedures such as laparoscopic cholecystectomy and lymph node dissection. Therefore when a surgical procedure is indicated, I evaluate the feasibility of a laparoscopic procedure first. In some patients with extensive adhesions, or when these are suspected, it may be wise not to perform a laparoscopy. This is decided on an individual patient basis.

In patients who have complicated incontinence of which the stress component is only one among many, it may be difficult to decide whether surgery is indicated at all. A golden rule for this decision is not available, but I will operate if the bladder capacity is at least 400 cc and stress incontinence can be objectively noted at a filling of less than 400 cc. The presence of signs of urgency in addition to stress incontinence is not a contraindication to surgery. So-called mixed incontinence is challenging in view of an unpredictable outcome, which may not match the patient's expectations.

Surgical technique

Two large groups of incontent patients can be identified: those who have urinary incontinence only and those with incontinence and pelvic floor relaxation. The clinical and laboratory investigations will have delineated the extent of the pelvic floor relaxation and thereby dictate the extent of the surgery required. Patients under 40 years old are more likely to present with isolated urethrocele. Urethropexy would then be the only procedure to be performed. The older patient over 60 years of age is more likely to present with a combination of rectocele, enterocele, and cystocele. The stress incontinence may be occult or of secondary importance to the patient. In such a case, the surgical procedure is more elaborate. From a practical point the vaginal portion of the procedure is completed before the abdominal part is begun

The question of whether the uterus should be removed as part of the procedure is interesting. Intrinsically, the uterus is not involved in the pathophysiologic process of stress incontinence or pelvic floor relaxation, and thus it can be argued that there is no reason to remove it. In my experience anatomic structures are easier to identify when the uterus is left in place. The procedure itself is identical with or without the presence of the uterus. The description of the procedure that follows is written generically, ignoring the presence or absence of the uterus. When representing the successive steps of surgery graphically, it is easier to depict the pelvis without the uterus as the drawings are less crowded and easier to understand.

The vaginal part of the pelvic reconstruction may encompass a vaginal hysterectomy and/or anterior and posterior repair. It is not the objective of this chapter to provide a technical description of these well-known surgical procedures. Because of the importance of the posterior repair, salient points will be noted. The levator muscles must be carefully identified and dissected. The muscle plates are then approximated in front of the rectum, using several interrupted sutures tied under minimal tension. The posterior repair can be reinforced by inserting materials that will generate a dense layer of scar tissue. An interesting approach, published by Zacharin, is the use of the resected portion of the vaginal wall.[5] Instead of discarding the tissue, it can be used for interposition between the levator muscles and the vaginal wall. The devascularized tissue will necrose and induce an inflammatory reaction, increasing the deposition of granulation tissue. Vicryl mesh is another material that promotes ingrowth of fibroblasts.

Once the vaginal steps have been completed, a Foley catheter is inserted and the patient's legs are repositioned. Although time consuming, the patient must be correctly positioned prior to the laparoscopic part of the operation. The patient should be supine with the upper leg in continuity with the trunk. The knees are flexed to provide stability when the table is placed in the Trendelenberg position. The legs are in abduction to provide access to the vagina. In some way this position is similar to the "frog position." A roll of towels is placed underneath the patient's buttocks to optimize access to the cul-de-sac in preparation for the enterocele repair.

It should be stressed that approximation of the crura levatores is an integral part of an enterocele repair. Separation of the uterosacral ligaments, which is the most visible feature of an enterocele, is associated with separation of the crura levatores. The surgical reconstruction aims at bringing the support structures, namely the levatores ani and cardinal ligament complex, toward the midline, resulting in closure of the hernia—hence the emphasis on a good "posterior" repair.

The surgeon stands, if right handed, on the left side of the patient. All further descriptions are given with a right-handed operator in mind. A mirror image should be envisioned for a left-handed operator.

A total of four portals are used for the completion of enterocele repair and bladder neck suspension. The umbilical portal provides access for the laparoscope. Three additional portals will allow manipulation. A 10 mm suprapubic port is used for introduction of the suture material. Two 5 mm lateral ports are placed at the level of the iliac crests, some 3 to 4 cm medial.

Once the pneumoperitoneum has been established, the principal trocar and cannula is inserted intraumbilically and the laparoscope is passed. Adhesiolysis and enterolysis may be required to gain access to the cul-de-sac.

Enterocele repair. The enterocele repair is performed first, because access to the cul-de-sac is made difficult after a bladder neck suspension. The anatomic landmarks are the cul-de-sac, the uterosacral ligaments, the ureters, and the vagina. A forceps introduced into the vagina and pushed upward will stretch the uterosacral ligaments and highlight the edge of the "hernia" (Fig. 24-1). As a result of the posterior repair that has just been completed, the peritoneum of the cul-de-sac may already be open or detached from the underlying tissue planes.

There are five essential steps to laparoscopic enterocele repair: (1) excision of the hernial sac, (2) dissection of the bladder, (3) opening of the rectovaginal septum, (4) approximation of the uterosacral ligaments, and (5) colposuspension. These will now be described.

First the hernia sac is completely resected. The incision line follows the edge of the uterosacral ligaments, which describe an inverted U or horseshoe shape (Fig. 24-2). The peritoneum is completely dissected free from the loose connective tissue until it is attached to the anterior wall of the rectum only. This peritoneal flap is then excised from the rectum.

The bladder is dissected off the anterior wall of the vagina to isolate the upper third of the vagina completely (Fig. 24-3). This is especially important in patients who previously have undergone a hysterectomy and in whom the bladder bulges over the vaginal vault. The dissection of the vesicovaginal septum is important for gaining access to the cardinal ligaments, which are attached laterally into the side walls of the middle third of the vagina.

The rectovaginal septum is now bluntly opened. Due to

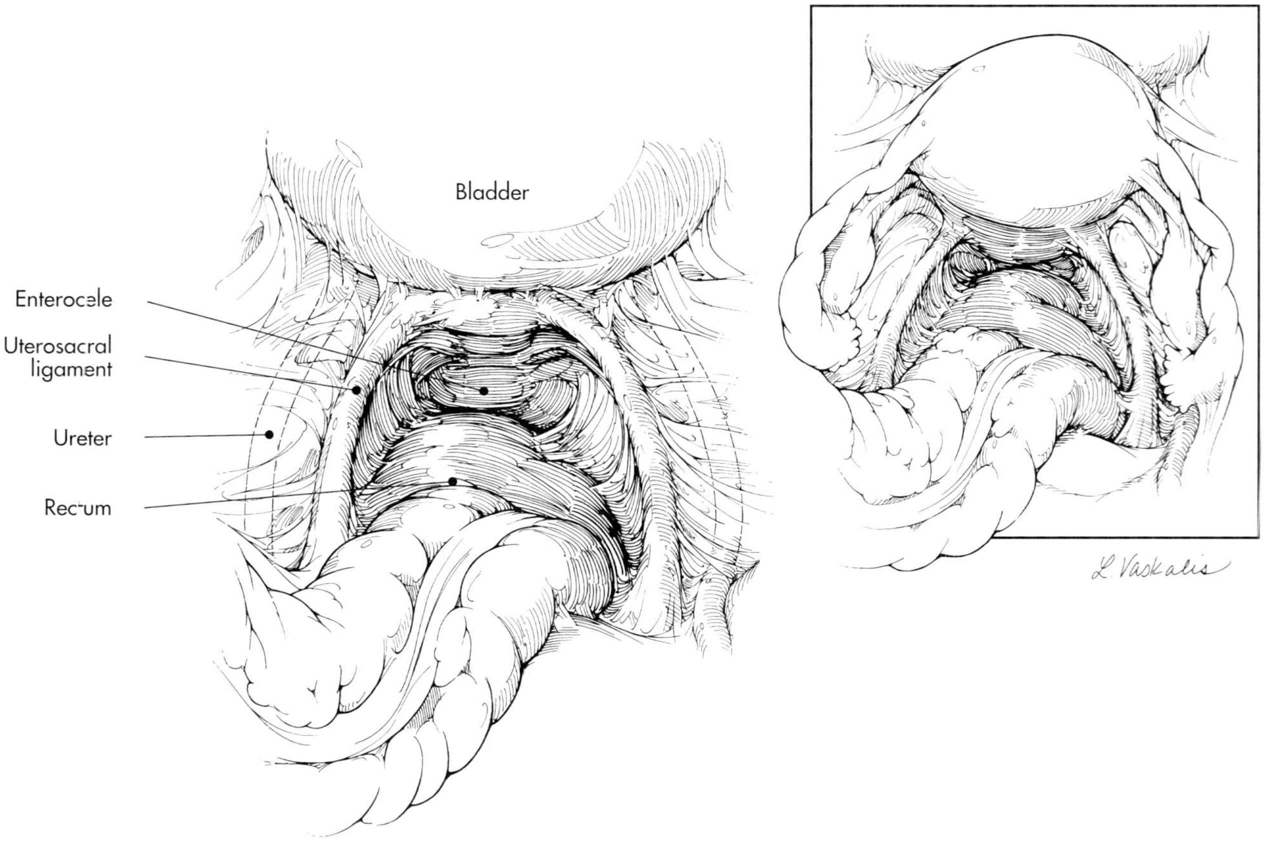

Fig. 24-1. Anatomic landmarks for the enterocele repair.

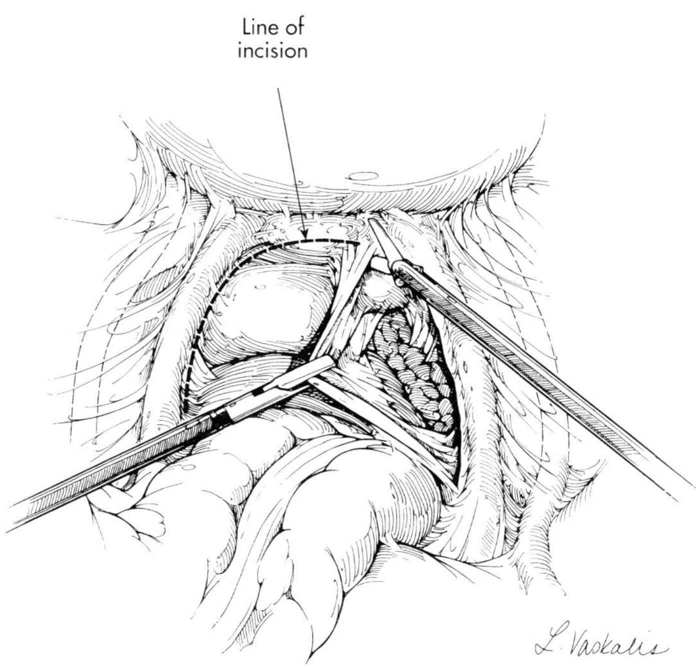

Fig. 24-2. Resection of the hernia sac.

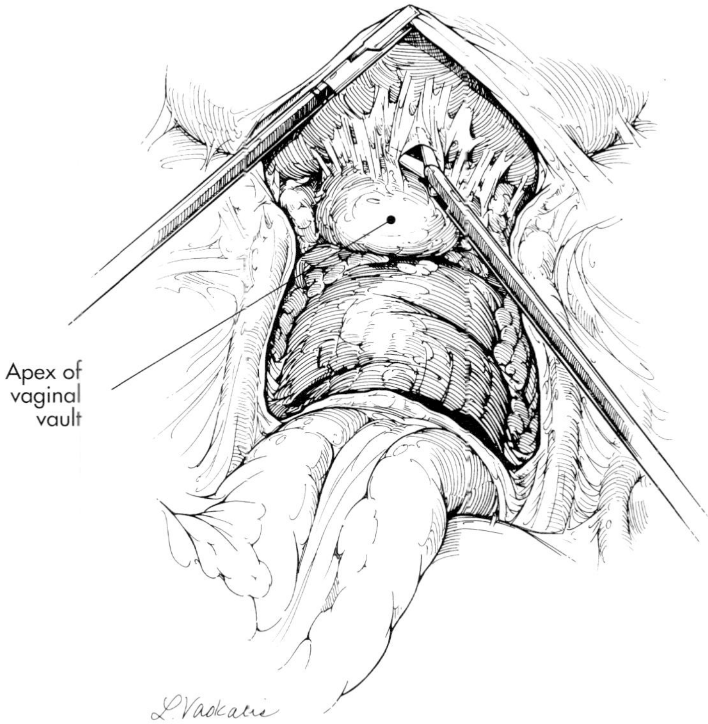

Fig. 24-3. Dissection of the bladder off the anterior vaginal wall.

the previously executed posterior repair, the dissection of the rectovaginal space is rather easy. The stitches in the levator muscles can be easily identified. In addition it is possible to add a suture in the levator plate at this time, if visual inspection from the abdominal side reveals insufficient approximation of the crura (Fig. 24-4). With regard to approximation of the muscles, it is likely that the length of the suture line is more important than the tightness of the stitches. The muscles should be approximated without excessive tension, even if they do not touch each other in the midline. Approximation of the fascial layer of the pelvic floor follows.

The first stitch is applied posteriorly in front of the dorsal insertion of the uterosacral ligaments. The needle is first driven through the right ligament, incorporating as much fascial tissue as possible, and then several times through the edge of the peritoneal resection at the level of the anterior wall of the rectum. Finally, the needle is passed through the left uterosacral ligament and the suture tied with an extracorporeal knot (Fig. 24-5). Care is taken not to strangle the rectum. Once the suture is tied, the positions of the ureters are checked. Invariably there is some degree of medial displacement. Should this be judged excessive, a relief incision into the peritoneum between the ligament and the ureter can be made.

Once the posterior border of the hernia has been closed, the large defect in the pelvic floor becomes apparent, between the uterosacral ligaments, the anterior wall of the rectum, and the posterior wall of the vagina. A forceps introduced into the vagina gently pushes the vaginal cuff upward to evaluate how far it reaches, without excess force being applied. The needle is passed through the right uterosacral ligament at the level where the vaginal cuff reaches. Then the needle catches the vaginal wall and the left ligament (Fig. 24-6). When this suture is tied, the vagina lies upon the approximated levator muscles and becomes suspended to the uterosacral ligaments. The vagina now occupies the space that was previously filled by the enterocele. This surgical procedure therefore reconstructs the rectovaginal septum because it reestablishes the anatomic relationship between vagina and rectum. Some degree of "overcorrection" is however unavoidable. Two or three more sutures are applied to close the defect completely.

One or two stitches are placed in front of the new position of the vaginal cuff and will provide some support for the bottom of the bladder. These stitches are placed immediately lateral to the vaginal wall, within the cardinal ligament complex and medial to the ureter (Fig. 24-7). To strengthen the vesicovaginal septum further, a Vicryl mesh may be interposed between the vagina and the bladder, on top of the sutures connecting the cardinal ligaments. The peritoneum of the bladder flap is loosely draped over the enterocele repair to finish the procedure.

Urethropexy. After completion of the enterocele repair, the urethropexy, if necessary, is performed. The landmarks are the left umbilical ligament, which delineates the lateral border of the dissection and the lateral edge of the bladder on the left. The pubic bone can be identified as a ridge at the bottom of this triangular space bounded by the left umbilical ligament and the bladder wall. The Foley catheter helps in locating the bladder. Filling the bladder is sometimes helpful in a patient with multiple previous operations.

Gentle probing with an ancillary instrument helps locate the pubic bone. The initial peritoneal incision is made above the pubic bone immediately medial to the left umbilical ligament (Fig. 24-8) in order to avoid the superior vesical pedicle. This pedicle runs anterior to the round ligament but slightly below the level of the pubic bone. The superior vesical pedicle is not easily recognized, but the venous plexus is significant and will bleed profusely if incised. Avoiding this vascular structure is important, because the bleeding it may cause will obscure the tissue planes and make the procedure difficult. The surgeon should strive to reach the pubic bone as quickly as possible. The distance between the peritoneum and the pubic bone is short, even in the obese patient. The dissection must remain in a plane perpendicular to the pubic bone. There is a tendency to shift toward the midline too early, leading to bladder injury.

Once the pubic bone is reached, the assistant will insert a blunt instrument into the incision and retract the bladder to the right. The space of Retzius is easily opened with mini-

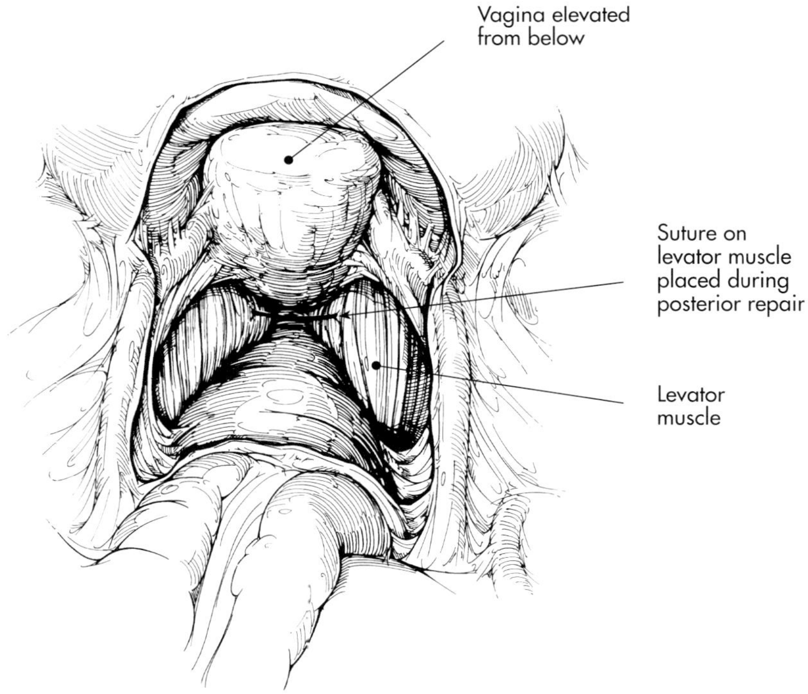

Fig. 24-4. Opening of the rectovaginal septum.

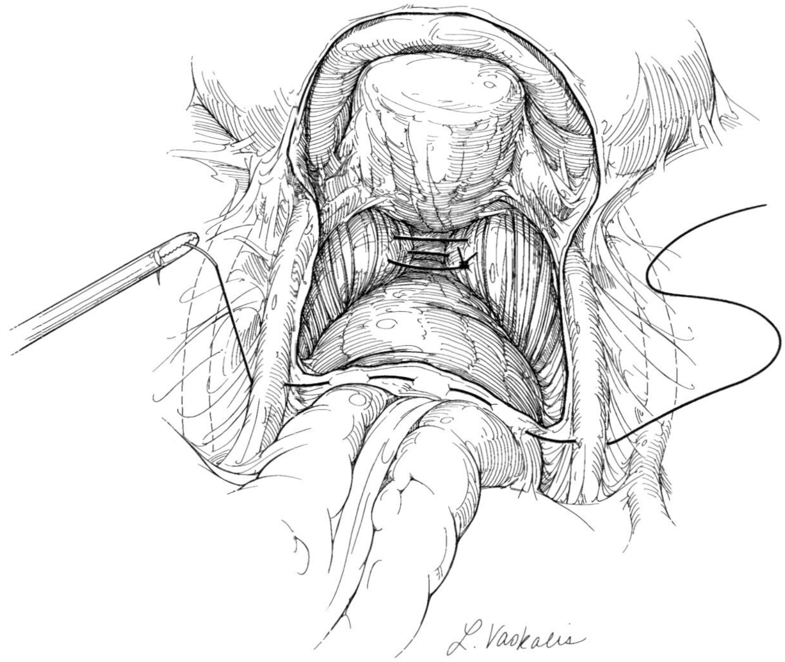

Fig. 24-5. First stitch of the enterocele repair.

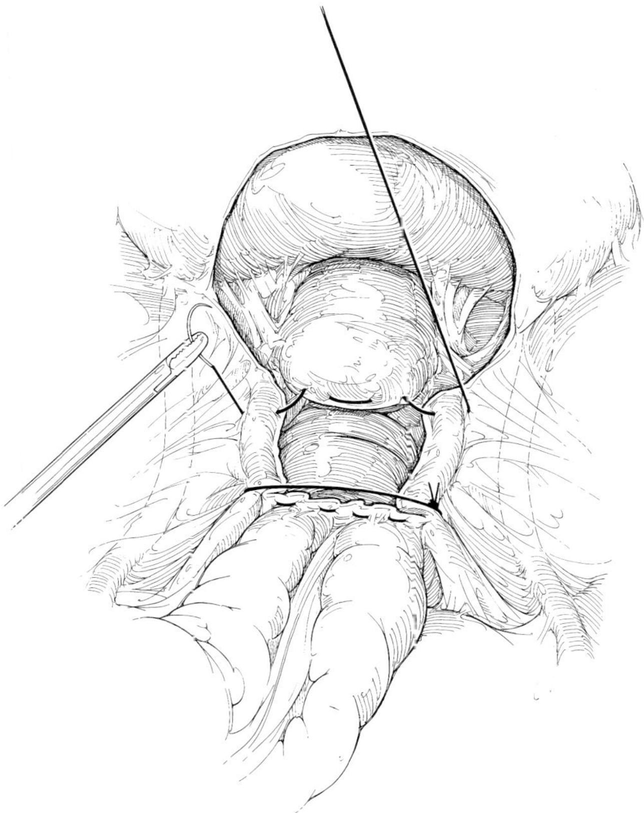

Fig. 24-6. Second stitch of the enterocele repair.

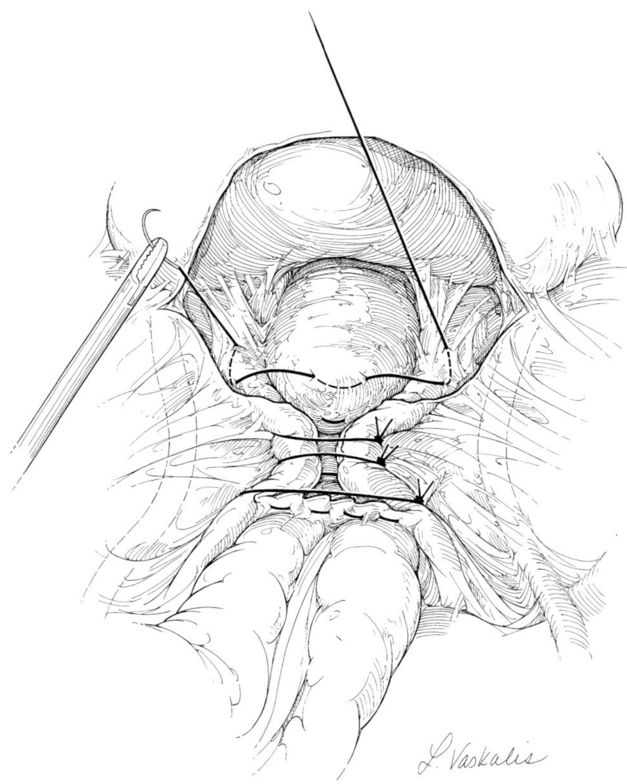

Fig. 24-7. Approximation of the cardinal ligaments.

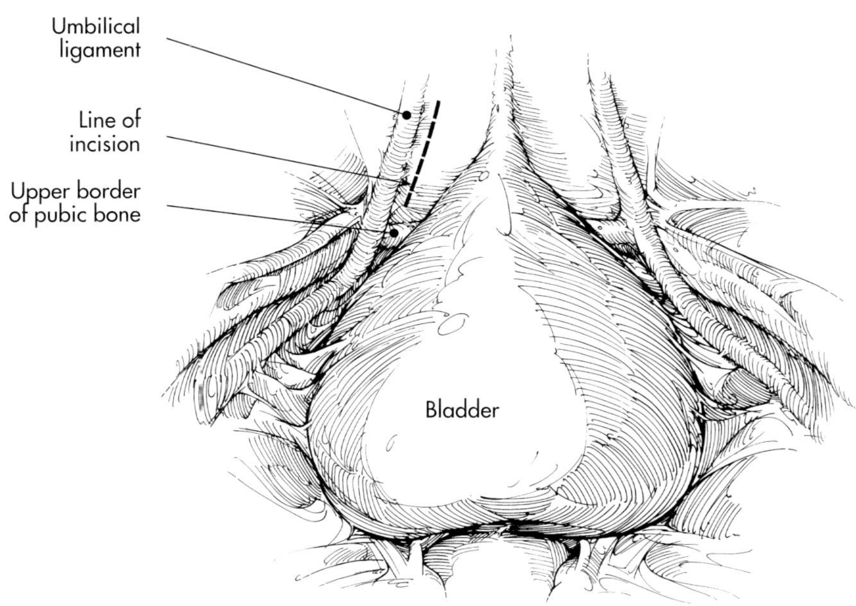

Fig. 24-8. Anatomic landmarks for the urethropexy.

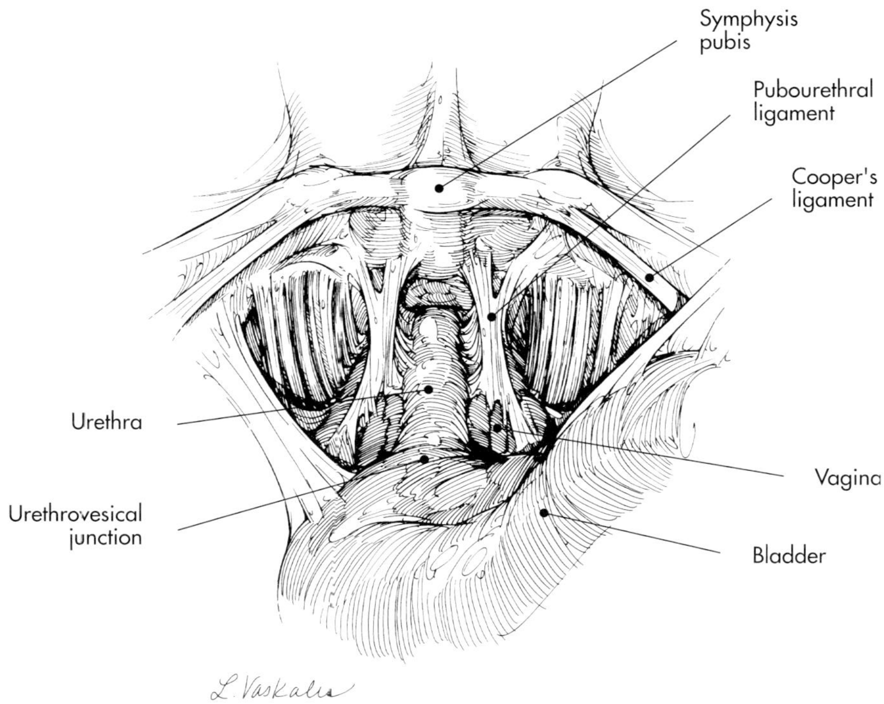

Fig. 24-9. Anatomy of the space of Retzius.

mal traction and some blunt dissection. The dissection is continued toward the right until the entire space is opened and all anatomic structures can be identified on both sides. The urachus is only seldom an obstacle to complete dissection of the operative field. The anatomic structures, which should be identified, are: the urethra, the bladder neck, the anterior wall of the bladder, the vaginal wall, the obturator muscles, the pubourethral ligaments, the pubic rami and symphysis, and the ligaments (Fig. 24-9). Identification of Cooper's ligaments still represents a challenge. A wide dissection of the pubic bone will facilitate identification of these ligaments.

Simultaneous vaginal examination during laparoscopic evaluation of the space of Retzius greatly facilitates identification of the pubourethral ligament, which is located at the level of the undersurface of the symphysis.

The foundation of the procedure is precise identification of the pubourethral ligament and incorporation of the ligament into the repair. The essential principle, on which the procedure is based, is the fact that the pubourethral ligament is the key to urinary continence and that laparoscopic urethropexy aims at shortening and strengthening that ligament to reduce mobility of the urethra. As a tribute to Dr. Zacharin, a true pioneer in pelvic reconstructive surgery, I call this procedure a modified Zacharin urethropexy.

The surgeon now places the left hand in the patient's vagina, thereby displacing the bladder neck toward the left of the patient to facilitate application of the right sided suture. The vaginal wall is only minimally elevated, otherwise the space between the vagina and the pubic bone is reduced to such an extent that it becomes difficult to introduce the needle in the correct position.

The needle and suture (Ethibond 2/0—36 inches) is introduced through the 10 mm cannula. The needle holder is passed through the left lateral portal, allowing optimal access to the space of Retzius. The needle is grasped and then guided into the space of Retzius. The right-sided stitch is placed first. The needle is passed through the fascia of the vaginal wall, alongside the urethra above the pubourethral ligament. The needle is driven through the fascia and through the pubourethral ligament. The needle is then passed through the ipsilateral Cooper's ligament (Fig. 24-10). If this is impossible the suture must be placed in the posterior perichondrium of the pubic symphysis. An extracorporeal knot is made with minimal traction on the suture. The objective of the suture is to shorten the ligament slightly and to immobilize the urethra but not to elevate the urethra into an unnatural position, which would lead to chronic retention. Manipulation of the bladder neck with the left hand in the patient's vagina will allow the surgeon to evaluate the amount of elevation. The surgeon should perform a manual evaluation of the bladder neck to confirm correct positioning. Elevation of the urethra during actual suturing can then be performed by an assistant to free both the surgeon's hands. The left-sided suture is placed in a similar fashion.

For reinforcement, a strip of Vicryl mesh is sutured in place between the pubourethral ligament and Cooper's liga-

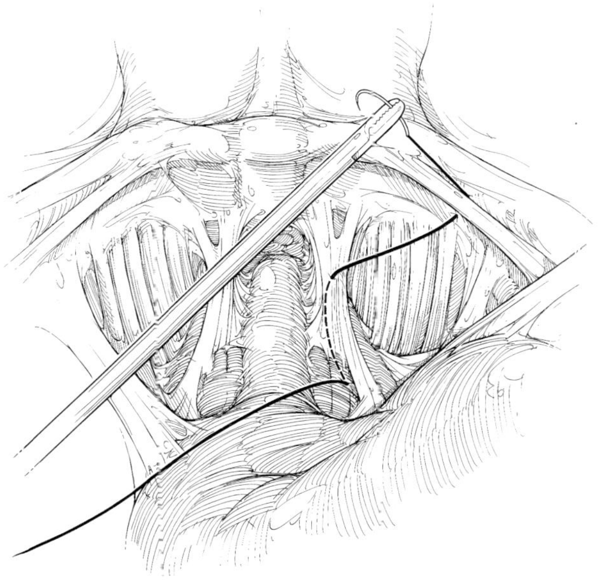

Fig. 24-10. Placement of the right-sided stitch.

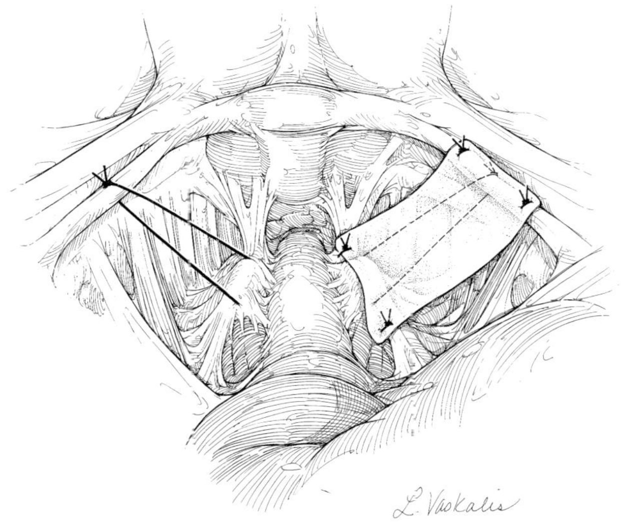

Fig. 24-11. Placement of the mesh.

ment on each side (Fig. 24-11). The purpose of the mesh is to promote ingrowth of fibrocytes and thus increase the amount of scarring.

It will be obvious in some patients, once the space of Retzius is opened and dissected, that the vagina is detached from the side wall, presenting the lateral defect described previously. I recommend repairing the defect with sutures, approximating the lateral vaginal wall and the obturator muscle. These lateral defects can be uni- or bilateral.

The peritoneal defect may be closed with one or two sutures.

Complications

We have performed laparoscopic urethropexy in approximately 125 patients. Inability to complete the procedure under laparascopic control occurred in two instances early in our experience.

Bladder injury during dissection occurred in four instances, two early in our experience and two later. The latter cases were repeat interventions in which the dissection of the space of Retzius was anticipated to be difficult. Three of these bladder lacerations were repaired under laparoscopic control. The first, which occurred in the second patient undergoing the procedure, was repaired by laparotomy, because there was also difficulty in completing the actual procedure.

Further complications such as bleeding, infection, and injury to bowel or urinary structures other than the bladder did not occur but are a real possibility. Whether the incidence of this type of complication will be higher in patients treated with the laparoscopic approach versus the alternative routes remains to be seen.

The last category of possible complications is those that result from the suspension itself. The main complication is overcorrection, which requires long-term catheterization and possibly continuous self-catheterization on one hand and de novo bladder symptoms of the urgency type on the other. Overcorrection occurred in one patient who underwent a procedure in which the sutures were anchored in the symphysis. After approximately 3 months, she was able to void. Tallying urgency symptoms that occur de novo is somewhat more difficult because of their subjective nature. Many patients with preoperative mixed incontinence have difficulty understanding that the surgery did not cure them completely. This may lead to increased incapacitation by the urgency component, which in actuality remained unchanged or even improved. Nonetheless, de novo symptoms are real and therefore an integral concomitant of the treatment of urinary incontinence. The incidence of such symptoms was evaluated at 24% in a series of 42 patients. This incidence is comparable to the numbers reported for the classical procedures such as Marshall-Marchetti-Krantz[6] or Burch suspension.[7]

Results

A cohort of 42 patients was prospectively studied from June, 1991, until December, 1992. This provided a follow-up period of 8 to 26 months with a median of 18. The results have been published previously.[8] One patient was lost to follow-up and another presented with recurrence of symptoms less than 3 months after the procedure, which is therefore considered to be a failure. She has, however, staunchly refused to submit to objective testing. The remaining 40 patients are satisfied. Eight of them have re-

Table 24-1. Comparison of urogynecologic procedures

	Preperitoneal open	Preperitoneal closed	Transvaginal	Transperitoneal
Anatomic detail	Fair	Good	Fair	Best
Technical ease	Best	Fair	Good	Fair
Morbidity (pain)	Fair	Best	Good	Best
Complications	Good	Unknown	Good	Unknown
Simultaneous enterocele repair	Impossible	Impossible	Good	Best

sidual symptoms of stress, urgency, or a combination of both. In some cases the residual urgency had been predicted by the preoperative cystometrogram.

Definite comments about the validity of the procedure await the 5-year follow-up evaluation. It appears that thus far the results are comparable with those expected after classical interventions.

CONCLUSIONS

Urethropexy or colposuspension can be performed in different ways, giving more or less comparable results. These routes of access are the traditional suprapubic preperitoneal access, the endoscopic preperitoneal, and the laparoscopic. In addition to these, there is a myriad of so called "needle" suspension procedures, which in essence aim at reproducing a similar surgical result through vaginal access. The differences among those procedures, which are in great part subjective, are summarized in Table 24-1.

It is obvious that preperitoneal access excludes the performance of an enterocele repair at least by the abdominal route. This is the main reason why I prefer the transperitoneal approach, which in addition offers better visualization of the anatomic structures than the vaginal method.

The earlier literature has shown retropubic suspension to be superior to anterior colporrhaphy for the relief of stress urinary incontinence.[9,10] This would suggest that laparoscopic colpourethropexy should also give better results than the vaginal approach.

Like all of the surgical procedures described in this text, laparoscopic access for urologic procedures is associated with less discomfort and more rapid recovery for the patient but requires additional training of surgeons.

The future place of laparoscopy in urogynecology will be defined as more experience is gained, but preliminary results appear to be promising.

REFERENCES

1. Herzog AR, Fultz NH: Prevalence and incidence of urinary incontinence in community-dwelling populations. *J Am Geriatr Soc* 38:273, 1990.
2. Zacharin RF: Abdominoperineal urethral suspension in the management of recurrent stress incontinence of urine—a 15 year experience. *Obstet Gynecol* 62:644-654, 1983.
3. Moschcowitz AV: The pathogenesis, anatomy and cure of prolapse of the rectum. *Surg Gynecol Obstet* 15:7-21, 1912.
4. Nichols DH: Types of enterocele and principles underlying choice of operation for repairs. *Obstet Gynecol* 40:257-262, 1972.
5. Zacharin RF: The use of vaginal skin graft for the treatment of recurrent recto and cystocele. *Aust New Zeal J Obstetr Gynaecol* 32:146-149, 1992.
6. Marshall VF, Marchetti AA, Krantz KE: The correction of stress incontinence by simple vesico-urethral suspension. *Surg Gynecol Obstet* 88:509, 1949.
7. Burch JC: Urethro-vaginal fixation to Cooper's ligament for correction of stress incontinence, cystocele, and prolapse. *Am J Obstet Gynecol* 81:281, 1961.
8. Vancaillie TG, Schuessler W: Laparoscopic bladder neck suspension. *J Laparoendo Surg* 1:169, 1991.
9. Bergman A, Ballard CA, Koonings PP: Comparison of three different surgical procedures for genuine stress incontinence: prospective randomized study. *Am J Obstet Gynecol* 160:1102, 1989.
10. Bergman A, Koonings PP, Ballard CA: Primary stress urinary incontinence and pelvic relaxation: prospective randomized comparison of three different operations. *Am J Obstet Gynecol* 161:91, 1989.

Chapter 25

GYNECOLOGIC CANCER

Denis Querleu
Eric Leblanc

Staging procedures for gynecologic malignancy often require surgical intervention and may become major operative procedures. In this chapter the techniques of laparoscopic lymphadenectomy will be described. Lymphadenectomy may also be considered as part of surgical therapy of gynecologic cancer. Staging procedures may thus be used in conjunction with surgical removal of the primary tumor. This applies to endometrial and possibly to early ovarian cancers, with a combination of a laparoscopic staging procedure and vaginal or laparoscopic hysterectomy. When radical hysterectomy is required, in particular for cervical cancer, classical vaginal surgery may follow laparoscopic staging.[1] Techniques of laparoscopic or laparoscopically assisted radical hysterectomy have also been described. These techniques for radical surgery of cancer are still investigational, but their feasibility has been demonstrated by several teams.[2-5] In addition, laparoscopic surgery may be used for ovarian transposition, sparing ovarian function in young women with pelvic and abdominal malignancy requiring irradiation.

LYMPHADENECTOMY

Lymphadenectomy can be part of staging or therapeutic surgical procedure.

Technique of laparoscopic pelvic lymphadenectomy

Only the techniques specific to the pelvic lymphadenectomy will be described. Positioning of the patient and a description of intraabdominal examination have been given in Chapter 12. Two ancillary 5 mm portals in the right and left lower quadrants (approximately 4 cm above the inguinal ligament and lateral to the inferior epigastric vessels) and an additional 10 mm portal in the midline 3 cm above the symphysis pubis are made (Fig. 25-1).

Interiliac lymphadenectomy is first performed as follows: The external iliac vessels and umbilical artery are identified under the peritoneal surface. The procedure begins with incision of the pelvic peritoneum between the round and infundibulopelvic ligaments, parallel to the axis of the external iliac vessels. The round ligament is grasped with a forceps, and the peritoneum is cut then easily pulled apart to open the whole area between the round and infundibulopelvic ligaments. Next the paravesical space is entered and widened by blunt dissection between the umbilical artery medially and the external iliac vessels laterally (Fig. 25-2). To achieve this, the instrument grasping the round ligament is released, closed, and placed in the paravesical space, pushing the umbilical artery medially to open the paravesical space. It is recommended that the paravesical space be opened down to the level of the pelvic floor, well under the level of the obturator pedicle. This is usually achieved without any significant bleeding. The bottom of the paravesical space will then be used to store the dissected nodes before removal, avoiding potential contamination of the peritoneal cavity by metastatic cells, as well as the small amount of lymphatic fluid and blood from the dissection area, leaving the operative field always clear.

The cellulolymphatic area below the external iliac vein is then clearly visible and safely dissected. An anterior obturator vein is usually present, joining the external iliac vein to the main obturator veins. This vessel may be dissected free or cut between clips or after electrodesiccation with bipolar forceps. The obturator nerve is identified and dissected caudally to the point at which it leaves the pelvis. The inferior aspect of the external iliac veins is separated by blunt dissection with a closed forceps. The fatty tissue between the obturator nerve and the external iliac vein is then grasped with a grasping forceps and thoroughly sepa-

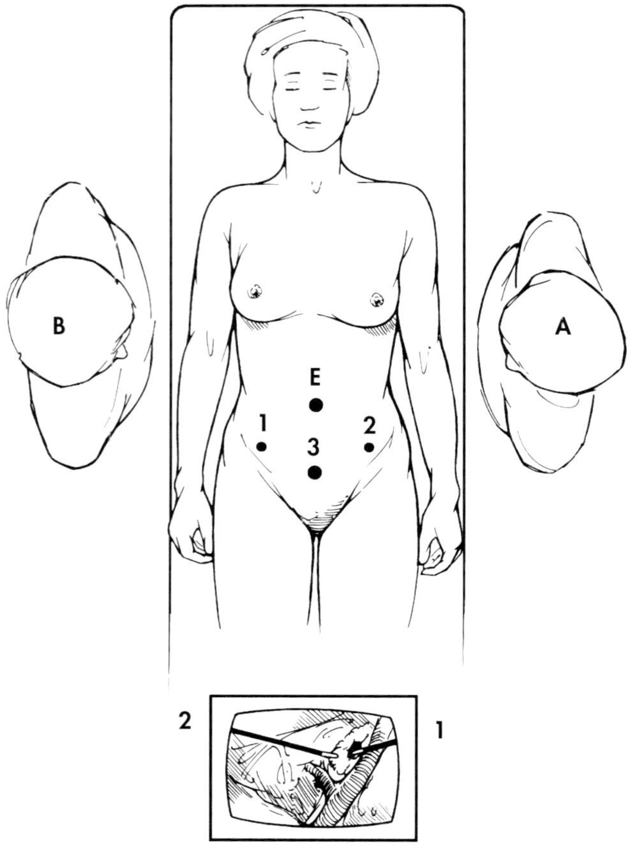

Fig. 25-1. Operating room set-up for laparoscopic pelvic lymphadenectomy, ovarian transposition, or laparoscopic preparation for radical hysterectomy. The senior surgeon **(A)** stands at the left side of the patient, the first assistant **(B)** on the right side. This position is ideal for working on the right pelvic wall and may be suitable for working on the left pelvic wall. The surgeons may have to shift to work on the left pelvic wall. The screen is placed at the feet of the patient. If two screens are available, they can be placed beside the legs of the patient, facing each surgeon. The endoscope *(E)* is introduced through the umbilicus. Two 5 mm portals *(1* and *2)* are placed 5 cm above the inguinal canals. One 10 mm portal *(3)* is placed in the midline 3 cm above the symphysis pubis.

rated from the pelvic wall by blunt dissection with the tip of an instrument held by the other hand (Fig. 25-3). At this point, the pelvic bone and the internal obturator muscle are exposed. The caudal part of the connective tissue pedicle is then detached from the area of the obturator foramen and the femoral canal. This is achieved by gentle traction. The tissue flap is firmly grasped and moved cranially, then carefully dissected bluntly from the external iliac vein and artery laterally and the umbilical artery medially.

At this point, the cellulolymphatic flap is attached only in the hypogastric bifurcation area. It is gently separated by traction and blunt dissection from the external and internal iliac artery up to the level of the division of the common iliac artery. Two methods can be used to achieve this goal: the surgeon can either follow the umbilical artery as a guide to the division of the anterior trunk of the hypogastric artery or follow the external iliac artery. In both cases, the medial aspect of the external iliac vein must be identified and carefully freed. The operation is complete only if the angle between the internal and external iliac artery is dissected.

The nodes located below the external iliac vein must also be removed. The vein can either be retracted against the pelvic wall or it can be dissected free from the pelvic wall (Fig. 25-4). The excised nodes are then extracted from the abdomen by means of the Dargent forceps through the 10 mm cannula that had been placed suprapubically in the midline. Hemostasis is confirmed. A minimal amount of blood may have to be aspirated. The same procedure is performed on the opposite side. At the end of the procedure, the peritoneum is left open to allow drainage of the lymphatic fluid into the abdominal cavity. No drain is left in place.

In some instances, removal of the nodes located outside the interiliac area may be indicated. Removal of nodes lateral to the external iliac artery requires blunt dissection between the psoas muscle and the external iliac artery, taking care not to injure the psoic artery. Removal of common iliac nodes requires the placement of an incision in the parietal peritoneum above the infundibulopelvic ligament. The ureter must be identified and displaced. Removal of presacral nodes requires extension of the peritoneal incision up to the level of the promontory and the identification of the middle sacral vessels and the left common iliac vein.

Technique of low paraaortic lymphadenectomy

The video monitor is placed at the head of the operating table, and the surgeon either stands on the side of the patient or preferably between her legs (Fig. 25-5). Although some surgeons advise a suprapubic approach, we use a transumbilical approach for the placement of the endoscope. Three additional portals are necessary (Fig. 25-5): the first designed to accommodate a 5 mm cannula to the right of the umbilicus, the second (5 or 10 mm) on the left side and the third for a 10 mm cannula midway between the umbilicus and the symphysis pubis. The two 5 mm portals are used for the introduction of scissors, forceps, bipolar forceps, and suction-irrigation cannulas. The 10 mm portal on the left side also permits the use of an endoretractor (Endoretract USSC, Norwalk, Conn.). The last 10 mm port may be used for standard 5 mm instruments with the help of an adaptor. This portal also permits the use of a clip applicator when necessary and the extraction of the nodes.

The surgeon holds the instruments introduced through the right paraumbilical and the lower (suprapubic) portals. The assistants hold the endoscope and the instrument introduced through the left paraumbilical portal (Fig. 25-5). The operating table is placed in a 10 degree Trendelenberg position and tilted to the left. The bowel is gently retracted toward the left upper quadrant. The aorta is identified under the peritoneum, up to the level of the mesenteric root.

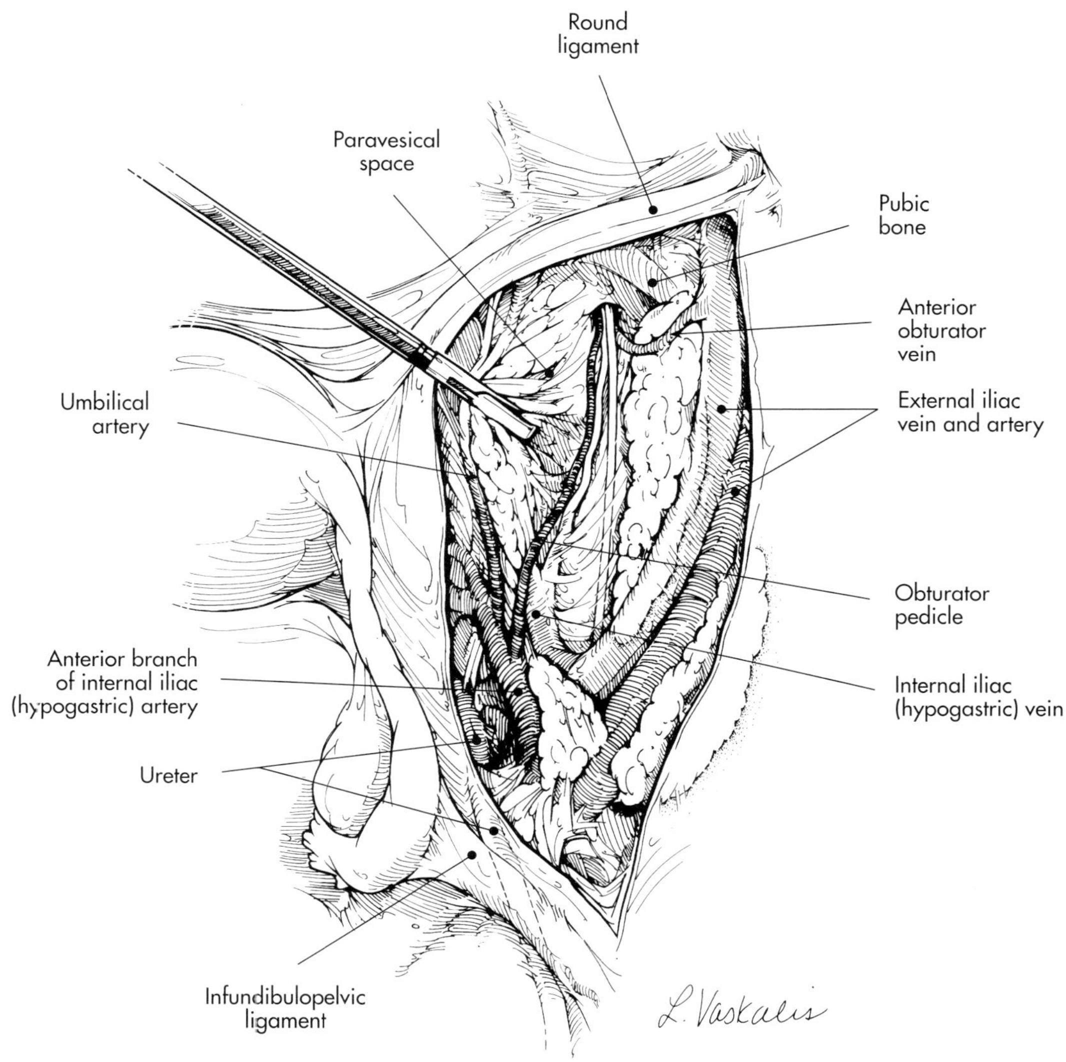

Fig. 25-2. Landmarks for laparoscopic pelvic lymphadenectomy *(right side)*. The pelvic peritoneum has been opened between the round ligament and the infundibulopelvic ligament. The ureter is left at a distance from the operative field. The paravesical space is developed by blunt dissection laterally to the umbilical artery and medially to the external iliac vein. The landmarks for interiliac dissection are the external iliac vein, the pubic bone, the obturator pedicle, the anterior branch of the internal iliac artery, the external iliac artery. Care must be taken to avoid injury to the anterior obturator vein and to the hypogastric veins. The obturator and medial external ilial lymph nodes are located under the external iliac vein and above the obturator pedicle. The hypogastric nodes are located between the external and internal iliac arteries. The nodes lateral to the external iliac artery may also be easily removed. The common iliac nodes are usually removed during the para-aortic step of the operation but may be reached through this incision of the pelvic peritoneum.

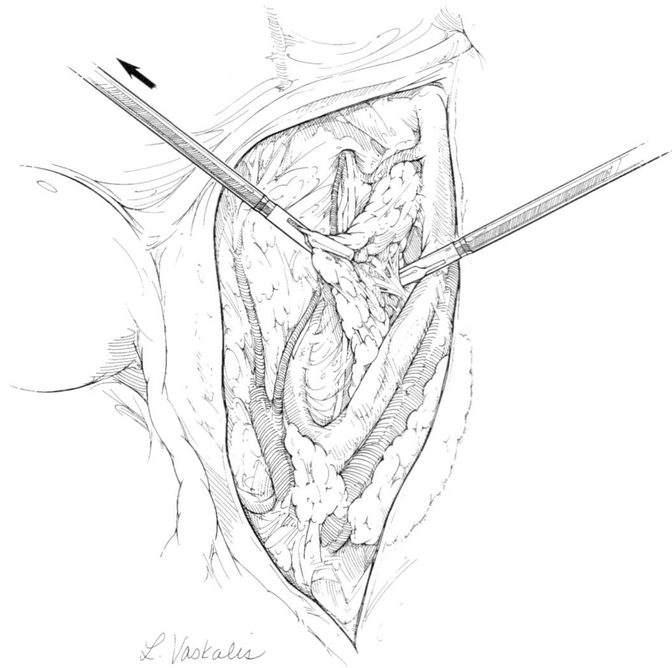

Fig. 25-3. Dissection of the obturator nodes *(right side)*. After identification of the obturator pedicle and of the inferior aspect of the external iliac vein, the lymphatic fat pad is grasped with a forceps held with the left hand. The obturator nerve, the anterior obturator vein, and the external iliac vein are freed by blunt dissection with the tip of a closed forceps or of a suction irrigation cannula. Blunt dissection is performed by a movement of the instrument parallel to the axis of the vessels.

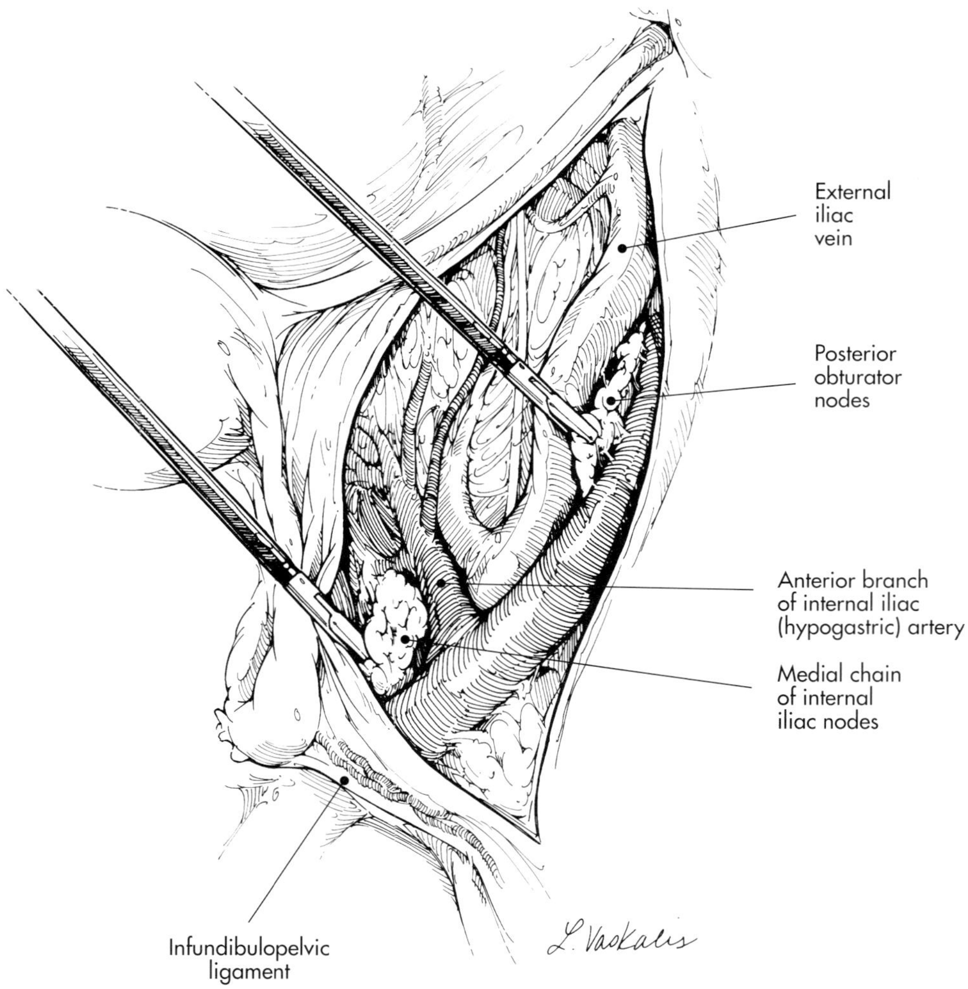

Fig. 25-4. Laparoscopic pelvic dissection, final view *(right side)*. At the end of the laparoscopic pelvic dissection, the surgeon must be able to identify the anterior branch of the hypogastric artery, to move the external iliac vein medially from the pelvic wall, to locate and remove the posterior obturator nodes under the external iliac vein, to retract the infundibulopelvic ligament cephalad and identify, if necessary, the medial chain of the internal iliac nodes up to the level of the sacral promontory.

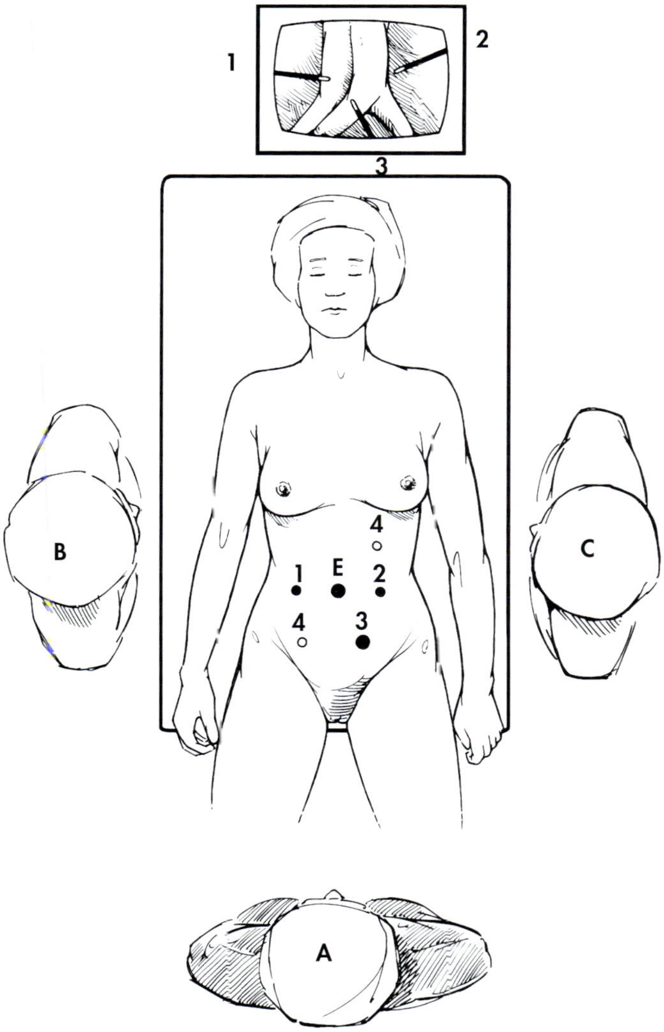

Fig. 25-5. Operating room setup for para-aortic dissection. The legs of the patient are placed at 0 degree extension, with a 30 degree angle between them. The surgeon *(A)* stands between the legs of the patient, the first assistant *(B)* at the right side. The nurse or a junior assistant *(C)* may stand at the left side. Alternately, the surgeon may stand at *B* and the first assistant at *A*. The screen is placed at the head of the patient and the videocamera is oriented to show the large vessels vertically, the lower part of the aorta being shown at the lower part of the screen. Two 5 mm ports *(1,2)* are placed 10 cm lateral to the umbilicus. A 10 mm port *(3)* is placed in the midline or slightly lateral (on the right for a right-handed surgeon). The endoscope *(E)* is introduced through the umbilicus. Additional ports *(4)* may be necessary in the left upper quandrant (for retraction of the bowel or biopsies of the diaphragmatic peritoneum) or in the right lower quandrant (for the introduction of additional instruments).

The posterior peritoneum is incised over the lower 5 cm of aorta and the first 2 cm of the right common iliac artery. The left margin of the incision is grasped by the assistant with forceps and retracted laterally to the patient's left side, ensuring in most cases the retraction of the bowel (Fig. 25-6). If this is not sufficient to move the bowel away, an incision in the left upper quadrant is necessary to introduce an additional instrument to retract the bowel loops. The anterior aspect of the aorta and of the vena cava are identified and freed by blunt dissection. The retroperitoneal space is thus developed beneath the root of the mesentery up to the transverse duodenum.

The retroperitoneal space is then developed laterally under the right and left mesocolon, and the psoas muscles are easily reached. The lumbar ureters and ovarian vessels are usually lifted along with the ascending and descending colon and readily identifiable under the mesocolon. The tip of the endoscope is placed in the retroperitoneal field. The anterior aspect of the aorta is freed up to the level of the inferior mesenteric artery. The vena cava is identified at the right side of the aorta. Its anterior aspect is easily freed. Its right aspect is identified. All the landmarks for low paraaortic dissection are thus in view.

The paraaortic cellulolymphatic pads are now ready for removal. The left lateroaortic, the precaval, interaorticocaval, and laterocaval nodal areas may be separately freed from the large vessels and removed (Fig. 25-7).

Throughout the operation, blunt dissection with the closed end of atraumatic forceps or with the tip of the suction irrigation cannula (used at the same time to clear the operative field when necessary) seems to provide the safest way of freeing the cellulolymphatic flaps. Electrosurgery with monopolar or bipolar scissors may also be used. As soon as part of a flap is freed from the great vessels, it may be firmly grasped with a forceps and elevated to show its posterior aspect, overlying the vessels or the prevertebral plane. Care must be taken during dissection from the great vessels. All of the small vessels going to or coming from the major vessels must be electrodesiccated with bipolar forceps or occluded using clips. The lumbar veins must be identified, particularly beneath the aorta, just in front of the prevertebral fascia. When moderate bleeding occurs, the surgeon must remain calm and use compression with the tip of a closed atraumatic forceps or the aspiration irrigation cannula. The bleeding stops either spontaneously or after hemostasis has been secured with clips or electrodesiccation.

Technique of infrarenal paraaortic dissection

Paraaortic node dissection for staging ovarian carcinomas must be extended to the level of the renal vein and include removal of the nodes related to the origin of the ovarian vessels.

The operation begins as a low para-aortic dissection. The instrument introduced through the left portal, held by the assistant, is then placed in the middle retroperitoneal space, lifting the transverse duodenum.

Further dissection is carried out to identify the left renal vein. The dissection proceeds up to the origins of the ovarian arteries. Both ovarian arteries have to be divided once occluded by electrodesiccation (see Fig. 25-6 and 25-7).

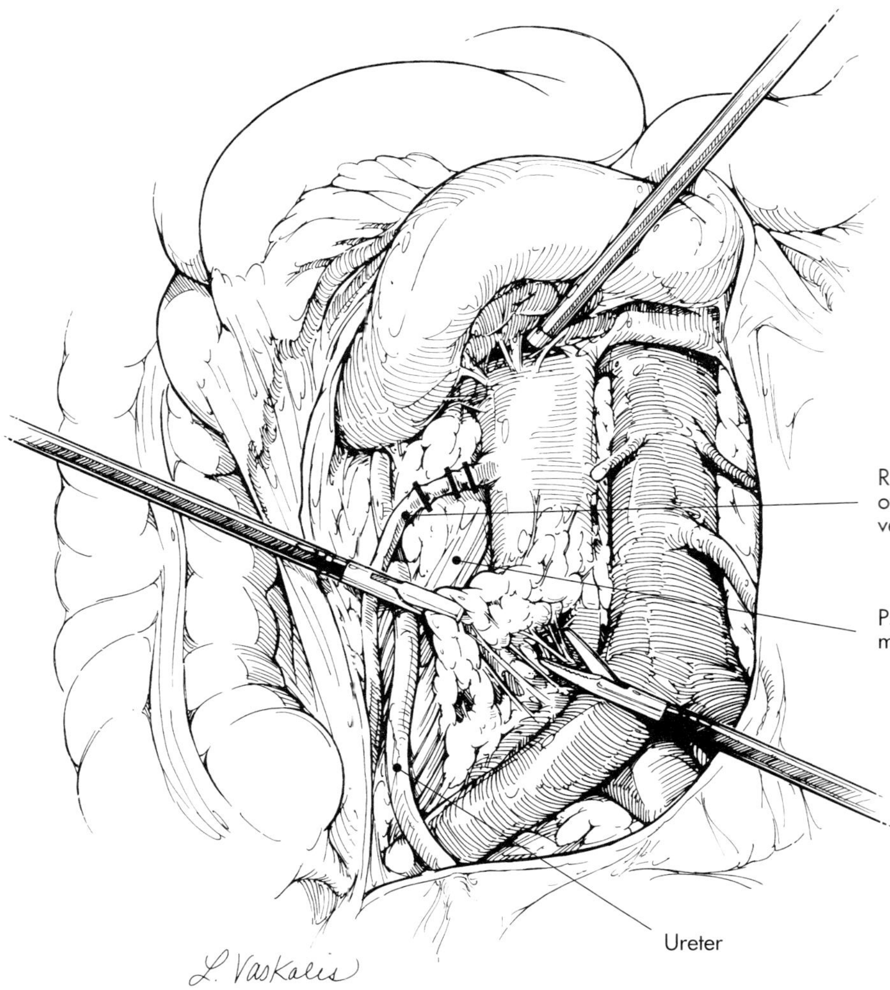

Fig. 25-6. Access to the para-aortic area and dissection of the laterocaval and precaval nodes. The posterior peritoneum has been opened along the right common iliac artery and the aorta, up to the level of the transverse duodenum. The instrument introduced through port 1 (see Fig. 26-5) is used to develop the retroperitoneal space on the right side, showing the ovarian vein, the ureter, and the psoas muscle. The same instrument is later used to grasp the nodes. The instrument introduced through port 2 moves the mesentery root upward or alternately may be used to clean the operative field by irrigation and suction. Scissors or instruments for blunt dissection are introduced through port 3. This port is also used to introduce bipolar or current clips. The placement of clips on the ovarian vein is shown.

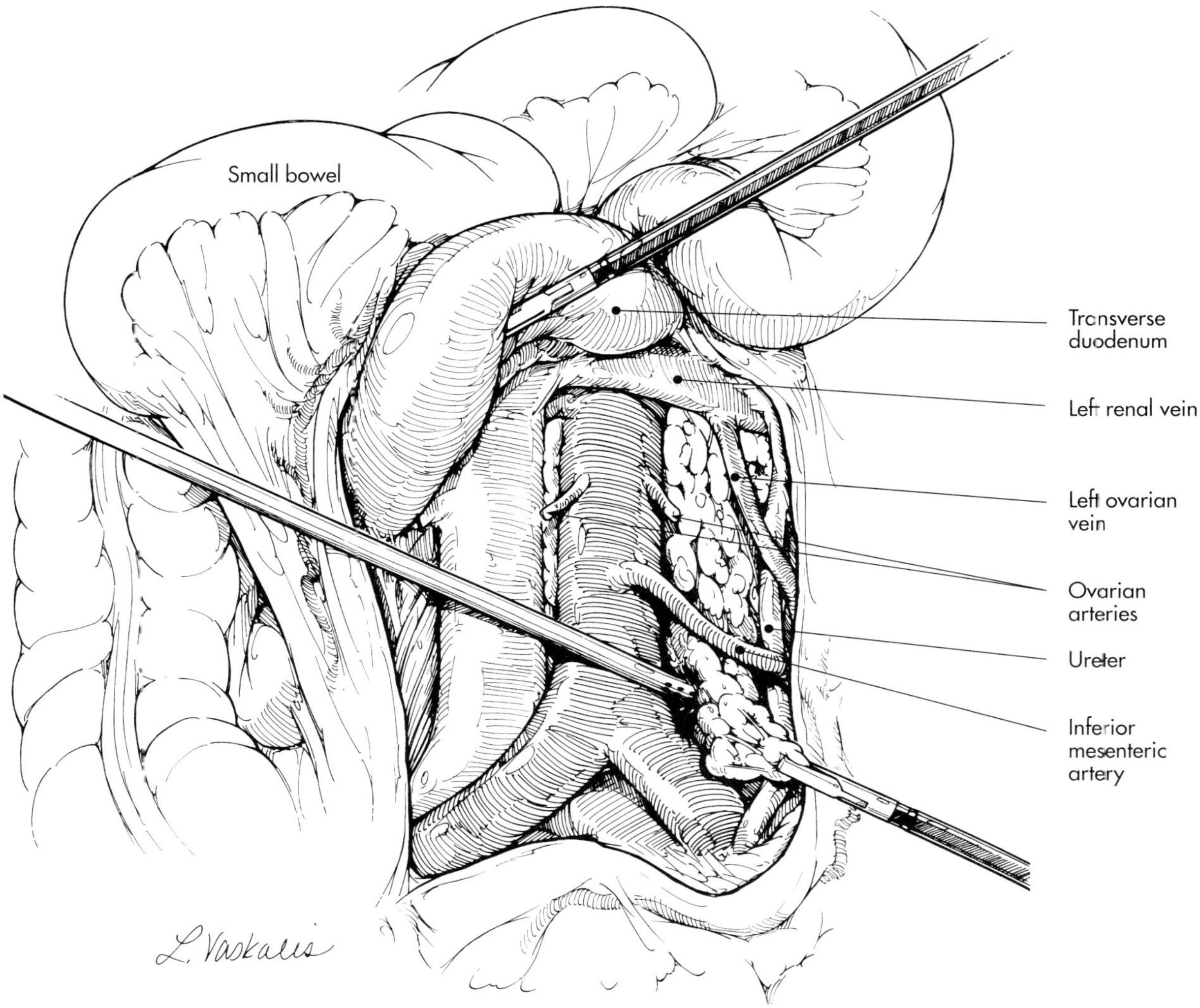

Fig. 25-7. Dissection of the left lateroaortic nodes. Port 2 (see Fig. 26-5) is used to grasp the left aspect of the peritoneal incision or later to lift the transverse duodenum. Opening the upper part of the dissection and retracting the bowel exposes the left renal vein. The small bowel loops are gently placed in the left upper quadrant. An instrument introduced through port 1 is used to secure hemostasis and for sharp or blunt dissection. Dissection of nodes with the tip of the suction cannula is shown. Instrument 3 is used to develop the retroperitoneal space and to identify the ureter and the inferior mesenteric artery and later to grasp the nodes. The ovarian arteries have been cut after electrodesiccation to open the upper part of the operative field. It is then possible to identify the lateral part of the left renal vein and the left ovarian vein.

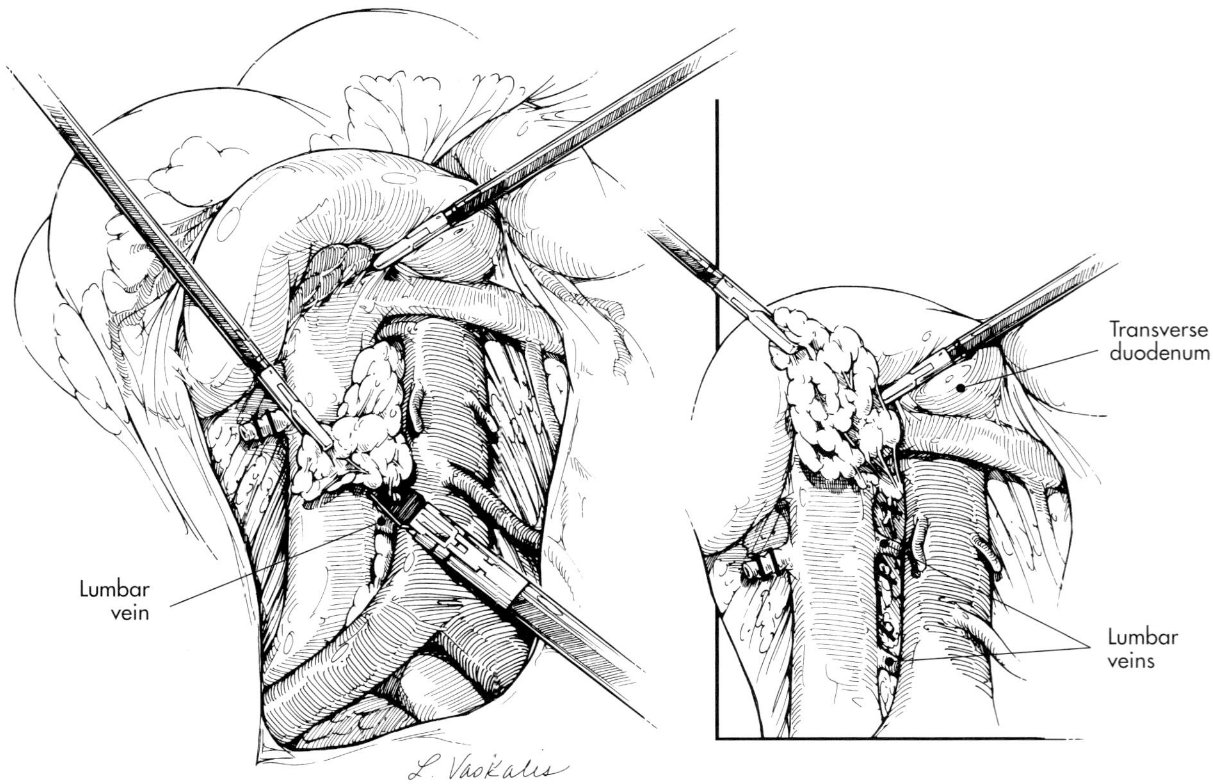

Fig. 25-8. Dissection of the interaorticocaval area. Instrument 2 (see Fig. 25-5) retracts the transverse duodenum and shows the medial part of the left renal vein. Instrument 1 lifts the nodes, showing the posterior attachments to the prevertebral fascia. Care must be taken to avoid injury of the lumbar veins. Instrument 3 is used for hemostasis and/or sharp dissection. The placement of clips is shown. Blunt dissection is not recommended in this area. *(Inset)* The final step of the dissection is shown: the lymphatic pad is lifted and the last attachment to the angle between the vena cava and the left renal vein is freed.

This step is essential to allow elevation of the peritoneum and the viscera, providing space for a true panoramic endoscopic view of the retroperitoneal space and giving access to the left renal vein. The endoretractor (introduced through a 10 mm left portal) at this stage is most helpful in exposing the operative field.

Sampling of the laterocaval fat pad may require section of the cephalic end of the right ovarian vein. The vein is dessicated using bipolar current; then three clips are used, two near the vena cava and one lateral to the section. The right lumbar ureter, the psoas muscle, the right lumbar veins, and the right aspect of the vena cava are thoroughly identified, allowing the removal of the laterocaval nodes.

The left side of the aorta is freed distal and proximal to the origin of the inferior mesenteric artery. The left ovarian vein and the left lumbar ureter are identified. The left lateroaortic nodes are now ready for removal by blunt dissection. The cephalic end of the left ovarian vein may have to be divided between clips (Fig. 25-7). Usually, identification of the place where the left ovarian vein empties into the left renal vein is enough, as the nodes are located medially to the ovarian vein.

The procedure is completed with the removal of the precaval, preaortic, and interaorticocaval nodes. The cellulolymphatic flap is grasped and moved away from the vessels and from the prevertebral fascia. In the area between the aorta and the vena cava, two or three lumbar veins are present. Injury to these is a serious complication. To avoid this injury, the interaorticocaval flap is separated from the prevertebral plane using clips and scissors, beginning at the caudal part of the dissection. At the end of the dissection, the interaorticocaval flap is perpendicular to the axis of the great vessels. It is detached from the left renal vein, again using clips to secure hemostasis (Fig. 25-8).

Interiliac lymphadenectomy by retroperitoneal approach

After some historic attempts at elective node sampling using modified mediastinoscopes, Dargent and Salvat[6] were the first to use a panoramic retroperitoneal approach for pelvic lymphadenectomy. They have been performing interiliac dissection. This technique is being replaced, even by these authors, by the transumbilical approach. Indeed, the transumbilical transperitoneal approach that we have been using since 1988 is simpler to perform and allows us to complete not only an interiliac dissection but also a number of additional staging or therapeutic procedures. However, the retroperitoneal technique may still have to be used when the laparoscopic approach is contraindicated or impossible due to intraperitoneal adhesions.

The description of Dargent's technique follows.[1,6] The operation begins with a 3 cm transverse incision 3 cm above the symphysis pubis. The space of Retzius is opened with the finger, and the two Cooper ligaments are palpated. The preperitoneal and retroparietal spaces are then digitally developed on both sides of the midline. The laparoscopic 10 mm cannula is introduced in the preperitoneal space, a continuous suture is placed on the cutaneous opening to avoid a loss of gas, and CO_2 insufflated through the sheath of the cannula.

The videoendoscope is introduced. Three ancillary portals are made, one in the midline in the infraumbilical area and two in the right and left inguinal areas. The middle and the right instruments are used for the dissection of the right side, the middle and the left instruments for the dissection of the left side. One of the instruments is used to retract the peritoneal sac upward. The other one allows the surgeon to identify and bluntly free the external iliac vessels up to the level of the bifurcation of the common iliac artery and the obturator nerve. The nodal tissue is prepared but not completely separated from the vessels. It will be removed later with the help of the coelioextractor. The 5 mm cannula trocar is replaced by a 10 mm cannula to accommodate this instrument.

Dargent has performed this operation more than 200 times. The node yield from the interiliac region is the same as that obtained by laparotomy, six to seven nodes on each side. The survival of patients with stage IB and IIA cervical cancers treated by a radical vaginal hysterectomy combined with a retroperitoneal endoscopic lymphadenectomy is excellent (95% 3-year survival in node-negative patients). However, the laparotomy rate is high (5% overall, 14% in previously operated patients), compared with the zero laparotomy rate that we have observed in a large series of laparoscopic lymphadenectomies (see below).

Complications of laparoscopic lymphadenectomy

Potential complications of lymphadenectomy include hemorrhage secondary to laceration of the external iliac vein, vena cava, or the inferior mesenteric artery. Ureteral injury may occur during pelvic or para-aortic dissection by laparotomy and is certainly a potential hazard of laparoscopic lymphadenectomy.

A high proportion of complications has been observed in the early experience of urological teams.[7,8] Kavoussi et al., in 1993, reported the combined experience of eight medical centers.[7] The procedure was impossible in 16 of 372 patients due to technical difficulties or to obesity. Fifty-five complications occurred; 13 of them required open surgery. Vascular, bowel, bladder, or ureteral injury were encountered. Deep venous thrombosis occurred in five cases, functional or mechanical bowel obstruction in seven. The difficulties of managing male patients with urologic malignancy may partially explain these rather poor results. The male urologic patient is on average older, the anatomy is different, the areolar tissues are usually dense, and a history of previous surgery is more frequent. However, the authors note the effects of the learning curve, with a high proportion of complications occurring in their early experience. The overall complication rate was as low as 3% in the later cases in their series. Urologic surgeons reproduced the technique used by experienced laparoscopic gynecologists and had to learn laparoscopic surgery. The same learning curve applies to gynecologic oncologists.

The early experience of gynecologists is different. However, significant numbers of cases were published only by teams experiences both in oncologic surgery and in laparoscopic surgery. The complication rate was very low in Childers et al. series.[9] In 61 cases considered candidates for para-aortic lymphadenectomy, these authors failed to perform the procedure in only four instances and observed no significant postoperative complication.

In our series of 166 cases, only seven intraoperative complications were observed. One patient did not tolerate the prolonged pneumoperitoneum and we had to abandon the procedure after removal of only three nodes. In an other case, bleeding from the umbilical artery required bipolar desiccation of the vessel. In a third case, injury to an epigastric artery at the site of an ancillary portal required repair. In one patient venous bleeding in the left paravesical space was controlled by compression with the endoscopic forceps. In a fifth woman venous bleeding near the origin of the right ovarian vein was observed during a right infrarenal node sampling. Tearing of the origin of the right ovarian artery in another patient led to pulsatile bleeding from the aorta; the complication was managed by application of bipolar current. Finally, one injury to the external iliac vein has been laparoscopically controlled and treated by an over and over suture with nonabsorbable thread. No unintended laparotomy was necessary during the period under consideration.

When laparoscopic pelvic lymphadenectomy was performed as the only procedure, the postoperative period was uneventful and the patients were discharged from the surgical ward the following day in all but one case. In this patient, a spontaneously resolving pelvic hematoma was observed 5 days after laparoscopic pelvic lymphadenectomy and radium application. Two pelvic lymphocysts were observed, and ecchymosis of the flank was observed in two cases of paraaortic lymphadenectomy.

Careful patient selection is required. Obese patients, in whom para-aortic or even pelvic dissection is problematic even by laparotomy and those with extensive intraabdominal adhesions or with severe respiratory or cardiovascular disease should be excluded. This also applies to patients with positive fine needle aspiration of metastatic nodes detected by noninvasive procedures such as lymphangiography or CAT scan. Laparoscopic lymphadenectomy is a true surgical operation, with potential complications. Patients must be aware that an unintended laparotomy may have to be performed.

TOTAL HYSTERECTOMY

The recent advances in laparoscopic surgery have included developments in the concept of laparoscopic hysterectomy (LH) or laparoscopically assisted vaginal hysterectomy (LAVH). Vaginal hysterectomy may also be used and is our first choice for hysterectomy in benign conditions. In oncology, it is important to avoid manipulation or morcellation of the uterus or ovaries, and some part of the operation must be done laparoscopically to avoid any trauma to the diseased uterus or ovary. The vaginal surgeon will favor the shorter and cheaper LAVH, in which only the upper uterine ligaments are divided laparoscopically, leaving all the subsequent steps for the vaginal approach.

Laparoscopically assisted vaginal hysterectomy

The set-up is the same as that used for pelvic node dissection. In uterine disease, the uterus is not cannulated. To divide the ovarian ligaments, some authors use sutures, staplers, or clips. We use bipolar electrodesiccation. On each side, the adnexa is grasped and brought medially. The ureter is identified under the peritoneum but not dissected. The ovarian ligament is skeletonized by incision of its peritoneal surface, to enable more efficient electrodesiccation of its vessels using bipolar forceps. Current is applied and the vessels are gradually occluded and divided. All of the vessels must be secured before completing the division of the whole ligament. The round ligament is divided with scissors after bipolar electrodesiccation or divided using a monopolar electrode which achieves hemostasis simultaneously. The peritoneum between the round and ovarian ligaments is incised.

The upper pedicles of the uterus having been secured and divided, the procedure is completed vaginally. The patient is placed in full lithotomy position. The vagina is incised, the pouch of Douglas is opened, and the vesicouterine space is bluntly developed. Retractors are placed in the pouch of Douglas and in the vesicouterine space. The cardinal and uterosacral ligaments are secured and divided. The vesicouterine pouch is entered and the uterine arteries are secured and divided (see Chapter 22). The uterus and ovaries (if they have also been excised) can then be pulled out of the pelvis. The peritoneum and vagina are closed from below.

LAPAROSCOPIC RADICAL HYSTERECTOMY (LRH) AND LAPAROSCOPICALLY ASSISTED RADICAL VAGINAL HYSTERECTOMY (LARVH)

Laparoscopic radical hysterectomies[2,3] and laparoscopically assisted radical vaginal hysterectomies[4,5] were described a few years after the first reports of laparoscopic lymphadenectomy.

The term "radical" hysterectomy includes many different operations.[10] We use only two terms, referring to two operations that are different in radicality. "Proximal" or "modified" radical hysterectomy refers to those procedures in which only the proximal part of the parametria is excised medially to the level of the ureters and corresponds to the Piver type 2 or 3. "Distal" or "classical" radical hysterectomy is the procedure that removes the entire parametria, up to their insertion to the pelvic side wall, and corresponds to the Piver type 4.

In the first cases of laparoscopic radical hysterectomy (LRH) presented in the literature, early (IA) cervical cancers were removed by a procedure reproducing modified radical hysterectomy.[2,3] A pelvic lymphadenectomy was performed, with or without limited para-aortic node sampling. The ovarian, uterine, and cervical pedicles were dessicated with bipolar current and divided with the carbon dioxide laser or with scissors. The ureters were unroofed, the rectovaginal and vesicovaginal spaces were developed, and the parametria were cut laparoscopically. The vagina and some part of the remaining paracolpos was incised vaginally. However, the radicality of the procedure was less than ideal. These operations are similar to extrafascial simple hysterectomies and are adequate for the treatment of early (IA2) cervical cancers. The procedure takes much longer when performed by laparoscopy (up to 420 minutes).

In laparoscopically assisted radical vaginal hysterectomy (LARVH), an oncologic surgeon familiar with both laparoscopic surgery and radical vaginal hysterectomy is able to take advantage of the benefits of both routes in the same patient. Laparoscopic surgery is well suited to lymph node dissection and gives a direct view of the ureters and of the origin of the uterine arteries. Vaginal surgery allows precise incision of the vaginal cuff. Both routes may be used for the section of parametria at the appropriate level to ensure a true radical excision (Fig. 25-9). The combination of these two approaches may prove to be the most logical technique for surgical therapy of cervical carcinomas in the future, avoiding the discomfort of both laparotomy and of perineotomy.

Surgical technique of modified radical hysterectomy

"Proximal" or modified radical hysterectomy is indicated for early (stage IB, less than 2 cm wide or not exceeding 10 cc, or stage IB, after primary brachytherapy*) may be performed by laparoscopy. The laparoscopic approach effectively follows the steps of the technique used at laparotomy. The basic difference between the two techniques is in the way hemostasis is achieved.

We believe that the same operation may be done more quickly, more easily, and more radically using concurrent laparoscopic and vaginal approaches. Ureteral dissection and lymphadenectomy are effected by laparoscopy; incision

*Radium or cesium therapy.

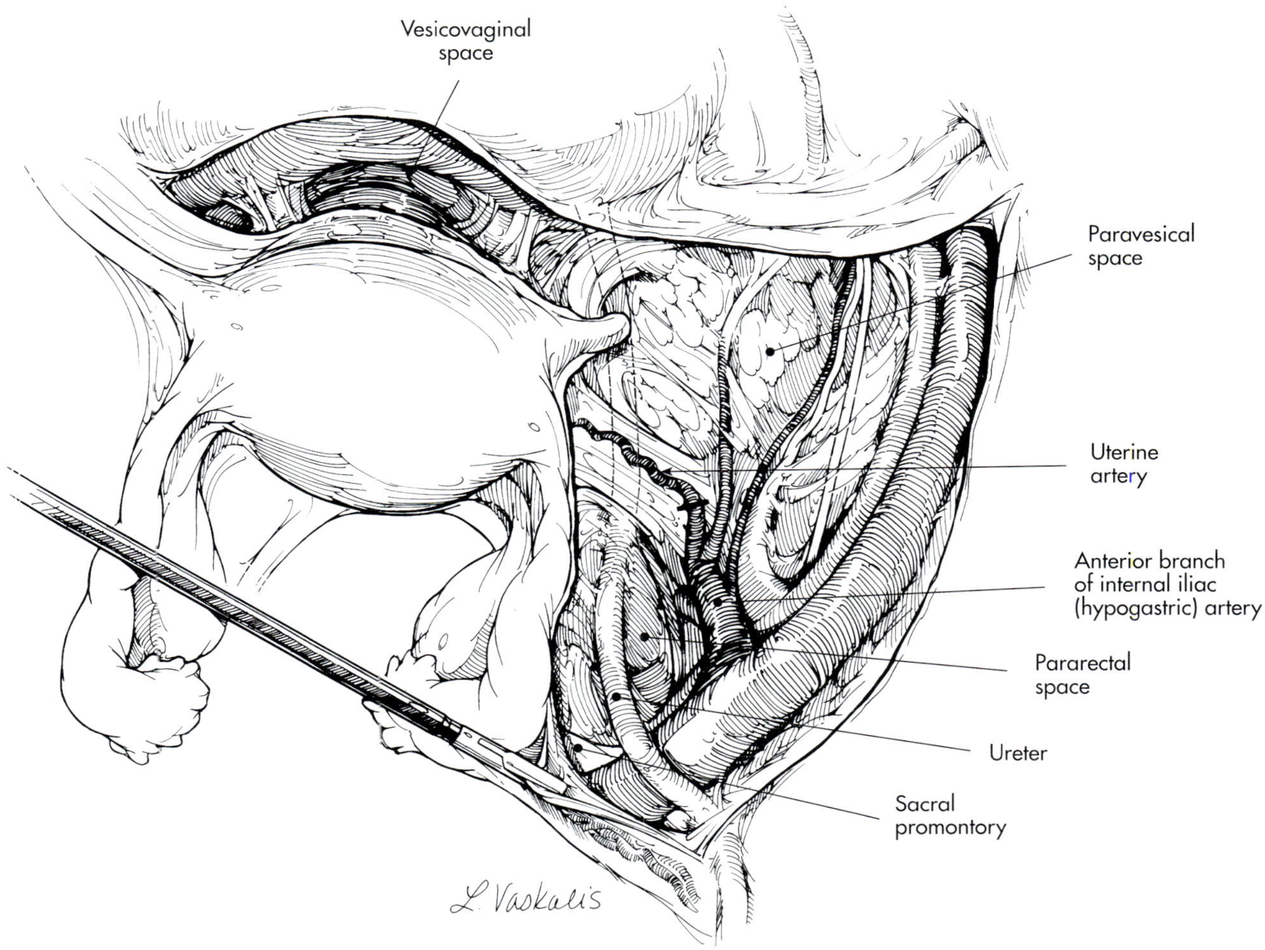

Fig. 25-9. Laparoscopic preparation for radical hysterectomy. The laparoscopic technique for radical hysterectomy is similar to the standard laparotomy technique. The surgeon must identify and develop the paravesical space by blunt dissection, the pararectal space, and the vesicovaginal space. The uterine artery or the anterior branch of the hypogastric artery are divided after hemostasis has been secured. The ureter is freed from the vagina, the overlying uterine artery, and the underlying cardinal ligament. The lateral pelvic peritoneum is incised; the medial aspect of the incised peritoneum is grasped. The ureter is identified from the iliac vessels and the promontory area to its crossing of the uterine artery. All these steps are quite easy to accomplish under laparoscopic visualization.

of the vaginal cuff and section of the proximal parametria are performed by the vaginal route.[4] A description of this technique follows.

Bilateral pelvic lymphadenectomy and, when required, para-aortic dissection are performed first (see above). The portals for this part of the operation will be used for the preparation of the vaginal radical hysterectomy. The ureter is identified at the point at which it crosses the iliac vessels. The ovarian ligaments (in cases of salpingo-oophorectomy) or the uteroovarian vessels (in cases of ovarian conservation) and the round ligaments are cut. The broad ligaments are incised.

The ureter is identified from the pelvic brim to the level of the uterine artery (Fig. 25-10). For this purpose, the incised posterior leaf of the broad ligament is grasped and brought medially, showing the ureter running on the deep surface. The ureter is easily moved by gentle blunt dissection. Its crossing of the uterine artery is identified. A clear, magnified view of the posterior opening of the ureteral tunnel is usually obtained.

Separation of the ureter from the uterine artery may be accomplished in two ways. The ureteral tunnel may be delineated with the help of a laparoscopic dissector (Microfrance, Bourbon-l'Archambault, France), then the uterine

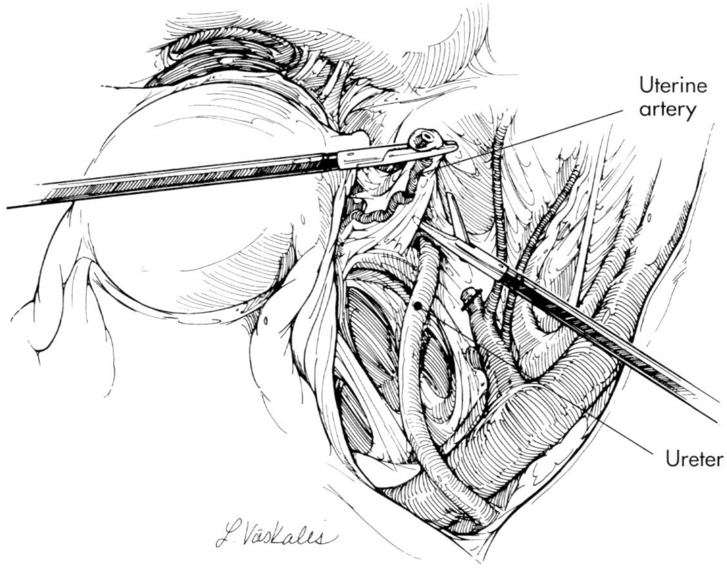

Fig. 25-10. Laparoscopic separation of the ureter and uterine artery. The ureter can be unroofed by section of the uterine pedicle above it. The technique shown in this illustration is probably safer. The uterine artery is divided. Its medial stump is grasped and brought medially, uncovering the ureter. The ureter is freed by sharp dissection; bipolar electrodesiccation of uterine veins overlying the ureter may be necessary.

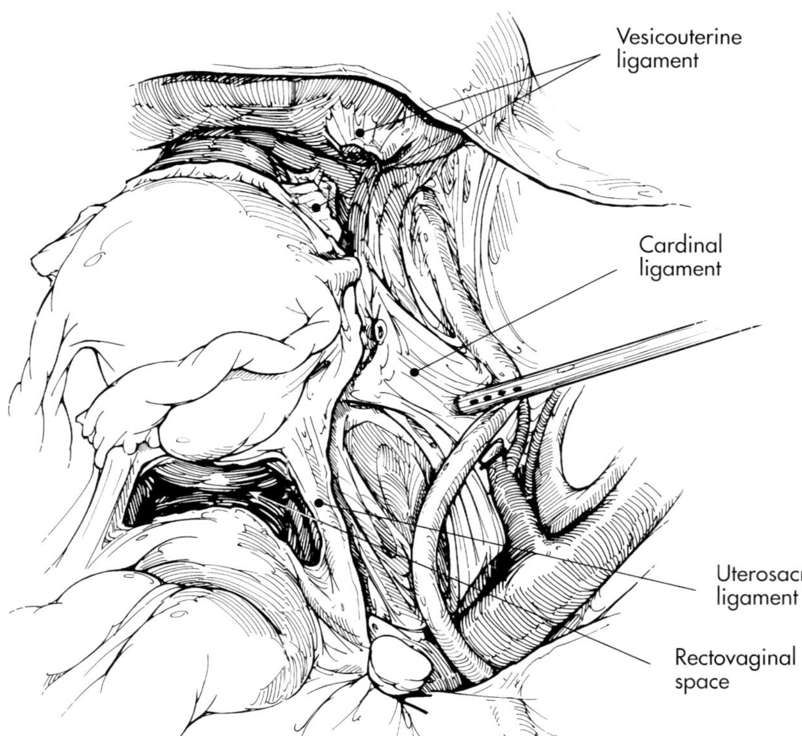

Fig. 25-11. Laparoscopic dissection of the terminal ureter. After unroofing the ureter, the vesicouterine ligament is divided to free the terminal ureter and the bladder base from the cervix. The ureter is moved laterally by blunt dissection, revealing the underlying cardinal ligament. The rectovaginal space is developed between the uterosacral ligaments. The proximal part of the cardinal ligament is thus ready for division, and a modified radical hysterectomy is completed. These last steps may be accomplished by laparoscopy or per vagina, defining laparoscopic radical hysterectomy and laparoscopically assisted radical hysterectomy, respectively.

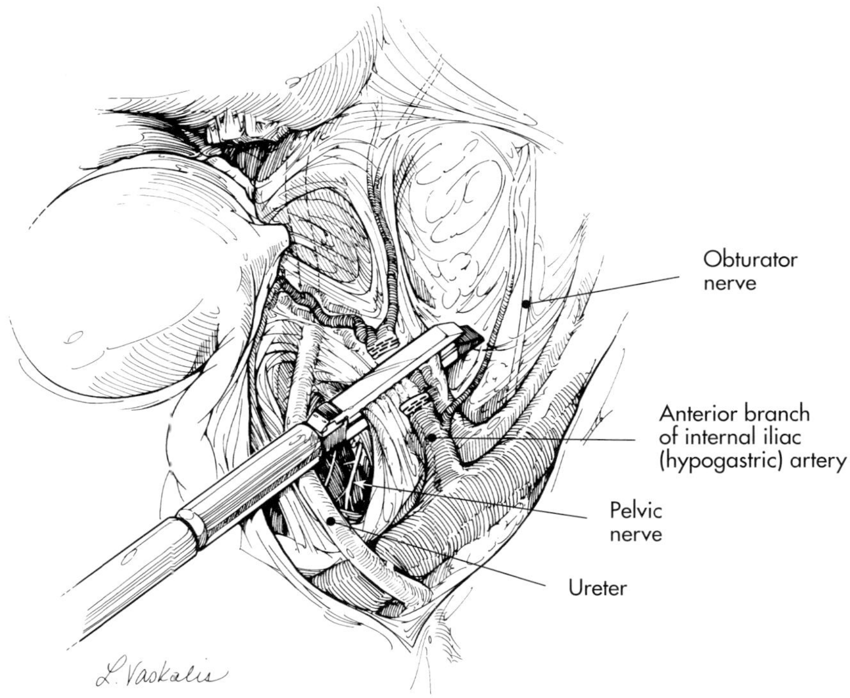

Fig. 25-12. Laparoscopic transection of the cardinal ligament at the pelvic wall. The paravesical and pararectal spaces have been developed. The pelvic nerve has been identified and may be preserved with the goal of reducing the rate of postoperative urinary retention. The anterior branch of the hypogastric artery has been divided with a shot of the GIA stapler. The stapler is then placed around the pelvic insertion of the cardinal ligament, taking care not to include the ureter or the obturator nerve. Transection of the cardinal ligament at this point defines radical hysterectomy. The operation may be completed vaginally (Dargent technique of "coeliio-Schauta") or by laparoscopy.

pedicle is cut after bipolar desiccation or placement of clips. We prefer the following method: The origin of the uterine artery is identified at the level of the anterior branch of the hypogastric artery (this artery has been identified during the lymphadenectomy). It is skeletonized by blunt dissection in order to place clips or, preferably, to apply bipolar current. The visceral stump of the uterine artery is then grasped and brought medially to display the ureter. Bipolar current may have to be applied to uterine veins running above the ureter (Fig. 25-10).

After unroofing, further separation of the ureter is obtained by section of the cephalic part of the vesicouterine ligament (Figs. 25-11 and 25-12). The bladder base and the terminal ureter are then freed from the cervix. Finally, the ureter is further mobilized from the cervix and vagina by blunt dissection. It must be entirely freed from the vaginal wall to ensure the safety of the vaginal step of the operation: only the properly freed terminal ureters can be moved away by a retractor placed under the bladder base. At this point, the LARVH operation will differ from the LRH operation. In the LRH operation, the cardinal ligament should be electrodesiccated or stapled and divided 2 cm from the cervix after further laparoscopic separation of the bladder and rectum and laparoscopic division of the uterosacral ligaments (Fig. 25-12). In the LARVH operation, the operation is completed vaginally (Figs. 25-13 and 25-14).

The vaginal operation begins with the incision of the vagina and the division of the proximal parametrium. No perineal incision is required. The vagina is grasped with forceps and incised circumferentially 2 to 3 cm from the fornices or at the level required by the lesion (the normal vagina can be delineated by iodine application). A vaginal cuff is formed with Krobak forceps, as described for classical vaginal radical surgery.[11] The vesicovaginal and rectovaginal space are developed by blunt dissection. The pararectal spaces are entered. The uterosacral ligaments are then identified and divided, improving the mobility of the cervix.

The paravesical spaces are entered and partially developed on each side. After a limited opening is made in the paravesical space, the ureter can be palpated between two fingers, one placed in the paravesical space and the second one in the vesicovaginal space. The lower and medial part of the vesicouterine ligament is then divided, under the level of the ureteral "knee" (see Fig. 25-13).

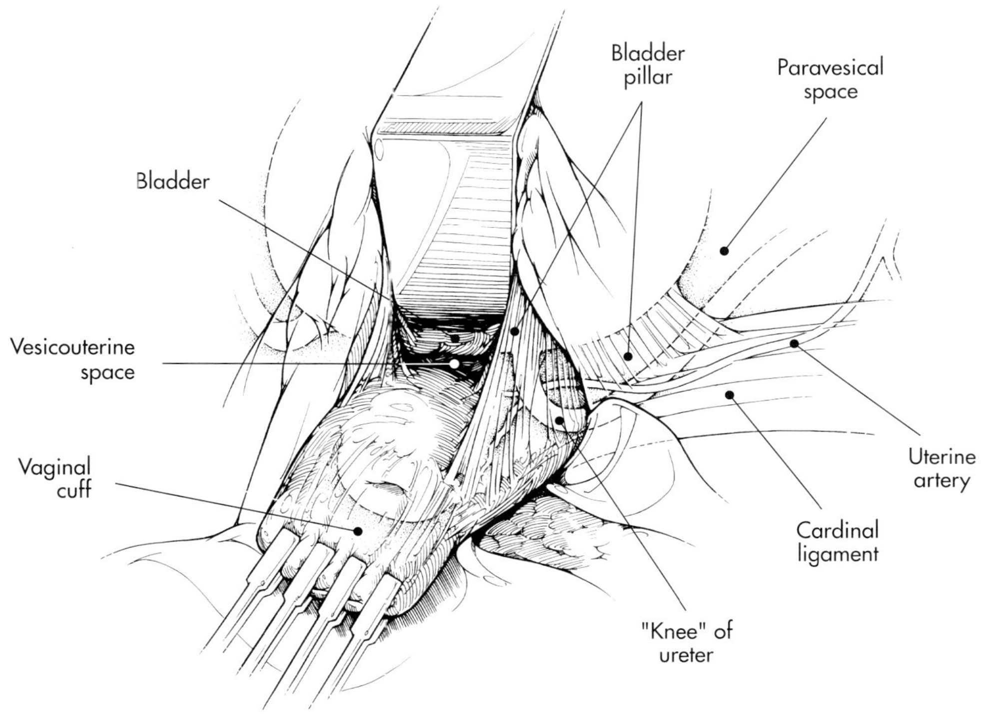

Fig. 25-13. The anatomic landmarks of the Schauta technique. We recommend ending the operations of radical or modified radical hysterectomy by the vaginal route. This method is shorter, but requires training in radical vaginal surgery. After incision of the vagina at the required distance from the cervix, a vaginal cuff is created with forceps. The paravesical space and the vesicouterine space are opened. Traction on the vaginal cuff and simultaneous retraction of the bladder by a retractor in the opposite direction distorts the anatomy. The uterer is pulled downward as it is attached to the bladder pillar, joining the cardinal ligament to the bladder. The lower point of the ureter is called the knee. The uterine artery seems to come into the operative field from this knee. The ureter is identified by palpation and freed after section of the external and internal part of the bladder pillar. After laparoscopic preparation, this operation is made easier due to dissection of the ureter (Querleu technique) or to section of the cardinal ligament (Dargent technique).

The cardinal ligaments are then divided at the required level, about 2 cm lateral to cervix. The left side is usually divided first. A retractor is placed under the left part of the bladder base, lifting the already separated ureter. Two clamps are placed on the proximal parametrium. The right parametrium is prepared and cut in the same fashion. Finally, the peritoneal cul-de-sacs are entered and the specimen is removed. The vesical and rectal peritoneum are approximated in the midline. The vagina is closed, leaving a rubber tube for drainage.

Surgical technique of classical radical hysterectomy

In our version of the operation, the laparoscopic part of the procedure includes lymphadenectomy, division of the ovarian vessels and the origin of the uterine arteries, and dissection of the ureter down to the level of the bladder (Fig. 25-14, *A*). The vaginal step of the operation is completed as already described, but the parametria are divided at their insertion on the pelvic wall.

In the Dargent version of the operation,[5] the ureter is identified but not dissected laparoscopically. The paravesical and pararectal spaces are developed laparoscopically. The pelvic nerve is identified in the pararectal space and may sometimes be left intact to spare the patient the usual voiding difficulties associated with radical hysterectomy. The anterior branch of the hypogastric artery and the pelvic wall insertion of the parametria are divided by the use of a stapler (Fig. 25-14, *C*). The operation is then completed vaginally. The vagina is incised, the uterosacral ligaments are divided, and the paravesical and pararectal spaces are entered according to the classical Schauta-Amreich technique.[11] The ureters are palpated in the vesicovaginal pillars (Fig. 25-13). The medial and lateral part of the pillars are then divided and the ureters are fully dissected. The uterine artery is grasped and dissected up to its origin. The operation ends with the division of the ovarian ligaments. The degree of radicality is impressive. Due to the primary section of the cardinal ligaments, the vaginal dissection of the

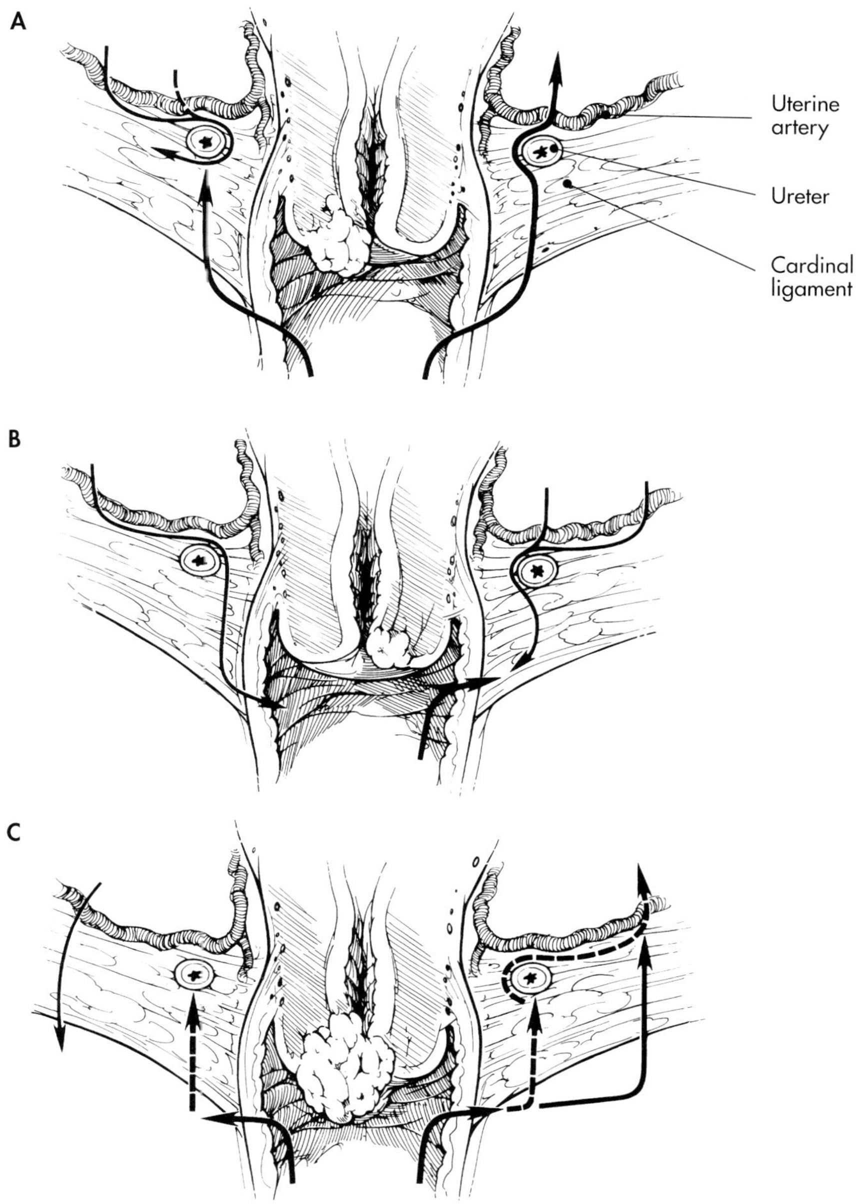

Fig. 25-14. Sketch representation of different radical hysterectomy techniques. The arrows coming from above show the laparoscopic steps of the operation, the arrows coming from below show the vaginal steps. **A,** Modified radical hysterectomy (MRH). On the right side of the drawing, the standard vaginal MRH (Schauta-Stoeckel technique). On the left side, Querleu's laparoscopically assisted vaginal technique, with section of the uterine artery at its origin *(full line)* or at the level of its crossing of the ureter *(dotted line)*. **B,** Modified radical hysterectomy. On the right side of the drawing, the technique described by Canis et al. and by Nezhat et al. Some part of the operation is done vaginally after partial section of the proximal part of the cardinal ligament. On the left side of the picture, a theoric sketch of the full laparoscopic operation. **C,** Radical hysterectomy. On the right side of the drawing, the standard Schauta-Amreich technique, with freeing the ureter and the uterine artery *(dotted line),* then section of the distal part of the cardinal ligament *(full line).* On the left side of the drawing, the laparoscopically assisted (Dargent) technique, with primary section of the cardinal ligament by laparoscopy, then vaginal separation of the ureter from the bladder pillar *(dotted line).*

ureters is amazingly easy and bloodless. A Schuchardt perineal incision is avoided in all cases, reducing the discomfort of the postoperative period.

Radical hysterectomy with partial cystectomy (type 5) is rarely carried out. In one of our cases, a laparoscopic dissection of bowel adhesions and of both ureters allowed us to perform a safe removal of a cervical stump using the vaginal route. The involvement of the detrusor muscle by the malignancy required partial cystectomy that was performed from below during the vaginal step of the operation.

Results of LRH and LARVH

Nezhat et al. have reported their experience of 19 cases, including 10 IA2 cervical cancers but also 8 stage IB and one IIA patients.[12] One procedure was converted to laparotomy. The average operative time was 315 minutes for LRH and 163 minutes for LARVH, suggesting that this method is probably the best choice for modified radical hysterectomies. There were two minor postoperative complications (one urinary tract infection, one incisional bleeding). The postoperative hospital stay averaged 2.1 days.

Querleu has operated upon eight cases between November, 1990, and December, 1992.[13] He successfully completed all eight radical hysterectomies—four modified, three distal, one with cystectomy. In all except the carcinoma of the cervical stump with no visible uterine artery, the ureters were dissected and the uterine arteries divided laparoscopically. The distal cardinal ligaments were divided laparoscopically in one case and vaginally in two. The proximal cardinal ligaments were divided vaginally in all modified operations. A perineal incision was avoided in all cases. The operative blood loss was less than 300 ml in six cases, but two cases required transfusions for blood loss over 1000 ml. No unintended laparotomy was required. The average operative time was 277 minutes, including lymphadenectomy, frozen section examination, and radical hysterectomy. The average postoperative stay was 4.1 days in standard cases, 5.25 if the case with bladder opening is included. No major complication and, particularly, no lymphocyst, no ureteral injury, and no urinary retention of more than 3-day duration occurred. A recurrence after a 2-year disease-free interval occurred in one case. A posterior exenteration had to be performed for a pelvic posterior growth involving the rectum. Since the publication of this experience, further follow-up of the patients is available. The patient who experienced pelvic recurrence died 3 years after the initial operation. All the other patients are doing well.

SALPINGO-OOPHORECTOMY

Salpingo-oophorectomy may be performed laparoscopically using bipolar current, ligatures, or stapling. We use the less expensive and less time-consuming bipolar method. The adnexa is grasped with one instrument. Traction in the appropriate direction exposes the ovarian ligament. The ureter is identified and the ovarian vessels are skeletonized to obtain the best effects from electrodessication. Bipolar current is applied to the ovarian vessels as they are gradually divided; additional electrodessication may have to be applied to the stumps. The peritoneum is incised on both leaves of the broad ligament, from the ovarian ligament to the uterine cornua. The adnexa is elevated and is now attached only by the utero-ovarian vessels and ligament. This pedicle is divided after hemostasis has been secured by the use of bipolar current or endoloops. The adnexa is removed within the protection of an endoscopic bag (see Chapter 17).

OMENTECTOMY

Partial omentectomy or infracolic omentectomy may be performed laparoscopically using electrosurgery and scissors. The surgeon stands between the legs of the patient and looks at the screen placed at the head of the table. The omentum is gradually divided by multiple applications of bipolar or monopolar current followed by section with scissors. In infracolic omentectomy, an excellent view of the inferior aspect of the transverse colon is given by a section of the avascular peritoneum of the superficial layers of the greater omentum. The omentum is stored in the pouch of Douglas or in a paracolic gutter. It may removed vaginally along with the uterus or through a minilaparotomy incision.

OVARIAN TRANSPOSITION

Indications

Ovarian conservation is possible and even advisable during therapy of most early cervical carcinomas, as ovarian metastases are quite rare in epidermoid cervical cancers without macroscopic implants on the ovarian surface. In some patients with cervical or vaginal cancer, external radiotherapy may be recommended. When the patient is premenopausal, pelvic radiotherapy results in the loss of endocrine ovarian function. A dose of 8 grays (Gy) to the ovaries is enough to suppress ovarian function in 70% of patients under 40 and in 100% of patients over 40. On the other hand, ovarian function is retained in about 80% of cases after ovarian transposition.[14] The only known adverse effect of ovarian transposition is the high rate of occurrence of functional ovarian cysts.

Many younger patients present with lymphomas, nongynecologic pelvic tumors, or vaginal or cervical tumors (clear-cell adenocarcinomas, rhabdomyosarcoma, endodermal sinus tumor). Some of these lesions are curable by conservative surgery, radiotherapy, chemotherapy, or a combination of methods. Future fertility should be conserved and the ovaries may have to be displaced out of the irradiation fields. Pregnancy may later be achieved by in vitro fertilization.

Surgical technique

To reduce the amount of exposure to the ovaries during pelvic irradiation, both adnexae must be displaced. In high ovarian transposition, the ovaries are placed laterally and

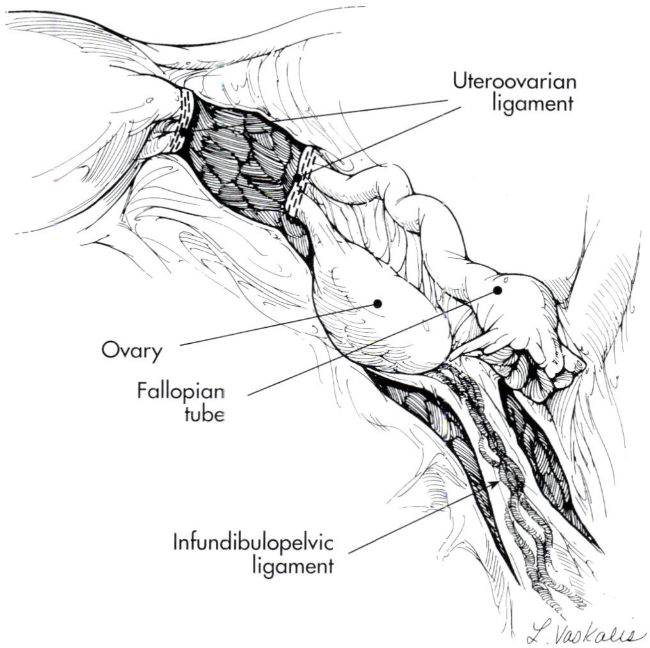

Fig. 25-15. Preparation for adnexal transposition. The uteroovarian ligament and tube have been divided with a stapler. The ovary and the tube are vascularized by the infundibuloovarian vessels. The peritoneum is incised on the lateral and medial side of the infundibulopelvic ligament.

cranially, in the paracolic gutters. In posterior oophoropexy, the ovaries are placed behind the uterus.

High ovarian transposition. When the ovarian transposition is performed by laparotomy, the ovaries and their blood supply from the infundibulopelvic ligaments are preserved. The uteroovarian vessels are ligated and divided at the uterine cornua; the peritoneum is incised on both leaves of the broad ligaments then on both sides of the infundibulopelvic ligaments. The adnexae are then mobilized and sutured, without any torsion of the ovarian vessels, in the paracolic gutters. Both ovaries are tagged with metallic clips for later radiologic localization.

Endoscopic techniques for ovarian suspension to the anterior abdominal wall, with or without section of the uteroovarian vessels have been described.[14] We use a method quite similar to the standard laparotomy technique.

The uteroovarian ligament and fallopian tube are first secured and divided with the use of bipolar current, sutures, or automatic stapling devices (Fig. 25-15). The use of staplers is recommended because they obtain precise hemostasis on both sides of the divided area. The adnexa is grasped with forceps. The avascular area of the broad ligament under the uteroovarian ligament is identified. A short incision is made at this level on both sides of the broad ligament to ensure proper placement of the stapler, parallel to the axis of the uterus and well above the uterine artery. The stapler is applied to the uteroovarian ligament and tube and is fired. The peritoneum is incised with endoscopic scissors on the medial and lateral sides of the broad ligament up to the level of the common iliac vessels. The ureter is identified at its crossing of the iliac vessels. The incisions are extended for 3 to 4 cm in the iliac area. The adnexa is now free.

Both adnexae are placed on the anterolateral part of the paracolic gutter, taking care to avoid torsion of the pedicle (Fig. 25-16, *A* and *B*). The adnexa must be approximated to the peritoneum of the paracolic gutter. Clips are not suitable for correct and solid fixation. Staples or endoscopic sutures may be used. We prefer to use a peritoneal bridge.

A 3 cm incision is made in the upper paracolic gutter, approximately 3 to 4 cm above the upper end of the initial peritoneal incision. A tunnel between the two incisions is made by blunt dissection, creating a peritoneal bridge. The adnexa is grasped, passed under the bridge and brought again into the peritoneal cavity through the upper incision. The adnexa is thus maintained in high position and at the same time a physiologic retroperitoneal position of the ovarian vessels is obtained (Fig. 25-16).

Additional clips are placed to localize the lower part of the ovary for later dosimetry. No peritoneal repair is necessary.

Posterior oophoropexy. A variant of high ovarian transposition has been described in patients with Hodgkin's disease, in whom the ovaries may be placed posterior to the uterus. When this kind of oophoropexy is performed before irradiation, approximately 60% of women retain ovarian function.[15] This procedure is simple to perform laparoscopically. A silk suture on a needle is passed through the uteroovarian ligaments, adjacent to the ovaries, and into the uterine seromuscularis. The ovaries are tied together and marked with staples.

This procedure is simpler than the high ovarian transpo-

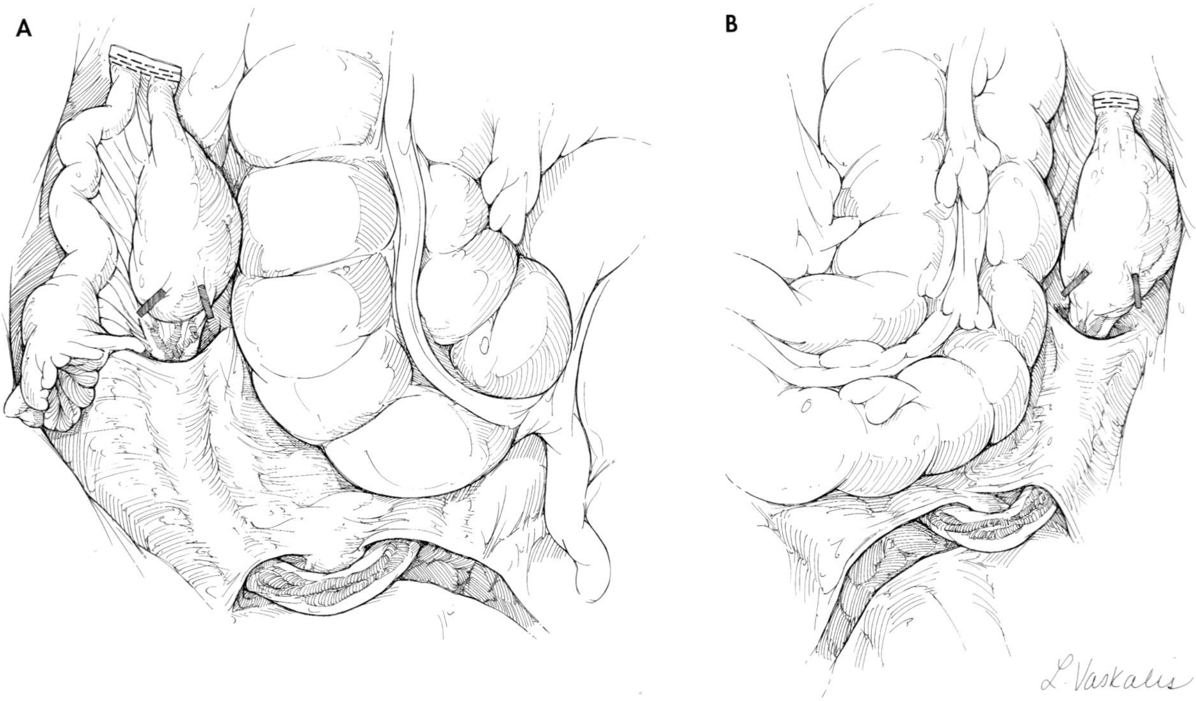

Fig. 25-16. Ovarian transposition. The ovaries are brought into the paracolic gutters. A tunnel has been created under the peritoneum of the lower part of the paracolic gutter. The adnexa *(left side)* or the ovary alone *(right side)* are passed under the tunnel. Clips are put on the ovaries for later radiologic identification.

sition but is less efficient for protection of the ovaries. It is obviously inapplicable when direct irradiation of the central pelvis is planned. We thus prefer high ovarian transposition in all cases.

LAPAROSCOPIC SURGICAL THERAPY OF EARLY OVARIAN CARCINOMA

History and general principles

Laparoscopic surgical therapy of advanced ovarian carcinomas is obviously impossible. However, this approach may be used in early ovarian carcinomas, provided that the intact ovarian tumor can be removed vaginally along with the uterus. Reich et al. reported a case of laparoscopic surgery for ovarian carcinoma,[16] showing that a number of goals of surgery for ovarian tumors, such as omentectomy, peritoneal sampling, and cytology, as well as appendectomy, may be achieved laparoscopically. They were unable to evaluate the para-aortic lymph nodes. Nezhat et al.[17] described attempting laparoscopically assisted surgery of a borderline ovarian tumor. As para-aortic lymphadenectomy up to the level of the left renal vein is an essential part of the surgical staging of early ovarian carcinomas, failure to complete comprehensive staging represents a potential risk of undertreatment and would preclude a laparoscopic approach in the surgical therapy of this condition. We have operated on one patient with granulosa cell tumor of the ovary fulfilling all the requirements of oncologic surgery.

Laparoscopic surgery may also be useful in the further management of patients referred with a diagnosis of early ovarian carcinoma and unsatisfactory staging and/or incomplete surgery. We have operated on five patients in whom restaging was indicated and performed at the same time laparoscopic contralateral salpingo-oophorectomy and/or hysterectomy, omentectomy, and appendectomy.[18]

Laparoscopic surgical management of the ovarian mass

The laparoscopic surgeon must be able to diagnose and appropriately manage unsuspected ovarian cancer, as when the preoperative work-up including ultrasonography, Doppler imaging, and plasma Ca-125 measurements has suggested the presence of a benign condition.

Whereas laparoscopy is a reliable tool for the diagnosis of early ovarian carcinoma,[19] any delay between diagnosis and therapy, improper staging, peritoneal spillage, or abdominal wall contamination with tumor cells may reduce the effectiveness of surgical therapy.[20]

The risk of abdominal wall involvement by tumoral implants has been documented,[21] and contact between the abdominal wall and an ovarian tumor must be avoided by the use of endoscopic bags or, if not available, by using a sterile surgical glove fashioned into a bag by placing a purse string suture at the cuff. Larger specimens may be removed by extending one of the incisions. There is evidence that integrity of the capsule is of no prognostic importance,[22,23] provided that spillage of tumor cells in the pelvis is followed by immediate and abundant peritoneal washing. It is recommended that oophorectomy be used or salpingo-oophorectomy rather than cystectomy for the management of ovarian cysts in menopausal patients to avoid cystic rupture during dissection.

The standards of management of ovarian tumors by laparoscopy include:

1. Careful examination of the external surface of the tumor
2. Manipulation of the ovary or cyst with a minimum of spillage; if spillage occurs, the procedure must be concluded with extensive peritoneal lavage
3. If aspiration of the cyst contents is planned, this must be done with great care, with direct puncture of the cyst by a 5 mm trocar, immediate aspiration, and several lavages of the cyst
4. Avoidance of any contact between the tumor and the abdominal wall
5. Liberal use of salpingo-oophorectomy with no attempt to dissect the lesion in postmenopausal patients or in the presence of a suspicious mass in younger patients
6. Use of frozen section examination, recognizing the limits of accuracy of this technique
7. Immediate definitive therapy of the ovarian carcinoma by either laparotomy or laparoscopy and, if immediate therapy is not possible, the delay between the diagnostic laparoscopy and definitive surgery should be minimal

Surgical treatment of a suspicious or malignant ovarian tumor usually involves total abdominal hysterectomy and bilateral salpingo-oophorectomy. Unilateral salpingo-oophorectomy may be undertaken as an interim measure when the diagnosis is uncertain, if informed consent for a more extensive procedure has not been obtained, and in selected younger patients who wish to preserve fertility.

The laparoscopic techniques of LH and LAVH are applicable to early ovarian carcinomas. It is, however, essential to emphasize the need for the removal of the unruptured tumor to minimize the risk of a graft of tumor cells. The tumor may be removed through the vaginal opening, along with the uterus. The vaginal route is adequate if the ovaries are mobilized by previous section of the ovarian and broad ligaments, and if the size of the ovary is approximately less than 6 cm, or can be reduced after aspiration of its content. In every case, the ovary should be protected by an endoscopic bag before attempted removal.

Elective laparoscopic unilateral salpingo-oophorectomy for early ovarian carcinoma is possible, in theory, in younger patients. In fact, laparotomy is preferable when the preoperative workup suggests malignancy, as minilaparotomy incisions are not suitable for removal of obviously malignant ovarian tumors.

A role for diagnostic unilateral salpingo-oophorectomy can be envisioned in the case of an unexpected suspicious unilateral mass in pre- or postmenopausal patients, if the operation can be performed with no spillage or abdominal wall contamination and a specimen for frozen section and definitive pathologic examination can be obtained. Surgical therapy can then be properly tailored. If the tumor is found to be benign, the limited laparoscopic operation is the best choice. If the tumor is malignant, proper staging and, in parous patients, radical surgery is indicated.

The occasional place for laparoscopic unilateral cystectomy is when a cyst is found in a young patient and there is limited small intracystic growth, providing the cyst can be removed within the protection of an endoscopic bag. When frozen section examination confirms the diagnosis of cancer, salpingo-oophorectomy is completed.

The rationale for staging procedures has been described in Chapter 12. Adequate staging is most important for early ovarian cancer, especially when the disease is apparently limited to one ovary. In such cases, inadequate surgical exploration may ignore peritoneal or nodal involvement and consequently lead to undertreatment. Examination of the entire peritoneum, diaphragmatic, and hepatic surfaces, sampling of the peritoneal fluid, multiple punch biopsies of the peritoneal lining, omentectomy, and pelvic and para-aortic infrarenal lymphadenectomy are feasible by laparoscopic means. All these procedures have been described in this chapter or in Chapter 12. Appendectomy is also described in Chapter 23.

The role of laparoscopy in ovarian cancer is primarily diagnostic. Laparoscopic surgical treatment of ovarian carcinomas is still investigational and should be limited to institutions or surgeons with considerable expertise in gynecologic oncology and operative laparoscopy and applied only to highly selected cases. The case of previously untreated tumors is quite rare. Only patients with early ovarian carcinomas should be offered treatment by operative laparoscopy. If unsuspected abdominal implants are found or if, during comprehensive staging, removal of the tumor without rupture appears impossible, it is absolutely necessary to move to open surgery. In many other instances, the diagnosis of ovarian carcinoma is made from specimens from ovarian cystectomy, unilateral (salpingo)oophorectomy, or hysterectomy with unilateral or bilateral salpingo-oophorectomy. Such patients are usually referred to gynecologic oncologists for additional surgical staging and treatment. Additional surgery may include total hysterectomy and contralateral salpingo-oophorectomy, which may be carried out laparoscopically, provided the contralateral ovary is not affected and there are no peritoneal implants.

Laparoscopic debulking of advanced ovarian cancer

Some authors are investigating the role of neoadjuvant chemotherapy. Inoperable patients are given chemotherapy and, after an average of three courses, the clinical response is evaluated. Obviously nonresponders are spared more therapeutic attempts. In responders, a second-look procedure is done, usually after three courses of chemotherapy, to assess the operability of the tumor. In operable patients, second-line surgery is undertaken. Some authors are investigating the feasibility of laparoscopic debulking surgery (i.e., omentectomy) in this context. (Surwit and Childers: personal communication.)

LAPAROSCOPICALLY ASSISTED VAGINAL HYSTERECTOMY IN STAGE I ENDOMETRIAL CARCINOMAS

Principles of therapy

As the surgical therapy of stage I endometrial cancer does not require radical hysterectomy, the technique of standard vaginal, laparoscopic, or LAVH may be applied. Childers and Surwit described the first two cases in the English literature.[24]

Salpingo-oophorectomy is required and may be done vaginally. However, since ligation and section of the infundibulopelvic ligaments by this route may prove difficult, on occasion the laparoscopic approach may facilitate the procedure. In this regard, laparoscopy may be undertaken as the first step of the operation (Chapter 22).

Laparoscopy offers the additional benefit of allowing staging. Examination of the ovaries and of the pelvic peritoneum, peritoneal fluid sampling for cytologic examination, examination of the liver surface, and, when necessary, pelvic or para-aortic lymphadenectomy may be completed at the same time.

Both pelvic and para-aortic lymphadenectomy may be performed laparoscopically even in obese patients.[9] However, the indication for and extent of lymphadenectomy is controversial and must be balanced with the cost and risk of the procedure. Although some investigators advise pelvic and para-arotic dissection, many feel that lymphadenectomy should be tailored according to the risk of node involvement (see Chapter 12, Fig. 12-2). In stage IA, grade 1 patients, lymphadenectomy is not required. In other patients, pelvic lymphadenectomy yields a significant rate of node involvement and may benefit the patient. Usually, an obturator and medial external iliac dissection is done, although some advise full pelvic dissection. In the para-aortic area, node sampling only is standard and full dissection is not required. As the risk of aortic node involvement is minimal (2%) when the pelvic nodes are intact, para-aortic node sampling is required only in patients with pelvic node involvement. Frozen section examination may thus be useful to indicate the need for para-aortic dissection.

Primary laparoscopic surgery

Primary laparoscopic surgery is undertaken particularly when lymphadenectomy is clearly needed (grade 2 or 3 adenocarcinoma, myometrial involvement suspected in preoperative workup). Staging surgery is performed first. Laparoscopic division of the infundibulopelvic ligaments facilitates the subsequent vaginal portion of the operation.

Secondary laparoscopic surgery

In some cases, laparoscopy may be used to complement vaginal hysterectomy. When the preoperative workup, including ultrasonography and magnetic resonance imaging, suggests a IA tumor, vaginal hysterectomy is done first. If macroscopic and/or frozen section examination of the hysterectomy specimen reveals myometrial invasion, laparoscopic lymphadenectomy is carried out. If the ovaries cannot be removed vaginally, laparoscopic surgery may be used to remove the ovaries.

The same principles apply to unsuspected endometrial cancers found in hysterectomy specimens. Secondary laparoscopic surgery is used in such cases for further staging and/or bilateral oophorectomy.

TREATMENT OF CERVICAL CANCERS

The techniques of laparoscopic surgery may be applied to the treatment of cervical cancers at various stages (Fig. 25-17).

Simple hysterectomy or conization alone is indicated in IA2 cervical cancers. When lymphadenectomy is indicated (depth of invasion between 3 and 5 mm or lymphatic invasion), it may be done laparoscopically in combination with vaginal hysterectomy or as a complement to a diagnostic conization or simple hysterectomy.

Proximal (modified) radical hysterectomy is indicated for early invasive cervical cancer (IB tumor not exceeding 2 cm or 10 cm^3.) This volume may be obtained after brachytherapy or the tumor may be small indicating primary radical hysterectomy. Vaginal radical hysterectomy, LRH, or LARVH with pelvic (interiliac) lymphadenectomy may be used. Para-aortic dissection is indicated, in our experience, only in the pelvic node-postitive patient.

Distal (classical) radical hysterectomy is indicated in larger but still nonbulky IB, IIA, or proximal IIB tumors not previously submitted to radiation therapy. Vaginal procedures may be used for tumor volumes up to 4 cm or 50 cm^3. We advise the use of the Dargent LARVH if the pelvic and para-aortic lymphadenectomy does not yield positive nodes.

As bulky tumors (more than 4 cm or 50 cm^3) are not suitable for a primary vaginal approach, we use laparoscopic surgery only for staging in such cases (see Chapter 12).

When obviously diseased nodes are found, the question is to remove or to leave them for later irradiation. We feel

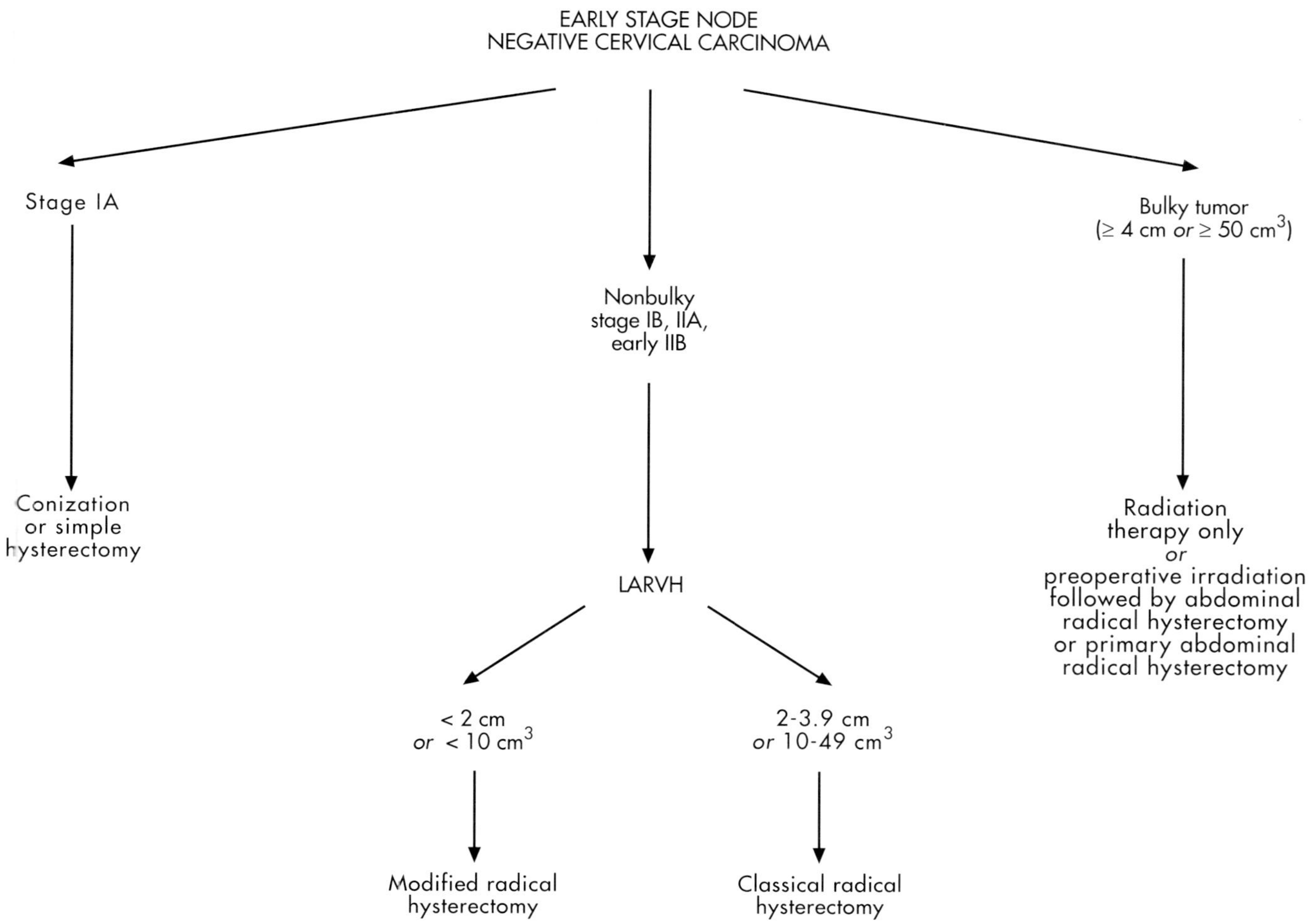

Fig. 25-17. Indications for radical hysterectomy in early stage node-negative cervical carcinoma.

that many enlarged nodes may be safely removed laparoscopically, provided they do not involve the iliac vessels. The therapeutic role of node debulking surgery is however questionable.

REFERENCES

1. Dargent D: Laparoscopic surgery and gynecologic cancer. *Curr Opinion Obstet Gynecol* 5: 294-300, 1993.
2. Canis M, Mage G, Wattiez A, et al: La chirurgie endoscopique a-t-elle une place dans la chirurgie radicale du cancer du col utérin? (letter). *J Gynecol Obstet Biol Repr* 19:921, 1990.
3. Nezhat CR, Burrell MO, Nezhat FR, et al: Laparoscopic radical hysterectomy with paraaortic and pelvic node dissection. *Am J Obstet Gynecol* 166:864-865, 1992.
4. Querleu D: Hystérectomies de Schauta-Amreich et Schauta-Stoeckel assistées par coelioscopie. *J Gynecol Obstet Biol Repr* 20:747-748, 1991.
5. Dargent D, Mathevet P: Hystérectomie élargie laparoscopico-vaginale. *J Gynecol Obstet Biol Repr* 21:709-710, 1992.
6. Dargent D, Salvat J: L'envahissement ganglionnaire pelvien. Paris, 1989, Medsi.
7. Kavoussi LR, Sosa E, Chandhoke P, et al: Complications of laparoscopic pelvic lymph node dissection. *J Urol* 149: 322-325, 1993.
8. Burney TL, Campbell EC, Naslund MJ, JACOBS SC. Complications of staging laparoscopic pelvic lymphadenectomy. *Surg Laparosc Endosc* 3:184-190, 1993.
9. Childers JM, Hatch KD, Tran An, Surwit EA; Laparoscopic para-aortic lymphadenectomy in gynecologic malignancies. *Obstet Gynecol* 82:741-747, 1993.
10. Piver MS, Rutledge F, Smith JP: Five classes of extended hysterectomy for women with cervical cancer. *Obstet Gynecol* 44:265-267, 1974.
11. Reiffenstuhl G, Platzer W: Atlas of vaginal surgery. Vol 1. Philadelphia, 1975, WB Saunders.
12. Nezhat CR, Nezhat FR, Burrell MO, et al: Laparoscopic radical hysterectomy and laparoscopically assisted vaginal radical hysterectomy with pelvic and paraaortic dissection. *J Gynecol Surg* 9:105-120, 1993.
13. Querleu D: Laparoscopically-assisted radical vaginal hysterectomy. *Gynecol Oncol* 51:248-254, 1993.
14. Prouvostma, Canis M, LE Bouedec G, et al: Transposition ovarienne per-coelioscopique avant curiethérapie dans les cancers du col utérin stade IA et IB. *J Gynecol Obstet Biol Repr* 20:361-365, 1991.
15. Williams RS, Mendenhall N: Laparoscopic oophoropexy for preservation of ovarian function before pelvic node irradiation. *Obstet Gynecol* 80:541-543, 1992.

16. Reich H, McGlynn F, Wilkie W: Laparoscopic management of stage I ovarian cancer. *J Reprod Med* 35: 601-605, 1990.
17. Nezhat C, Nezhat F, Burrell M: Laparoscopically assisted hysterectomy for the management of a borderline ovarian tumor: a case-report. *J Laparoendosc Surg* 2:167-169, 1992.
18. Querleu D, Leblanc E: Laparoscopic infrarenal node dissection in the restaging of carcinomas of the ovary and fallopian tube. *Cancer* 1994. (In press.)
19. Mage G, Canis M, Manhes H, et al: Laparoscopic management of adnexal cystic masses. *J Gynecol Surg* 6:71-79, 1990.
20. Maiman M, Seltzer V, Boyce J: Laparoscopic excision of ovarian neoplasms subsequently found to be malignant. *Obstet Gynecol* 77:563-566, 1991.
21. Hsiu J, Given F, Kemp G. Tumor implantation after diagnostic laparoscopic biopsy of serous ovarian tumors of low malignant potential. *Obstet Gynecol* 68:905-935, 1986.
22. Sevelda P, Vavra N, Schemper M, Salzer H: Prognostic factors for survival in stage I epithelial ovarian carcinoma. *Cancer* 65:2349-2352, 1990.
23. Dembo AJ, Davy M, Stenwig AE, et al: Prognostic factors in patients with stage I epithelial ovarian cancer. *Obstet Gynecol* 75:263-273, 1990.
24. Childers JM, Surwit EA: Combined laparoscopic and vaginal surgery for the management of stage I endometrial cancer. Two case reports. *Gynecol Oncol* 45:46-51, 1992.

Chapter 26

COMPLICATIONS AND THEIR MANAGEMENT

Laparoscopy permits thorough inspection of the abdominal and pelvic cavities, which gives it its important diagnostic function. Laparoscopy also provides the means of access for a variety of surgical procedures.

Complications may arise from the steps that are necessary to perform a laparoscopy and from the procedure carried out using laparoscopy as a means of access. The true incidence of complications is unknown since the vast majority are not reported.

Querleu et al. have studied laparoscopic complications.[1] The study comprised two phases of 2 years each. The first of these phases was retrospective and the second prospective. Their study was confined to complications that resulted in an unintended laparotomy. There were no statistical differences between the results of the first and second phase of the study. The data were derived from seven centers chosen "on the basis of large experience with these techniques." The exclusivity of the centers reporting and the similar rates of complications that resulted in unintended laparotomy in both the retrospective and prospective phases of the study give it great credibility. Reports from retrospective surveys of the individual members of an association are much less reliable as reporting is frequently incomplete[2,3] and inaccurate.

Over the 4 years that encompassed both the retrospective and prospective phases of the Querleu et al. study,[1] the rates of complications that resulted in an unintended laparotomy were as follows: 1.7 per thousand for diagnostic laparoscopy, 0.4 per thousand with minor (minimal adhesiolysis, ablation of minimal endometriosis, ovarian biopsy or puncture, tubal sterilization and assisted reproduction) procedures, 4.8 per thousand when major surgical procedures (extended adhesiolysis, tuboplasty, uterine suspension, surgery for tubal pregnancy, salpingitis, and moderate or severe endometriosis) were carried out, and 8.9 per thousand with advanced surgical procedures (hysterectomy, adnexectomy, myomectomy, bladder neck suspension, lymphadenectomy). One death occurred in the "major surgical" group following trauma to a major vessel.

Laparoscopy is the most frequently performed gynecologic procedure. "The vast applications and frequency of usage of laparoscopy demand that it be associated with the absolute minimum rate of complications."[4] This is particularly important when the procedure is being performed simply for diagnostic purposes.

Laparoscopy has the potential of causing a multitude of complications. The extent of these complications varies greatly from the minor to the major and may even prove fatal. Complications may be associated with every step of the laparoscopic procedure.

The complications associated with laparoscopy are similar whether the procedure is diagnostic or undertaken to provide access necessary to perform a gynecologic operation. The complication rate is increased, as would be expected, when surgical procedures are performed. The necessary dissection, ligation, division, and use of energy sources such as electricity and lasers all pose risks. Since every step necessary to perform a laparoscopy may result in complications, these will be discussed first.

COMPLICATIONS ASSOCIATED WITH THE PERFORMANCE OF LAPAROSCOPY

Failure to complete the procedure

Although failure to complete the procedure rarely causes significant morbidity, it should be regarded as a complication. By far the most common reason for failure is the inability to establish a proper pneumoperitoneum.[5] This tends to occur in the very obese patient or when the tentative or inexperienced surgeon fails to place the Veress needle in the proper space.

Extensive intra-abdominal or intrapelvic adhesions can greatly limit the view. The strategies to deal with this situation have been described in Chapter 5.

Introduction of the pneumoperitoneum

Extraperitoneal insufflation. If the tip of the Veress needle remains in the preperitoneal space, emphysema will be created, stripping the peritoneum from the overlying muscles (Fig. 26-1). The unwary can be misled because this will eventually lead to the disappearance of liver dullness. Palpation of the abdomen may elicit a sensation of crepitus. Bubbles in the blood at the incision are another indication that preperitoneal insufflation may be occurring. If it is recognized early that the tip of the Veress needle is misplaced, the CO_2 line should be disconnected. The inflow tap is left open and the abdomen gently compressed to expel as much CO_2 as possible. The needle is removed and reintroduced, either at the original or an alternative site (see Chapter 5).

Often the complication will not be recognized until the telescope is passed through the principal cannula. Observation should begin as the telescope is inserted. The typical spider's web appearance of the effects of preperitoneal gas will readily be visible. As soon as it is recognized, the telescope should be advanced no further to avoid stripping even more of the peritoneum. The telescope should be removed and as much CO_2 as possible encouraged to escape. It may be advantageous to leave the cannula in place as the Veress needle is introduced at an alternative site. If the needle is correctly placed, the pressure of the intraperitoneal CO_2 will force the remaining preperitoneal gas through the cannula.

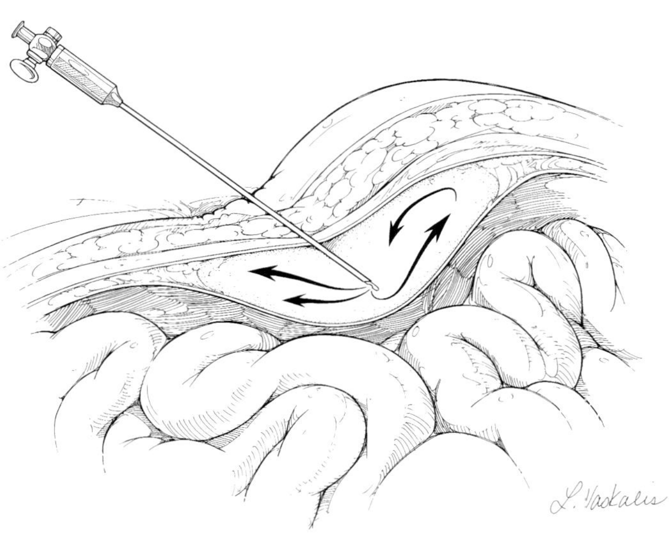

Fig. 26-1. Extraperitoneal insufflation.

Mediastinal emphysema. Gas inadvertently insufflated into the preperitoneal space may enter the mediastinum. Extensive mediastinal emphysema will compromise cardiac function. The anesthetist may evince concern. There will be loss of dullness to percussion over the precordium and auscultation may reveal muffling of the heart sounds.

The laparoscopy should be abandoned immediately and as much gas as possible evacuated. Any necessary supportive measures should be instituted and the patient kept under close observation until it is clear that the gas has been absorbed.

Pneumothorax. Only if an upper abdominal site is chosen for the insertion of the Veress needle will this complication occur. If such a site has been selected, the needle must be directed away from the diaphragm. The anesthetist may notice difficulty ventilating the patient. There will be increased tympanism and a decrease in the audible intensity of the breath sounds on the affected side. There may be a contralateral mediastinal shift.

The procedure must be abandoned immediately and the gas allowed to escape. Initially the tap of the Veress needle is shut until the gas tubing can be placed underwater to allow the gas to escape but prevent room air from being sucked into the pleural cavity.

Further management will depend upon the patient's condition. Some may require simple observation. Only the more severely affected may need assisted ventilation or even the placement of a pleural drainage tube.

Pneumo omentum. If, during insufflation somewhat higher than usual pressures are recorded, it should be suspected that the tip of the Veress needle has entered the omentum. The needle should be withdrawn slightly or the anterior parietes grasped and shaken. Either maneuver is often sufficient to dislodge the omentum and insufflation pressure will fall to normal.

Fortunately this is almost always a very minor complication and the typical appearances of gas bubbles between the leaves of the omentum will be noted when the telescope is inserted. The condition is almost always innocuous and resolves spontaneously.

Penetration of a hollow viscus. The bladder, stomach, or bowel may all be penetrated by the Veress needle. The surgeon must always ensure that the bladder is empty prior to starting. If pneumaturia is noted the Veress needle should be withdrawn for a few centimeters. Such a complication is not an indication to abandon the procedure but rather to evaluate the dome of the bladder very carefully when the telescope is introduced.

An upper abdominal site of insertion or overdistention of the stomach during induction of anesthesia can put the stomach at risk. This is particularly so following a difficult endotracheal intubation. The surgeon should always percuss the upper abdomen. If increased tympanism is noted the stomach contents should be aspirated with a nasogastric tube before the pneumoperitoneum is induced.

The syringe test, described in Chapter 5, usually allows early recognition that the stomach or bowel has been penetrated. The syringe test is not infallible, however. If the abdomen distends asymmetrically or there is belching or passing of flatus coincident with induction of the pneumoperitoneum, entry into the gastointestinal tract should be suspected. If a needlescope is available it can be inserted through the outer shaft of the Veress needle to permit immediate inspection of the site of entry. Direct visualization can be used to position the Veress needle correctly. If a needlescope is not available, insufflation should be discontinued, the gas line disconnected, and as much gas as possible allowed to escape. The pneumoperitoneum should then be reestablished. As soon as the laparoscope is inserted through the principal cannula, the site of any suspected penetration must be examined thoroughly. Simple needle penetrations require a period of observation for any signs of developing peritonitis.

Occasionally the tip of the needle can tear the bowel. In these circumstances it will be necessary to repair the rent either laparoscopically (see Chapter 18) or by laparotomy.

Through and through injuries are more likely to be extensive, particularly at the exit site. It is vital therefore that both sides of any damaged bowel be examined thoroughly.

Blood vessel injuries. The omental and mesenteric blood vasculature may be traumatized by the Veress needle or it may enter any of the major abdominal or pelvic vessels.

These are serious complications and may be avoided by elevating the anterior wall and ensuring that the Veress needle is inserted toward the hollow of the sacrum exactly in the midline. Only that portion of the needle necessary to enter the peritoneal cavity should be inserted. It must be emphasized that thin subjects, infants, and adolescents are at particular risk of vascular injuries.

The first indication that such an event may have occurred is the appearance of blood at the hub of the Veress needle when the syringe test is performed. The needle should be withdrawn slightly, its position retested, and an adequate pneumoperitoneum established. As soon as the laparoscope is inserted, a thorough inspection must be carried out to evaluate the nature of any vessel damage. Minor bleeding or a small nongrowing hematoma may be ignored but should be reexamined once the laparoscopic procedure has been completed to ensure there is no further bleeding or growth of the hematoma. Major bleeding or formation of a rapidly growing hematoma requires immediate surgical intervention and arrest of the hemorrhage. If a large vessel has been injured, a vascular surgeon should be consulted immediately.

Gas embolism. If vessel penetration by the Veress needle has gone unnoted and gas insufflation has been instituted, intravascular passage of carbon dioxide will lead to gas embolism, an event that may be fatal. Aspiration of the syringe prior to connecting the gas line should guard against this fortunately rare occurrence.

Transuterine insufflation enjoyed a short vogue. It has now been discontinued because the incidence of severe morbidity and mortality from gas embolism was unacceptably high.

Should embolism occur, the anesthetist will note that the patient is experiencing cardiorespiratory difficulty. A mill wheel murmur will be heard over the precordium. The patient should be placed in the left lateral decubitus position and an immediate cardiac puncture performed to release gas from the right atrium. Fortunately this maneuver is almost invariably successful.

Puncture of liver and spleen. These organs can be injured when the Veress needle is inserted in the upper abdomen or if they are enlarged because of disease. An exceedingly high insufflation pressure would be recorded. The Veress needle should be withdrawn and reinserted. Once again the surface of the liver and/or spleen should be inspected as soon as the laparoscope is in position. Palpation and percussion of the abdomen prior to insertion of the Veress needle, particularly if there is any suggestion of organomegaly, should ensure that this complication does not occur.

Introduction of the principal and ancillary trocars

Sharp tips of the trocars, particularly the principal trocars, will give rise to the most severe injuries that occur during a performance of laparoscopy. The measures necessary to avoid trocar injuries have been described in Chapter 5. Damage caused by the principal trocar may be unavoidable as its insertion is by necessity, blind. Injuries essentially should never happen during insertion of ancillary trocars as their entry to the abdomen can be kept under direct vision.

If accidents do occur, there may be bleeding from the abdominal wall, perforation of a hollow viscus, laceration of blood vessels, or injury to the liver or spleen. Management will be dependent upon the severity of the damage that has been caused.

Bleeding from the abdominal wall. Superficial bleeding can usually be controlled with an external suture or with a pressure dressing.

Preperitoneal and intraperitoneal bleeding may occur from the site of ancillary puncture, particularly if the inferior epigastric vessel is damaged.[6] Blood will be noticed running down the cannula, or an abdominal wall hematoma may be seen to be developing. Minor injuries tend to be self-limiting. If the bleeding does not stop or the hematoma continues to increase in size, either the incision must be extended and the bleeding vessel identified and ligated or a curved needle can be introduced down the ancillary puncture site and manipulated with laparoscopic instruments so that a suture can be placed under direct laparoscopic control.

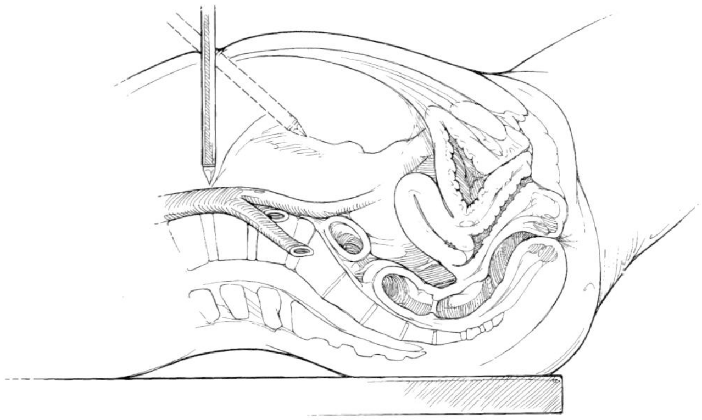

Fig. 26-2. Injury to major vessels. The great vessels can be punctured if the principal trocar and cannula are introduced vertically and not in the direction of the hollow of the sacrum.

Blood vessel injuries. Trocar injuries to small blood vessels may be self-limiting or, as for example in the case of omental vessels, may be controlled by electrodesiccation. If mesenteric vessels have been damaged the vitality of the bowel may be at risk. Treatment of such injuries usually will require blood transfusion, vascular repair, and, where indicated, bowel resection. Appropriate surgical consultation is recommended in all instances. Injury to major vessel may occur and severe hemorrhage usually ensues (Figs. 26-2 and 26-3). The aorta, inferior vena cava, and iliac arteries and veins may all be at risk. To avoid injury to such vessels the following precautions must be taken:

1. There must be adequate pneumoperitoneum.
2. The operating table must be kept horizontal until the principal trocar and cannula have been inserted. The Trendelenberg position alters the relationship of the sacrum and aorta to the umbilicus, narrowing the distance between them, and placing the vessels at risk. It is the surgeon's responsibility to direct when the position of the table should be altered.
3. The trocar must be sharp and inserted smoothly. Dense scars may cause resistance. Overcoming this resistance may result in sudden uncontrolled entry into the peritoneal cavity. Of even greater importance, they may deflect the trocar and cannula from the critically important plane and angle of insertion.
4. Meticulous attention must be paid to the plane and angle of insertion of the principal trocar and cannula.

Sagittal insertion with no deviation from this plane will protect the iliac vessels in the lateral part of their courses. An angle of insertion of 45 degrees (toward the hollow of the sacrum) should protect the aorta and vena cava and origins of the common iliac vessels. If the umbilicus is normally sited this is usually the case. The umbilicus can be abnormally sited in obese patients and those with extensive scarring. It is safer to palpate the apices of the iliac crests that identify the level of the fourth lumbar vertebra. The bifurcation of the aorta lies at this level in the vast majority of individuals. Once the probable site of the bifurcation has been established, the angle of insertion can be adjusted to ensure that the sharp tip of the trocar is kept well away from this region.

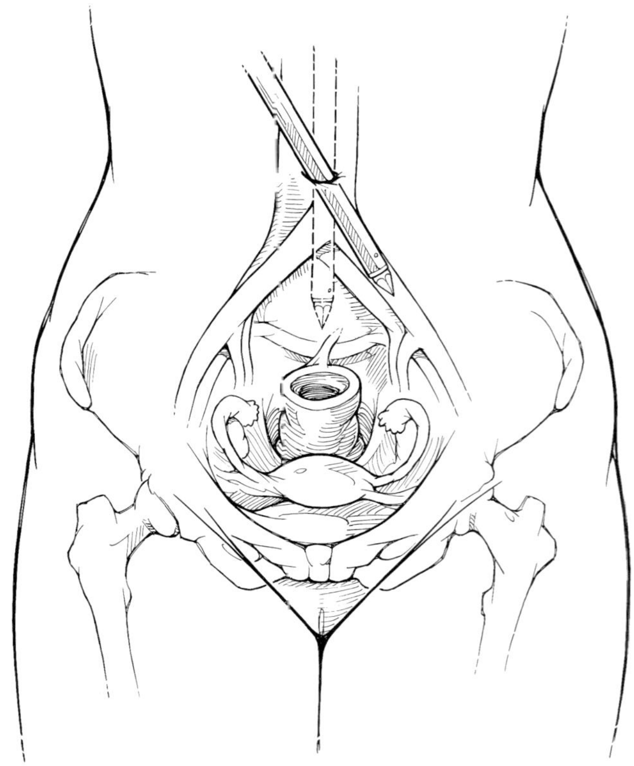

Fig. 26-3. Injury to major vessels. Iliac vessels can be punctured if the principal trocar and cannula are not introduced in the sagittal plane.

Should injury to a major vessel occur, blood may be seen in the cannula as the telescope is inserted. Frank intraperitoneal bleeding may be noted. Often, however, a large retroperitoneal hematoma ensues, the first indication of which may be a precipitous fall in blood pressure. If there is any reason to suspect injury to a major vessel, there is no room for half measures. While the anesthetist is inserting central venous lines and arranging for blood to be made available, the surgeon must stop the bleeding. Access to the site of injury is gained immediately through a midline incision and pressure applied to arrest the hemorrhage. As these first aid measures are being instituted, emergency consultation is sought with a vascular surgeon.

Once the vessel has been repaired it is incumbent upon the surgical team to ensure that no collateral damage has occurred to any other intra-abdominal organs.

Injury to a hollow viscus. The hollow viscera can be injured by the principal or ancillary trocar. The resulting le-

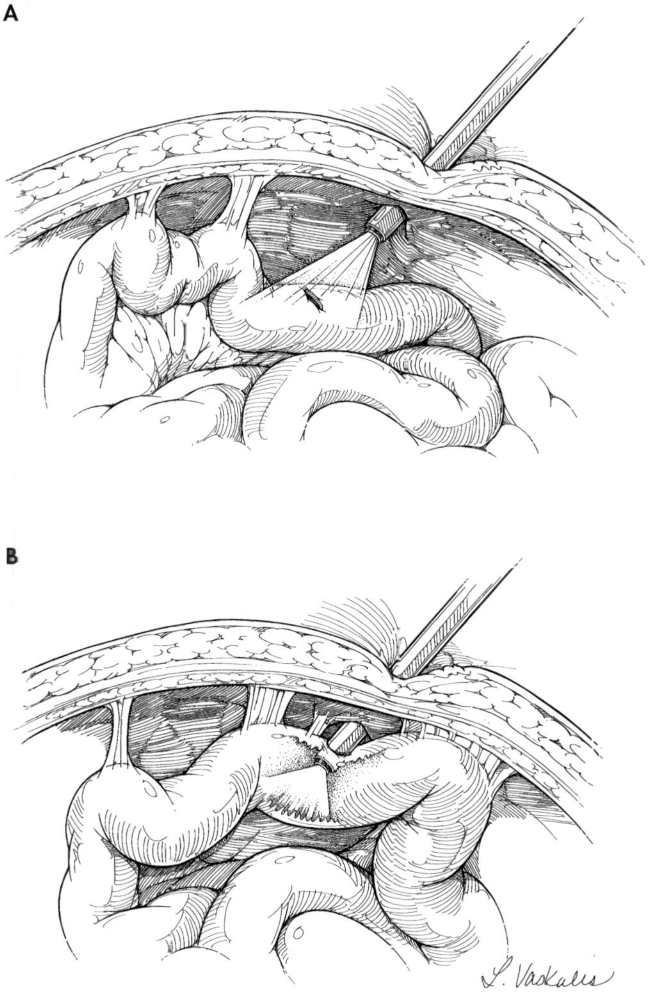

Fig. 26-4. Bowel injury with the principal trocar and cannula. **A,** If the bowel has been perforated and has slipped off the cannula, the defect may be observed at the time of the initial survey. **B,** If the bowel has been entered and the cannula has remained in situ, the mucosa will be visible as soon as the laparoscope is introduced.

sions range in severity from bruising or tearing of the serosa to complete penetration. If the lumen is entered the viscus may slip off the cannula (Fig. 26-4, *A*), the cannula may remain within the viscus (Fig. 26-4, *B*), or the bowel may be impaled so that the cannula has exited through the opposite wall (Fig. 26-5). This last injury is difficult to recognize if the bowel is impaled by the principal cannula. If at any time a fecal smell is noted as gas escaped from any of the canulas, damage to the large bowel should be suspected.

When the principal cannula remains within the lumen of the viscus, the mucosal pattern will be instantly apparent as the telescope is introduced. If the viscus has slipped off there may be evidence of bleeding or peritoneal soiling with gastrointestinal contents. It is sound practice to introduce

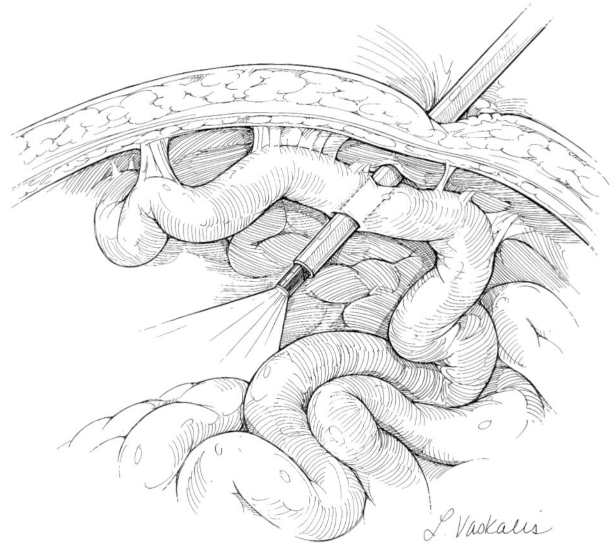

Fig. 26-5. Bowel injury with the principal trocar and cannula. If the bowel has been transfixed by the cannula, this will not be apparent when the laparoscope is introduced.

the principal trocar and cannula with the patient still in the horizontal position and immediately to inspect the line of introduction when the telescope is introduced, thus enabling the surgeon to recognize immediately that damage has been caused.

Minor injuries are self-limiting and probably require no treatment. They should be reinspected at the close of the procedure. The fundus of the uterus can be punctured and usually bleeds, although this bleeding is usually self-limiting. If bleeding persists, electrodesiccation will usually cause it to stop. The blood should be lavaged from the pelvis. Lacerations of the bladder can be sutured and an indwelling catheter left in situ.

The most serious injuries are those to stomach and bowel. Management will depend on the location and extent of the damage. In many instances it will be possible to carry out closure laparoscopically as has been discussed in Chapter 18. If the surgeon wishes to repair the defect by laparotomy, the laparoscope should be left in the viscus. This will permit the area of damage to be identified instantly and allow repair to be carried through a well-placed minilaparotomy incision. The principles of management include closure of the defect in two layers, in such a way to avoid postoperative stenosis, extensive peritoneal lavage, and drainage when appropriate. If the affected organ is the large bowel, cultures should be taken and intensive antibiotic therapy instituted. The most severe injuries to the small bowel may require resection of the damaged segment and end-to-end anastomosis. Severe large bowel injuries may require the performance of a temporary defunctioning colostomy.

If it is strongly suspected that perforation has occurred,

but is not possible to identify the site by laparoscopy, it is safer to err on the side of caution and perform a laparotomy to examine the entire gastrointestinal tract.

On occasion it may not be recognized that the bowel has been entered. Peritonitis will occur and these patients will become extremely ill, their illness becoming apparent after they awake from the anaesthetic.

Injuries to liver and spleen. Fortunately these injuries are very rare and vary from minor bruising or puncture to penetration to laceration. The latter will be associated with hemorrhage and will require prompt surgical repair.

COMPLICATIONS THAT MAY OCCUR WITH BOTH DIAGNOSTIC AND OPERATIVE LAPAROSCOPY

Certain complications may be associated with both diagnostic and operative laparoscopy.

Cervical laceration

Cervical lacerations are relatively frequent occurrences and are caused by tearing the tenaculum free from the cervix. In every case of laparoscopy in which a tenaculum has been used, at the close of the procedure the cervix should be inspected to ensure that it is dry. If bleeding is occurring, either from the tenaculum puncture or from a laceration, it may be controlled by compression, electrocoagulation, or suturing with an absorbable suture.

Uterine perforation

Uterine perforation may be caused by the uterine cannula or if dilation and curettage is performed. The area of puncture will be instantly apparent at the time of laparoscopy and the degree of trauma and amount of bleeding can easily be assessed. In most cases the bleeding will be self-limiting; if it is not, injection of dilute vasopressin solution, laparoscopic coagulation, or suturing may be required.

Shoulder pain

Carbon dioxide is converted to carbonic acid. The carbonic acid is an irritant to the diaphragm, which shares the same nerve supply as the shoulders, and the pain is referred to the shoulders. While of little significance it is troubling to the patient. The more gas that can be expelled at the close of the procedure and the less room air that is allowed to enter through the canula, the less will the patient experience this symptom.

Pelvic inflammatory disease

Any uterine manipulation will be associated with a low but unavoidable risk of recrudescence of acute pelvic inflammatory disease. Should such an event occur, antibiotic therapy will be required; details are described in Chapter 10.

Incisional hernia

Failure to remove the principal cannula with the valve open can create suction, thus drawing a loop of bowel or omentum into the umbilical incision. The risk of incisional hernia increases in direct proportion to the size of the cannula inserted. While incisions for portals under 8 mm in size may be simply approximated with Steri-strips or superficial sutures, it is prudent to approximate the fascia of entry sites 8 mm or larger. The rate of this complication has increased with the use of larger portals for operative laparoscopy.[7] It will present with early or delayed postoperative pain at the site of the incision and may require surgical correction.

Explosion

Explosions will not occur during diagnostic laparoscopy. Any electrosurgery used during operative procedures is an incandescent source. This in itself does not pose any difficulties, nor does it pose difficulties if carbon dioxide is used as a distention medium. If either air or nitrous oxide have been used they will support combustion. This physical property becomes very important if the bowel has been perforated and methane gas has entered the peritoneal cavity.

Other injuries

Careless positioning of the patient can lead to damaged soft parts, vessels, and nerves. The hands are vulnerable to the moving parts of the table. Placing the patient in the deep Trendlenberg position can cause traction injuries of the brachial plexuses.[8] The use of leg stirrups carries its own risk; femoral neuropathy has been reported.[9] The leg veins can be compressed leading to deep venous thrombosis. The peroneal nerve is susceptible to pressure injury, leading to a complaint of foot drop postoperatively. If the patient is roughly handled when the legs are placed in stirrups, back injury can occur.

Anesthesia-related complications

Although these complications fall within the purview of the anaesthetist, the surgeon should be familiar with them. They include postoperative myalgia, cardiac arrhythmias, and aspiration of gastric contents. Local and parenteral anesthetic agents also carry their own risks.

Myalgia. Succinylcholine, which is used as a muscle relaxant, is associated with postoperative muscle cramps, particularly in patients who suffer from cholinesterase deficiency and have difficulty metabolizing this compound. The establishment of spontaneous respiration may also be delayed in such patients, who will require prolonged assisted ventilation.

Cardiac arrhythmias. The combination of increased intra-abdominal pressure and the use of the Trendelenberg position will reduce pulmonary excursion. Carbon dioxide, if absorbed, may lead to hypercarbia. The combination of poor tidal flow and metabolic hypercarbia will lead to a rise in the arterial P_{CO_2}, an event that may induce cardiac arrythmia. This risk is further exaggerated if Halothane is used as the anesthetic agent. For this reason it is advised that patients undergoing laparoscopy should be intubated and maintained with assisted ventilation.

Aspiration of gastric contents. Any general anesthetic can be complicated by regurgitation and aspiration of the gastric contents. Laparoscopy does not differ from other surgical procedures in this respect.

Complications associated with local anesthesia and parenteral agents. A small number of patients will be hypersensitive to local anesthetic agents. The effect of these agents may be augmented by the administration of parenteral hypnotic and analgesic medications. The use of Ketamine, Valium, and Droperidol may lead to hallucinations.

COMPLICATIONS ASSOCIATED WITH OPERATIVE PROCEDURES

Any woman who is undergoing operative laparoscopy is exposed to all the hazards of laparoscopy that have just been described. In addition, each of the following surgical steps—dissection and section, securing pedicles and blood vessels, and the use of electrical and laser energy—may cause a variety of complications. While specific procedures may carry greater risks of specific complications that have been described in the preceding chapters, a ureter is no less tied nor a hemorrhage no less profuse whether the operation being performed was an adnexectomy for endometriosis or hysterectomy. These surgical mishaps occur irrespective of the mode of access. Infection can follow a laparotomy just as virulently as it does from a laparoscopy.

The principles of prevention, recognition, and management of surgical complications are the same whether a given procedure is being performed vaginally, by laparoscopy, laparotomy, or minilaparotomy.

Three major types of complications will be encountered: hemorrhage, injuries to the gastrointestinal tract, and genitourinary tract injuries (see box). In addition, the longer the time taken for operative procedures, the greater volume of gas flow. The use of copious amounts of irrigation solutions may predispose the patient to more anesthetic complications and hypothermia. Lowering of the core temperature is prevented by the use of warming mattresses and gas warmers and by ensuring that cold irrigation solutions are not used. Peripheral nerves are at risk of compression injuries because of the need to keep the patient in stirrups or in the deep Trendelenberg position. Clearly, attention must be paid to proper positioning.

Complications associated with operative laparoscopy

Vascular

Hemorrhage
- Early
- Delayed

Hematoma
- Early
- Delayed
- Infected

Gastrointestinal

Perforation of stomach

Small and large bowel injury
- Recognized immediately
- Late presentation
- Fecal peritonitis

Genitourinary

Perforation of the bladder

Ureter
- Division
- Occlusion
- Necrosis
- Infection

Anesthetic

- Cardiac arrhythmias
- Aspiration of gastric contents
- Myalgia

Infection

Others

- Hypothermia
- Nerve injury
- Thrombosis
- Gas embolism
- Hernia

Hemorrhage

Bleeding may be immediate or delayed and results from injury to a blood vessel or use of ineffective methods or techniques for securing hemostasis. The need to transfuse the patient with crystalloid solutions or blood will depend upon the rapidity of the bleeding and the degree of shock.

Immediate bleeding. Frank hemorrhage, continuous oozing, or expanding hematoma formation should be instantly apparent. They result from trauma to a vessel; inadequate occlusion of a vessel irrespective of the method used prior to division; or blunt dissection. Prevention hinges upon delicate dissection, identification of any vessels that may be at risk, and the proper occlusion of any vessel to be divided. Treatment should be immediate and requires that the source of the bleeding be stopped.

Irrigation will greatly assist in identification of the bleeding site. It may be necessary first to secure temporary hemostasis by exerting pressure, either by compressing the vessel with the tip of a blunt instrument or by grasping it with forceps. The method used to achieve permanent occlusion will depend on the size and site of the vessel. Small ones can be electrodesiccated. Larger ones must be ligated, suture ligated, or clipped. Electrical energy should not be used in close proximity to vital structures. Hemorrhage is a potentially life-threatening situation. If it becomes apparent that laparoscopic means are failing to control the bleeding, a laparotomy incision should be made and the hemorrhage stopped.

Continuous oozing from raw areas may be coming from identifiable vessels that can be dealt with individually. General capillary weeping is usually responsive to injection of a dilute vasopressive solution.

Hematomas may be retroperitoneal or within the abdominal wall. It will be necessary to incise the peritoneum to identify and deal with the bleeding vessel if a retroperitoneal hematoma is expanding rapidly.

Delayed bleeding

Delayed bleeding will occur when a pedicle has been poorly secured. Oozing that was not visible at the time of the surgery can start to appear once the effects of any vasopressive solutions have worn off or the tamponade effect of the pneumoperitoneum has been removed after the abdomen has been deflated. For these reasons it is prudent, at the end of any operative procedure, to reduce the intraabdominal pressure and to flood the operative site with irrigation fluid. All pedicles should be inspected. Small oozing vessels can be identified and spot desiccated. Larger vessels or pedicles must be ligated, suture ligated, or clipped.

It may not become apparent until some time postoperatively that intrapelvic or intra-abdominal bleeding has occurred. The patient may show evidence of hypotension and tachycardia. She may be pale and sweating. The abdomen may be distended. Bowel sounds may be absent. Blood or serosanginous fluid may be seen escaping from abdominal or vaginal incisions. Management will be dependent upon the amount of time that has elapsed, the patient's condition, and the probable site of bleeding.

As a general rule, if less than 24 hours have passed, the patient is obviously ill, and the hematocrit values are falling, it will be appropriate to reoperate to find and occlude the vessel. The method of access will depend on the condition of the patient and the apparent severity of the bleeding. If doubt exists it is safer to proceed directly to laparotomy. Obvious vaginal cuff bleeding will be dealt with vaginally.

If bleeding has ocurred more than 24 hours postoperatively, it is not usually possible to find the vessel or vessels responsible. The patient should be followed with serial evaluation of the hematocrit values and CT scans to assess the size of the hematoma. Repeated blood transfusion may be required. If there is any reason to suspect that a coagulopathy is developing, consultation should be sought. If it is apparent that the bleeding is continuing, embolization of the internal iliac vessels under ultrasonic guidance should be considered. These pelvic hematomas are prone to becoming infected. Any such abscesses should be drained (see Chapter 16).

Gastrointestinal injury

Injuries may occur to small or large bowel. The damage may be nonperforating or perforating and may be recognized at the time of surgery or may become apparent some time postoperatively. If it is anticipated that large bowel is at risk, the bowel should be prepared preoperatively with GoLytely. Adhesions from the bowel should never be torn free but rather divided. Electrical energy should not be used in close proximity to bowel.

Nonperforating trauma. These lesions are usually noticed when endometriosis has been dissected from the surface of the bowel. If they are noted at surgery they should be oversewn (see Chapter 18). It is probable that many such defects go undiscovered and give rise to no further problems. They do have the potential for late perforation, however. This is particularly true of injuries which have resulted from electrical trauma (see below).

Perforating trauma. The bowel can be breached inadvertently during dissection of adhesions or excision of lesions of the bowel wall. These perforations are usually immediately apparent. Suspected perforation of the large bowel can often be identified by flooding the pelvis with irrigation solution and insufflating air per rectum.

Small holes can be closed with a purse string suture. A reinforcing second-layer closure should be placed.[10] Larger rents should be closed in two layers in such a way to ensure that the long axis of the suture line lies in the transverse axis of the bowel to prevent stricture formation[11] (see Chapter 18). Thorough lavage must be performed to remove all bowel contents that have spilled into the peritoneal cavity. Material should be aspirated and sent for culture. A course of broad-spectrum antibiotics should be started immediately. Drainage may be necessary.

Obvious electrical or thermal injuries must be dealt with immediately. The spread of damage is much greater than the area of blanching and can create a large area of necrosis leading to delayed perforation of the bowel. When an obvious and persistent blanched area(s) is apparent, the bowel must be excised for 5 cm on either side of the margins of the damaged site and an end-to-end anastomosis performed (Fig. 26-6).[10]

If an injury has ocurred and has not been recognized, the patient in whom full thickness perforation has been missed will be acutely ill in the immediately postoperative period. Electrical injuries may not declare themselves until several days later when the devitalized bowel wall perforates.

These patients complain of increasing abdominal pain, nausea, and vomiting. They are usually febrile. Tachycardia, hypotension, and sweating are usually observed. The abdomen is tender and rigid. The x-ray sign of free air un-

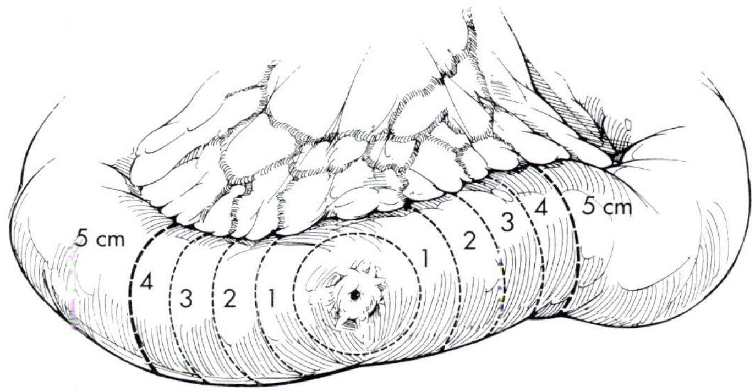

Fig. 26-6. Electrical injury to the bowel. The spread of damage is much greater than the initial area of blanching and can result in a large area of necrosis. Excision of a generous segment on each side of the injury site is required.

der the diaphragm is unreliable because there may be residual gas from the pneumoperitoneum for up to 48 hours postoperatively.

This is a potentially life-threatening complication and must be managed accordingly. We agree with the dictum of Soderstrom et al. that, "A patient who has increasing postoperative pain following a laparoscopy has a bowel perforation until proven otherwise."[10] A general surgeon should be consulted. The perforation must be identified and repaired. On occasion it may be necessary to perform a temporary defunctioning colostomy or ileostomy. Antibiotic therapy is indicated.

Genitourinary injury

Injuries may occur to the bladder or ureter and may be recognized at once or may have delayed presentations. The urinary tract is susceptible to infection.

Bladder. Perforation of the bladder will occur either as a result of dissecting it free from the cervix or during removal of a lesion from the dome. Particular care must be taken when bladder dissection is performed in patients who have sustained retrocystic uterine scars, which occur following cesarean section, some myomectomies, and some metroplasties. In such high-risk cases, instillation of 60 cc of dilute methylene blue solution into the bladder prior to dissection will permit instant recognition if perforation occurs (see Chapter 22). The appearance of methylene blue will alert the surgeon. If this precaution has not been taken, the pelvis can be flooded with irrigation solution and air instilled into the bladder through a catheter. Bubbles in the fluid will betray the site of perforation.

Such perforations should be oversewn in one or two layers and the air/fluid test repeated or more methylene blue solution instilled to confirm the integrity of the repair. A Foley catheter is left in place for 10 to 14 days and removed at the time of the cystogram, which is performed to confirm the integrity of the bladder wall. Oral sulphonamides or antibiotics are given while the catheter is in situ.

Delayed perforation can be identified postoperatively.[14] When the trauma has been electrical or thermal, symptoms may not present until several days later. The leakage of urine into the peritoneal cavity will give rise to pain, bloating, and fever. Hematuria may be present. Consultation should be sought with a urologist. Diagnosis may require the performance of cystography, cystoscopy, and/or laparoscopy. If a laparoscopy is indicated, the site of the defect is sought by the instillation of methylene blue into the bladder. Cystoscopy is usually reserved for those cases in which there is concern that a ureter is involved.

Those perforations that have been identified in the early postoperative period and are not due to thermal or electrical injury can be managed in the same way as those noted intraoperatively (see above).

Just as with bowel, electrical or thermal damage to the bladder will create an area of necrosis that will extend beyond the margins of the visible defect. These patients will require wide excision of the involved area and repair of the resulting wound. An indwelling catheter and antibiotic coverage will be required.

Ureter. The ureter has always been the rock upon which gynecologists have come to grief. Because of its proximity to the operative site at both the pelvic brim and at the level of the uterine arteries, it is particularly prone to damage. In addition, disease processes that distort the normal anatomic relationships and congenital anomalies may distance the ureter from its normal position. The first and absolute principle to be observed is to identify the structure, even if preliminary dissection is required. In cases in which difficulty is anticipated, it may be advisable first to place ureteric catheters to facilitate identification. Illuminated ureteric catheters are also available for this purpose.

Great care must be taken when dissecting close to the ureter. It is possible to damage the vascular supply. The ureter can also be transected, included in a suture or staple, or devitalized with electrical energy. Thus three injuries may result: division, occlusion, and necrosis. All of these may be recognized intraoperatively or may not present until the postoperative period.

Every endeavour should be made to note ureteric injury intraoperatively. Dr. Thomas Green of Boston was widely quoted when he remarked, "The venial sin is injury to the ureter; the mortal sin is failure of recognition."[12]

If transection is noted or suspected, intravenous injection of indigo carmine will soon result in visible leakage of the compound from the proximal end. The area at which it is believed that trauma has occurred should be dissected free and closely scrutinized. A cleanly cut ureter can be immediately repaired. A ureteric stent is inserted under cystoscopic guidance and maneuvered from the lower end into the upper end with laparoscopic grasping forceps. The ureter is sutured with 4-0 polydioxanone. The stent is left in place for 2 weeks and removed at the time of retrograde pyelography, which should demonstrate water-tight integrity."[12]

If it is recognized that a suture has been placed in such a way as to include the ureter, the stitch should be immediately removed. If the suture was placed to occlude a pedicle, division may result in bleeding and thus it will be necessary to reocclude the pedicle. The rest of the operation is concluded and then the ureter is inspected to ensure that normal peristalsis is occurring and that there is no obvious sign of injury to the ureter. It may be necessary to dissect the ureter to facilitate this thorough inspection.

If the ureter has been stapled it will inevitably have been divided. The stapled portion must be excised and an immediate anastomosis performed (see Chapter 18). If the trauma has ocurred close to the bladder, a laparotomy and ureterocystostomy may be performed. Electrical injuries will mandate wide excision of the devitalized portion and repair.

Unfortunately these injuries are not always noted intraoperatively. Such patients will present later either complaining of the effects of leakage of urine into the peritoneal cavity or the sequelae of ureteric obstruction. In the former case the symptoms will be similar to those described above, which occur when an injury to the bladder has not been recognized.

Urologic consultation is sought. Diagnosis is made by intravenous pyelography and/or intravenous injection of indigo carmine and paracentesis 1 hour later when the dye will have had time to stain the peritoneal fluid. The ureter must be repaired, although on occasion some have been managed sucessfully by the cystoscopic placement of ureteric stents combined with drainage. This latter approach leads to a prolonged recovery period. If the injury is the result of electrodesiccation there can be extensive destruction of tissue. Treatment is more difficult. A few patients have had to undergo nephrectomy.[13]

Ureteric obstruction usually presents with flank pain and fever. Intravenous pyelography or ultrasonography will show the presence of a hydronephrosis of the affected side. A urologic consultation should be sought. Attempts to carry out retrograde ureteric catheterization will fail at the level of the obstruction. The obstruction may be due to tissue edema or angulation of the ureter due to tissue tension, sutures, or staples.[14] Percutaneous nephrostomy is indicated if it is suspected that the obstruction may be self-correcting, otherwise the obstructed section must be excised and the ureter repaired, either as a primary approach or when it becomes apparent following nephrostomy that ureteric function has not returned.

Infection

Urinary tract infection (UTI) is an unavoidable risk of gynecologic surgery. Laparoscopic surgery confers no special protection. The investigation and management of UTI is no different, regardless of the route of access by which the surgery has been performed.

CONCLUSIONS

In an ideal world complications would never arise. In day to day practice they are unavoidable and in laparoscopic practice may be results of the laparoscopy itself or of the procedure for which laparoscopy has provided the means of access. It is the responsibility of every surgeon to keep the rate of maloccurrences to an absolute minimum. To do so only fully trained surgeons should carry out procedures with which they are thoroughly familiar. A procedure should not be undertaken unless the physician can deal with any complication that might arise or have ready access to skilled consultants. High-risk situations should be identified and any particular risk anticipated. Meticulous adherence to the details of proper technique is essential to prevent complications.

The surgeon must be able to recognize complications as soon as they have occurred or, in the event this has not been possible, be able to make the diagnosis rapidly. Once the diagnosis has been established, surgeons, either by virtue of their own training or with the help of consultants, must repair the damage to keep the suffering and disability of the patient to an absolute minimum.

REFERENCES

1. Querleu D, Chevallier L, Chapron C, Bruhat MA: Complications of gynaecological laparoscopic surgery. A French multicentre collabortive study. *Gynaecol Endo* 2:3-6, 1993.
2. Mintz M: Le risque et la prophylaxie des accidents en coelioscopie gynécologique. Enquête portant sur 100.000 cas. *Gyn Obst Biol Repr* 5:681-695, 1976.
3. Lehmann-Willenbrock E, Riedel H-H, Mecke H, Semm K: Pelviscopy/laparoscopy and its complications in Germany, 1949-1988. *J Rep Med* 37:671-677, 1992.
4. Gomel V, Taylor PJ, Yuzpe AA, Rioux JE: Laparoscopy and hysteroscopy in gynecologic practice. Chicago 1986, Year Book.
5. Soderstrom RM, Butler JC: A critical evaluation of complications in laparoscopy. *J Rep Med* 10:245-248, 1973.
6. Hurd WW, Pearl ML, DeLancey JOL, et al: Laparoscopic injury of abdominal wall blood vessels: a report of three cases. *Obstet Gynecol* 82:673-6, 1993.
7. Kadar N, Reich H, Liu CY, et al: Incisional hernias after major laparoscopic gynecologic procedures. *Am J Obstet Gynecol* 168:1493-5, 1993.
8. Romanowski L, Reich H, McGlynn F, et al: Brachial plexus neuropathies after advanced laparoscopic surgery. *Fertil Steril* 60:729-732, 1992.
9. Hershlag A, Loy RA, Lavy G, DeCherney AH: Femoral neuropathy after laparoscopy, a case report. *J Rep Med* 575-576.
10. Soderstrom RM, Levinson C, Levy B: Complications of operative laparoscopy: In Soderstrom RM, editor: Operative Laparoscopy. New York, 1993, Raven Press.
11. Reich H, McGlynn F, Budin R: Laparoscopic repair of full-thickness bowel injury. *J LaparoEndo Sur* 1:119-122, 1991.
12. Gomel V, James C: Intraoperative management of ureteral injury during operative laparoscopy. *Fertil Steril* 55:416-419, 1991.
13. Grainger DA, Soderstrom RM, Schiff SF, et al: Ureteral injuries at laparoscopy: insights into diagnosis, management, and prevention. *Obstet Gynecol* 75:839-843, 1990.
14. Woodland MB: Ureter injury during laparoscopy-assisted vaginal hysterectomy with the endoscopic linear stapler. *Am J Obstet Gynecol* 167:756-7, 1992.

Chapter 27

FUTURE DIRECTIONS

A cursory glance at the table of contents of this book should serve to reveal the enormous advances that have taken place in the last decade in laparoscopy, particularly in laparoscopic surgical techniques. In fact, it would take less space to list the gynecologic procedures that cannot be performed laparoscopically than to list those that can. This revolution in minimal access surgery is being mirrored in almost all of the surgical disciplines.

It is now time to consider the future, a notoriously difficult task, yet one that must be addressed. The course will be charted by the inevitable coming together of forces internal and external to our discipline. While it is not possible to predict with total accuracy where this course will lead, it is possible to examine these influences and to suggest how the future will unfold.

Internal forces will include (1) The innate drive of the innovator, in the words of the early pioneers of the space program, "to push the envelope." Even 10 years ago the concept of laparoscopic hysterectomy was inconceivable. (2) The "me too" effect, whereby once a procedure has been described by an innovator the gynecologist feels pressure to introduce it into daily practice. It is to be hoped, (3) our willingness to appraise critically the outcome of any new techniques.

External forces will include (1) the rate of technologic change, (2) the effects of costs, (3) the influence of regulatory bodies, and (4) the way in which consumer pressure can subtly, or indeed not so subtly, influence medical practice.

This chapter will address these issues.

INTERNAL INFLUENCES

Role of the innovator

The range of gynecologic operations is limited. With the exceptions of tubotubal anastomosis and the field of oncology, areas that even now are under intense examination by innovative laparoscopic surgeons, it is difficult to see how the ambit of laparoscopic gynecologic procedures can be expanded further, at least in the adult patient. Much work remains to be done in pediatric endoscopy and in our ability to intervene in utero.

The "me too" effect

The rapidity of dissemination of laparoscopic technology has been amazing. Much credit must go to such organizations as the American Association of Gynecologic Laparoscopists (AAGL). Unfortunately, some would consider the spread of new techniques to have been somewhat precipitant. Practicing physicians are no less susceptible to the need to "Keep up with the Joneses,"—the "me too" effect. Operations are being performed that, while technically feasible, have not been submitted to rigorous scrutiny to determine their efficacy or if they are indeed superior to the older methods.[1] This issue will be discussed further in the next section and the section dealing with the possible effects of regulatory bodies.

Critical appraisal

Any critical appraisal of laparoscopic surgery must consider the following questions:

Have the indications been properly developed?

Are the rates of complications, not only in the hands of virtuosi surgeons but in the hands of ordinary practitioners, well documented and do they compare favorably with the rates for the same procedure carried out by more traditional means?

Is the procedure cost effective?

How effective is the procedure in producing the desired outcome?

Do other treatment options exist that might spare the patient any surgical intervention?

These questions will now be considered. Space precludes

full discussion of every possible laparoscopic procedure. Illustrative examples will be used.

Indications. Let us take the case of myomectomy. Infertility and habitual abortion are often cited as indications for the performance of myomectomy. The laparoscopic approach to this procedure has been described in Chapter 19. It is clear that laparoscopic myomectomy is limited to those lesions that are of reasonable size and that are predominantly subserous. Is such intervention warranted in infertile patients and those complaining of habitual abortion?

Myomata occur in 20% to 30% of women over the age of 30.[2] Eighty-nine percent of such women will have delivered at least on infant at term.[3] This same cohort study was unable to demonstrate any significantly increased risk of abortion when women with fibroids were compared with matched controls.

Vercellini et al.[4] have summarized data collected from 13 published series of myomectomies, all of which were performed to correct infertility. One hundred seventy-two (55%) of 314 women so treated did conceive. Regrettably, all of the studies used the patients as their own controls. As such it is not possible to determine how many women would have conceived if no surgery had been performed. Until a randomized prospective study of myomectomy vs. expectant treatment is conducted, and with sufficient numbers to have the statistical power to detect no difference if none exists, the question of whether or not infertility constitutes a valid indication for myomectomy, laparoscopic or otherwise, will remain unanswered.

Complications. The exact rates of complications can be determined only by examination of data derived from large numbers of cases. True appreciation of complication rates is extremely difficult to determine. Those surgeons who are least likely to comply with voluntary requests to report their procedures and complications may well be those with the highest rates.

An excellent start has been made by Querleu et al.[5] A multicenter study was conducted in seven major French centers. Seventeen thousand, five hundred twenty-one cases were reported. Of these cases, 8343 were diagnostic and 9187 were operative. These operative procedures included lysis of adhesions, surgery for ectopic pregnancy, salpingectomy, distal tuboplasty, ovarian cystectomy, conservative surgery for pelvic inflammatory disease, endometriosis, and more complex procedures. There were no deaths in the diagnostic group and one in the operative group following a trocar injury to a major vessel. There were 48 major complications that led to unintended laparotomy, a rate of 5.23 per 1000. These are very valuable data, which were discussed in greater detail in Chapter 26. It is to be hoped that similar data will become available from every center (not only select ones) and that the true rates and types of complications for specific procedures will soon be known

Cost-benefit ratio. It is argued convincingly that one of the major advantages of minimal access surgery is cost saving. This argument was challenged by Summit et al.[6] A randomized prospective study comparing laparoscopic-assisted vaginal hysterectomy (LAVH) with vaginal hysterectomy was performed. Fifty-six women were enrolled. Twenty-seven underwent the former procedure and 29 the latter. The outcomes of interest that were studied included mean length of operating room time, complications, amount of pain medication required, and cost. The mean operating room time for LAVH was 120 minutes compared with 65 minutes for vaginal hysterectomy. Significantly more analgesia was required for the LAVH group. The difference in cost was startling. A vaginal hysterectomy cost $4891, an LAVH $7,905. It would seem that transforming a vaginal hysterectomy into an LAVH is not cost effective. This may well change as surgeons become more experienced in the laparoscopic method and reduce the operating time considerably. This study did not address the question of the relative benefits of converting a procedure that could have been performed only abdominally to an LAVH.

Hidden costs may accrue to laparoscopic surgery. An informal survey carried out in the Province of British Columbia has unveiled no less than nine cases of transection of the common bile duct that occurred during laparoscopic cholecystectomy. All of these patients have required further surgery, two having to undergo liver transplantation. The medicolegal costs have yet to be determined but will be considerable and indeed may exceed the savings that have accrued from the introduction of the technique.

When cost is considered, questions must be asked about a further phenomenon—questions which at present remain unanswered. Is it possible that patients who might well have decided that they were unwilling to undergo extensive surgery might now be more amenable to accepting what some, incorrectly, refer to as a "minimally invasive" procedure? Certainly an increasing number of requests for endometrial ablation are coming from women who, far from having heavy periods, simply do not wish to tolerate the inconvenience of menstruation. Is it possible that an increased volume of laparoscopic procedures may reduce any costs saved per individual case?

There remains one final factor in the cost-benefit equation. While it may be argued that a given procedure is less expensive than one carried out through a laparotomy incision, if the efficacy of either in producing the desired outcome is in doubt it may well be that any monies expended are simply being wasted.

Outcome. Two examples will serve to illustrate why evaluation of outcome is so critical to defining the future place of laparoscopic surgery: the treatment of ectopic pregnancy (see Chapter 14), and the role of surgical management of the Revised American Fertility Society (RAFS)[7] stages 1 and 2 endometriosis for the treatment of infertility.

The very satisfactory outcomes following laparoscopic surgery for tubal ectopic pregnancy are well documented. Except under exceptional circumstances, it is difficult today to justify submitting such a patient to laparotomy. Endometriosis presents a more puzzling picture.

It is still not clear whether or not surgical treatment of RAFS stages 1 and 2 endometriosis will improve the pregnancy rate. A beneficial effect has been suggested by one study of treatment-dependent vs. treatment-independent pregnancies in such patients.[8] No difference in the pregnancy rates was noted when patients treated by laparoscopy or laparotomy were compared.[9] While both of these studies would support the concept that laparoscopic treatment is as equally efficacious as laparotomy and that there is a measurable improvement in the pregnancy rate, further work is required to confirm these findings.

Treatment options. It has been remarked that any surgical procedure represents a failure of less invasive therapy. Just as laparoscopic surgery is replacing many traditional operations, it is reasonable to hope that any therapeutic option that is equally or more effective, less invasive, carries a lower rate of complications, and is less expensive should replace laparoscopy.

Ectopic pregnancy can serve as an example of how such treatments might evolve. When 100 patients were treated with systemically administered methotrexate, 96 were considered to have been treated successfully.[10] Only five experienced side effects. The recurrence rate of ectopic pregnancy among those who conceived was 10%. Whether this option or the direct injection of the gestational sac under ultrasonographic guidance[11] will ultimately replace laparoscopic surgery remains to be seen.

Already in vitro fertilization (IVF) (see Chapter 15) is becoming a viable alternative to tubal surgery for the infertile woman with damaged tubes, particularly when it is now possible to predict with reasonable accuracy the relative likelihood of success for a given individual woman.[12]

Unpredictable advances can occur at any time in other branches of medicine or the basic sciences. Although the early promise was not fulfilled that gonadotropin-releasing hormone agonists would render surgical management of fibroids obsolete, who can predict when some other compound, perhaps related to one that interferes with the action of epidermal growth factor, will not appear?

Thus the future will be influenced by factors that are clearly under the control of the medical profession. How we choose to direct our efforts will be to some extent in our own hands. Properly conducted observational studies of large numbers of patients and prospective randomized clinical trials must be conducted. Whether or not we have the will and resources to carry out such research and the integrity to modify our practices in the light of the answers that will be forthcoming remains to be seen.

At the end of the twentieth century the practice of medicine is no longer strictly a concern of the providers of the services. Those external forces that will play an increasing role will now be discussed.

EXTERNAL INFLUENCES

Technologic change

The rate of technologic change increases exponentially. A consideration of Chapter 8 gives some indication of developments in documentation and visualization systems that already are beginning to appear. Virtual reality is being explored as a surgical training method. Robotic scalpels are being designed that one day may be more accurate than the trained surgical hand and less susceptible to injuries with the attendant risks to the surgeon.

Newer methods of suturing, ligating, and stapling will be developed and by their application reduce the time taken to perform a given procedure. True minimal access surgery will be a reality only if large pieces of excised tissue can be removed without resorting to extending an abdominal incision or opening the posterior fornix. Electrically driven coring devices are under production. One has a cutting cylinder that is introduced through a 14 mm cannula and driven by an externally sited microengine. The instrument has been used successfully to deal with large fibroids.[13]

Costs

Cost will undoubtedly be a limiting factor that will influence the introduction of some of these advances. While it may be possible to develop a budget with which to purchase a new endoscope with the ability to generate three-dimensional images, the higher resolution monitors needed for such a system may make the total set-up unaffordable. Many of us will have to adopt the attitude of Max Aitken, who for his efforts in the British Ministry of Aircraft Production in the Churchill cabinet, was ennobled as Lord Beaverbrook. He markedly increased the delivery of fighter airplanes to the squadrons during the Battle of Britain by application of the philosophy that "excellence is the mortal enemy of the merely very good." Those who must foot the bills for a three-dimensional display will have to be convinced that it is infinitely superior to the older units, not only in the opinion of the surgeon but as demonstrated by measurably improved outcomes.

Regulatory bodies

It is surprising that, in an era in which no drug can be introduced into daily practice without satisfying long and rigorous scrutiny by the Food and Drug Administration in America and the Health Protection Branch in Canada, new surgical procedures seem to be immune from such evaluation. The Australian Institute of Health and Welfare has just produced a detailed analysis of "Technologies for the treatment of menorrhagia and uterine myomas."[14] The document runs to some 74 pages and is replete with tables of cost-benefit analysis. Earlier in this chapter the place of laparoscopic myomectomy was questioned. The Australian report concludes, "Since the procedure is used mainly for small subserous myomas which are usually asymptomatic, it is not necessarily useful as a primary treatment at present." It would be naive to believe that much more intensive evaluations will not be carried out by comparable bodies and that in the foreseeable future no new techniques will be permitted to enter routine practice without approval by some statutory body.

Consumer pressure

Patients or, if you prefer (and certainly many of them prefer) the designation, "consumers of health care" are no longer passive recipients of our advice. They expect to be informed and to play much more active roles in the definition of their treatment. The enormous effect of AIDS and breast cancer activists is already being felt. Single disease special interest groups are proliferating rapidly. Many are remarkably well informed. Many are not, and the ease with which public opinion can be swayed by vocal spokespersons and the media cannot be underestimated. Already we are being asked to perform endometrial ablations in totally inappropriate circumstances because someone has extolled the virtues of the technique on a television talk show. The indication for LAVH, just as it was with certain laser procedures in the past, might well be to preserve a surgeon's practice rather than the fact that it is so demonstrably better than a vaginal hysterectomy.

CONCLUSIONS

By the very nature of its subject this chapter has been speculative. It has been an attempt, by extrapolating from present knowledge, to identify some of those forces that will mold the way in which laparoscopy will develop. Predictions rarely are completely fulfilled but it is nevertheless reasonable to hope that the combination of internal and external forces will create an environment in which laparoscopy will continue to evolve and that invalid procedures will become footnotes to medical history. Valid procedures and technologic advances will continue to allow us to offer our patients the benefits of endoscopic surgery, a field that undoubtedly represents the surgery of the future.

REFERENCES

1. Gomel V: Operative laparoscopy: time for acceptance. *Fertil Steril* 52:1-11, 1989.
2. Vollenhoven BJ, Lawrence AS, Healy DL: Uterine fibroids: a clinical review. *Br J Obstet Gynaecol* 97:285-298, 1990.
3. Ross RK, Pike MC, Vessey MP, et al: Risk factors for uterine fibriods: reduced risk associated with oral contraceptives. *Br Med J* 293:359-362, 1986.
4. Vercellini P, Bocciolone L, Rognoni MT, Bolis G: Fibroids and infertility. In Shaw RW, editor: Advances in Reproductive Endocrinology, Uterine fibroids, time for review, New Jersey, 1992, The Parthenon Publishing Group.
5. Querleu D, Chevallier L, Chapron C, Bruhat MA: Complications of laparoscopic surgery. A French multicentre collaborative study. *Gynaecol Endosc* 2:3-6, 1993.
6. Summitt RL Jr, Stovall TG, Lipscomb GH, Ling FW: Randomized comparison of laparoscopy-assisted vaginal hysterectomy with standard vaginal hysterectomy in an outpatient setting. *Obstet Gynaecol* 80:895-901, 1992.
7. American Fertility Society: Revised classification of endometriosis. *Fertil Steril* 43:351, 1985.
8. Tulandi T, Mouchawar M: Treatment-dependant and treatment-independent pregnancy in women with minimal and mild endometriosis. *Fertil Steril* 56:790, 1991.
9. Grant NF: Infertility and endometriosis: comparison of outcomes with laparotomy versus laparoscopic techniques. *Am J Obstet Gynecol* 166:1072-1073, 1992.
10. Stovall TG, Ling FW, Buster JE: Outpatient chemotherapy of unruptured tubal pregnancy. *Fertil Steril* 51:435-438, 1989.
11. Feichtinger W, Kemeter P: Conservative treatment of ectopic pregnancy by transvaginal aspiration under sonographic control and injection of methotrexate. *Lancet* 1:381-382, 1987.
12. Gomel V: Distal tubal occlusion. *Fertil Steril* 49:946-948, 1988.
13. Steiner RA, Wright E, Tadir Y, Haller U: Electrical cutting device for laparoscopic removal of tissue from the abdominal cavity. *Obstet Gynecol* 81:471-474, 1993.
14. Hirsch NA: Technologies for the treatment of menorrhagia and uterine myomas. HealthCare Technology Series Number 10, Canberra, 1993, Australian Government Publishing Service.

INDEX

A

AAGL; *See* American Association of Gynecologic Laparoscopists[1]
Abdomen
inspection, palpation and percussion of, 59
Abdominal closure, 63, 64
Abdominal masses
diagnostic laparoscopy and, 66
Abdominal scars
tender masses in
as indication of endometriosis, 133, 134
Abdominal surgeries
prior
as relative contraindication
for diagnostic laparoscopy, 69
Ablation
endometrial
as alternative to hysterectomy, 242
of uterosacral ligaments
in endometriosis, 205
Abortion
acute pelvic pain and, 119
tubal, 163, 165
Abscesses
tubo-ovarian
ruptured
laparoscopic management of, 185, 186
Abscesses, pelvic; *See* Pelvic abscesses
Acetyl salicylic acid
in treatment of endometriosis, 127
Acquired lesions
intrapelvic
as cause of chronic cyclic pain, 128
laparoscopy and, 128
uterine
as cause of chronic cyclic pain, 128
hysterosalpingography and, 128
hysteroscopy and, 128
Active electrode trauma; *See* Electrode trauma
Adenocarcinomas
clear-cell
laparoscopic lymphadenectomy, 146
Adenomyosis; *See* Acquired lesions, uterine
Adhesiolysis, 83, *84*, 85
endometriosis and, 203, 204
preceding laparoscopic hysterectomy, 244
Adhesions; *See also* Periadnexal adhesive disease
intra abdominal
diagnostic laparoscopy and, 66, 67
intraluminal
identified through hysterosalpingography, 105*T*, 106

Italicized number denotes a page with an illustration; italicized *T* denotes a page with a table.

Adhesions—cont'd
omental
endoscopic survey and, 112
pelvic
chronic acyclic pain and, 129
periadnexal
treated by salpingo-ovariolysis, *171*, 172
prevention of, 87
Adler, D. H.
history of laparoscopy, 3
Adnexa
tender
as indication of endometriosis, 133
Adnexectomies
history of laparoscopy, 3
for removal of cystic ovarian tumors, 195
results of, 195
with sutures or ligatures, 195
through electrodesiccation, 195
AFS; *See* American Fertility Society
Albano, V.
history of laparoscopy, 2
Albucasis
history of electrosurgery, 26
Alternate ground site burns
ESUs in prevention of, 40*T*, 41
Alternating current
effect on cells, 30, *31*, 32
Amenorrhea
laparoscopy and, 110
American Association of Gynecologic Laparoscopists
training, 6
American Fertility Society
classification of distal tubal disease, 107, 108*T*, 176
classification system of endometriosis, 136
credentialling guidelines
operative endoscopy, 7, 8
American Society of Anesthesiologists
patient classification system, 71, 72
Aminoglycoside
postoperative treatment of PID, 186
Ammeters
large vessel hemostasis and, 38, 39
Amoxicillin/clavulanic acid
in treatment of PID, 123
Ampullary occlusions
identified through hysterosalpingography, 105*T*, 106
Anaprox; *See* Naproxen sodium
Anastomosis
tubocornual, 105
tubotubal
microsurgery compared to laparoscopy, 176
results of, 178
for sterilization reversal, 176

Anastomosis—cont'd
tubotubal—cont'd
technique, *177*, 178
Anderson, E. T.
history of electrosurgery, 27
history of laparoscopic sterilization, 149
history of laparoscopy, 2, 3
Anesthesia
equipment, 72
general
diagnostic laparoscopy and, 58
in operative laparoscopy, 73, 74
local
diagnostic laparoscopy and, 58
for tubal sterilizations, 73
Anovulation
causes of, 110
Appendectomies
endometriosis and, 209
intracorporeal, *261*, *262*
results of, 263
laparoscopically assisted, 4, 260, *261*
results of, 263
Appendicitis
anatomy of the appendix, 259
danger to female reproductive organs, 259
as differentiated from PID, 259
laparoscopic diagnosis of, 124, 259
symptoms of, 259
Appendix
anatomy of, 259, *260*
Argon beam coagulators, 24, 37, *38*
for laparoscopic fulguration, 39
presacral neurectomy and, *233*, 234
Argon lasers, 51, 52
for tissue coagulation in laparoscopy, 53
Armboards, 13, 14
Arrhythmias, cardiac; *See* Cardiac arrhythmias
Arylpropionic acid derivatives
in treatment of primary dysmenorrhea, 126*T*, 127
ASA; *See* American Society of Anesthesiologists
Aspiration
cystic ovarian tumors and, 191, 192
gastric
as complication of laparoscopy, 305
needles and, 20, 21
Aspirin
in treatment of primary dysmenorrhea, 126*T*, 127
Assisted reproductive technologies (ART)
GIFT, PROST, and ZIFT, 179, 180

B

Babylonian Talmud
history of laparoscopy, 1

Back injuries
  as complication of laparoscopy, 304
Bacteroides
  as cause of PID, 121
Bailey, Gregory J., 96
Bardenheuer, R.
  history of electrosurgery, 27
Barnes, A. C.
  history of laparoscopic sterilization, 149
  history of laparoscopy, 2, 3
Basov, Nikolai G.
  history of laser surgery, 44
Beer
  history of electrosurgery, 27
Bellina, J. H.
  history of laser surgery, 44
Benzoic acid derivatives
  in treatment of primary dysmenorrhea, 126*T*, 127
Bernkeim, B. M.
  history of laparoscopy, 2
Biopsy forceps, 24
  Palmer drill, 24
    in laparoscopic sterilization, 150
Biopsy specimens
  of endometriosis, 135
    appearance of, 202*T*, 203
  during endoscopic examination
    of ovarian tumors, 138, 140
Black coagulation; *See* Fulguration
Bladder
  care of, 59
  dysfunction
    as symptom of endometriosis, 133
  injuries
    as complication of laparoscopy, 300, 301
    electrical
      as complication of operative laparoscopy, 307
  relationship to pelvic floor, 265
  surgery of
    in endometriosis, 209, *210*
Bleeding; *See also* Hemorrhages; Hemostasis
  abdominal wall
    as complication of laparoscopy, 301
  gastrointestinal
    as symptom of endometriosis, 133
  urinary
    as symptom of endometriosis, 133
  uterine
    as contraindication for
      hysterosalpingography, 101
Blood clotting
  heparin and, 87
Blood vessels
  already divided
    producing hemostasis in, 75-77
  injuries to
    as complication of laparoscopy, 301, *302*, 304
  intact
    producing hemostasis in, 75
Body weight extremes; *See also* Obesity; Thin patients
  as relative contraindication
    for diagnostic laparoscopy, 69
Bonney test
  for stress incontinence, 268
Bosch, P. F.
  history of electrosurgery, 27
  history of laparoscopy, 2, 3
Bovie
  history of electrosurgery, 27
Bowel
  dysfunction
    as symptom of endometriosis, 133
  injuries
    as complication of laparoscopy, 300-304, *303*
    as complication of operative laparoscopy
      electrical, 306
      nonperforating, 306
      perforating, 306
Bowel disease
  inflammatory
    as relative contraindication
      for diagnostic laparoscopy, 69
Bozzini, P.
  history of laparoscopy, 1
Braces
  shoulder, 13, 14
Brachial plexus injuries
  as complication of laparoscopy, 304
Bridges, W. B.
  history of laser surgery, 44
Bruhat, M. A.
  history of laparoscopy, 3
  history of laser surgery, 44
Bupivacaine
  during LAVH, 250
  in operative laparoscopy, 73
  in surgical treatment of uterine retroversion, 237
Burns
  alternate ground site
    ESUs in prevention of, 40*T*, 41
  from dispersive electrodes
    cause and prevention, 40*T*, 42*T*
  intestinal
    laser surgery and, 54
Butyrophenones
  in treatment of primary dysmenorrhea, 126*T*, 127

C

CA-125 antigen
  elevated levels of
    as indication of endometriosis, 134
Cables; *See* Fiberoptic cables; Fluid-filled cables
Calibrated uterine resection tool (CURT)
  in subtotal laparoscopic hysterectomy, 254, *255*, *256*
Cameras
  video
    endoscopic light generators and, 92
Canadian Consensus Conference on Endometriosis
  conference proceedings, 133
Cancers, cervical; *See* Cervical cancers
Cancers, genital; *See* Genital cancers
Cannulas, 15
  ancillary, 20
    introduction of, 63, *64*
  Cohen, 15, *16*
  disposable, 20
  fiberglass, 18
  Heinkel-Semm dilator and, 20
  metal, 18
  principal, 18-20
    introduction of, 61, *62*
  suction/irrigation, 20, 21
  valves and, 18, 19
Capacitive coupling
  cause and prevention, 40*T*, 41, 42*T*
  prevention shields and monitors, 43
Carbonization, 32
Carcinomas
  cervical
    FIGO classification of, 142*T*
  endometrial
    classification of, 143, 146*T*
    diagnostic laparoscopy and, 143, 146
  ovarian
    laparoscopic lymphadenectomies, 138, 141
  vaginal
    laparoscopic lymphadenectomy and, 146
  vulvar
    laparoscopic lymphadenectomy, 146
Cardiac arrhythmias
  as complication of laparoscopy, 304, 305
Cardiorespiratory disease; *See also* Respiratory complications
  major contraindications
    for diagnostic laparoscopy, 69
CAT scans
  deficiencies in testing for endometriosis, 134
Cautery
  differentiated from electrosurgery, 26
CCD chips
  in video cameras, 93, 94
Cefotaxime
  in treatment of pelvic abscesses, 182
Cefotaximine
  postoperative treatment of PID, 186
Cefotetan
  in treatment of PID, 123
Cefoxitin
  postoperative care, 185
  in treatment of PID, 123, 183
Ceftriaxone
  in treatment of PID, 123
Celioscopy
  history of laparoscopy, 1
Centers for Disease Control and Prevention
  recommendations for treatment of PID, 123
Cephalosporin
  in laparoscopic hysterectomy, 243
  postoperative treatment of PID, 186
  in treatment of PID, 123
Cervical cancers
  FIGO classification of, 142*T*, 143
  treated by LARVH, 296
  treated by LRH, 296, 297
Cervical carcinomas
  FIGO classification of, 142*T*
  laparoscopic lymphadenectomy and, 142, 143
    history of, 143
    technical considerations, 143
Cervical lacerations
  as complication of laparoscopy, 304
Cervical stenosis; *See* Acquired lesions, uterine
Cervix lesions
  colored
    as indication of endometriosis, 133, 134
Cetoperazone
  postoperative treatment of PID, 186
Charge-coupled device chips; *See* CCD chips
Chlamydia trachomatis
  as cause of pelvic inflammatory disease, 121
Chloramphenicol
  in treatment of pelvic abscesses, 182
Cholecystectomy
  by laparoscopy, 4
Cholecystitis
  acute
    laparoscopy in diagnosis of, 125
Chorionic gonadotropin; *See also* β hCG assay; GnRH agonists; GnRH analogues
  in inducing ovulation, 199

Citrovorum
  in tubal pregnancy, 158
Cittadini, E.
  history of laparoscopy, 2
Clindamycin
  in treatment of pelvic abscesses, 182
  in treatment of PID, 123, 183
Clips; *See also* Filshie clips; Hulka clip
  to produce hemostasis, 75
Clomiphene
  in inducing ovulation, 199
CO lasers, 52
CO_2 lasers
  as cutting tool, 53
Coagulation; *See also* Endocoagulation; Thermocoagulation; White coagulation
  laser surgery and, 50, 51
  of tissue
    by electrosurgery, 32, 33, 34-38
    in laparoscopy
      argon lasers and, 53
Cohen, Melvin R.
  history of laparoscopy, 2
Cohen cannulas, 15, *16*; *See also* Cannulas
Colitis
  ulcerative
    as relative contraindication
      for diagnostic laparoscopy, 69
Colonic lesions
  anterior
    endometriosis and, 214
Colpotomies
  for removal of large specimens, 84
  in treatment of pelvic abscesses, 183
Computer-assisted tomography scans; *See* CAT scans
Congenital lesions
  as cause of chronic cyclic pain, 128
Contraceptives
  oral
    in treatment of primary dysmenorrhea, 126
Contraindications
  major
    for diagnostic laparoscopy
      cardiorespiratory disease, 69
      hernias, 69
      ileus-intestinal obstructions, 69
      inexperienced surgeon, 69
      peritonitis, 69
  relative
    for diagnostic laparoscopy
      body weight extremes, 69
      displaced or enlarged organs, 70
      inflammatory bowel disease, 69
      intrauterine pregnancy, 69
      large intra-abdominal masses, 70
      prior abdominal surgeries, 69
      regional ileitis, 69
      ulcerative colitis, 69
Controllers
  camera, 94
    frame rates, 94
Cornual occlusion
  laparoscopy timing and, 113
Cornual polyps; *See* Intramural polyps
Cornual pregnancies; *See also* Pregnancies
  operative laparoscopy and, 165, 166
Corpus luteum
  bleeding
    acute pelvic pain and, 122, 124
Costs
  of laparoscopy, 310, 311
C-reactive protein values
  PID and, 122
Credentialling, 7-12
  grandfather clause, 12
Cul-de-sac
  differentiated from enterocele, 266
  in endometriosis
    indicated by tender nodularity of, 133
    restoration of, 205, *206*
  relationship to pelvic floor, 266
Culdocentesis
  PID and, 122
Current
  effect on temperature rise in tissues, 28
Current density; *See* Power density
Current diversion
  alternate ground site burns
    cause and prevention, 40*T*, 41
CURT; *See* Calibrated uterine resection tool
Cushing
  history of electrosurgery, 27
Cutting, 32, *33*, 34-38
Cystectomies
  for treatment of ovarian cancers, 295
Cystic ovarian tumors; *See* Ovarian tumors, cystic
Cystographies
  in diagnosis of bladder injuries, 307
Cystometrograms
  as test for stress incontinence, 268
Cystoscopies
  in diagnosis of bladder injuries, 307
  as test for cystic ovarian tumors, 191, 192
  as test for stress incontinence, 268

D

Danazol
  as treatment for uterine lesions, 128
  in treatment of endometriosis, 203
D'Arsonval, Arsene
  history of electrosurgery, 26
deForest
  invention of vacuum tube, 26, 27
Dehiscence
  uterine
    as complication of laparoscopic myomectomy, 227
Dehydration, 32
Dermoid cysts; *See* Teratomas, benign
Desiccation, 32, *33*, 34-38
  in laparoscopic sterilization, 150
  small vessel hemostasis and, 39
Desormeaux, A. J.
  history of laparoscopy, 1
Dextran
  to prevent adhesion formation, 87
DHE; *See* Dihydro porphyrin ether
Diagnostic laparoscopy; *See* Laparoscopies, diagnostic
Diaphragms
  endometriosis and, 214
Dihydro porphyrin ether
  in endometriosis, 216
Diode sensors, hole accumulator; *See* HAD sensors
Direct coupling
  cause and prevention, 40T, 41, 42*T*
  prevention shields and monitors, 43
Dispersive electrodes; *See* Electrodes, dispersive
Dissection
  adhesiolysis, 83, *84*, 85
  blunt, 82
Dissection—cont'd
  hydrodissection, 82, 83
  sharp, 82
Distal tubal disease
  American Fertility Society classification of, 107, 108*T*
  as identified through hysterosalpingography, 105*T*, 107
  as identified through laparoscopy, 105*T*, 111
Distal tubal occlusion
  prognosis for pregnancy
    when treated by fimbrioplasty, 175
    when treated by microsurgery, 176
    when treated by salpingo-ovariolysis, 175
    when treated by salpingostomy, 176
  treated by salpingostomy, 172, 173, *174*, 175
Distension media, *37*, 38
Diverticulitis
  Meckel's
    laparoscopy in diagnosis of, 125
Documentation
  definition of, 89
  documentation system, 93, 94, 96
  purpose of, 89, 90
  video
    archiving of, 96, 97
    guidelines for, 97
    legal status, 91
    technical aspects of, 91-93
Dornier Medical Systems, 52
Doxycycline
  postoperative care, 185
  in treatment of PID, 123, 183
Doyen, E.
  history of electrosurgery, 26
Doyle, J. B.
  history of LUNA, 230
Dysmenorrhea
  as cause of chronic cyclic pelvic pain, 125
  LUNA and, 230, 232, 233
  presacral neurectomy and, 233-235
  primary
    endometriosis and, 127
    pathophysiology of, 125, 126
    treatment of, 126, 127
  secondary
    causes of, 127
    endometriosis and, 127
    IUDs and, 127
    prostaglandins and, 127
    treatment of, 127, 128
  as symptom of endometriosis, 133
Dyspareunia
  PID and, 121

E

Ectopic pregnancies; *See also* Tubal pregnancies
  diagnosis of, 120
  differential diagnosis of, 119, 120
  symptoms of, 120
  tests for, 120
Edison, Thomas
  history of laparoscopy, 1
Edwards
  history of laparoscopy, 3
Egypt
  history of electrosurgery, 26
Einstein, Albert
  history of laser surgery, 44
Electrical energy
  principles of, 27-32
Electricity
  properties of, 28

Electrode trauma
increased zone of effect
cause and prevention, 40*T*
unintended activation
cause and prevention, 39, 40*T*
unintended arcing to adjacent structures
cause and prevention, 40*T*
Electrodes
dispersive, 36
fulgurating, 36
shields and monitors
in prevention of capacitive or direct coupling, 43
tissue proximity, 36
Electrodesiccation
in adnexectomy, 195
to produce hemostasis, 75
tube, 160
Electromagnetic waves
role in laser physics, 44-48
Electromicrosurgery, 38
Electrosurgery
in coagulation of tissue, 32, *33*, 34-38
complications of, 39, 40*T*, 42
definition of, 26
differentiated from cautery, 26
history of, 26
in laparoscopic sterilization, 150, 152
bipolar, 150, 152
thermocoagulation, 152
unipolar, 150
desiccation and transection, 150
desiccation only, 150
principles of, 26
safety considerations in, 43, 44
in tubal pregnancy
salpingectomies and, 160
segmental excisions and, 160, 163, *164*
in vaporization of tissue, 32, *33*, 34-38
Electrosurgical generators; *See* ESUs
Electrosurgical instruments
introduction of, 62, 63
Electrosurgical lasers, 24
Embolisms, gas; *See* Gas embolisms
Emphysema
mediastinal
as complication of laparoscopy, 300
Endocoagulation, 24, 55; *See also* Coagulation; Thermocoagulation
development of, 3
for salpingectomy
in tubal pregnancy, 160
Endodermal sinus tumors
laparoscopic lymphadenectomy and, 146
Endoloop; *See* Roeder loop
Endometrial ablation
as alternative to hysterectomy, 242
Endometrial carcinomas
classification of, 143, 146*T*
diagnostic laparoscopy and, 143, 146
Endometrial hyperplasia
as alternative to hysterectomy, 242
as indication for hysterectomy, 241
Endometrial secretory protein PP14
evaluation of levels of
as indication of endometriosis, 134
Endometriosis
American Fertility Society classification system of, 136
appendectomy and, 209
biopsy specimens, 135, 202*T*
chronic acyclic pelvic pain and, 129
endoscopic survey and, 112
Endometriosis—cont'd
gastrointestinal, 209, 211, *212*, 213, 214
genitourinary, 205, 207, 209
identified through hysterosalpingography, 105*T*, 106
as indication for hysterectomy, 241
infertility and, 100
laparoscopic surgery for
conservative
of the diaphragm, 214
general principles, 202, 203
of the nonreproductive organs, 205, 207, 209, 211, 214
results of, 216
overview, 201
of the reproductive organs, 203-205
results of, 214, 216*T*
radical, 201
laparoscopy and, 134, 135
morphologic appearance
of adhesions, 136
of ovarian endometriomata, 136
of superficial implants, 135, 136
presacral neurectomy and, 233
prevalence of, 133
symptoms of, 133, 134
tests for, 134
Endometrium antibodies
evaluation of levels of
as indication of endometriosis, 134
Endopouch, 25
for removal of large specimens, 86, 87
Endoretractor
use in laparoscopy, 138
Endoscope
light transmission and, 96
Endoscopic imaging
future of, 97
Endoscopic surveys; *See also* Laparoscopic surveys
endometriosis and, 112
omental adhesions and, 112
in oncology, 138
periadnexal adhesive disease and, 112
Endoscopies
laser
training and credentialling, 12
operative
credentialling guidelines
American Fertility Society, 7, 8
Society of Reproductive Surgeons, 7, 8
training in Canada, 9-11
training in U.S., 6-9
Energy
role in laser physics, 46
Enterocele
differentiated from cul-de-sac, 266
Epinephrine
during LAVH, 250
to produce hemostasis, 74
Episiotomy scars
tender masses in
as indication of endometriosis, 133, 134
Equipment
general, 13, 14
storage, 14
Erbium:YAG lasers, 52
Erythrocyte sedimentation rate (ESR)
PID and, 122
Escherichia coli
as cause of PID, 121
ESR; *See* Erythrocyte sedimentation rate (ESR)
ESUs, *28*, 29, *30*; *See also* Solid-state generators
ESUs—cont'd
in operative laparoscopy, 73
output, 34
in prevention of alternate ground site burns, 40*T*, 41
Explosions
as complication of laparoscopy, 304
laser surgery and, 54

F

Fabricant, V. A.
history of laser surgery, 44
Fallopian tubes
injury to
infertility and, 100, 101
Falloppius, 100
Falope rings
in laparoscopic tubal sterilization, 154
Faradic effect, 32
Femoral neuropathy
as complication of laparoscopy, 304
Fenamates
in treatment of primary dysmenorrhea, 126T, 127
Fenestration
cystic ovarian tumors and, 191, 192
Fertility-promoting surgery
laparoscopy
fimbrioplasty, 172, *173*
general principles of, 169, 170
retrograde salpingostomy, 175
salpingo-ovariolysis, *171*, 172
salpingostomy, 172, 173, *174*, 175
microsurgery
general principles of, 169
Fervers, C.
history of electrosurgery and, 27
history of laparoscopy, 2
Fever
PID and, 121, 122
Fiberoptic cables, 15
Fibertome lasers, 52
Fibrin
pelvic abscesses and, 187
Fibroids, ovarian; *See* Ovarian fibroids
Fibroids, uterine; *See* Uterine, fibroids
FIGO classification
of cervical carcinomas staging, 142*T*
of ovarian cancer staging, 139, 140
Filshie clips; *See also* Clips
in laparoscopic tubal sterilization, 152-154
Fimbrioplasty
fertility-promoting surgery
treatment of tubal phimosis/prefimbrial phimosis, 172, *173*
history of laparoscopy, 3
Fire hazards
laser surgery and, 54
FIT CCDs
in video cameras, 94
Fluence
laser beams and, 48
Fluid-filled cables
alcohol, 15
Forceps
biopsy, 24, 150
Frangenheim hook punch, 150
grasping, 21, 23, 62, 63
Fourestier, N.
history of laparoscopy, 2
Fowler's position, 13, 62, 63
Frame interline transfer CCDs; *See* FIT CCDs
Frangenheim, H.

Frangenheim, H.—cont'd
  history of electrosurgery and, 27
  history of laparoscopy, 2
Frangenheim hook punch forceps
  in laparoscopic sterilization, 150
Franklin, Benjamin
  history of electrosurgery, 26
Fulgurating electrodes; *See* Electrodes, fulgurating
Fulguration, *33*, 34-38
  achieved through argon beam coagulators, 39
  development of, 26
  small vessel hemostasis and, 39

G

Gamete intrafallopian transfer (GIFT), 80, 179
Gargiulo, T.
  technique for treatment of uterine retroversion, 238, 239
Gas embolisms
  as complication of laparoscopy, 301
Gasless laparoscopies; *See* Laparoscopies, gasless
Gastric aspiration; *See* Aspiration, gastric
Gastrointestinal bleeding
  as symptom of endometriosis, 133
Gastrointestinal injuries
  as complication of operative laparoscopy, 306, *307*
General anesthesia; *See* Anesthesia, general
Generators, electrosurgical; *See* ESUs
Genetic history
  as indication of endometriosis, 133
Genital cancers
  as indication for hysterectomy, 241
Genital tract infection, lower; *See* Lower genital tract infection
Genitourinary injuries
  as complication of operative laparoscopy, 307
Gentamicin
  in treatment of PID, 123
GIFT; *See* Gamete intrafallopian transfer (GIFT)
Gilliam suspension technique
  as treatment for uterine retroversion, 236, 237
Glaziu, A.
  history of laparoscopy, 2
Glucagon
  in treatment of tubocornual spasms, 105
GnRH agonists; *See also* β hCG assay; Chorionic gonadotropin
  in treatment for uterine lesions, 128
  in treatment of uterine fibroids, 222
GnRH analogues; *See also* β hCG assay; Chorionic gonadotropin
  in treatment of endometriosis, 203
Goggles, safety
  laser surgery and, 53, 54
Gomel, Victor
  history of laparoscopy, 3
Gonadal dysgenesis
  anovulation and, 110
Gonadotrophin-releasing hormone agonists; *See* GnRH agonists
Gonadotropin therapy
  laparoscopy before, 110
Gonorrhea, neisseria; *See* Neisseria gonorrhea
Gordon, J. P.
  invention of masers, 44
Grandfather clause
  credentialling and, 12
Grasping forceps, 21, 23
  alligator, 23
  claw, 23
Grasping forceps—cont'd
  introduction of, 62, 63

H

HAD sensors
  in video cameras, 94
Harmonic scalpels, 54, 55
β-hCG assay; *See also* Chorionic gonadotropin; GnRH agonists; GnRH analogues
  as test for ectopic pregnancy, 120
Heinkel-Semm dilator
  cannulas and, 20
Hemophilus influenzae
  as cause of PID, 121
Hemorrhages; *See also* Bleeding
  delayed bleeding
    as complication of laparoscopy, 306
  immediate bleeding
    as complication of laparoscopy, 305, 306
Hemostasis; *See also* Bleeding; Blood vessels
  large vessel
    white coagulation and, 38
  in operative laparoscopy, 74-82
  small vessel
    desiccation and, 39
    fulguration and, 39
Heparin
  to decrease blood clotting, 87
Hepatomegaly
  diagnostic laparoscopy and, 66
Hernias
  diaphragmatic
    major contraindication
      for diagnostic laparoscopy, 69
  incisional
    as complication of laparoscopy, 304
  large abdominal
    major contraindication
      for diagnostic laparoscopy, 69
Hippocrates
  history of electrosurgery, 26
Hole accumulator diode sensors; *See* HAD sensors
Holmium:YAG lasers, 52
Hopkins, H.
  history of laparoscopy, 2
HSG; *See* Hysterosalpingographies
Hulka clip; *See also* Clips
  in laparoscopic tubal sterilization, 152
Hulka uterine manipulator
  postpartum, 15
Human chorionic gonadotropinassay; *See* β hCG assay
Hydatid cysts of Morgagni; *See* Paraovarian cysts
Hydrocortisone acetate
  to prevent adhesion formation, 87
Hydrocortisone succinate
  in fertility-promoting procedures, 172
  to prevent adhesion formation, 87
Hydrodissection, 82, 83
Hydrosalpinx
  treatment by salpingostomy, 172, 173, *174*, 175
Hypermenorrhea
  as symptom of endometriosis, 133
Hyperplasia, endometrial; *See* Endometrial hyperplasia
Hysterectomies
  abdominal, 242, 243, 295
  indications for, 241, 242
  laparoscopic, 4
    debulking of ovarian cancers, 296
Hysterectomies—cont'd
  laparoscopic—cont'd
    laparoscope insertion and survey, 244
    LARVH
      in treatment of cervical cancers, 296
    LAVH
      compared to vaginal hysterectomy, 257
      results of, 257
      technique, 249-252, 286
      for treatment of ovarian cancers, 295
    LRH
      modified radical technique, 286, *287-289*
      results of, 292
      technique, 290, *291*
      in treatment of cervical cancers, 296, 297
    LRVH
      modified radical technique, 289, *290*, *291*
      results of, 292
      in treatment of ovarian cancers, 296
    preoperative preparation, 243, 244
    subtotal
      auxilliary cervical procedures, 254
      Semm's technique, 254, *255*, *256*
      technique, 252, 253, *254*
    total
      as an alternative to abdominal hysterectomy, 243
      technique, 244, *245-250*
    treatment of additional lesions, 244
    for treatment of ovarian cancers, 295
  precautions with, 241, 242
  radical
    technique, 290, *291*
  subtotal, 242, 243
  total, 242, 243
  for treatment of uterine lesions, 128
  vaginal, 242, 243
    compared to LAVH
      complications of, 257
      results of, 257
    contraindications to, 243
Hysterosalpingographies
  compared with laparoscopy, 109, 110
  complications of, 103, 104
  contraindications for, 101
  in diagnosis of uterine fibroids, 221
  as indication for laparoscopy, 111
  infertility and, 101-109
  limitations of, 107
  oil-based media and, 102
  radionuclide, 109
  technique, 102, *103*, *104*
  timing of, 101, 102
  tubal abnormality identification, 104, 105*T*, 106, 107
  tubal pregnancy and, 157, 158
  uterine abnormality identification, *104*, *105*
  uterine lesion identification, 128
  water-soluble media and, 102
Hysteroscopies
  as alternative to hysterectomy, 242
  intrauterine lesions and, 110
  uterine fibroid diagnosis, 221
  uterine fibroids and, 220
  uterine lesion identification, 128

I

Ibuprofen
  in treatment of secondary dysmenorrhea, 127
Ileitis
  regional
    laparoscopy in diagnosis of, 125

Ileitis—cont'd
regional—cont'd
as relative contraindication
for diagnostic laparoscopy, 69
Ileus-intestinal obstructions
severe
major contraindication
for diagnostic laparoscopy, 69
Illumination
of imaging systems (documentation), 91, 92
Imaging
static
electronic, 96
video
frame grabbing, 96
Imaging equipment, 72, 73
Imaging systems (documentation)
illumination and, 91, 92
Impedance
effect on temperature rise in tissues, 28
Implants
peritoneal
in endometriosis
excision or destructive of, *202*, 203
In vitro fertilization (IVF), 179, 180
Incontinence
stress
Bonney test for, 268
cystometrogram as test for, 268
cystoscopy as test for, 268
pathophysiology of, 266, 267
patient interview, 267
physical examination, 267, 268
Q-tip test for, 268
surgery for
contraindications, 268
technique, 268, *270-273*
Indoleacetic acid derivatives
in treatment of primary dysmenorrhea, 126*T*, 127
Indomethacin
in treatment of endometriosis, 127
Infertility
assessment of tubal and peritoneal factors, 110
endometriosis and, 100, 133
endoscopic survey in, 111, 112
fallopian tube patency and, 100, 101
hysterosalpingography and, 101-109
laparoscopy and, 109-113
LPD and, 100
LUF syndrome and, 99, 100
ovulation assessment and, 99, 100
preliminary investigation, 99
sperm antibodies and, 101
sperm-cervical mucus interaction and, 100
Institute Rizzoli
history of laparoscopy, 1
Instrument tables
in operative laparoscopy, 73
Instruments
pretesting of, 58, 59
removal of, 63, 64
Insufflation
testing of, 60, 61
Insufflators, 14
in operative laparoscopy, 73
preoperative testing of, 57
Interstitial pregnancies; *See* Cornual pregnancies
Intestinal burns
laser surgery and, 54
Intestinal complications
laparoscopic treatment of, 4
Intra-abdominal masses
large
as relative contraindication
for diagnostic laparoscopy, 70
Intraluminal adhesions
identified through hysterosalpingography, 105*T*, 106
Intramural polyps
identified through hysterosalpingography, 105*T*, 106
Intrapelvic lesions; *See* Acquired lesions, intrapelvic
Intrauterine devices; *See* IUDs
Intrauterine diseases
laparoscopy timing and, 113
Intrauterine lesions
hysteroscopy and, 110
Isthmic occlusion
identified through hysterosalpingography, 105*T*, 106
IUDs
PID and, 121
secondary dysmenorrhea and, 127
IVF; *See* In vitro fertilization (IVF)

J

Jacobaeus, H. C.
history of laparoscopy, 1
Jacob-Palmer laparoscope, 17, *18*
Jellett, H.
history of LUNA, 230

K

Kalk, H.
history of laparoscopy, 2
Kapandji, M.
technique for treatment of uterine prolapse, *239*
Kapany
history of laparoscopy, 2
Kelling, G.
history of laparoscopy, 1
Knot pushers
Clarke, 80
Roeder, 80
Knotting techniques
extracorporeal, 78, *79*, 80
intracorporeal, *81*
slip, 78, *79*, 80
surgical, *80*
KTP lasers, 51
for cutting in laparoscopy, 53

L

Laparoscopes
operating, 17, 18
45-degree angle eyepiece, 17, 18
90-degree angle eyepiece, 17, 18
Jacob-Palmer, 17, *18*
Laparoscopic surveys, 63; *See also* Endoscopic surveys
Laparoscopic uterosacral nerve ablation (LUNA)
complications of, 232, 233
history of, 230, 232
results of, 232*T*
technique, 232
Laparoscopically assisted radical vaginal hysterectomies (LARVH); *See* Hysterectomies, laparoscopic, LARVH
Laparoscopically assisted vaginal hysterectomies (LAVH); *See* Hysterectomies, laparoscopic, LAVH
Laparoscopies; *See also* Video laparoscopies
acute pelvic pain and, 124
chronic acyclic pelvic pain and, 128, 129
compared with hysterosalpingography, 109, 110
in diagnosis of bladder injuries, 307
diagnostic
abdominal masses and, 66
acute appendicitis and, 124, 259, 260
acute cholecystitis and, 125
acute perihepatitis and, 125
anesthesia and, 58
contraindications for, 68, 69
major, 69
relative, 69, 70
gasless, 64, 65
indicated for ovarian cancers, 141
pediatric, 65, 66
distal tubal disease and, 108*T*, 111
endometrial carcinomas and, 143, 146
endometriosis and, 134, 135
future directions of
internal and external influences, 309-312
gasless, 64, 65
in gynecologic oncology
general principles of, 137, 138
history of, 1-4, 2
identification of intrapelvic lesions, 128
as indicated by hysterosalpingography, 111
indications for, 68, 110, 111
infections
surgical
management of complications, 308
infertility and, 109-113
lymphadenectomy and
with cervical carcinomas, 142, 143
history of, 143
technical considerations, 143
management of complications
anesthesia-related
cardiac arrhythmias, 304, 305
gastric aspiration, 305
myalgia, 304
back injuries, 304
blood vessel injuries, 304
brachial plexus injuries, 304
cervical lacerations, 304
deep venous thrombosis, 304
explosion, 304
femoral neuropathy, 304
incisional hernias, 304
nerve injuries, 304
PID, 304
from pneumoperitoneum introduction
bladder injuries, 300, 301
blood vessel injuries, 301
bowel injuries, 300, 301
extraperitoneal insufflation, *300*
gas embolisms, 301
incompletion of procedure, 299
liver injuries, 301
mediastinal emphysema, 300
pneumo-omentum, 300
pneumothorax, 300
spleen injuries, 301
stomach injuries, 300, 301
shoulder pain, 304
from trocar introduction
abdominal wall bleeding, 301
blood vessel injuries, *302*
bowel injuries, *303*, 304
liver injuries, 304
spleen injuries, 304

Laparoscopies—cont'd
management of complications—cont'd
from trocar introduction—cont'd
stomach injuries, 303, 304
uterine injuries, 303, 304
Meckel's diverticulitis and, 125
menstrual cycle timing and, 113
neoplasia and, 137-148
open, 64
ovarian tumors and, 139-142
hazards of, 139
preoperative evaluation, 139
patient positioning for, 58
PID and, 122
precautions with pregnancy, 119-121
preoperative equipment check, 57
preoperative evaluation, 57
primary dysmenorrhea and, 127
principles of, 57-67
proximal tubal disease and, 111
regional ileitis and, 125
role in ovarian cancers, 294-296
second-look procedures
with ovarian cancers, 141, 142
surgical
fertility-promoting procedures, 169-180
history of, 2-4
management of complications
gastrointestinal injuries, 306, *307*, 308
genitourinary injuries, 307
hemorrhages, 305, 306
urinary tract infections, 308
operating room setup, 72, 73
patient selection, 71
placement of secondary portals, 74
preoperative preparation, 71, 72
principles of, 71-74
safety precautions, 74
stratification by surgical complexity, 11, 12
technique, 74-78, 80-84, 86, 87
technique, 58-65
tubal disease and, 110
urogynecology and, 265
LARVH; *See* Hysterectomies, laparoscopic, LARVH
Laser beams
incident angle of, 51
properties of, 46-48
Laser endoscopies; *See* Endoscopies, laser
Laser physics
principles of, 44, *45*, 46-48
Laser surgery
complications of, 54
history of, 44
safety considerations in, 53, 54
tissue effects of, 49-51
Lasers
argon, 51, 52
for tissue coagulation in laparoscopy, 53
CO, 52
CO_2
as cutting tool, 53
electrosurgical, 24
erbium:YAG, 52
fibertome, 52
holmium:YAG, 52
introduction of, 62, 63
KTP, 51
for cutting in laparoscopy, 53
Nd:YAG, 51
laparoscopy and, 53
myolysis and, 226
in operative laparoscopy, 73
Lasers—cont'd
optical
history of laser surgery, 44
Lavage
pelvic, 87
Lavage equipment
in operative laparoscopy, 73
Laval University
courses in laparoscopy, 3
LAVH; *See* Hysterectomies, laparoscopic, LAVH
Leiomyomata uteri; *See* Uterine, fibroids
Lesions
acquired
intrapelvic
as cause of chronic cyclic pain, 128
laparoscopy and, 128
uterine
as cause of chronic cyclic pain, 128
hysterosalpingography and, 128
hysteroscopy and, 128
colonic
anterior
endometriosis and, 214
colored cervix
as indication of endometriosis, 133, 134
colored umbilicus
as indication of endometriosis, 133, 134
colored vaginal
as indication of endometriosis, 133, 134
colored vulva
as indication of endometriosis, 133, 134
congenital
as cause of chronic cyclic pain, 128
intrauterine
hysteroscopy and, 110
rectal
anterior
endometriosis and, 211
circumferential
endometriosis and, 211, *212*, *213*, 214
Levy, B. S.
history of electrosurgery and, 27
LGTI; *See* Lower genital tract infection
Lidocaine
during LAVH, 250
in operative laparoscopy, 73
in surgical treatment of uterine retroversion, 237
Ligatures
in adnexectomy, 195
to produce hemostasis, 75-77
Light amplification by the stimulated emission of radiation; *See* Lasers
Light bulbs
mercury vapor, 14, 15
xenon, 14, 15
Light emission
stimulated, 45, 46
Light generators, endoscopic
video cameras and, 92
Light sources, 14, 15
for photographic and video capability, 96
Liston, W. A.
history of laparoscopy, 3
Lithotomy position, 13, 58
Liu, Y. S.
history of laser surgery, 44
Liver injuries
as complication of laparoscopy, 301, 304
Lloyd-Davis stirrups, 13, 58
Local anesthesia; *See* Anesthesia, local
Lower genital tract infection
as contraindication for hysterosalpingography, 101
Lower genital tract infection—cont'd
preceding PID, 121
LPD; *See* Luteal phase defect (LPD)
LRH; *See* Hysterectomies, laparoscopic
LUF syndrome; *See* Luteinized unruptured follicle (LUF) syndrome
LUNA; *See* Laparoscopic uterosacral nerve ablation
Luteal phase defect (LPD)
infertility and, 100
Luteinized unruptured follicle (LUF) syndrome
infertility and, 99, 100
Lymphadenectomies
laparoscopic
of cervical carcinomas, 142, 143, 296, 297
history of, 143
of clear-cell adenocarcinomas, 146
complications of, 285, 286
of endodermal sinus tumors, 146
of endometrial carcinomas, 138, 141
infrarenal para-aortic
technique, 281, *282-284*
interiliac
retroperitoneal approach, 284, 285
low para-aortic
technique, 278, 281, *282*, *283*
ovarian carcinomas and, 138, 141, 296
para-aortic, 4
pelvic, 4
of rhabdomyosarcomas, 146
technique, 277, 278, *279*
of vaginal carcinomas, 146
of vulvar carcinomas, 146

M

Macromorcellators; *See also* Morcellators
for removal of large specimens, 86
Magnetic resonance imaging scans; *See* MRIs
Maiman, Theodore H.
invention of optical lasers, 44
Majoli uterine manipulator, 15, *16*
Manipulators
external, 15
uterine
Majoli, 15, *16*
Valtchev, 15, *16*
Marcaine
in LAVH, 250
in operative laparoscopy, 73
in surgical treatment of uterine retroversion, 237
Masers
history of laser surgery, 44
Meckel's diverticulitis
laparoscopy in diagnosis of, 125
Mefenamic acid
in treatment of primary dysmenorrhea, 126*T*, 127
Menopause
premature
anovulation and, 110
Menorrhagia
as symptom of endometriosis, 133
Menstruation
cycle
laparoscopy timing and, 113
disorders
as indication for hysterectomy, 241
retrograde
acute pelvic pain and, 122, 124
Metal oxide semiconductor chips; *See* MOS chips
Methotrexate
in cornual pregnancy, 166
treatment of trophoblast, 166
in tubal pregnancy, 158, 159

Metronidazole
  in treatment of PID, 123, 183
    postoperative, 186
Microendoscopes
  endometriosis and, 216
Microsurgery
  for distal tubal occlusions
    prognosis for pregnancy, 176
  fertility-promoting
    general principles of, 169
  for tubotubal anastomosis, 176
Microwave amplification by the stimulated emission of radiation; *See* Masers
Minnesota Multiphasic Personality Inventory (MMPI)
  chronic acyclic pelvic pain and, 130
Mittelschmerz
  acute pelvic pain and, 122, 124
  as cause of chronic cyclic pelvic pain, 125
MMPI; *See* Minnesota Multiphasic Personality Inventory
Monitors
  analog, 94, 96
  digital, 94, 96
Monitors, electrode; *See* Electrodes, shields and monitors
Morcellation
  for removal of large specimens, 86
Morcellators; *See also* Macromorcellators
  tissue, 25
MOS chips
  in video cameras, 93, 94
MRIs
  deficiencies in testing for endometriosis, 134
  in diagnosis of uterine fibroids, 221
Multimedia presentations, 94
Myalgia
  as complication of laparoscopy, 304
Mycoplasma hominis
  as cause of PID, 121
Myolysis
  as alternative to hysterectomy, 242
  in treatment of uterine fibroids, 226
Myomas; *See* Uterine, fibroids
Myomectomies
  abdominal
    results, 219, 220
    technique, 219
  as alternative to hysterectomy, 242
  laparoscopic
    advantages and disadvantages of, 220
    indications and contraindications to, 220, 221
    intraoperative complications of, 227
    postoperative procedures, 227
    preoperative evaluation, 221
    results of, 227
    technique, 222, *223-225*, 226

N

Naprosyn; *See* Naproxen sodium
Naproxen
  in treatment of secondary dysmenorrhea, 127
Naproxen sodium
  in treatment of primary dysmenorrhea, 126*T*, 127
Narcoleptic agents
  in operative laparoscopy, 73
National Television Standards Committee (NTSC)
  video format, 93
Nd: YAG lasers, 51
  laparoscopy and, 53
Nd: YAG lasers—cont'd
  myolysis and, 226
Needles
  aspiration, 20, 21
  curved, 76, 77, *79*
  straight and ski, 76, 77, *78*
  Veress, *17*
    introduction of, 59.60, *61*
    pretesting of, 58, 59
    sites for, 59, *60*, 61
  Veress-Frangenhem
    in pediatric laparoscopy, 17, 65, 66
Negative metal oxide semiconductor chips; *See* NMOS chips
Neisseria gonorrhea
  as cause of PID, 121
Neodymium:yttrium-aluminum-garnet lasers; *See* Nd: YAG lasers
Neoplasia
  diagnostic laparoscopy and, 137-148
Nephrectomies
  in treatment of ureter injuries, 308
Nephrostomies
  percutaneous
    in treatment of ureter injuries, 308
Nerve injuries
  as complication of laparoscopy, 304
Nerve supply
  of the pelvis, 115, 116
Neurectomies
  presacral
    history of, 233
    results of, 234
    surgical anatomy of, 229, 230, *231*
    technique, 233, 234
      using the argon beam coagulator, *233*, 234
    in treatment of endometriosis, 205, 233
    in treatment of PID, 233
Neuromuscular stimulation, 32
Neuwirth, R. S.
  history of electrosurgery and, 27
  history of laparoscopy, 3
Newman
  history of laparoscopy, 1
Nezhat, C.
  history of laparoscopy, 4
Niddah Treatise
  history of laparoscopy, 1
Nifedipine
  in treatment of primary dysmenorrhea, 127
Nitze, M.
  history of laparoscopy, 1
NMOS chips
  in video cameras, 93, 94
Nordentoeft
  history of laparoscopy, 2
NTSC; *See* National Television Standards Committee (NTSC)

O

Obesity; *See also* Body weight extremes
  diagnostic laparoscopy and, 65
Occlusion, cornual; *See* Cornual occlusion
Occlusion, distal tubal; *See* Distal tubal occlusion
Occlusion, isthmic; *See* Isthmic occlusion
Ofloxacin
  in treatment of PID, 123
Omental adhesions
  endoscopic survey and, 112
Omentectomies
  technique, 292
Oncology, gynecologic
  diagnostic laparoscopy in
    general principles of, 137, 138
Oophorectomies
  history of laparoscopy, 3
  with ovarian cancers, 296
  removal of cystic ovarian tumors
    results of, 195
Oophoropexies
  posterior
    as treatment for ovarian cancers, 293, 294
Operating laparoscopes; *See* Laparoscopes, operating
Operating room setups
  for operative laparoscopy, 72, 73
Operating tables, 13, 14
Optical lasers
  history of laser surgery, 44
Oral contraceptives
  in treatment of primary dysmenorrhea, 125
Organomegaly
  diagnostic laparoscopy and, 66
Organs
  displaced or enlarged
    as relative contraindication for diagnostic laparoscopy, 70
Orosomucoid
  PID and, 122
Ovarian cancers, 286
  early
    laparoscopic operative therapy for, 294-296
  indications for laparoscopy, 141
    precautions with second-look procedures, 141, 142
  staging of
    FIGO classification, 139, 140
    general principles of, 139
  treated by LAVH, LARVH, or LRH, 286, *287*
  treated by lymphadenectomy
    infrarenal para-aortic, 281, *282*, *283*, 284
    interiliac
      by retroperitoneal approach, 284, 285
    laparoscopic pelvic, 277, 278, *279*, *280*
    low para-aortic, 278, 281, *282*, *283*
Ovarian carcinomas
  laparoscopic lymphadenectomies, 138, 141, 296
Ovarian cystectomies, 192, *193*
  intact cyst removal, 192, 193, *194*
    of benign teratomas, 193, 195
Ovarian drilling
  in polycystic ovarian syndrome, 198, 199
Ovarian electrocautery; *See* Ovarian drilling
Ovarian endometriomata
  morphologic appearance of lesions, 136
Ovarian fibroids
  removal of, 84, 86, 87
Ovarian hyperstimulation
  acute pelvic pain and, 122, 124
Ovarian torsion
  adnexectomy and, 196
Ovarian transposition
  indications for, 292
  posterior oophoropexy, 293, 294
  technique, 292, *293*, *294*
Ovarian tumors; *See also* Teratomas
  acute pelvic pain and, 122, 124
  cystic, 189
    benign neoplastic
      removal of, 84, 86, 87
    diagnostic ultrasound, 189, 190
    laparoscopic management of, 190-197
      adnexectomy, 195

Ovarian tumors—cont'd
laparoscopic management of—cont'd
aspiration, cystoscopy and fenestration, 191, 192
differentiation between benign and malignant, 190, 191
in endometriosis, 204, 205
general principles of, 190, 191
oophorectomy, 195
preoperative evaluation, 189
serum CA 125 levels and, 190
as indication for hysterectomy, 241
laparoscopy
diagnosis of, 139
precautions of, 139
preoperative evaluation, 139
Oviduct abnormalities; *See* Tubal abnormalities
Ovulation assessment
infertility and, 99, 100

P

Pain
shoulder
as complication of laparoscopy, 304
as symptom of endometriosis, 133
PAL; *See* Phase Alternation Line (PAL)
Palmer, R.
history of electrosurgery and, 27
history of laparoscopic sterilization, 149
history of laparoscopy, 2, 3
Palmer drill
biopsy forceps
in laparoscopic sterilization, 150
Panteleoni, D.
history of laparoscopy, 1
Para-aortic lymphadenectomies
by laparoscopy, 4
Paraovarian cysts
laparoscopic surgery and, 197, 198
Patient selection
for operative laparoscopy, 71
PCO; *See* Polycystic ovarian syndrome
PD; *See* Power density
Pediatric laparoscopies
diagnostic, 65, 66
Veress-Frangenhem needles in, 17, 65, 66
Pedicles
securing of
to produce hemostasis, 75
Pelvic abscesses
fibrin and, 187
laparoscopic diagnosis of
cost effectiveness of, 187
postoperative care, 185
preoperative preparation, 183
prognosis for, 186, 187
rationale for, 187
technique, 183, 184, 185
medical therapy, 182
surgical treatment of, 183
Pelvic adhesions
chronic acyclic pain and, 129
Pelvic floor relaxation; *See* Incontinence, stress
Pelvic infections
as indication for hysterectomy, 241
Pelvic inflammatory disease; *See also* Salpingitis
as complication of laparoscopy, 304
as contraindication for hysterosalpingography, 101
as differentiated from appendicitis, 259
dyspareunia and, 121
etiology of, 121
fever and, 121, 122
Pelvic inflammatory disease—cont'd
hysterosalpingography identification of, 105T, 107
incidence of, 121
IUDs and, 121
laparoscopic diagnosis of, 122, 181, 182
perihepatitis and, 121
sexual transmission of, 121
symptoms of, 119, 120, 121, 122
tests for, 122
treated by presacral neurectomy, 233
treatment of, 122, 123
Pelvic lymphadenectomies
by laparoscopy, 4
Pelvic pain
acute
bleeding corpus luteum and, 122, 124
differential diagnosis of, 118
immediate action, 118, 119
laparoscopy and, 124
mittelschmerz and, 122, 124
nonreproductive causes of, 118, 124, 125
ovarian cyst complications, 122, 124
ovarian hyperstimulation and, 122, 124
ovarian tumors and, 122, 124
PID and, 121, 122
pregnancy disorders and, 119-121
ultrasonography and, 124
chronic
acyclic
endometriosis and, 129
laparoscopy and, 128, 129
management of, 130
organic causes of, 128
pelvic adhesions and, 129
psychogenic causes of, 129, 130
cyclic
causes of, 125, 126-130
differential diagnosis of, 117
menstrual cycle and, 117
menstruation
retrograde and, 122, 124
patient history and, 117
perception of, 116
physical examination and, 117, 118
referred, 116
splanchnic, 116
Pelvic tuberculosis; *See* Tuberculosis, pelvic
Peptococci
as cause of PID, 121
Peptostreptococci
as cause of PID, 121
Percutaneous drainage
treatment of pelvic abscesses, 183
Periadnexal adhesions
treated by salpingo-ovariolysis, *171*, 172
Periadnexal adhesive disease; *See also* Adhesions
endoscopic survey and, 112
as indicated by laparoscopy, 111
Perihepatitis
acute
laparoscopy in diagnosis of, 125
PID and, 121
Perineal care, 59
Peripheral leukocyte count (WC)
PID and, 122
Peritoneal implants
in endometriosis
excision or destructive of, *202*, 203
Peritonitis
major contraindication
for diagnostic laparoscopy, 69
Phase Alternation Line (PAL)
video formats, 93
Phillips, Jordan
founder of AAGL, 3
Phimosis
hysterosalpingography identification of, 105*T*, 107
prefimbrial
treated by fimbrioplasty, 172, *173*
Photodynamic therapy
endometriosis and, 216
Photographic film (documentation)
sensitivity of, 91, 92
Physical examination
pelvic pain and, 117, 118
PID; *See* Pelvic inflammatory disease
PIXELs
in video cameras, 94
Pneumo-omentum
as complication of laparoscopy, 300
Pneumoperitoneum
induction of, 59-61
Pneumoperitoneum machines; *See* Insufflators
Pneumothorax
as complication of laparoscopy, 300
Polycystic ovarian syndrome
laparoscopic drilling and, 198, 199
Pompeii
history of laparoscopy, 1
Ponstan; *See* Mefenamic acid
Postoperative care
after laparoscopic myomectomies, 227
with cefoxitin, 185
with doxycycline, 185
of pelvic abscesses
after laparoscopic diagnosis, 185
of PID
with aminoglycoside, 186
with cefotaximine, 186
with cephalosporin, 186
with cetoperazone, 186
with metronidazole, 186
of tubal pregnancy
after operative laparoscopy, 166
Potassium-titanyl-phosphate lasers; *See* KTP lasers
Power, F. H.
history of laparoscopic sterilization, 149
history of laparoscopy, 2
Power density
role in electrosurgery, 34, *35*, 36
role in laser surgery, 47-50
PP14; *See* Endometrial secretory protein PP14
Preceptorships, 7-12
Prefimbrial phimosis
treated by fimbrioplasty, 172, *173*
Pregnancies
acute pelvic pain, 119-121
complications of
as indication for hysterectomy, 241
as contraindication for hysterosalpingography, 101
intrauterine
diagnostic laparoscopy and, 66
relative contraindication for, 69
precautions with laparoscopy, 119-121
Premature menopause
anovulation and, 110
Premenstrual spotting
as symptom of endometriosis, 133
Preoperative equipment check, 57
Preoperative evaluation, 57
of cystic ovarian tumors, 189

Preoperative evaluation—cont'd
  for laparoscopic myomectomies, 221
  by laparoscopy
    of ovarian tumors, 139
  of ovarian tumors
    by laparoscopy, 139
Preoperative preparation, 71, 72
  for laparoscopic hysterectomies, 243, 244
  of pelvic abscesses
    by laparoscopic diagnosis, 183
Preoperative testing
  of insufflators, 57
Presacral nerves
  anatomy of, 229, 230, *231*
Probes, 20
  introduction of, 62, 63
  rectal, 15
Prognosis for pregnancy
  distal tubal occlusion
    when treated by microsurgery, 176
Prohhorov, Aleksandr M.
  history of laser surgery, 44
Pronuclear stage embryos (PROST), 179, 180
  assisted reproductive technologies (ART), 179, 180
PROST; *See* Pronuclear stage embryos (PROST)
Prostaglandins
  primary dysmenorrhea and, 126
  secondary dysmenorrhea and, 127
  synthetase inhibitors
    primary dysmenorrhea and, 126*T*
Protective eye wear
  laser surgery and, 53, 54
Proximal tubal disease
  as identified through laparoscopy, 111
Pyelographies
  in diagnosis of ureter injuries, 308

Q

Q-tip tests
  for stress incontinence, 268
Querleu, D.
  complications of laparoscopy, 310

R

Recamier, R.
  invention of speculum, 1
Recording systems
  video
    endoscopic, *92*, 93
Rectal lesions
  anterior
    endometriosis and, 211
  circumferential
    endometriosis and, 211, *212*, *213*, 214
Rectal probes, 15
Rectum
  relationship to pelvic floor, 266
Redi, R.
  history of laparoscopy, 1
Regional anesthesia; *See* Anesthesia, local
Regulations
  lack of in laparoscopy, 311
Reich, H.
  history of laparoscopy, 4
REM; *See* Return electrode monitor
Resistance
  effect on temperature rise in tissues, 28
Respiratory complications; *See also* Cardiorespiratory disease
  laser surgery and, 54
Retractors, 20
Return electrode monitor
  in prevention of dispersive electrode burns, 42
Rhabdomyosarcomas
  laparoscopic lymphadenectomy and, 146
Rioux, Jacques E.
  history of laparoscopic sterilization, 150
  history of laparoscopy, 3
Rivere
  history of electrosurgery, 26
Roeder loop
  for ligating, 24
  in oophorectomy and adnexectomy
    of cystic ovarian tumors, 195
  to produce hemostasis, 75, 76, *77*
  in salpingectomy
    of tubal pregnancy, 160
Ruggi, J.
  history of LUNA, 230

S

Safety
  in electrosurgery, 43, 44
  in laser surgery, 53, 54
  in operative laparoscopy, 74
Salpingectomies
  history of laparoscopy, 3
  tubal pregnancy and, 160, *161*, *162*
    electrosurgical, 160
    by endocoagulation, 160
Salpingitis, 122; *See also* Pelvic inflammatory disease
Salpingitis isthmica nodosa (SIN)
  hysterosalpingography identification of, 105*T*, 106
Salpingography
  selective, 107, 109
Salpingo-oophorectomies
  bilateral, 242, 295
  technique, 292
  in treatment of ovarian cancers, 295
Salpingo-ovariolysis
  fertility-promoting, *171*, 172
  history of laparoscopy, 3
Salpingostomies
  fertility-promoting surgery, 172, 173, *174*, 175
  history of laparoscopy, 3
  retrograde
    fertility-promoting surgery, 175
  treatment of distal tubal occlusion, 172, 173, *174*, 175
Salpingotomies
  linear
    for tubal pregnancy, 163, *165*
Scalpels, harmonic; *See* Harmonic scalpels
Scars, abdominal; *See* Abdominal scars
Scars, episiotomy; *See* Episiotomy scars
Schawlow, Arthur L.
  history of laser surgery, 44
Scissors
  disposable, 24
  heavy duty, 25
  hook, 23
  introduction of, 62, 63
SECAM: *See* Sequence de Couleurs Avec Memoire (SECAM)
Second-look laparoscopy
  after myolysis, 242
  with ovarian cancers, 296
Sedimentation rate, erythrocyte; *See* Erythrocyte sedimentation rate (ESR)
Segmental excisions
  in tubal pregnancy
    with sutures, 160, 163
    through electrosurgery, 160, 163, *164*
Semm, Kurt, 55
  endocoagulation and, 24
Semm, Kurt—cont'd
  history of laparoscopy, 3, 4
  laparoscopic hysterectomy and, 254, *255*, *256*
  macromorcellators and, 86
Sensors, hole accumulator diode; *See* HAD sensors
Sequence de Couleurs Avec Memoire (SECAM) video formats, 93
Serum antichymotrypsin
  PID disease and, 122
Serum CA 125 levels
  in diagnosis of cystic ovarian tumors, 190
Serum progesterone assays
  as test for ectopic pregnancy, 120
Sexual transmission
  of PID, 121
Shapiro, H. I.
  history of laparoscopy, 3
Shields, electrode; *See* Electrodes, shields and monitors
Shoulder braces, 13, 14
Shoulder pain
  as complication of laparoscopy, 304
SIN; *See* Salpingitis isthmica nodosa (SIN)
Sinus tumors, endodermal; *See* Endodermal sinus tumors
Society of Obstetricians and Gynaecologists of Canada
  training guidelines, 9-11
Society of Reproductive Surgeons
  credentialling guidelines
    operative endoscopy, 7, 8
Soderstrom, R. M.
  history of electrosurgery and, 27
  history of laparoscopy, 3
Solid-state generators; *See also* ESUs
  history of electrosurgery and, 27
Spasms
  tubocornual
    during hysterosalpingography, 105
Speculum
  Recamier, R., 1
Sperm antibodies
  infertility and, 101
Sperm-cervical mucus interaction
  infertility and, 100
Splanchnoscopy
  history of laparoscopy, 1
Spleen injuries
  as complication of laparoscopy, 301, 304
Splenomegaly
  diagnostic laparoscopy and, 66
Spotting
  premenstrual
    as symptom of endometriosis, 133
Spray coagulation; *See* Fulguration
Stapling devices, 25
  for securing of pedicles, 81, 82
Static imaging
  electronic, 96
Steiner, O. P.
  history of laparoscopy, 1
Steptoe, Patrick C.
  history of laparoscopy, 2, 3
Sterilization
  laparoscopic
    biopsy forceps in, 150
    desiccation and, 150
    electrosurgery and, 150, 152
    Frangenheim hook punch forceps and, 150
    history of, 149, 150
    thermocoagulation and, 152
  reversal of, 112, 113
    by tubotubal anastomosis, 176

Stirrups
  Lloyd-Davis, 13, 58
Stomach injuries
  as complication of laparoscopy, 300, 301, 303, 304
Streptococci
  nonhemolytic
    as cause of PID, 121
Stress incontinence; *See* Incontinence, stress
Stromme, W. B.
  history of tubal pregnancy, 157
β-subunit human chorionic gonadotropin assays; *See* β hCG assay
Succinylcholine
  myalgia and, 305
Suction equipment, 14
  in operative laparoscopy, 73
Supracervical hysterectomies; *See* Hysterectomies, laparoscopic, subtotal
Suprapubic bladder neck suspension
  by laparoscopy, 4
Surgical team, 72
Sutures
  in adnexectomy, 195
  needles and, 76-78
  to produce hemostasis, 75, 77, 78
  for segmental excisions
    in tubal pregnancy, 160, 163
Suturing equipment, 24, 25

T

Tables
  operating, 13, 14
TAH/BSO
  treatment of pelvic abscesses, 183
Tait, R. L.
  history of tubal pregnancy, 157
Talmud, Babylonian
  history of laparoscopy, 1
Telescopes; *See also* Laparoscopes
  combined with operating instruments, 18
  diagnostic, 17
  with double posts, 18
  integrated bundle, 18
  introduction of, 62
  lensless, 18
  operating, 17, 18
  pretesting of, 59
  steam autoclavable, 18
Telesurgery
  future of endoscopic imaging, 97
TEM; *See* Transverse electromagnetic mode
Temperature
  of tissues, 28
Teratomas; *See also* Ovarian tumors
  benign
    ovarian cystectomy and, 193, 195
  removal of, 84, 86, 87
Tetracycline
  postoperative treatment of PID, 186
Thermal injuries, 37
Thermocoagulation; *See also* Coagulation; Endocoagulation
  electrosurgery
    in laparoscopic sterilization and, 152
  in laparoscopic sterilization, 152
Thin patients; *See also* Body weight extremes
  diagnostic laparoscopy and, 65
Thoyer-Rozat, J.
  history of laparoscopy, 2
Three-dimensional videos, 96
Three-stitch technique
  in treatment of uterine retroversion, 238, *239*
Thrombosis
  deep venous
    as complication of laparoscopy, 304
Tissue
  absorbance, 50, 51
  electrode proximity, 36
  exposure time, 51
  impedance or resistance, 36
  large
    removal of, 84, 86, 87
  small
    removal of, 83, 84
  time on or near, 37
Tolfenamic acid
  in treatment of endometriosis, 127
Total abdominal hysterectomy and bilateral salpingo-oophorectomy (TAH/BSO); *See* TAH/BSO
Townes, Charles H.
  invention of masers, 44
Training
  operative endoscopy
    Canada, 9-11
    U.S., 6-9
  videotapes/videodisks and, 90
Transabdominal incisions
  for removal of large specimens, 84, 86
Transabdominal ultrasound
  as test for ectopic pregnancy, 120
Transvaginal ultrasound
  as test for ectopic pregnancy, 120
Transverse electromagnetic mode
  role in laser surgery, 48-50
Trap-door valves
  cannulas and, 19
Trendelenburg position, 2, 13, 62, 63, 74
Trocars
  ancillary
    introduction of, 63, *64*
  disposable, 20
  principal, 19, 20
    introduction of, 61, *62*
Trophoblast
  methotrexate and, 158, 166
  tubal pregnancy and, 158-160
Trumpet valves
  cannulas and, 18, 19
Tubal abnormalities
  of the ampulla
    hysterosalpingography identification of, *106*
  of the infundibulum
    hysterosalpingography identification of, 107, 108*T*
  of the intraperitoneal spread
    hysterosalpingography identification of, 107, 108*T*
  of the isthmus
    hysterosalpingography identification of, *106*
  of the tubocornual region
    hysterosalpingography identification of, 105*T*, 106
Tubal cannulation, 107, 109
Tubal disease
  laparoscopy and, 110
Tubal phimosis
  treated by fimbrioplasty, 172
Tubal pregnancies; *See also* Ectopic pregnancies
  conservative surgical management of, 166, 167
  diagnostic laparoscopy and, 157, 158
  expectant management of, 157, 158
  history of, 157
  hysterosalpingography and, 157, 158
Tubal pregnancies—cont'd
  identified through hysterosalpingography, 105*T*, 106
  laparotomy and, 159
  local medical therapy, 158, 159
  medical treatment of, 158, 159
  minilaparotomy and, 159
  operative laparoscopy and
    cornual pregnancy, 165, 166
    general principles of, 159, 160
    linear salpingotomy, 163, *165*
    postoperative care, 166
    salpingectomy, 160, *161*, *162*
    segmental excisions, 160, 163, *164*
    tubal abortions, 163, 165
    tube electrodesiccation, 160
Tubal sterilization
  laparoscopic
    electrosurgical techniques, 150, 152
    falope rings and, 154
    filshie clips and, 152-154
    history of, 149
    hulka clips and, 152
    mechanical techniques, 152-154
    reversal of, 154, 155
  local anesthesia for, 73
Tuberculosis, pelvic
  identified through hysterosalpingography, 107
Tubocornual anastomosis, 105
Tubocornual spasms
  during hysterosalpingography, 105
Tubotubal anastomosis
  microsurgery compared to laparoscopy, 176
  results of, 178
  for sterilization reversal, 176
  technique, *177*, 178
Tumors, endodermal sinus; *See* Endodermal sinus tumors
Tumors, ovarian; *See* Ovarian tumors

U

Ultrasonographies
  acute pelvic pain and, 124
  in diagnosis of ureter injuries, 308
  in diagnosis of uterine fibroids, 221
  as test for ectopic pregnancy, 120
Ultrasound
  deficiencies in testing for endometriosis, 134
  in diagnosis of cystic ovarian tumors, 189, 190
Umbilicus lesions
  colored
    as indication of endometriosis, 133, 134
University of British Columbia
  courses in laparoscopy, 3
Ureter
  injuries
    as complication of operative laparoscopy, 307, 308
  surgery of
    in endometriosis, 207, *208*, 209
Urethra
  relationship to pelvic floor, 265, 266
Urethral disease
  intrinsic
    as contraindication for stress incontinence, 268
Urethropexies
  complications of, 275
  results of, 275, 276
  as treatment for stress incontinence, 269, 271, *273-275*
Urinary bleeding
  as symptom of endometriosis, 133

Urinary complications
  laparoscopic treatment of, 4
Urinary incontinence; *See* Incontinence, stress
Urinary tract infections
  as complication of operative laparoscopy, 308
Urogynecology
  laparoscopy and, 265
  technique, 265-275, 276*T*
Uterine
  abnormalities
    hysterosalpingography identification of, *104*, *105*
  bleeding
    as contraindication for hysterosalpingography, 101
  corpus
    removal of, 84, 86, 87
  fibroids
    abdominal myomectomy and, 219, 220
    hysteroscopic surgery and, 220
    as indication for hysterectomy, 241
    intramural
      laparoscopy and, 222-224, *225*
    medical treatment of, 221, 222
    myolysis as treatment for, 226
    subserous
      laparoscopy and, 222, *223*
    symptoms of, 221
    treated by GnRH agonists, 222
  perforations and punctures
    as complication of laparoscopy, 303, 304
  prolapse
    as indication for hysterectomy, 241
    ventrofixation and, 239
  retroversion
    Gilliam suspension technique and, 236, 237
    three-stitch technique and, 238, *239*
    Webster-Baldy suspension technique and, 237, 238
Uterine lesions; *See* Acquired lesions, uterine
Uterine manipulators
  Majoli, 15, *16*
  Valtchev, 15, *16*
Uteroligamentous fixation
  in treatment of uterine prolapse, *239*
Uterosacral ligaments
  ablation of
    in endometriosis, 205
  anatomy of, 229, 230, *231*
  tender nodularity of
    as indication of endometriosis, 133
Uterus
  fixed retroversion of
    as indication of endometriosis, 133
  punctures
    as complication of laparoscopy, 303
  tender nodularity of
    as indication of endometriosis, 133
UTI; *See* Urinary tract infections

V

Vacuum tubes
  invention of, 26, 27
Vagina
  relationship to pelvic floor, 266
Vaginal carcinomas
  laparoscopic lymphadenectomy and, 146
Vaginal hernias; *See* Enterocele
Vaginal lesions
  colored
    as indication of endometriosis, 133, 134
Valtchev uterine manipulator, 15, *16*
Valves
  cannulas and, 18, 19
    pretesting of, 59
  with malleable diaphragm
    cannulas and, 19
  trap-door
    cannulas and, 19
  trumpet
    cannulas and, 18, 19
Vaporization
  electrosurgery and, 32, *33*, 34-38
  laser surgery and, 50, 51
Vasopressin
  to produce hemostasis, 74
Ventrofixation
  in treatment of uterine prolapse, 239
Ventroscopies
  history of laparoscopy, 1
Ventrosuspension
  in treatment of uterine retroversion, 236-239
Veress, J.
  history of laparoscopy, 2
Veress needles, *17*
  introduction of, 59, 60, *61*
  pretesting of, 58, 59
  sites for, 59, *60*, 61
Veress-Frangenhem needles
  in pediatric laparoscopy, 17, 65, 66
Video cameras
  endoscopic light generators and, 92
  solid state, 93, 94
Video documentation
  archiving of, 96, 97
  guidelines for, 97
  legal status, 91
  technical aspects of, 91-93
Video documentation system, 93, 94, 96
Video formats
  National Television Standards Committee (NTSC), 93
  Phase Alternation Line (PAL), 93
Video imaging
  frame grabbing, 96
Video laparoscopies; *See also* Laparoscopies
  history of laparoscopy, 4
Video recording systems
  endoscopic, *92*, 93
Videodiscs
  for archival of medical records, 96, 97
  laser, 94, *95*
  training and, 90
Videotapes
  magnetic, 94
  training and, 90
Virtual reality systems
  in future training, 97
Voltage
  effect on temperature rise in tissues, 28
von Ott, D. O.
  history of laparoscopy, 1
Vulmiere, J.
  history of laparoscopy, 2
Vulva lesions
  colored
    as indication of endometriosis, 133, 134
Vulvar carcinomas
  laparoscopic lymphadenectomy and, 146

W

Warming pads, 14
Webster-Baldy suspension technique
  as treatment for uterine retroversion, 237, 238
Weight, body; *See* Body weight extremes
Wesley, John
  history of electrosurgery, 26
Wheeless, C. R.
  history of laparoscopy, 3
White coagulation, 31, 32; *See also* Coagulation
  discovery of, 26
  large vessel
    hemostasis and, 38
Wyeth
  history of electrosurgery, 27

X

Xylocaine
  during LAVH, 250
  in operative laparoscopy, 73
  in surgical treatment of uterine retroversion, 237

Z

Zacharin, Robert
  history of stress incontinence and, 266
Zeiger, H. J.
  invention of masers, 44
ZIFT; *See* Zygote intrafallopian transfer (ZIFT)
Zollikoffer, R.
  history of laparoscopy, 2
Zygote intrafallopian transfer (ZIFT), 179, 180